WITHDRAWN
WRIGHT STATE UNIVERSITY LIBRARIES

DRUG RESISTANCE IN LEUKEMIA AND LYMPHOMA III

ADVANCES IN EXPERIMENTAL MEDICINE AND BIOLOGY

Editorial Board:
NATHAN BACK, *State University of New York at Buffalo*
IRUN R. COHEN, *The Weizmann Institute of Science*
DAVID KRITCHEVSKY, *Wistar Institute*
ABEL LAJTHA, *N. S. Kline Institute for Psychiatric Research*
RODOLFO PAOLETTI, *University of Milan*

Recent Volumes in this Series

Volume 448
COPPER TRANSPORT AND ITS DISORDERS: Molecular and Cellular Aspects
Edited by Arturo Leone and Julian F. B. Mercer

Volume 449
VASOPRESSIN AND OXYTOCIN: Molecular, Cellular, and Clinical Advances
Edited by Hans H. Zingg, Charles W. Bourque, and Daniel G. Bichet

Volume 450
ADVANCES IN MODELING AND CONTROL OF VENTILATION
Edited by Richard L. Hughson, David A. Cunningham, and James Duffin

Volume 451
GENE THERAPY OF CANCER
Edited by Peter Walden, Uwe Trefzer, Wolfram Sterry, and Farzin Farzaneh

Volume 452
MECHANISMS OF LYMPHOCYTE ACTIVATION AND IMMUNE REGULATION VII:
Molecular Determinants of Microbial Immunity
Edited by Sudhir Gupta, Alan Sher, and Rafi Ahmed

Volume 453
MECHANISMS OF WORK PRODUCTION AND WORK ABSORPTION IN MUSCLE
Edited by Haruo Sugi and Gerald H. Pollack

Volume 454
OXYGEN TRANSPORT TO TISSUE XX
Edited by Antal G. Hudetz and Duane F. Bruley

Volume 455
RHEUMADERM: Current Issues in Rheumatology and Dermatology
Edited by Carmel Mallia and Jouni Uitto

Volume 456
RESOLVING THE ANTIBIOTIC PARADOX:
Progress in Understanding Drug Resistance and Development of New Antibiotics
Edited by Barry P. Rosen and Shahriar Mobashery

Volume 457
DRUG RESISTANCE IN LEUKEMIA AND LYMPHOMA III
Edited by G. J. L. Kaspers, R. Pieters, and A. J. P. Veerman

A Continuation Order Plan is available for this series. A continuation order will bring delivery of each new volume immediately upon publication. Volumes are billed only upon actual shipment. For further information please contact the publisher.

DRUG RESISTANCE IN LEUKEMIA AND LYMPHOMA III

Edited by

G. J. L. Kaspers
R. Pieters and
A. J. P. Veerman

University Hospital Vrije Universiteit
Amsterdam, The Netherlands

KLUWER ACADEMIC / PLENUM PUBLISHERS
NEW YORK, BOSTON, DORDRECHT, LONDON, MOSCOW

Library of Congress Cataloging-in-Publication Data

Drug resistance in leukemia and lymphoma III / edited by G.J.L.
  Kaspers, R. Pieters, and A.J.P. Veerman.
       p.   cm. -- (Advances in experimental medicine and biology ; v.
  457)
     "Proceedings of the Third International Symposium on Drug
  Resistance in Leukemia and Lymphoma, held March 4-7, in Amsterdam,
  the Netherlands"--T.p. verso.
     Includes bibliographical references and index.
     ISBN 0-306-46055-6
     1. Leukemia--Molecular aspects--Congresses.   2. Lymphomas-
  -Molecular aspects--Congresses.   3. Drug resistance in cancer cells-
  -Congresses.   I. Kaspers, G. J. L., 1963-   . II. Pieters, R.
  III. International Symposium on Drug Resistance in Leukemia and
  Lymphoma (3rd : 1998 : Amsterdam, Netherlands)   IV. Series.
     [DNLM: 1. Leukemia--drug therapy congresses. 2. Lymphoma--drug
  therapy congresses. 3. Drug Resistance, Neoplasm--physiology
  congresses.   WH 250 D794 1999 / W1 AD559 v.457 1999]
  RC643.D77 1999
  616.99'419'061--dc21
  DNLM/DLC
  for Library of Congress   98-43929
                                                                     CIP

Proceedings of the Third International Symposium on Drug Resistance in Leukemia and Lymphoma,
held March 4 – 7, 1998, in Amsterdam, The Netherlands

ISBN 0-306-46055-6

© 1999 Kluwer Academic / Plenum Publishers, New York
233 Spring Street, New York, N.Y. 10013

10 9 8 7 6 5 4 3 2 1

A C.I.P. record for this book is available from the Library of Congress.

All rights reserved

No part of this book may be reproduced, stored in a retrieval system, or transmitted in any form or by any means, electronic, mechanical, photocopying, microfilming, recording, or otherwise, without written permission from the Publisher

Printed in the United States of America

PREFACE

Cellular drug resistance is a major limitation to the success of chemotherapy of leukemia and lymphoma. The importance of this has now been recognized by both clinicians and scientists. It is of utmost importance to bridge the gap between laboratory and clinic in this field of research. This is the main purpose of the series of International Symposia on Drug Resistance in Leukemia and Lymphoma. These are held every three years in Amsterdam, The Netherlands, since 1992. This book contains the proceedings of the third of these meetings, organised in 1998.

The book covers all important aspects of drug resistance in leukemia and lymphoma, both in the form of extensive reviews as in manuscripts describing original data. General mechanisms of resistance are discussed, including the drug resistance related proteins p-glycoprotein, MRP (multi-drug resistance protein) and LRP (lung resistance protein), and the role of glutathione and glutathione-S-transferases. Moreover, more drug type-specific mechanisms of resistance are a topic, such as for glucocorticoids and antifolates. Much information is provided on apoptosis and its regulators, and on the results of cell culture drug resistance assays. Several papers focus on the modulation or circumvention of drug resistance.

All together, the book contains more than 60 chapters with an extensive amount of information on all aspects of drug resistance in leukemia and lymphoma. It can be recommended to scientists, laboratory researchers, and clinicians.

CONTENTS

Section I. Drug Resistance Related Proteins and Glutathione

1. MDR1/P-gp Expression as a Prognostic Factor in Acute Leukemias 1
   Jean-Pierre Marie and Ollivier Legrand

2. Clinical Significance of P-Glycoprotein (P-gp) Expression in Childhood Acute
   Lymphoblastic Leukemia: Results of a 6-Year Prospective Study 11
   Catharina Dhooge and Barbara De Moerloose

3. Prognostic Value of P-gp Expression and Related Function in Childhood Acute
   Leukemia 21
   Z. Karakaş, L. Ağaoğlu, S. Erdem, G. Yanikkaya Demirel, M. Arasa,
   F. Süzergöz, G. Deniz, S. Anak, and G. Gedikoğlu

4. Comparison of P-Glycoprotein Expression and Function with *in Vitro* Sensitivity
   to Anthracyclines in AML 29
   Alena W. Elgie, Jean M. Sargent, Christine J. Williamson,
   Grazyna M. Lewandowicz, and Colin G. Taylor

5. Quinine Improves Results of Intensive Chemotherapy (IC) in Myelodysplastic
   Syndromes (MDS) Expressing P-Glycoprotein (PGP): Updated Results of
   a Randomized Study 35
   E. Wattel, E. Solary, B. Hecquet, D. Caillot, N. Ifrah, A. Brion, N. Milpied,
   M. Janvier, A. Guerci, H. Rochant, C. Cordonnier, F. Dreyfus, A. Veil,
   L. Hoang-Ngoc, A. M. Stoppa, N. Gratecos, A. Sadoun, H. Tilly, P. Brice,
   B. Lioure, B. Desablens, B. Pignon, J. P. Abgrall, M. Leporrier,
   B. Dupriez, D. Guyotat, P. Lepelley, and P. Fenaux

6. Treatment of Poor Prognosis AML Patients Using PSC833 (Valspodar) plus
   Mitoxantrone, Etoposide, and Cytarabine (PSC-MEC) 47
   R. Advani, G. Visani, D. Milligan, H. Saba, M. Tallman, J. M. Rowe,
   P. H. Wiernik, J. Ramek, K. Dugan, B. Lum, J. Villena, E. Davis,
   E. Paietta, M. Litchman, A. Covelli, B. Sikic, and P. Greenberg

7. Assessment of P-Glycoprotein Expression by Immunocytochemistry and Flow
   Cytometry Using Two Different Monoclonal Antibodies Coupled with
   Functional Efflux Analysis in 34 Patients with Acute
   Myeloid Leukemia 57
   S. Poulain, P. Lepelley, N. Cambier, A. Cosson, P. Fenaux, and E. Wattel

8. Preliminary Immunocytochemical Studies of MDR-1 and MDR-3 Pgp
   Expression in B-Cell Leukaemias 65
   Annemarie Larkin, Elizabeth Moran, Denis Alexander, and Martin Clynes

9. A Mutation in the Promoter of the Multidrug Resistance Gene (*MDR*1) in
   Human Hematological Malignancies May Contribute to the Pathogenesis
   of Resistant Disease 71
   Deborah Rund, Idit Azar, and Olga Shperling

10. Reproducible Flow Cytometric Methodology for Measuring Multidrug
    Resistance in Leukaemic Blasts 77
    M. Pallis, J. Turzanski, S. Langabeer, and N. H. Russell

11. Natural Fluorescence Imaging of Leukemic Cells for Studying Uptake and
    Retention of Anthracyclines 89
    M. Monici, F. Fusi, P. Mazzinghi, A. Degli Innocenti o Nocentini,
    I. Landini, I. Banchelli, B. Bartolozzi, V. Santini, and P. A. Bernabei

12. Artificial Neural Networks as Versatile Tools for Prediction of
    MDR-Modulatory Activity 95
    C. Tmej, P. Chiba, K.-J. Schaper, G. Ecker, and W. Fleischhacker

13. Discordance of P-Glycoprotein Expression and Function in Acute Leukemia ... 107
    Barbara De Moerloose, Catharina Dhooge, and Jan Philippé

14. Multidrug Resistance Related Proteins in Primary Cutaneous Lymphomas 119
    Christian W. van Haselen, Marcel J. Flens, Rik J. Scheper,
    Paul van der Valk, George L. Scheffer, Johan Toonstra, and
    Willem A. van Vloten

15. The Lung Resistance Protein (LRP) Predicts Poor Outcome in Acute Myeloid
    Leukemia 133
    Robert Pirker, Gudrun Pohl, Thomas Stranzl, Ralf W. Suchomel,
    Rik J. Scheper, Ulrich Jäger, Klaus Geissler, Klaus Lechner, and
    Martin Filipits

16. MRP Expression in Acute Myeloid Leukemia: An Update 141
    Martin Filipits, Thomas Stranzl, Gudrun Pohl, Ralf W. Suchomel, Sabine
    Zöchbauer, Raoul Brunner, Klaus Lechner, and Robert Pirker

17. Evidence for Functional Discrimination between Leukemic Cells
    Overexpressing Multidrug-Resistance Associated Protein and
    P-Glycoprotein 151
    Zineb Benderra, Hamid Morjani, Aurélie Trussardi, and Michel Manfait

Contents

18. Both Pgp and MRP1 Activities Using Calcein-AM Contribute to Drug
    Resistance in AML 161
    Ollivier Legrand, Ghislaine Simonin, Jean-Yves Perrot, Robert Zittoun, and
    Jean-Pierre Marie

19. Absolute Levels of MDR-1, MRP, and BCL-2 mRNA and Tumor Remission in
    Acute Leukemia 177
    T. Köhler, S. Leiblein, S. Borchert, J. Eller, A.-K. Rost, D. Laßner, R. Krahl,
    W. Helbig, O. Wagner, and H. Remke

20. Multidrug Resistance Protein MRP1, Glutathione, and Related Enzymes:
    Their Importance in Acute Myeloid Leukemia 187
    Dorina M. van der Kolk, Edo Vellenga, Michael Müller, and
    Elisabeth G. E. de Vries

21. Glutathione and the Regulation of Cell Death 199
    A. G. Hall

22. Evidence for the Involvement of the Glutathione Pathway in Drug Resistance in
    AML 205
    J. M. Sargent, C. Williamson, A. G. Hall, A. W. Elgie, and C. G. Taylor

23. Glutathione in Childhood Acute Leukaemias 211
    P. Kearns, R. Pieters, M. M. A. Rottier, A. J. P. Veerman, K. Schmiegalow,
    A. D. J. Pearson, and A. G. Hall

Section II. Apoptosis and Cell Death Regulations

24. Apoptosis: Molecules and Mechanisms 217
    Marina Konopleva, Shourong Zhao, Zhong Xie, Harry Segall, Anas Younes,
    David F. Claxton, Zeev Estrov, Steven M. Kornblau, and Michael Andreeff

25. Activation of Apoptosis Pathways by Anticancer Drugs 237
    Klaus-Michael Debatin

26. BCL-2 Stimulates Apoptin®-Induced Apoptosis 245
    Astrid A. A. M. Danen-Van Oorschot, Alex J. van der Eb, and
    Mathieu H. M. Noteborn

27. CD95 (Fas/Apo-1) Antigen Is a New Prognostic Marker of Blast Cells of Acute
    Lymphoblastic Leukaemia Patients 251
    A. Yu. Baryshnikov, E. R. Polosukhina, N. N. Tupitsin, N. V. Gavrikova,
    L. Yu. Andreeva, T. N. Zabotina, S. A. Mayakova, V. I. Kurmashov,
    A. B. Syrkin, Z. G. Kadagidze, D. Yu. Blochin, and Yu. V. Shishkin

28. Inhibition of Fas/Fas-Ligand Does Not Block Chemotherapy-Induced Apoptosis
    in Drug Sensitive and Resistant Cells 259
    Deborah S. Richardson, Paul D. Allen, Stephen M. Kelsey, and
    Adrian C. Newland

29. Effects of PARP Inhibition on Drug and FAS-Induced Apoptosis in Leukaemic Cells 267
   Deborah S, Richardson, Paul D. Allen, Stephen M. Kelsey, and Adrian C. Newland

30. Apoptotic Fraction in Childhood ALL Assessed by DNA *in Situ* Labelling Is Ploidy Independent 281
   Allen F. Pyesmany, Lynne M. Ball, Margaret Yhap, M. Henry, Krista Laybolt, D. Christie Riddell, and Dick van Velzen

31. PCNA Bearing Structures Are Retained in Apoptotic Phase of Childhood ALL Cell Cycle 289
   Lynne M. Ball, Christopher L. Lannon, Margaret Yhap, Allen F. Pyesmany, M. Henry, Krista Laybolt, D. Christie Riddell, and Dick van Velzen

32. Apoptosis Corrected Proliferation Fraction in Childhood ALL Is Related to Karyotype 297
   Lynne M. Ball, Allen F. Pyesmany, Margaret Yhap, Christopher L. Lannon, M. Henry, Krista Laybolt, D. Christie Riddell, and Dick van Velzen

33. Proliferation and Apoptosis Does Not Affect Presenting White Cell Count in Childhood ALL 305
   Allen F. Pyesmany, Lynne M. Ball, Margaret Yhap, M. Henry, Krista Laybolt, D. Christie Riddell, and Dick van Velzen

34. Apoptosis by Anthracyclines at Therapeutic Concentrations in MDR1+ Human Leukemic Cells 313
   Barbara Chiodini, Renato Bassan, and Tiziano Barbui

35. BCL-2 Expression in Childhood Leukemia versus Spontaneous Apoptosis, Drug Induced Apoptosis and in Vitro Drug Resistance 325
   E. G. Haarman, G. J. L. Kaspers, R. Pieters, C. H. van Zantwijk, G. J. Broekema, K. Hählen, and A. J. P. Veerman

36. Comparison of BCL-2 and Bax Protein Expression with *in Vitro* Sensitivity to Ara-C and 6TG in AML 335
   S. E. Balkham, J. M. Sargent, A. W. Elgie, C. J. Williamson, and C. G. Taylor

37. Synthetic Cyclin Dependent Kinase Inhibitors: New Generation of Potent Anti-Cancer Drugs 341
   Marián Hajdúch, Libor Havlíček, Jaroslav Veselý, Radko Novotný, Vladimír Mihál, and Miroslav Strnad

38. Factors Contributing to the Resistance to Apoptosis Induced by Topoisomerase I Inhibitors in Vincristine Resistant Cells 355
   Valérie Palissot, Aurélie Trussardi, Marie-Claude Gorisse, and Jean Dufer

39. Two Distinct Modes of Oncoprotein Expression during Apoptosis Resistance in Vincristine and Daunorubicin Multidrug-Resistant HL60 Cells 365
   Rajae Belhoussine, Hamid Morjani, Reynald Gillet, Valérie Palissot, and Michel Manfait

Section III. Risk Factors and Cell Culture Assays

40. Genetic Abnormalities and Drug Resistance in Acute Lymphoblastic Leukemia .. 383
    Ching-Hon Pui and William E. Evans

41. Resistance Testing and Mechanisms of Resistance in Childhood Leukemia:
    Studies from Amsterdam 391
    R. Pieters, G. J. L. Kaspers, N. L. Ramakers-van Woerden, M. L. den Boer,
    M. G. Rots, Ch. M. Zwaan, E. G. Haarman, and A. J. P. Veerman

42. Pharmacokinetics of Anticancer Drugs *in Vitro* 397
    Alexandra Wagner, Georg Hempel, Gumbinger H. G., Heribert Jürgens, and
    Joachim Boos

43. Down Syndrome and Acute Myeloid Leukemia: Lessons Learned from
    Experience with High-Dose Ara-C Containing Regimens 409
    Yaddanapudi Ravindranath and Jeffrey W. Taub

44. Cellular Drug Resistance in Childhood Acute Myeloid Leukemia:
    A Mini-Review with Emphasis on Cell Culture Assays 415
    G. J. L. Kaspers, Ch. M. Zwaan, R. Pieters, and A. J. P. Veerman

45. Is in Vitro Sensitivity of Blast Cells Correlated to Therapeutic Effect in
    Childhood Acute Lymphoblastic Leukemia? 423
    Britt-Marie Frost, Rolf Larsson, Peter Nygren, and Gudmar Lönnerholm

46. In Vitro Cytotoxic Drug Activity and in Vivo Pharmacokinetics in Childhood
    Acute Myeloid Leukemia 429
    Gudmar Lönnerholm, Britt-Marie Frost, Rolf Larsson, E. Liliemark,
    Peter Nygren, and Curt Peterson

47. Prognosis in Adult AML Is Precisely Predicted by the Disc-Assay Using the
    Chemosensitivity-Index C_I 437
    Peter Staib, Bernd Lathan, Timo Schinköthe, Sabine Wiedenmann,
    Bernhard Pantke, Thomas Dimski, Dimitris Voliotis, and Volker Diehl

48. Drug Resistance Testing of Acute Myeloid Leukemia in Adults Using the MTT
    Assay 445
    N. Stute, T. Köhler, L. Lehmann, W. Wetzstein, and G. Ehninger

49. MTT Assay for Drug Resistance in Childhood Acute Leukemia and Effect of
    Cyclosporin and Interferon: A Preliminary Report 453
    Zeynep Karakaş, Leyla Ağaoğlu, Serap Erdem, Sema Anak,
    Ayşegül Hacıbektaşoğlu, and Gündüz Gedikoğlu

50. Differential Antileukemic Activity of Prednisolone and Dexamethasone in
    Freshly Isolated Leukemic Cells 459
    Vladimír Mihál, Marián Hajdúch, Věra Nosková, Gabriela Feketová,
    Kassmine Jess, Libuše Gojová, Ivo Kašpárek, Jan Starý, Bohumír Blažek,
    Dagmar Pospíšilová, and Zbynik Novák

51. Activity of Vinorelbine on B-Chronic Lymphocytic Leukemia Cells *in Vitro* ... 473
    P. A. Bernabei, I. Landini, B. Bartolozzi, I. Banchelli,
       A. Degli Innocenti o Nocentini, and V. Santini

52. Studies of Some Mechanisms of Drug Resistance in Chronic Myeloid Leukemia
       (CML) 477
    Anna G. Turkina, Natalia P. Logacheva, Tatjana P. Stromskaya,
       Tatjana N. Zabotina, Sergei V. Kuznetzov, Kuralay K. Sachibzadaeva,
       Akshin Tagiev, Vacheslav S. Juravlev, Nina D. Khoroshko,
       Anatoly Y. Baryshnikov, and Alla A. Stavrovskaya

53. Clinical Sensitivity to Anthracyclines in Ph/BCR+ Acute Lymphoblastic
       Leukemia 489
    Renato Bassan, Ama Z. S. Rohatiner, Alessandro Rambaldi, Teresa Lerede,
       Eros Di Bona, Maxine Carter, Giuseppe Rossi, Enrico Pogliani,
       Giorgio Lamberteghi-Deliliers, Piero Fabris, Adolfo Porcellini,
       T. Andrew Lister, and Tiziano Barbui

54. Differential Kinetics of Drug Resistance in Human Leukaemic Cells Measured
       by SCGE/CLSM 501
    Lynne M. Ball, Christopher L. Lannon, G. Ross Langley, Allen F. Pyesmany,
       Margaret Yhap, and Dick van Velzen

55. Demonstration of Differences in Drug Resistance by Direct Testing of DNA
       Excision Repair Activity following Standard and Liposomal Daunorubicin
       Exposure in Normal Paediatric Marrow Using High Resolution CLSM ... 509
    Christopher L. Lannon, Lynne M. Ball, Allen F. Pyesmany, Margaret Yhap,
       G. Ross Langley, and Dick van Velzen

56. Microsatellite Instability Assessment in Prediction of Drug Resistance in
       Childhood Burkitt's and Large Cell Diffuse Malignant Non-Hodgkin
       Lymphoma (MNHL) 517
    Margaret Yhap, Allen F. Pyesmany, Lynne M. Ball, D. Christie Riddle,
       Jiang Mu, and Dick van Velzen

57. High Resolution Confocal Laser Scanning Microscopy Analysis of DNA
       Excision Repair Capability in Small Volume Marrow Samples Exposed to
       DNA Directed Treatment Moieties 527
    Christopher L. Lannon, Lynne M. Ball, Allen F. Pyesmany, Margaret Yhap,
       Ross Langley, and Dick van Velzen

Section IV. Antifolates

58. Defining the Optimal Dosage of Methotrexate for Childhood Acute
       Lymphoblastic Leukemia: New Insights from the Lab and Clinic 537
    William E. Evans, Ching-Hon Pui, and Mary V. Relling

Contents

59. Mechanisms of Methotrexate Resistance in Acute Leukemia:
    Decreased Transport and Polyglutamylation 543
    Richard Gorlick, Peter Cole, Debabrata Banerjee, Giuseppe Longo,
    Wei Wei Li, Daniel Hochhauser, and Joseph R. Bertino

60. Lack of Cross-Resistance between Prednisolone and Methotrexate in Childhood
    Acute Lymphoblastic Leukemia? A Preliminary Analysis 551
    I. R. H. J. Hegge, G. J. L. Kaspers, M. G. Rots, G. Jansen, R. Pieters, and
    A. J. P. Veerman

Section V. Nucleoside Analogues and Growth Factors

61. New Developments in the Treatment of Acute Myeloid Leukemia 557
    Mariëlle Smeets, Theo de Witte, Netty van der Lely, Reinier Raymakers, and
    Petra Muus

62. Aphidicolin Markedly Increases the *in Vitro* Sensitivity to Ara-C of Blast Cells
    from Patients with AML 567
    J. M. Sargent, A. W. Elgie, C. J. Williamson, and C. G. Taylor

63. Common Resistance Mechanisms to Nucleoside Analogues in Variants of the
    Human Erythroleukemic Line K562 571
    Charles Dumontet, Evelyne Callet Bauchu, Krystyna Fabianowska,
    Michel Lepoivre, Dorota Wyczechowska, Frédérique Bodin, and
    Marie Odile Rolland

64. Expression of DNA Mismatch Repair Proteins in Acute Lymphoblastic
    Leukaemia and Normal Bone Marrow 579
    E. C. Matheson and A. G. Hall

65. Effects of CSFS and Their Combinations with Chemotherapeutic Agents (Ch)
    on Leukemic Blasts (LB) in Children (MTT-Assay) 585
    E. Litvinova, K. Gurova, K. Chimishkian, and G. Mentkevich

Section VI. Glucocorticoids

66. Glucocorticosteroid Therapy in Childhood Acute Lymphoblastic Leukemia 593
    Paul S. Gaynon and Aaron L. Carrel

67. Glucocorticoid Induced Apoptosis in Leukemia 607
    Lou A. Smets, Gajja Salomons, and Joop van den Berg

68. Glucocorticoid Resistance and the AP-1 Transcription Factor in Leukemia 615
    S. Bailey, A. G. Hall, A. D. J. P. Pearson, M. M. Reid, and C. P. F. Redfern

Section VII. Asparaginase

69. The Three Asparaginases: Comparative Pharmacology and Optimal Use in
    Childhood Leukemia 621
    Barbara L. Asselin

Index 631

MDR1/P-GP EXPRESSION AS A PROGNOSTIC FACTOR IN ACUTE LEUKEMIAS

Jean-Pierre Marie and Ollivier Legrand

Service d'Hématologie Biologique de l'Hôtel-Dieu
Formation de Recherche Associé Claude Bernard
Université Paris VI. Hôtel-Dieu
75181 Paris Cedex 04, France

Keywords: AML, ALL, MDR1/P-gp, LRP, MRP, prognostic.

1. ABSTRACT

P-glycoprotein (P-gp) is often expressed (40–50%) on leukemic cells at diagnosis in acute myelogenous leukemia (AML), and is even more frequently present after treatment failure. Several large cohorts of newly diagnosed AML patients treated with a classical anthracycline + standard doses of cytosine arabinoside were tested for the prognosis value of MDR1 phenotype, and demonstrated an high correlation between a significant increase of MDR1 gene expression and treatment failure (or, better, drug resistance).

This P-gp(+) drug resistance could be due either to a particular phenotype of bad prognosis AML, as it is suggested by the association of myelodysplasia, complex karyotype and advanced age with MDR1 phenotype, or due primarily to the active efflux of anthracyclines and VP16 in P-gp (+) leukemic cells. Several observations tend to confirm the functional role of the P-gp in clinical drug resistance: (i) using multivariate analysis, MDR1 phenotype appears to be an independent variable, as potent (or higher) as karyotype and age for predicting *in vivo* drug resistance; (ii) the prognostic value is limited to the CD34(+)/P-gp(+) phenotype, wich is linked to a functional P-gp; (iii) the *in vitro* sensitivity to anthracyclines and VP16 is highly correlated with P-gp expression. All these data argue for an early use of P-gp modifier agents in the treatment of AML.

The role of the MDR1 gene in ALL resistance is controversial and marginal compared to the sensitivity of ALL blasts to glucocorticoids, and the frequency of MDR1 phenotype is low at diagnosis, and is increasing only after repetitive chemotherapies.

Drug Resistance in Leukemia and Lymphoma III, edited by Kaspers *et al.*
Kluwer Academic / Plenum Publishers, New York, 1999.

Table 1. Resistance genes in AML

	AML<55 yr 349 pts	AML>55yr 203 pts	Reccurent AML 93 pts	CML - BC 52 pts
P-gp	37%	73%	46%	84%
MRP	10%	10%	33%	14%
LRP	44%	56%	81%	60%

According to C. Willman, Sem Hematol 34, supp 5 Oct 1997.

2. INTRODUCTION

Twenty years after the description of P-gp by V Ling, the prognostic value of this "resistance" protein remains questionable in the large majority of cancer. This is due to the heterogeneity of techniques used for measuring P-gp, the threshold for defining "positivity", and the type of clinical response.

The publication of several consensus concerning the measurement of MDR1/P-gp[1,2] permitted the re-examination of prognostic role of this gene expression in acute leukemia. This is of importance for defining the strategies of induction and consolidation treatment in these diseases, where P-gp modulators as cyclosporin A, quinine and PSC833 were tested since several years.

3. EXPRESSION OF MDR1/P-GP IN ACUTE LEUKEMIA

It was emphasized that the methods used for MDR1/P-gp detection are of critical importance, because of the relatively low level of protein/activity found in the leukemic cells compared to the resistant cell lines used as control. If only the studies with validated (reproducible) techniques for MDR1/P-gp measurement are retained for a retrospective analysis, few data are available except in adult AML. For these reasons, some studies representing milestones, or reporting data in rare diseases like ATL will be considered, despite the lack of proof of reproducibility.

The MDR phenotype confered by the expression of the *mdr* 1 gene could be "disease related", i.e. present from the onset of the overt disease, or "treatment related", i.e. absent at diagnosis, but more and more frequently observed during the course of the disease, mainly after repeated chemotherapy.

The high frequency of MDR1/P-gp in untreated adult AML argues for the constitutive expression of this phenotype in this disease, with a rather low incidence of selection or upregulation at relapse (Table 1). On the other hand, childhood and adult acute lymphoblastic leukemias express this phenotype in a small proportion of cases at diagnosis, and only multiple relapses exhibited measurable MDR1/P-gp expression.[3] One exception in this setting is the adult T leukemia-lymphoma (ATL), with leukemic cells showing a high frequency of P-gp cells at diagnosis.[4]

3.1. Adult Acute Myelogenous Leukemia

Since 1981, many studies reported an high frequency of *mdr 1* gene expression in acute myelogenous leukemia. The large multicentric studies showed between 1/3 to 1/2 of "positive" cases at diagnosis (Table 1), whatever the technique used, and even more in the elderly patients. The major influence on prognosis was on the induction treatment failure

Table 2. MDR1 in adult AML: prognostic role

Authors	No pts.	Techniques	CR/resist.	DFS
Campos et al.	150	Flow Cytom.(MRK16)	p=0.00001*	p=0.05*
Nüssler et al.	166	Flow Cytom.(C219/4E3)	p=0.002*	NT
Hunault et al.	110	ARN/MRK16	Resist: p=0.00001*	NT
vdHeuvel-E.	130	I C C	p= 0.01*	NT
Del Poeta et al.	158	Flow C (C219+JSB1)	p=0.001*	p=0.02
According to consensus (2 techniques):				
Leith et al.	211(65a)	Flow C (MRK16)+ function	p=0.004* Resist: p=0.0007*	NS
Willman	352(Aa)	Flow C(MRK16)+ function	p=0.012* Resist: p=0.0007*	NT
Legrand et al.	52	Flow C (UIC2)+ function	Resist: p=0.03	NT

* Multivariate analysis.

and overal survival, but not on the disease free survival, raising the question of either the functionality of the P-gp in residual leukemic cells, or the role of high dose chemotherapy during consolidation (high dose cytarabine or high dose cyclophosphamide/TBI). In monoparametric analysis, MDR1 phenotype was as potent as "bad" cytogenetics (del 5,7,11q.2.3, t(9;22)), age, and secondary leukemia. In multivariate analysis (Table 2), MDR1 phenotype was an independent predictive factor of treatment failure, more or equally potent than cytogenetics and age. In our study, cytogenetic appeared of importance only in the MDR1(-) group of patients.[5]

This poor prognosis of the patients with AML expressing MDR1 phenotype could be due either to a particular immature phenotype of leukemia, or to the direct effect of the P-gp efflux pump on the leukemic drug resistance to anthracyclines and etoposide, or both.

3.1.1. Factors Associated with MDR1 Phenotype in AML. The SWOG group described as first the strong association of MDR1 phenotype and age. We confirmed these data, with a less strong correlation. Elderly leukemia is associated with increasing proportions of secondary leukemia and "bad" cytogenetics (Figure 1).[6]

The immature CD34 phenotype is strongly linked with P-gp. This was first emphasized by te Boekhorst et al.,[7] and confirmed by all studies using sensitive antibodies against CD34. The function of the P-gp is strictly correlated with CD34, and the poor prognostic significance attributed to this phenotype could be due to the active drug efflux

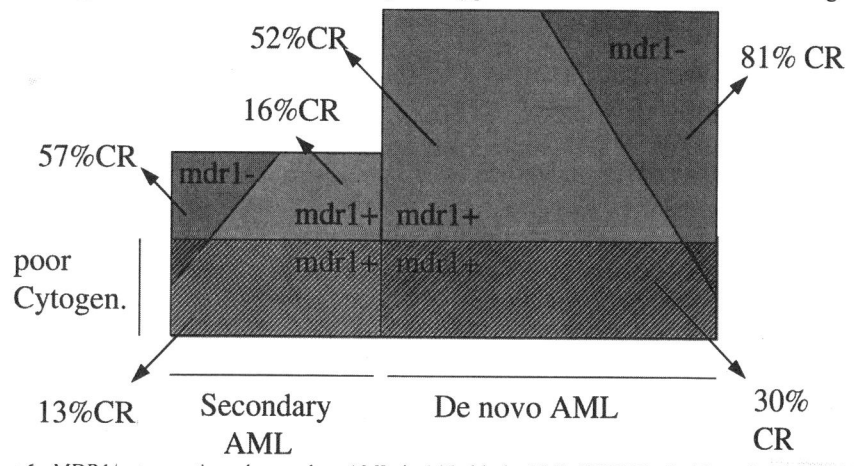

Figure 1. MDR1/cytogenetic and secondary AML in 146 elderly AML (SWOG). (Leith et al., Blood 1997.)

Table 3. Multivariate analysis in elderly AML (SWOG)

	Treatment Failure	Resistance to treatment
Cytogenetics	0.0031	0.017
Secondary leukemia	0.0035	0.11
MDR1/P-gp	0.004	0.0007

According to Leith et al., Blood, 1997.

of a functional P-gp. In multiparametric analysis for prognostic factors including these 2 parameters, only P-gp, but not CD34, appears to be significant.

The immature phenotype of P-gp cells is mirrored by the absence of P-gp in AML3: this was confirmed by all studies until now.

The MDR phenotype is also frequent in myelodysplastic syndrome (MDS) and secondary leukemia and blast crisis of CML, both diseases known to be of particularly bad prognosis.

Te Boekhorst et al.,[9] observed that the MDR1 phenotype was associated with an high autonomous in vitro leukemia growth, by itself a bad prognostic parameter.

All these data confirmed the frequent expression of MDR1/P-gp in a large subset of leukemia patients with known factors of bad prognostic significance.

3.1.2. Relationship between MDR1 Phenotype and in Vivo/in Vitro Drug Resistance. A functional P-gp is able to decrease the anthracyclines and etoposide (but no cytarabine) intracellular concentration within the leukemic cell. Therefore, P-gp have to be related to the in *vitro/in vivo* drug sensitivity. In our experience, using MTT assay for in vitro sensitivity of the fresh AML cells, MDR1/P-gp expression is correlated with DNR and VP16 LC50, but not cytarabine LC50 (manuscript in preparation). Clinically, the resistance to a classical 3+7 treatment is better correlated to P-gp than the global "treatment failure", including death during aplasia (Table 3).[6] Interestingly, Nüssler et al showed that the predictive potency of P-gp positivity observed in the 166 patients treated with a classical 3+7 treatment was completely lost in the 63 patients treated with intermediate doses of cytarabine.[10]

These data tend to support the active role of a functional P-gp in anthracycline resistance, and to encourage the use of P-gp modulators in AML, even in first phase.

3.1.3. Role of Other Proteins Involved in MDR Phenotype in Adult AML. More discordant results were published concerning the incidence and the role of MRP expression in AML (Table 4): the range of MRP expression is narrow compared to P-gp, and a basal expression is found in all cases. A possible bias in the published studies is the high expression of this protein in normal mononuclear cells,[11] representing a risk of contamination of the sample, except if a double labelling is monitored by flow cytometry.

Ten to thirty percent of the patients presented a "high" expression. The prognostic value of MRP is probably marginal, but could be additional and could explain some rhodamine efflux in P-gp(-)/efflux (+) cases. The best sensitive technique for this monitoring is the use of calcein efflux (modified by specific modulator like probenicid).[12]

The role of LRP/MVP was recently investigated with different techniques, and with different results (Table 5). List at al, using immunocytochemistry, showed a strong correlation between LRP expression and treatment failure,[13] as Pirker with RT-PCR.[14] On the other hand, Leith et al.,[15] and Legrand et al.,[12] using flow cytometry (and RT-PCR for Legrand), were unable to demonstrate any relation between LRP and treatment failure in the

Table 4. MRP in adult AML

Authors	No. patients	Techniques	CR	DFS	O S
Hart et al. (1994)	33	RT-PCR	NS	NT	NT
Zhou et al. (1995)	58	RT-PCR	Resist (p=0.005)	NT	NT
Filipits et al. (1997)	80	I C C	NS	NT	NS
Legrand et al. (1997)	53	RT-PCR/Flow C function (Calcein AM)	NS p=0.03	NT NT	NT NT
Leith et al. (ASH97)	352	Flow cytometry	Resist: NS	NT	NT

same category of patients. Using retrospectively immunocytochemistry with LRP56 antibody on the same leukemic samples, Legrand et al observed a relationship between LRP expression and a lower overall survival (manuscript in preparation), raising the question of a threshold for positivity, more easy to observe with immunocytochemistry.

Using MTT assay for testing in vitro drug resistance in fresh leukemic samples, we were unable to show any relationship between the expression of MRP or LRP and LC50 of anthracyclines or etoposide (manuscript in preparation).

We therefore concluded that, in adult AML, the major protein involved in clinical resistance to anthracycline is the P-gp, and that this protein is often associated with other factors of bad prognostic significance.

3.2. Childhood AML

Until now, only 2 studies used 2 methods of analysis according to consensus (Table 6). The number of patients studied is low, and showed a global incidence of MDR1/P-gp (+) lower than in adult AML (13% to 30%), and none of them showed a correlation between MDR1/P-gp and prognosis (CR, OS, DFS). Evenmore, Pearson et al. described a close association between the expression of P-gp and the t(8;21), given as a good prognostic factor in adult AML.[16] This association was not showed in the adult cases tested by the same authors.

3.3. Childhood Acute Lymphoblastic Leukemia (ALL)

Except for one study using criticable methodology,[17] the incidence of *mdr* 1 overexpression in untreated patients with ALL was generally found to be low (<10%) at diagnosis and even at relapse (Table 7), except during the latest stage of the disease, when a clinical drug resistance is usually observed.

Table 5. LRP in adult AML

Authors	No pts	Techniques	CR	DFS	OS
List et al. (1996)	87	I C C (LRP56)	p=0.002	NS	NS
Hart et al. (1997)	33	RT-PCR	p=0.03	NT	NT
Pirker et al. (1997)	86	I C C (LRP56)	p=0.01	NS	p=0.006
Legrand et al. (1997)	90	RT-PCR/FlowC	Resist : NS	NS	0.03/NS
		I C C(LRP56)	NS	NS	0.02
Leith et al. (ASH 97)	352	Flow C	Resist: NS	NT	NT

Table 6. MDR1 in childhood AML

Authors/Reference	Technique	Nb of cases(+) (Initial/Relapse)	Correlation with in vivo response (CR, OS, DFS)
vd Heuvel-E Br J. Haemat 97	ICC (C219 + C494)	13+/23 Initial	87% CR PN pooled with adults
Siever Leukemia 95	Flow Cytom. (20%)	17+/130 Initial	No correlations
Ivy Blood 96	Flow Cytom. + Rho	5+/23 Initial 5+/12 Relapse	Rho reversal higher in relapse (ALL+AML)
Pearson Leukemia 96	Flow Cytom. + DiOC2	6+/20 Flow C 9+/20 DiOC2	All P-gp (+) had t(8;21)
den Boer Blood 98	Flow Cytom. MTT	20 Initial 7 Relapse	Not related to drug resistance

The MDR phenotype is found only in ALL subgroup of CD7+/CD4-/CD8- ALL, wich is thought to originate from a hematopoietic stem cell.

The MDR1 phenotype was not predictive for induction treatment failure, whatever the method of detection used. This could be explained by the predominent place of corticosteroids as the major drug in ALL. On the other hand, two publications, using both immunocytochemistry, claimed an association between P-gp and a shorter overall survival: Goasguen tested only 36 children, and 73% of the 14 P-gp(+) in CR eventually relapsed, versus only 32% in the 22 P-gp(-) patients.[18] Sauerbray et al.[17] studied a high number of patients, and were able to run a multivariate analysis for predictive factors: the MDR1 phenotype was independently related to a poor prognosis. The two studies using flow cytometry and functional tests found few positive cases at diagnosis, and did not show any correlation between positivity and survival.[19,20]

We tested MDR1/P-gp expression with 4 techniques in 36 recently established ALL cell lines, retaining the phenotype and cytogenetic markers of the fresh leukemic cells, and observed a frequent overexpression of MDR1/P-gp, except in patients entered in CR.[21] The in vitro cultures probably selected clones prone to express P-gp.

Fewer publications concerned MRP in ALL, but all showed a measurable level of MRP at diagnosis, comparatively higher than in AML, and some cases showed an increase

Table 7. MDR1 in childhood ALL

Author Reference	Method	Nb(+) cases	Correlation with resistance
Kingreen Acute Leuk Sympo	ICC (1%(+))	3+/48 Initial 11+/47 Relapse	No correlation with clinical response
Ivy ASTRACT 93	RT-PCR	65+/213 Initial 12+/46 Relapse	No correlation with CR, OS and EFS
Sauerbray BrJC94	ICC (1+(+))	36+/104 Initial	independly related to a poorer survival
Ivy Blood 96	Flow Cytom. Rho	1+/30 Initial 10+/38 Relapse	Rho higher in relapse
Den Boer Blood 98	Flow Cytom MTT	100 Initial 27 Relapse	Not related to DNR drug resistance

Table 8. Adult ALL and MDR1/P-gp expression

Authors/Reference	Technique	Type AL	No+/Total tested	Prognostic role of P-gp
Kuwazuru Blood 90	Immuno-blotting C219	ATL	8+/20 Initial 6+/6 Relapse	Refractory to treatment
Goasguen Blood 93	I CC JSB1 and C219	Adult ALL	9+/23 Initial	56% CR vs 93%, p=0.05
Wattel Leukemia 95	Flow Cytom JSB1	Adult ALL	32+/50 Initial	No relation with %CR, OS and DFS

prognostic significance after treatment. The prognosis incidence of this expression is presently not demonstrated.

3.4. Adult Acute Lymphoblastic Leukemia (Table 8)

Several studies in ALL mixed some adult cases with childhood ALL. Very few data were dedicated to adult ALL,[18,22] and none of them fulfilled the criteria defined in the Memphis's consensus. Wattel et al, using flow cytometry of JSB1 (an internal epitope), observed a high proportion of positive cases before treatment (32/50), but did not found any correlation between this expression and CR rate, overall survival or disease free survival. In a small cohort of 23 adults tested by immunocytochemistry, Goasguen et al., were alone to describe a correlation between P-gp expression (9/23) and failure of complete remission.

The absence of large series tested with adequate methods precludes any conclusions concerning the prognostic significance of P-gp in adult ALL.

The Adult T Lymphome-Leukemia (ATL), of particular bad prognosis, was investigated by immunoblotting by Kuwasaru et al.,[4] and found to be positive in 8/20 at diagnosis, and in all 6 relapsed cases, refractory to polychemotherapy.

4. CONCLUSION

Until now, the only clear and reproducible results concerning clinical prognostic factors is the expression of MDR1/P-gp in adult AML. This gene is expressed in patients with frequently associated other "bad prognosis" parameters, but is the best predictive factor for in vivo resistance, when a "classical" (3+7) treatment is used.

The prognostic value of the other "resistance genes" (MRP, LRP) in AML, and of MDR1/P-gp and others in childhood AML and ALL is still not well defined, partly due to the methodology problems.

ACKNOWLEDGMENTS

The MDR1/P-gp experimental work was granted by Association Claude Bernard, Assistance-Publique -Hôpitaux de Paris, and the Association Contre le Cancer.

REFERENCES

1. Beck W, Grogan T, Willman C, Cordon-Cardo C, Parham D, Kuttesch J, Andreeff M, Bates S, Berard C, Boyett J, Brophy N, Broxterman H, Chan H, Dalton W, Dietel M, Fojo A, Gascoyne R, Head D, Houghton P, Srivastava D, Lehnert M, Leith C, Paietta E, Pavelic Z, Rimsza L, Ronnson I, Sikic B, Twentyman P, Warnke R, Weinstein R: Methods to detect P-glycoprotein-associated multidrug resistance in patients' tumors: consensus recommendations. Cancer Research 1996, 56:3010–3020.
2. Marie J, Huet S, Faussat A, Perrot J, Chevillard S, Barbu V, Bayle C, Boutonnat J, Calvo F, Campos-Guyotat L, Colosetti P, Cazin J, P dC, Delvincourt C, Demur C, Drenou B, Fenneteau O, Feuillard J, Garnier-Suillerot A, Genne P, Gorisse M, Gosselin P, Jouault H, Lacave R, Le Calvez G, Léglise M, Léonce S, Manfait M, Maynadié M, Merle-Béral H, Merlin J, Mousseau M, Morjani H, Picard F, Pinguet F, Poncelet P, Racadot E, Raphael M, Richard B, Rossi J, Schlegel N, Vielh P, Zhou D, Robert J: Multicentric evaluation of the MDR phenotype in leukemia. Leukemia 1997, 11:1086–1094.
3. Beck J, Handgretinger R, Dopfer R, Klingebiel T, Niethammer D, Gekeler V: Expression of mdr1,mrp,topoisomerase IIa/b and cyclin A in primary or relapsed states of acute lymphoblastic leukemia. British Journal of Haematology 1995, 89:356–363.
4. Kuwazuru Y, Hanada S, Furukawa T, Yochimura A, Sumizawa T, Utsunomiya A, Ishibashi K, Saito T, Uozumi K, Maruyama M, Ishizawai M, Arima T, Akiyama S: Expression of P-glycoprotein in adult T-cell leukemia cells. Blood 1990, 10:2065–2071.
5. Hunault M, Zhou D, Delmer A, Ramond S, Viguié F, Cadiou M, Perrot J, Levy V, Rio B, Cymbalista F, Zittoun R, Marie J: Multidrug resistance (MDR1) gene expression in acute myeloid leukemia: major prognosis significance for the in vivo drug resistance to induction treatment. Annals of Hematology 1997, 74:65–71.
6. Leith C, Kopecky K, Godwin J, McConnell T, Slovak M, Chen I, Head D, Appelbaum F, Willman C: Acute myeloid leukemia in the elderly: assessment of multidrug resistance (MDR1) and cytogenetics distinguishes biologic subgroups with remarkably distinct responses to standard chemotherapy. A Southwest Oncology Group study. Blood 1997, 89:3323–3329.
7. te Boekhorst P, de Leeuw K, Schoester M, Wittebol S, Nooter K, Hagemeijer A, Löwenberg B, Sonneveld P: Predominance of functional multidrug resistance (MDR-1) phenotype in CD34+ acute myeloid leukemia cells. Blood 1993, 82:3157–3162..
8. Pasman P, Schouten H: Multidrug resistance mediated by P-glycoprotein in haematological malignancies. Netherland Journal of Medicine 1993, 42:218–231.
9. te Boekhorst P, Löwenberg B, van Kapel J, Nooter K, Sonneveld P: Multidrug resistant cells with high proliferative capacity determine response to therapy in acute myeloid leukemia. Leukemia 1995, 9:1025–1031.
10. Nüssler V, Pelka-Fleischer R, Zwierzina H, Nerl C, Beckert B, Gieseler F, Diem H, Ledderose G, Gullis E, Sauer H, Willmans W: P-glycoprotein expression in patients with acute leukemia - clinical relevance. Leukemia 1996, 10, supp 3:S23-S31.
11. Legrand O, Perrot J, Tang R, Simonin G, Gurbuxani S, Zittoun R, Marie J: Expression of the multidrug resistance- associated protein (MRP) mRNA and protein in normal peripheral blood and bone marrow haematopoietic cells. British Journal of Haematology 1996, 94:23–33.
12. Legrand O, Simonin G, Perrot J, Zittoun R, Marie J: P-gp and MRP activities using calcein-AM are prognostic factors in adult myeloid leukemia patients. Blood 1998, 91:4480–4488.
13. List A, Spiers C, Grogan T, Johnson C, Roe D, Greer J, Wolff S, Broxterman H, Scheffer G, Scheper R, Dalton W: Overexpression of the major vault transporter protein lung-resistance protein predicts treatment outcome in acute myeloid leukemia. Blood 1996, 87:2464–2469.
14. Pirker R, Pohl G, Stranzl T, al e: Expression of the LRP predicts poor outcome in the de novo AML. Blood 1997, 90:suppl, 566a.
15. Leith C, Kopescky K, Chen I, al e: Frequency and clinical significance of expression of the multidrug resistance proteins, MDR1, MRP and LRP in AML patients less than 65 yo. Blood 1997, 90:suppl, 389a.
16. Pearson L, Leith C, Duncan M, Chen I, McConnel T, Trinkaus K, Foucar K, Willman C: MDR1 expression and functional dye/drug efflux is highly correlated with the t(8;21) chromosomal translocation in pediatric acute myeloid leukemia. Leukemia 1996, 10:1274–1282.
17. Sauerbrey A, Zintl F, Volm M: P-glycoprotein and glutathione S-transferase pi in childhood acute lymphblastic leukaemia. British Journal of Cancer 1994, 70:1144–1149.
18. Goasguen J, Dossot J, Fardel O, Le Mee F, L Gall E, Leblay R, Le Prisé P, Chaperon J, Fauchet R: Expression of the multidrug resistance P-glycoprotein (P-170) in 59 de novo acute lymphoblastic leukemia: prognostic implications. Blood 1993, 81:2394–2398.

19. Ivy S, Olshefski R, Taylor B, Patel K, Reaman G: Correlation of P-glycoprotein expression and function in childhood acute leukemia: a children's cancer group study. Blood 1996, 88:309–318.
20. den Boer M, Pieters R, Kazemier K, al e: Relationship between major vault protein/lung resistance protein, multidrug resistance-associated protein, P-glycoprotein expression, and drug resistance in childhood leukemia. Blood 1998, 91:2092–2098.
21. Brophy NA, Marie JP, Rojas VA, Warnke RA, Mcfall PJ, Smith SD, Sikic BI: Mdr1 gene expression in childhood acute lymphoblastic leukemias and lymphomas - a critical evaluation by four techniques. Leukemia 1994, 8:327–335.
22. Wattel E, Lepelley P, Merlat A, Sartiaux C, Bauters F, Jouet J, Fenaux P: Expression of the P-gp in newly diagnosed adult ALL: absence of correlation with response to treatment. Leukemia 1995, 11:1870–1874.

CLINICAL SIGNIFICANCE OF P-GLYCOPROTEIN (P-gp) EXPRESSION IN CHILDHOOD ACUTE LYMPHOBLASTIC LEUKEMIA

Results of a 6-Year Prospective Study

Catharina Dhooge[1] and Barbara De Moerloose[2]

[1]Department of Pediatrics
University Hospital
de pintelaan 185 B-9000 Gent, Belgium
[2]Research assistant of the Fund for Scientific Research (FWO), Flanders

Keywords: MDR, P-glycoprotein, childhood leukemia, immunocytochemistry.

1. ABSTRACT

P-glycoprotein (P-gp), a cellular drug-efflux pump is thought to be one of the major causes of multidrug resistance in malignancies. Since therapeutic strategies are being developed to circumvent drug resistance by inhibiting P-gp, prospective studies concerning the clinical relevance of P-gp in childhood leukemia are warranted. *Methods:* P-gp was studied in 102 consecutive cases of de novo childhood ALL and in 34 relapsed patients. An immunocytochemical technique with two monoclonal antibodies (C219,4E3) was used on bone marrow and blood smears. *Results:* 12/34 (35%) children were scored positive at relapse compared to 12/102 (12%) children with newly diagnosed ALL (p =0.006). No correlation between P-gp expression and clinical and hematological parameters was seen. All patients were treated according to the EORTC-CLCG protocols (survival at 5 years=85%). 20/102 patients relapsed. The mortality rate in the P-gp positive group was significantly worse (Logrank P=0.009) than in the P-gp negative patients. In the relapsed patient population 10/12 P-gp positive cases experienced an unfavourable outcome compared with 10/22 P-gp negative patients [Risk Ratio 2.21 (0.90–5.45)]. *Conclusions*: P-glycoprotein expression in newly diagnosed childhood ALL is an independent prognostic

Table 1. P-gp positive patients at diagnosis

Initials	Age at diagn Mo	Diagn	WBC	Bl0	Bl8	Risk	RF	P-gp BM C219	P-gp blood C219	P-gp BM 4E3	P-gp blood 4E3	resp	SEFS	Follow-up mo	Outcome
CA 1	61	1	7800	4130	330	1	1,42	2	2	1	2	CR	2	59	DEAD
CR 2	73	1	38800	28712	468	1	1,62	2	2	1	1	CR	1	62	ALIVE
BA 3	93	1	2600	26	0	1	0,39	2	0	1	0	CR	1	57	ALIVE
RD 4	34	1	18600	6138	680	1	1,00	2	2		2	CR	1	55	ALIVE
HKF 5	75	1	4700	0	0	1	0,85	2	0	2	0	CR	2	55	ALIVE
PA 6	7	1	178000	106800	4477	2	1,44	2	2	1	0	CR	1	23	DEAD
PM 7	40	2	46000	25920	3618	2	1,42	2	2	2	1	CR	1	50	ALIVE
RN 8	2	1	573000	435480	100	2	1,79	2	2	2	0	CR	2	5	DEAD
BJ 9	25	1	8500	3145	84	1	0,69	2	2	1	0	CR	2	35	ALIVE
DW 10	160	1	23300	9087	1512	2	1,50	2	2	2	2	CR	1	25	ALIVE
TP 11	27	1	49900	37425	76	1	1,61	2	0	2	2	CR	1	19	ALIVE
TP 12	45	1	310	40	0		—	0	0	2	0	—	2	0	DEAD

parameter for dismal outcome. P-gp positivity at relapse tends towards an adverse clinical outcome compared to the P-gp negative relapsed population

2. INTRODUCTION

Intensive treatment with anticancer agents and well designed chemotherapeutic strategies led to an important improvement in the cure for childhood leukemia. Chemotherapy failure in a minor group of childhood patients has been thought to be due to cellular drug resistance.[1] Few reports regarding MDR1 in childhood ALL are reported in the literature and contradictory results concerning the clinical application of P-GP are described.[2,3,4,5,6,7] Therefore we started a multicenter prospective study to investigate the presence of P-glycoprotein and its clinical implication in childhood ALL.

3. MATERIALS AND METHODS

3.1. Leukemia Cells from Patients

Between 1/10/1990 until the 30/9/1996 106 children (age 0–16) were admitted at the Department of Pediatrics of the University of Gent and at the Children's Hospital 'Reine Fabiola' in Brussel, Belgium with the diagnosis of de novo acute lymphoblastic leukemia (ALL). Of 102 children, smears of bone marrow (BM) and/or blood samples were prospectively evaluated for P-170 expression. Four children were exluded from the study because there was not enough material for P-170 immunocytochemical analysis.The diagnosis was based on standard morphology, cytochemistry and immunophenotyping of the blasts. DNA content and cytogenetics of the leukemic cells were studied in nearly all patients. In 13 patients, the diagnosis of T-ALL was made; 1 infant had a null cell Acute Leukemia; 88 children suffered from a non-B non-T ALL. Morphologic review by the pathologist for the EORTC-CLCG (European Organisation for Research and Treatment of Cancer - Childhood Leukemia Cooperative Group) confirmed the diagnosis in each case. All patients were treated according to the EORTC-CLCG (5883-58881) protocols, including vincristine and anthracyclines which are involved with MDR.

Pretreatment response to one week corticosteroids, calculation of the risk factor (RF) as defined by the protocol,[8] remission status (CR) and event free survival (EFS) are available for all patients (data not shown). All patients were seen on a regular basis at the pediatric hematology clinic. Mean time of follow-up is 46 months with a median of 47 months. We also examined 34 patients who were treated at our department for ALL during childhood and who subsequently relapsed. Patients' characteristics are listed in Table 2. In 17, slides from initial diagnosis together with slides at relapsed stage were available for MDR1 expression.Treatment at relapse was given according to the EORTC-CLCG protocols. At the time of evaluation, eight patients (case 1, 10, 13, 14, 18, 21, 23, 26) underwent a matched unrelated bone marrow transplantation (MUD); 4 patients received a transplant from a matched sibling (6, 16, 20, 25) and 2 autologous BMT were performed (case12,27). Smears of bone marrow and blood at diagnosis and in case of relapse were air-dried for 24 h, and then frozen at -20°C to increase permeability of the cell membrane. In case of CNS invasion, cytospins were made and stored at -20°C until use.

Table 2. Patients at relapse

Pat Init	Age diagn (mo)	Diagn	P-170 diagn	Time betw diag/rel	P-170 relapse	Follow-up (mo)	Therapy	Outcome
WD1	59	1	0	14	1	18	4	Dead
DMK2	66	1	0	39	2	105	1	Dead
PA3	27	1	0	19	2/2	128	1	Alive
PT4	32	1	0	42	1	126	1	Alive
RP5	56	3	0	102	1	223	1	Alive
BE6	29	1	0	32	2/2/2	59	3	Dead
ES7	68	1	0	43	1/1/1	147	1	Dead
HB8	111	1	0	60	2	111	1	Dead
ME9	164	1	1	5	2/2	11	1	Dead
DVK10	126	1	0	29	1	45	4	Dead
HS11	85	1	0	23	2	32	1	Dead
WS12	185	2	1	19	1/1	25	2	Dead
MK13	66	1	1	10	1/1	19	4	Dead
HT14	123	1	0	10	2	17	4	Dead
VS15	40	1	1	24	1	32	1	Dead
VPS16	42	1	0	39	2	89	3	Alive
DRK17	51	1	0	67	1	185	1	Alive
PA18	7	1	2	7	2/1	23	4	Dead
GD19	61	1	0	86	1	129	1	Alive
RN20	2	3	2	2	2	5	3	Dead
BS21	49	1	0	34	1/1	101	4	Dead
VK22	31	1	1	44	1	80	1	Alive
CA23	61	1	2	41	2/2/2	59	4	Dead
DBM24	125	1	1	33	1	56	1	Alive
MN25	173	1	1	24	2/2	34	3	Dead
CJ26	74	1	0	8	1	14	4	Dead
RZ27	99	1	1	33	1	61	2	Alive
BE28	118	1	1	47	1	48	1	Dead
VDSM29	74	1	1	35	1	37	1	Alive
DT30	107	2	1	32	1	33	1	Alive
BJ31	23	1	2	35	1	35	1	Alive
SS32	23	1	1	23	1	30	1	Alive
CP33	1	1	0	16	1	47	5	Dead
DWM34	41	1	1	48	1	47	1	Alive

Diagnosis:1=nonB nonT ALL;2=T-ALL;3=unclassified ;P-170: 1=negative;2= positive; 0=not done. P-170 at relapse: / subsequent relapses; bone marrow, cytospins of lumbar liquid Therapy:1=chemotherapy alone according to EORTC-CLCG;2= ABMT; 3= MSD BMT; 4= MUD; 5=other

3.2. Immunocytochemical Technique

An alkaline phosphatase-anti-alkaline phosphatase immunocytochemical assay (APAAP) with C219 (20µg/mL, Dako Corporation) and 4E3 (10 µg/ml Dako Corporation) was used.[9] After fixation in glutaraldehyde 0.0125% in Phosphate Buffered Saline (PBS – pH 7.2) for 30 sec. at 4°C, the slides were incubated with the monoclonal antibodies for 30 min at room temperature. The APAAP (APAAP-DAKOPATTS Glostrupp Denmark) staining procedure was executed as described by the manufacturer.[10] The sensitivity of the technique was improved by adding a tertiary layer of mouse anti-rabbit-antibodies plus APAAP complex after the use of rabbit anti-mouse antibodies.[11] In-vitro cultured cell-lines K-562 and its multidrug resistant clone (K-562/VLB) as well as slides without incubation with primary antibody were included in each experiment. The results were interpreted by three observers without knowledge of the patient's response to treatment. In agreement with the recommendations of the Memphis work shop,[12] no cutoff points were used and P-glycoprotein expression was scored as positive or negative on bone marrow and blood smears if a red staining pattern along the cell membrane was observed.

3.3. Statistical Methods

Mortality experience was estimated according the Kaplan-Meier procedure. Relative impact on mortality of baseline variables was expressed as Risk Ratio's (RR). Multivariate analysis was performed according to Cox proportional hazard modelling.

4. RESULTS

4.1. Cell Surface Reactivity of ALL Cells with Mab

4.1.1. Concordance between BM and Blood Smears. Three hundred fifty nine smears of bone marrow and blood were evaluated for P-gp at diagnosis. In 96 of 99 samples where BM and Blood smears were simultaneously examined, both BM and blood smears showed the same results (97% concordance). In the positive slides, using immunocytochemistry, a mean of 30% of the blast population was P-GP positive, reflecting the heterogeneity of the tumor cells.[13] As described previously[14,15] positive staining of normal myeloid precursor cells (CD34 positive cells) and in the neutrophils was observed in 40% of the examined samples. Normal and reactive lymphocytes were P-GP negative. Using this technique it was not possible to make a differentiation in intensity of the staining in order to use it as a (semi) quantitative method.

4.1.2. Feasability of the Technique. Three hundred eighty one smears of 102 children at diagnosis and hundred seventy one smears of 35 children at relapse were examined with the APAAP method which is a mean of 3.7 and 4.9 per patient respectively. Immunocytochemical analysis depends upon the observer's interpretation of the staining. In more than 80% of the slides, the 3 observers came to the same conclusions. In case of disagreement, other smears of the same patient (stored at the same time) were then analysed until a consensus was reached.

Using immunocytochemistry, it was possible to examine cytospins containing only few metastatic cells and with respect to the intact cell structure. 4 children with de novo ALL and 8 children at relapse had CNS invasion. Immunocytochemical analysis of cytospins containing metastastic disease revealed positive P-GP on the blasts in two (pat 3,8). We could not find a significant difference in staining intensity between diagnostic smears and slides at relapse.

4.2. Prognostic Value of P-gp Expression

4.2.1. P-gp Positivity at Initial Diagnosis. Twelve of 102 (12%) children expressed P-gp at diagnosis. The P-gp positive patients and their prognostic variables are listed in Table 1. Multivariate analysis showed that P-gp expression was independent of white blood-cell count (WBC), age, sex and risk factor (RF) (Table 3). 100/102 patients with de novo ALL achieved complete remission after induction therapy (98%). Twenty-one of 102 patients relapsed (20%). 74 of 90 P-gp negative cases are in CCR as compared with 7 of 12 P-gp positive cases.The mortality rate in the P-gp positive group was significantly worse (Logrank P=0.009) compared to the P-gp negative population (Figure 1). Event-free survival is 79 percent at 4 years (mean follow-up of 46 mo), overall survival at 5 years is 85 percent.

Table 3. Prognostic factors examined (N=102)

	%Dead	Mortality rate	RR_u*		RR_m**	
Age						
1–10 yrs	8.1 (7/87)	19.0	1		1	
<1 or >10 yrs	33.3 (5/15)	151.9	7.56 (2.21–25.83)	P=0.001	3.89 (0.94–16.13)	P=0.06
Sex						
F	13.7 (7/51)	34.7	1		1	
M	9.8 (5/51)	25.1	0.71 (0.22–2.23)	P=0.55	0.34 (0.08–1.40)	P=0.13
WBC						
≤ 100.000	7.7 (7/91)	18.7	1		1	
> 100.000	45.5 (5/11)	190.6	9.79 (2.91–32.92)	P=0.0001	8.13 (1.77–37.32)	P=0.007
Corticoresponse						
≤ 1000	9.7 (9/93)	24.1	1		1	
> 1000	33.3 (3/9)	110.9	4.38 (1.16–16.53)	P=0.03	1.24 (0.22–6.89)	P=0.81
DNA Index						
< 1.16 or > 1.60	7.3 (4/55)	22.2	1			
1.16–1.60	7.7 (1/13)	15.1	1.03 (0.12–9.26)	P=0.98		
PGP expression at diagnosis						
Neg	9.2 (8/87)	22.7	1		1	
Pos	33.3 (4/12)	108.7	4.31 (1.29–14.37)	P=0.02	3.19 (0.81–12.54)	P=0.10
P-gp expression at relapse						
Neg	45.5 (10/22)	78.0	1		1	
Pos	83.3 (10/12)	178.3	2.21 (0.9–5.45)	P=0.09	1.34 (0.51–3.51)	P=0.56

*RR_u: Univariate Risk Ratio (95% confidence interval and p-value)
**RR_m: Multivariately adjusted Risk Ratio (95% confidence interval and p-value) according to Cox proportional hazard modelling (DNA-index not included due to scarce information)

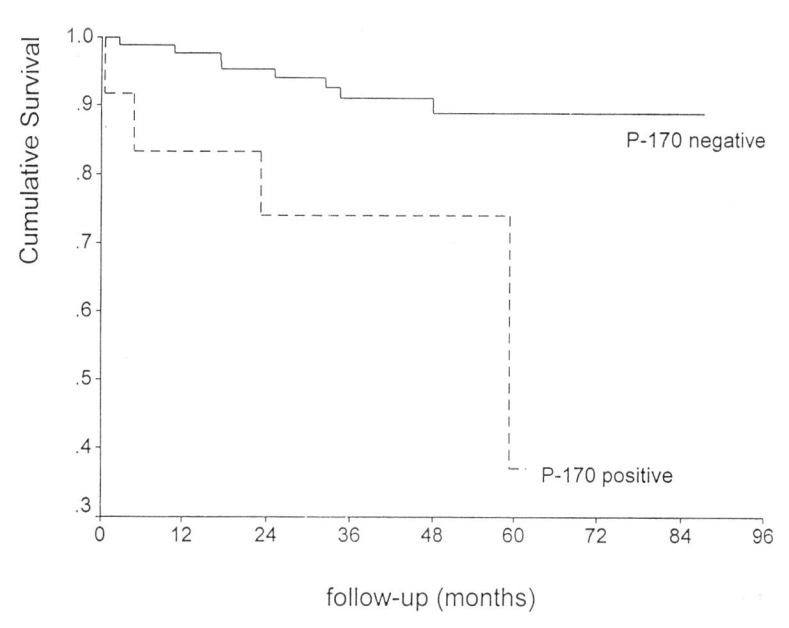

Figure 1. Kaplan-Meier patient's survival according to P-GP expression on leukemic blasts at diagnosis for all 102 children evaluated.

4.2.2. P-GP Positivity at Relapse. 12 of 34 (35%) were scored positive at relapse. This result is significantly higher than the initial percentage of positive cases at diagnosis ($X^2=7.62$ p=0.006). In the relapsed patient population, 10/12 P-GP positive cases experienced an unfavourable outcome compared with 10–22 P-GP negative patients [Risk Ratio 2.21 (0.90–5.45)] (Figure 2).

5. DISCUSSION

Few reports concerning the prognostic value of P-gp detection in childhood leukemia have been reported.[7,16,17] Our study showed that P-gp in newly diagnosed childhood ALL is rarely present on the leukemic cells (12%), in contrast to the AML where P-glycoprotein is present in up to 40–50% at diagnosis.[18,19,20]

However, among the different variables studied in our patient group, calculation of the relative impact on mortality clearly showed that P-gp expression was correlated with a significantly higher mortality risk (p=0.009). Moreover, in multivariate analysis, P-gp proved to be an independent prognostic factor.

In the relapsed patient population, the relative risk to experience a unfavourable outcome when P-gp was present, was two times higher (RR:2.21) compared to the P-gp negative relapsed patient group. These results support that not only the glycoprotein was present on the leukemic blasts but that the pump was functioning, resulting in multidrug resistance, both in de novo ALL as well as in the relapsed patients. Baines stressed the importance of longitudinal prospective studies using samples from the same patients before and after chemotherapy before any conclusions regarding the clinical implication of P-gp can be made. Our longitudinal prospective study with a 6 years follow-up clearly showed

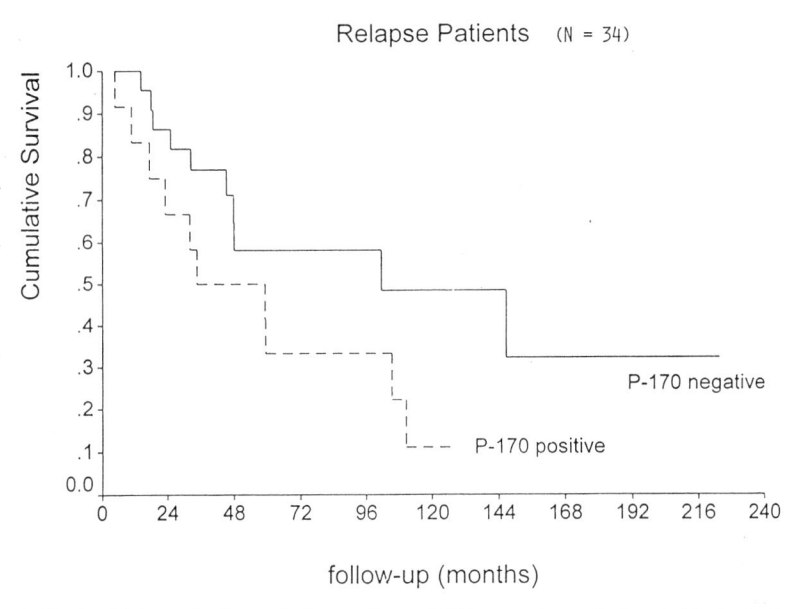

Figure 2. Kaplan-Meier patient's survival according to P-GP expression on leukemic blasts at relapse.

that P-gp expression remained negative in 85% of the relapsed patients who were P-gp negative at diagnosis. From these findings, we conclude that induction of MDR1 by previous chemotherapy is not likely to be the case in childhood ALL.

From a technical point of view, we found that immunohistochemistry, used as described above, was easily applicable, with good reproducability. Using a technique which shows the presence of the protein on each leukemic cell has some advantages, as was mentioned by others.[12,21,22] This technique offered the opportunity to examine cytospins of lumbar liquid containing only few tumor cells (< 5 cells/µL) as well as to detect heterogeneity of P-gp expression within a blastpopulation with respect to the intact cell structure, thus avoiding false positive interpretation.[11,13,14] Moreover, the fact that in our study population some patients with only 2 or 3% P-gp positive blasts at diagnosis subsequently relapsed, points towards the advantage of this technique to examine small numbers of intact cells with the MDR1 phenotype.

ACKNOWLEDGMENTS

This work was supported by a N.F.W.O. "Aspirant Kom Op".

REFERENCES

1. Kartner N, Ling V (1989) Multidrug Resistance in Cancer. Scientific American 26–33
2. Carulli G, Petrini M, Marini A, Ambrogi F (1988) P-glycoprotein in acute leukemia and in the blastic crisis of myeloid leukemia. N Engl J Med 319: 797–798
3. Kuwazuru Y, Yoshimura A, Hanada S, Utsunomiya A, Makino T, Ishibashi K, Kodama M, Iwahashi M, Arima T, Akiyama S (1990) Expression of the Multidrug transporter, P-Glycoprotein, in Acute Leukemia Cells and Correlation to Clinical Drug Resistance. Cancer 66: 868–873

4. Wattel E, Lepelley P, Merlat A (1995) Expression of the multidrug resistance P glycoprotein in newly diagnosed adult acute lymphoblastic leukemia: absence of correlation with response to treatment. Leukemia 9:1870–1874
5. Mizuno Y, Hara T, Nagata M, Tawa A, Tsuruo T, Ueda K (1991) Detection of multidrug-resistant protein, P-glycoprotein in childhood leukaemia and lymphoma. Eur J Pediatr 150: 416–418
6. Ubezio P, Limonta M, D'Incalci M, Damia G, Masera G, Giudici G, Wolverto J, Beck WT (1989) Failure to detect the P-glycoprotein multidrug resistant phenotype in case of resistant childhood acute lymphoblastic leukemia. Eur J Cancer Clin Oncol 25:1895–1899
7. Pieters R, Hongo T, Loonen AH (1992) Different types of non-P-glycoprotein mediated multiple drug resistance in children with relapsed acute lymphoblastic leukeamia. Br. J Cancer 65:691–697
8. Langermann H J, Henze G, Wulf M, Riehm H (1982) Abschatzung der Tumorzellmasse bei der akuten lymphoblastischen Leukamie im Kindersalter: prognostische Bedeutung und praktische Anwendung. Klin. Pediatr. 194: 209–213
9. Kartner N, Evernden-Porelle D, Bradley G, Ling V (1985) Detection of P-glycoprotein in multidrug-resistant cell lines by monoclonal antibodies. Nature 316: 820–823
10. Cordell JL, Falini B, Erber WN (1984) Immunoenzymatic labeling of monoclonal antibodies using immune complexes of alkaline phosphatase and monoclonal anti-alkaline phosphatase (APAAP) complexes. J Histochem Cytochem 32: 219–229
11. C Dhooge, De Moerloose B., De Potter C.(1994) Expression of the Multidrug Transporter, P-Glycoprotein, in Childhood Leukemia:A Prospective Clinical Study. International Journal of Pediatric Hematology/Oncology (1):311–314
12. Beck WT, Grogan TM, Willman CL (1996) Methods to detect P-Glycoprotein-associated Multidrug Resistance in Patients 'Tumors: Consensus Recommendations. Cancer Research 56:3010–3020
13. Knaust E, MacDonald P, Gruber A (1998) Heterogeneity in blast cell populations in acute myeloid leukemia (AML) affects accumulation abd efflux of daunorubicin. Leukemia 12 (2) 3rd Intern Symposium of Drug Resistance in Leukemia and Lymphoma:p10 (abstract)
14. List AF, Spier C, Greer J (1993) Phase I/II Trial of Cyclosporine as a Chemotherapy-Resistance Modifier in Acute Leukemia. Journal of Clinical Oncology 11(9):1652–1660
15. Schlaifer D, Laurent G, Chittal S, Tsuruo T, Soues S, Muller C, Charcosset J Y, Alard C, Brousset P, Mazerrolles C, Delsol G (1990) Immunohistochemical detection of multidrug resistance associated P-glycoprotein in tumour and stromal cells of human cancers. Br J Cancer 62, 177–182
16. Rothenberg ML, Mickley LA, Cole DE, Balis FM, Tsuruo T, Poplack D, Fojo AT (1989) Expression of mdr1/ P-170 gene in patients with acute lymphoblastic leukemia. Blood 74:1388–1395
17. Pui C-H (1995) Childhood Leukemias. The new England Journal of Medicine 332(24):1618–1630
18. Leith CP, Kopecky KJ, Godwin J (1997) Acute Myeloid Leukemia in the Elderly: Assessment of Multidrug Resistance (MDR1) and Cytogenetics Distinguishes Biologic Subgroups with Remarkably Distinct Responses to Standard Chemotherapy. A Southwest Oncology Group Study.Blood 89(9):3323–3329
19. Del Poeta G, Venditti A, Aronica G (1997) P-Glycoprotein expressiopn in de novo acute myeloid leukemia. Leukemia and Lymphoma 27:257–274
20. Van den Heuvel-Eibrinck M.M. , van der Holt B, Te Boekhorst P.A.W. (1997) MDR1 expression is an independent prognostic factor for response and survival in de novo acute myeloid leukemia Br. J. Haem. 99:76–83
21. Van der Heyden S, Gheuens E, De Bruijn E (1995) P-Glycoprotein: Clinical Significance and Methods of Analysis. Critical reviews in Clinical Laboratory Sciences 32(3):221–264
22. Chan HSL, Thorner PS, Haddad G (1995) Multidrug resistance in Malignancies of Children. International Journal of Pediatric Hematology/Oncology 2:11–29

3

PROGNOSTIC VALUE OF P-gp EXPRESSION AND RELATED FUNCTION IN CHILDHOOD ACUTE LEUKEMIA

Z. Karakaş,[1] L. Ağaoğlu,[1] S. Erdem,[2] G. Yanikkaya Demirel,[3] M. Arasa,[4] F. Süzergöz,[2] G. Deniz,[4] S. Anak,[1] and G. Gedikoğlu[5]

[1]Department of Pediatric Hematology/Oncology
[2]Department of Physiology
I.U. School of Medicine
[3]Pakize Tarzi Lab
[4]DETAE
[5]Our Children Leukemia Foundation
Capa 34390 Istanbul/Turkey

INTRODUCTION

Drug resistance is supposed to play an important role in the poor prognosis of part of the children with acute leukemia but the knowledge of drug resistance in these children is limited. Although increased expression of P-gp is found in some cases of childhood acute leukemia at initial presentation, the data are conflicting concerning the relation to clinical outcome.[4,5,9] Most of study on the subject has been accomplished on adults and children and due to variations in methods a consensus on the results has not been established yet. Many mechanisms are playing role in drug resistance, the need to evaluate the functional aspects together with P-gp levels has been reported.[4,6,8] The aim of this study is to evaluate the multidrug resistance in vitro and investigate the correlations with clinical findings. To evaluate the clinical importance of P-gp, its correlation with age, sex, morphology, immuno-phenotyping, hemogram, remission and outcome have been examined. We have measured the initial diagnosis, remission and relapse levels of P-gp by binding a specific monoclonal antibody (UIC2) and functional properties of the drug resistance with flow cytometry in childhood ALL and AML.

MATERIAL AND METHODS

Samples and Patients

This study has been accomplished on 92 cryopreserved bone marrow samples from 51 cases with acute leukemia and 10 bone marrow transplantation (BMT) donors which have been followed up at Pediatrics Hematology/Oncology Department of Istanbul University and Our Children Leukemia Foundation during the 22 months period from January 1996-October 1997.

P-gp was investigated using a monoclonal antibody (U1C2) directed against a cell surface epitope of the P-gp by flow cytometry with indirect fluorescence staining. Bone marrow aspirates from 92 children were evaluated (83 were eligible: an abnormal nonspecific binding was observed in 9 cases): 25 ALL, 12 AML, 11 relapsed patients (5 ALL, 6 AML), 16 ALL in remission, 9 AML in remission and 10 BMT donors (control group) were tested. Since normal bone marrow cells express P-gp; P-gp levels are evaluated as negative or positive. While the cut-off value changes with the monoclonal antibody and the method used; there is no consensus on the value. In several articles, over 5, 10, 20, 30% have been taken as the cut-off, generally values over the control group has been accepted as positive.[1,5] We have accepted the cut-off as two standard deviation value over the mean value which was >13.3%. For evaluation of functional properties of P-gp, intracellular Daunorubicin (DNR) and Rhodamine (Rho-123) accumulation is measured by flow cytometry and functional activity of P-gp by using CSA to block the efflux pump. P-gp activity was evaluated with below formula:

$$P\text{-gp activity} = \frac{DNR(Rho\text{-}123) + CSA - DNR(Rho\text{-}123) - CSA \times 100}{DNR(Rho\text{-}123) - CSA}$$

RESULTS

P-gp was positive in 44% of ALL, 75% of AML, 18.8% of remission ALL, 22.2% of remission AML cases. In all of the relapse cases, P-gp was positive (Figure 1). When P-gp positivity was correlated to all other clinical and laboratory prognostic factors, it was seen

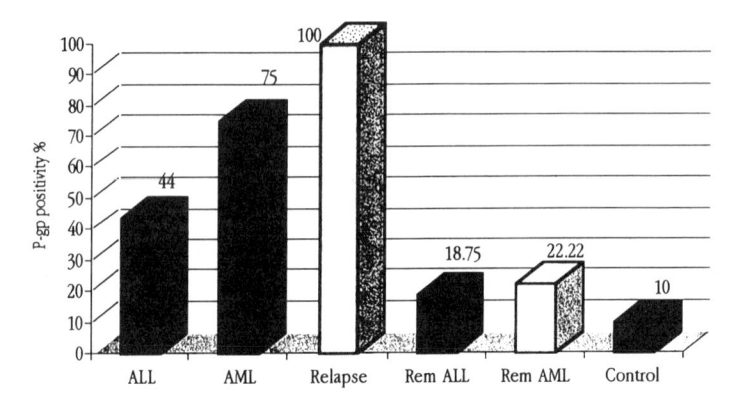

Figure 1. P-gp positivity in children with acute leukemia and control group.

Table 1. Relationship between P-gp positivity and other clinical prognostic factors

Features	ALL n	ALL n¹	ALL %¹	x^2	p	AML n	AML n	AML %	x^2	p
Age										
< 2	1	1	100			—	—	—		
2 - 9	19	7	36.8	2.18	0.33	7	4	57.1	2.85	0.09
≥9	5	3	60			5	5	100		
Sex										
Female	11	3	37.2	2.23	0.13	2	2	100	0.8	0.37
Male	14	8	51.7			10	7	70		
Hepatomegaly										
Positive	18	9	50	0.93	0.33	6	4	66.6	0.44	0.50
Negative	7	2	28.5			6	5	83.3		
Splenomegaly										
Positive	15	8	53.3	1.32	0.24	5	5	100	2.85	0.09
Negative	10	3	30			7	4	57.1		
LAP										
Positive	16	8	50	0.64	0.42	7	5	71.4	0.11	0.73
Negative	9	3	33.3			5	4	80		
Bleeding										
Positive	11	6	5.5	0.88	0.34	6	4	66.6	0.44	0.50
Negative	14	5	35.7		6	6	5	83.3		
Hct										
< 30	19	8	42.1	0.11	0.73	8	6	75	0.0	1
≥30	6	3	50			6	3	75		
Leukocyte										
< 50.000	20	7	35	3.28	0.06	9	7	77.7	0.14	0.70
≥ 50.000	5	4	80			3	2	66.6		
Platelet										
< 100.000	20	8	40	0.64	0.42	9	7	77.7	0.14	0.70
≥ 100.000	5	3	60			3	2	66.6		
FAB ALL										
L₁	19	9	43.3							
L₂	3	—	—	3.07	0.21	—	—	—	—	
L₃	3	2	66.6							
AML										
M₁						3	2	66.6		
M₂	—	—	—	—	—	4	3	75	44.4	0.21
M₄						4	4	100		

¹P-gp positivity

that P-gp positivity in ALL was independent from all other factors while in AML correlated to CD7, CD13 and CD34 (Table 1 and 2). Relation to survival in ALL and AML cases according to P-gp levels is shown in Figure 2 and 3. Functional activity of P-gp is shown on Table 3 and Figure 4 and 5.

DISCUSSION

In childhood acute leukemia, there is need for determining new predictive factors to be evaluated on individual basis and to foresee the relapses which is one of the main reasons of death in leukemia.[2]

Drug resistance is the most important and the most studied one of the predictive factors, recently.

Table 2. Relationship between P-gp and surface markers (CD)

Feature	ALL P-gp positivity n	n	%	x^2	p	AML P-gp positivity n	n	%	x^2	p
CD$_3$										
Positive	10	3	30	1.32	0.24	2	1	50	0.80	0.37
Negative	15	8	53.3			10	8	80		
CD$_5$										
Positive	11	4	36.3	0.46	0.49	1	–	0	3.27	0.07
Negative	14	7	50			11	9	81.8		
CD$_7$										
Positive	11	4	36.3	0.46	0.49	4	1	25	8.0	0.004
Negative	14	7	50			8	8	100		
CD$_{10}$										
Positive	16	5	31.2	2.93	0.08	–	–	–	–	–
Negative	9	6	66.6			12	9	75		
CD$_{19}$										
Positive	20	8	40	0.64	0.42	–	–	–	–	–
Negative	5	3	60			12	9	75		
CD$_{20}$										
Positive	4	2	50	0.06	0.79	1	1	100	0.36	0.54
Negative	21	9	42.8			11	8	72.7		
CD$_{22}$										
Positive	16	6	37.5	0.76	0.38	2	2	100	0.80	0.37
Negative	9	5	55.5			10	7	70		
CD$_{11b}$										
Positive	–	–	–	–	–	6	5	63.3	0.44	0.50
Negative	25	11	44			6	4	66.6		
CD$_{13}$										
Positive	14	2	14.2	0.06	0.79	6	3	50	4.0	0.04
Negative	11	9	81.8			6	6	100		
CD$_{14}$										
Positive	–	–	–	–		1	1	100	0.36	0.54
Negative	25	11	44			11	8	72.7		
CD$_{33}$										
Positive	14	2	14.2	0.06	0.79	12	9	75	–	–
Negative	11	9	81.8			–	–	–		
CD$_{34}$										
Positive	10	5	50	0.24	0.62	5	2	40	8.0	0.004
Negative	15	6	40			7	7	100		
HLADR										
Positive	19	7	36.8	1.64	0.19	12	9	75	–	–
Negative	6	4	66.6			–	–	–		
CD$_{45}$										
Positive	25	11	44	–	–	8	5	62.5	2.0	0.15
Negative	–	–	–			3	3	100		

There are many questions to be answered with the conflicts in present clinical studies. When our findings in this study are compared with present literature they have led us to the questions below.

Is the Resistance Related to P-gp Primary or Acquired?

Our results show that drug resistance related to p-glycoprotein can be primary and acquired resistance. P-gp was found to be positive at first diagnosed ALL and AML with

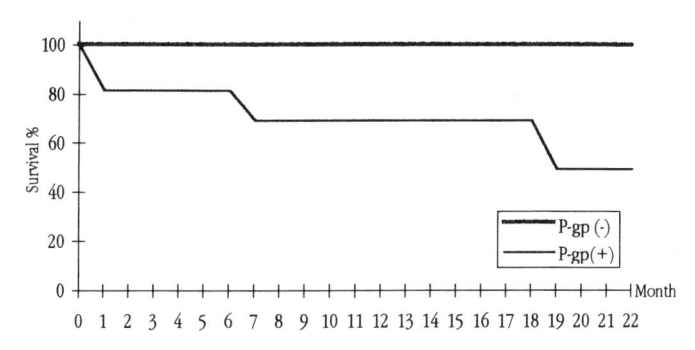

Figure 2. Survival in ALL patients relations to P-gp.

higher levels in AML (primary resistance).[6] In several published reports, P-gp is positive 10–36% in ALL, 13–71% in AML cases.[8] ALL has a better prognosis compared to AML and this may be due to cellular resistance.[7] The highest level of pgp were observed in relapsed patients. It may be due to their previous chemotherapy (acquired resistance).[4]

Is There a Prognostic Importance of P-gp Expression?

There are articles stating that P-gp positivity is related to prognosis and other stating that there is no correlation.[6] We think that conflicts are the results of different techniques, methods, and cut-off values.

What Is the Relation of P-gp with Other Prognostic Factors?

In studies of children and adults who had AML, it was reported that P-gp expression was positive at the onset of the disease, was increasing in relapse, comparatively lower in APL cases, was correlated to CD7 and CD34 positivities, respond to therapy and to chromosome anomalies, so it could be evaluated as an independent prognostic factor.[2-6] As will be observed with our results, P-gp expression is also a prognostic factor, evaluation of mdr phenotype by flow cytometry is an important indicator of therapy follow up. High relapse rate and short term survey have been reported in patients with P-gp positive ALL.[3]

Is There a Relation between P-gp Expression and Functions?

Intracellular drug concentration is regulated by other mechanisms than P-gp also and for this reason in researches for multidrug resistance together with protein levels and P-gp

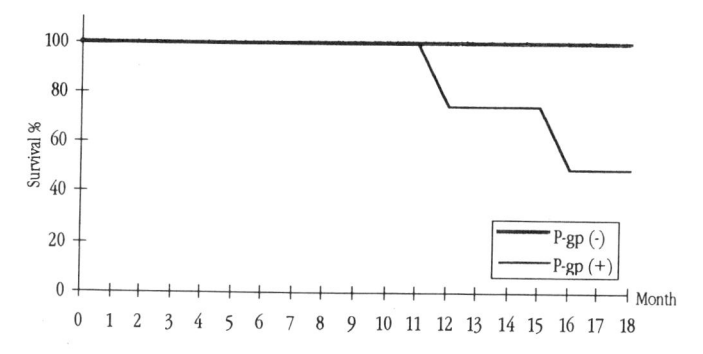

Figure 3. Survival in AML patients in relation to P-gp.

Table 3. Functional activity of P-gp

Functional activity	ALL Pgp (±) n %	ALL Pgp (-) n %	AML Pgp (±) n %	AML Pgp (-) n %	Relapse Pgp (±) n %	Relapse Pgp (-) n %	Total Pgp (±) n %	Total Pgp (-) n %
DNR								
Negative	4 (50)	8 (66.6)	2 (66.6)	1 (50)	5 (55.5)	—	11 (55)	9 (64.3)
Positive	4 (50)	4 (33.3)	1 (33.3)	1 (50)	4 (44.4)	—	9 (45)	5 (35.7)
< %50	3 (37.5)	3 (25)	1 (33.3)	—	1 (11.1)	—	5 (25)	3 (21.4)
≥ %50	1 (12.5)	1 (8.3)	—	1 (50)	3 (33.3)	—	4 (20)	2 (14.3)
Nonevaluable	3 –	2	6 –	1 –	2 —	—	14 —	—
Significance								
x^2/p	0.77	>0.05	2.23	>0.05			0.44	>0.05
Rho-123								
Negative	5 (45.4)	9 (75)	7 (63.6)	3 (2.72)	8 (80)	—	20	12
Positive	6 (54.5)	3 (25)	1 (9.1)	—	2 (20)	—	9	3
< %50	5 (45.4)	0 –	—	—	1 (10)	—	6	—
≥ %50	1 (9.1)	3 (25)	1 (9.1)	—	1 (10)	—	3	3
Nonevaluable	—	2 –	1	—	1	—	2	2
Significance								
x^2/p	8.04	<0.05					4.42	>0.05

function should be evaluated. Also, at first diagnosed ALL cases mean value of DNR levels was higher than AML ones but uncorrelated to P-gp levels. Rhodamine 123 accumulation was also higher in first admission ALL compared to AML, remission, relapse and control values but uncorrelated to P-gp levels.

A correlaton between the drug accumulation and P-gp expression was found which has led to explanation that non-functional P-gp (mutant form) and drug accumulation are not due to P-gp presence alone.[1,4,8]

What Is the Role of Membrane Transport Proteins Other Than P-gp?

The poor correlation between the P-gp expression and DNR transportation in AML blasts, led us to think about the presence of transportation molecules other than P-gp.[10]

The high level of non specific binding we have observed in nine of the patients were considered to be due to a non-P-gp molecule (MRP?). Non specific binding group were especially in high risk group 5 of these 9 patients (55.5%) had relapse and 6 (66.6%) were lost. It is been reported that MRP is increased in high risk patients and relapse. Also cyclosporine an effect the pump function with P-gp like proteins but this effect is minimal compared to P-gp.[6] It has been shown that MRP is increased during relapse. In our patients, we have observed functional activity in P-gp negative patients as well as the P-gp positive ones and could not detect a relation between the P-gp and functional activity.

We conclude that P-gp can be a good prognostic factor in leukemia but cannot explain the drug resistance alone.Other resistance mechanisms can be dominant under different conditions. To obtain a more clear picture of the situation efflux related to MRP should be evaluated also.[6]

Can Drug Resistance Be Prevented with Drug Resistance Regulators?

Although the P-gp was positive in all of our relapse patients, only 44.4% had functional activity. When the DNR levels were measured before and after cyclosporine only in

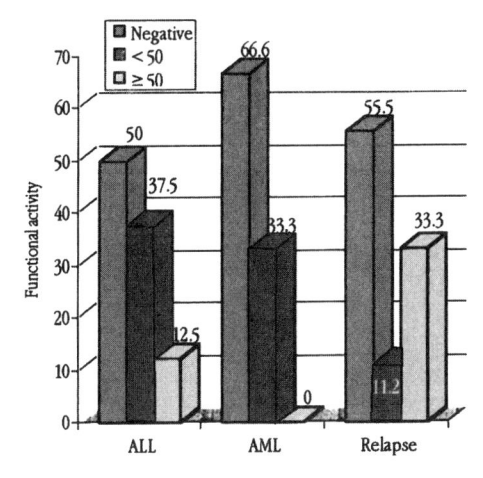

Figure 4. Functional activity evaluated with DNR.

first diagnosed ALL patients it had statistically important increase, in other groups did not have any effect. In our patient group who had non specific binding, P-gp functional activity was less than the other groups. This may be a supporting finding for the MRP presence for drug resistance which is effected from cyclosporine less compared to P-gp.

Will the P-gp Inhibition Contribute to Clinical Prognosis?

The clinical importance of the drug resistance is still not very well understood and even though there is research being done since 25–30 years, it has not taken its place in routine treatment protocols. To be able to detect the drug resistance before the beginning of treatment and use for treatment planning is the dream of the future.[6] The integration and correspondence of clinicians with basic scientists is necessary for developing of new treatment modalities for the benefit of drug resistant patients.[8]

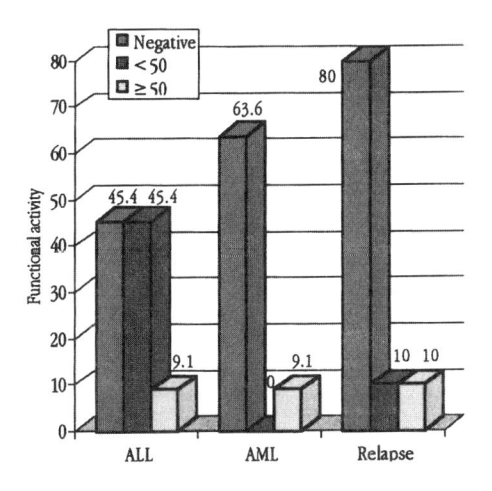

Figure 5. Functional activity evaluated with Rho-123.

REFERENCES

1. Bailly JD, Muller C, Jaffrezou JP, Demur C, Gassar G, Bordier C, Laurent G: Lack of correlation between expression and function of P-glycoprotein in acute myeloid leukemia cell lines. Leukemia 9(5):799–807, 1995.
2. Emura I, Naito M, Kakihara T, Wakabayashi M, Hayashi N, Chou T: Identification of Drug-Resistant myeloid leukemic cells by measurement of DNA Content, Nuclear Area and Detection of P-Glycoprotein. Cancer 77(5):878–887, 1996.
3. Goasquen JE, Dossot JM, Fardel O, Le Mee F, Le Gall E, Leblay R, Le Prise PY, Chaperon J, Fauchet R: Expression of the Multidrug Resistance-Associated P-Glycoprotein (P-170) in 59 Cases of De-Novo Acute Lymphoblastic Leukemia Prognostic implications. Blood 81(9):2394–2398, 1993.
4. Guerci A, Merlin JL, Missoum N, Fieldmann L, Marchal S, Witz F, Rose C, Guerci O: Predictive Value for Treatment Outcome in Acute Myeloid Leukemia of Cellular Daunorubicin Accumulation and P-Glycoprotein Expression Simultaneously Detemined by Flow Cytometry. Blood 85(8):2147–2153, 1995.
5. Ino T, Miyazaki H, Isogai M, Nomura T, Tsuzuki M, Tsuruo T, Ezaki K, Hirano M: Expression of P-Glycoprotein in De Novo Acute Myelogenous Leukemia at Initial Diagnosis: Results of Molecular and Functional Assays, and Correlation with Treatment Outcome. Leukemia 8(9): 1492–1497, 1994.
6. Ivy SP, Olshefski RS, Taylor BJ, Patel KM, Reaman GH: Correlation of P-Glycoprotein Expression and Function in Childhood Acute Leukemia: A Children's Cancer Group Study. Blood 88:309–318, 1996.
7. Kaspers GJ, Pieters R, Van Zantwijk CH, Van Wering ER, Veerman AJ : Clinical and cell biological features related to cellular drug resistance of childhood acute lymphoblastic leukemia. Leuk Lymphoma 19(5–6):407–416, 1995.
8. Pieters R, Hongo T, Loonen AH, Huismans DR, Broxterman HJ, Hahlen K, Veerman AJ: Different types of non-P-glycoprotein mediated multiple drug resistance in children with relapsed acute lymphoblastic leukemia. Br J Cancer 65(5):691–697, 1992.
9. Sievers EL, Smith FO, Woods WG, Lee JW, Bleyer WA, Willman CL, Bernstein ID: Cell surface expression of the multidrug resistance P-glycoprotein (P-170) as detected by monoclonal antibody MRK-16 in pediatric acute myeloid leukemia fails to define a poor prognostic group:a report from the Children's Cancer Group. Leukemia 9:2042–2048, 1995.
10. Xie XY, Robb D, Chow S, Hedley DW: Discordant P-glycoprotein antigen expression and transport function in acute myeloid leukemia. Leukemia 9:1882–1887, 1995.

COMPARISON OF P-GLYCOPROTEIN EXPRESSION AND FUNCTION WITH *IN VITRO* SENSITIVITY TO ANTHRACYCLINES IN AML

Alena W. Elgie, Jean M. Sargent, Christine J. Williamson, Grazyna M. Lewandowicz, and Colin G. Taylor

Haematology Research Department
Pembury Hospital
Pembury, Kent TN2 4QJ United Kingdom

Keywords: P-glycoprotein, Drug resistance, PSC833, GF120918, Resistance modulation, AML.

1. ABSTRACT

The importance of P-glycoprotein (P-gp) in AML has been well documented. Resistance to the anthracyclines can be overcome by several agents including Cyclosporin A (CsA), PSC833 and GF120918. We describe an investigation into the expression, using MRK16 and UIC2, and function of P-gp using daunorubicin with and without modulators by flow cytometric analysis on previously frozen blast cells from 27 patients with primary or secondary AML. We compared this with the *in vitro* chemosensitivity, using the MTT assay, of fresh blast cells from the same patients. Whilst we found a correlation between P-gp function using CsA and GF120918 and expression using MRK16 (p<0.05) and (p<0.02) respectively, we were unable to find any overall correlation between expression and function of P-gp with either *in vitro* sensitivity to the anthracyclines, previous treatment, or 1° or 2° disease. However it was possible to identify individual patients whose cells exhibited P-gp expression and function teamed with *in vitro* resistance to, and modification of, the anthracyclines. Furthermore, it is possible to identify which modulator had the greatest effect. The fact that we obtained higher indications of resistance reversal using the MTT assay along with finding P-gp expression and function in patients sensitive to the anthracyclines, suggests studies of P-gp should be teemed with chemosensitivity testing to identify specific patients who will benefit.

Drug Resistance in Leukemia and Lymphoma III, edited by Kaspers *et al.*
Kluwer Academic / Plenum Publishers, New York, 1999.

2. INTRODUCTION

One of the principal factors in therapy failure in acute myeloid leukaemia can be attributed to multidrug resistance. In recent years considerable attention has centred on the study of the multidrug resistance gene, *mdr-1*, which encodes the transmembrane protein P-170 or P-glycoprotein (P-gp). P-gp confers resistance to the vinca alkaloids, anthracyclines and epidophyllotoxins by actively effluxing drug from the cell.[1] Over expression of this gene has been found in *de novo* disease and in patients who have received previous treatment[2] and over expression of the protein has been found to result in poor prognosis and is associated with CD34+ cells.[3] It is possible to modulate this resistance using Cyclosporin A (CsA) and its analogue PSC833. It has been reported that PSC833 has greater effect than CsA.[4] A new agent, GF120918, has been reported as having good modulatory effects at 20nM.[5]

Our study centred on the analysis of P-gp expression using the MoAb's MRK16 and UIC2 which measure different epitopes of the protein. P-gp function was assessed by the accumulation of daunorubicin in the presence or absence of the modulators PSC833, CsA and GF120918. Where possible, correlation with the *in vitro* sensitivity to doxorubicin with and without the P-glycoprotein inhibitors was conducted.

3. METHODS

3.1. Patients

Peripheral blood or bone marrow was collected into citrate phosphate dextrose from 27 patients with AML, 23 with *de novo* disease (17 on first presentation and 6 on relapse) and 4 secondary to myelodysplasia or chronic granulocytic leukaemia. Of these 9 patients had received previous treatment. Blast cells were harvested using density gradient centrifugation, cells were washed in RPMI 1640, morphological assessment was made using the May Grünwald Giemsa stain and viability established using trypan blue dye exclusion. Final cell preparations contained greater than 80% blast cells, and viability of more than 90%. Final cell suspensions for the MTT assay at 1×10^6/ml were prepared in RPMI 1640 plus 10% FCS and antibiotics. Cells were prepared for cryopreservation in RPMI 1640 with 20% FCS and 10% DMSO until required for flow cytometry studies.

3.2. MTT Assay

Chemosensitivity testing was routinely conducted on all patients. Four dilutions of both daunorubicin (DNR) and doxorubicin (DOX) at 0.3–1.8µM, were made in RPMI 1640 plus 10% FCS and antibiotics. 100µl of cells at 1×10^6/ml were added to 100 µl of drugs at double strength, in triplicate in a microtitre plate. All experiments were controlled by cells in medium without drug. Plates were incubated for 48 hours at 37°C in 5%CO_2. Modification studies of drug + modulator were conducted using CsA its analogue PSC833 (Novartis Pharmaceuticals UK Ltd., Camberley, Surrey, UK) and GF120918 (GlaxoWellcome, Greenford, Middlesex, UK) at a fixed concentration of modifier (4 µM, 2 µM and 100nM respectively). Cells plus modulator alone controlled these experiments. Following 48hour incubation, medium +/- drugs was removed by flicking and each well was treated with 50 µl of 2mg/ml MTT in Hanks balanced salt solution without phenol red. Formazan crystals were dissolved in 100 µl of acid/alcohol (0.04N HCl in isopropanol). The plate was read on an Anthos 2001 plate reader at 570nm with a reference wavelength of 690nm. Patients were deemed sensitive if <30% of cells survived at 1.8 µM for both DOX and DNR. The LC_{50} (the concentration required to kill 50% of cells) was calculated and in some instances curves were extrapolated using our own customised software. Sensitivity ratios of the LC_{50} of drug/LC_{50} of drug + modulator were evaluated to measure the size of any modulatory effect.

3.3. P-gp Expression

Flow cytometric analysis of P-gp was performed using an indirect immunofluorescence staining technique with primary antibodies MRK16 (5 µg/ml) and UIC2 (8 µg/ml). Following thawing and overnight incubation to allow recovery, cells were washed in PBS with 1% foetal calf serum and 0.01% sodium azide ($PBS/FCS/NaN_3$) and incubated for 1 hour with MRK16 or UIC2 at room temperature. Cells were then washed twice in $PBS/FCS/NaN_3$ and incubated with FITC conjugated goat anti-mouse for 45 minutes at room temperature, following 2 further washes cells were analysed on a flow cytometer (Coulter Epics XL). Matched isotype controls of mouse IgG2a at the same protein concentration were used. Results were expressed as the ratio of the mean fluorescence of antibody labelled cells divided by that of the isotype control. Experiment were controlled using the DOX resistant K562R cell line.

3.4. P-gp Function

Cells in complete medium were incubated with and without modulating agents at concentrations determined by previous experiments (PSC 833 and CsA at 2 µM, GF120918 at 80 µM) for one hour. Daunorubicin (5 µM) was added for a further hour. Following 2 washes with PBS, the resultant drug accumulation was assessed on the flow cytometer and the ratio was calculated of the mean flourescence of cells with DNR/cells with DNR and modulator.

3.5. Evaluation and Statistics

Non-parametric methods were used where possible. Spearman's rank correlation co-efficient was used to compare fluorescence ratios and LC_{50} values. Mann Whitney U was used to compare groups of patients and the Wilcoxon signed rank test was used for paired data.

4. RESULTS

4.1. Chemosensitivity

The median LC_{50} for DNR was 0.355µM (range 0.177–3.546, n=27) and DOX 0.707µM (range 0.172–3.103, n=25). Using the method of assessment above we found 7/27 (26%) patients were resistant to DOX and 1/27 (3.7%) resistant to DNR. Overall there was a significant reduction (p=0.04) in the LC_{50} of DOX in blast cells co-incubated with CsA with a median sensitivity ratio of 1.77 (range 0.25–4, n=17). There was no correlation between the sensitivity ratio (DOX -/+ CsA) and either previous treatment or primary/secondary disease.

Table 1.

Modulator	Median of ratios	Range	n	Ratios ≤ 1	Ratios > 1
P-gp function					
CsA	1.12	0.19-2.4	24	8(33.3%)	16(66.6%)
PSC833	1.09	0.613-2.08	24	3(12.5%)	21(87.5%)
GF120918	1.06	0.21-1.64	24	9(37.5%)	15(62.5%)

Marker	Median of ratios	Range	n
P-gp Expression			
UIC2	1.085	0.88-1.71	23
MRK16	1.21	0.85-3.9	24

4.2. P-gp Function and Expression

The median ratio as assessed by flow cytometry for P-gp function is shown in Table 1. When we assessed ratios of greater than and equal to or less than 1 we found that incubation in PSC833 nearly always led to increased DNR accumulation compared to approximately 1/3 of samples for CsA and GF120918.

The results obtained for P-gp expression using UIC2 and MRK16 are shown in Table 1. We were able to establish a correlation between the functional assay using CsA and GF120918 and P-gp expression using MRK16 ($p<0.05$) and ($p<0.02$) respectively. Similarly we observed a significant correlation between the MTT assay sensitivity ratio generated by incubation in DOX -/+ CsA and the flow cytometric functional assay using GF120918 ($p<0.02$) and there was a trend towards significance with PSC.($p<0.1$). We were unable to correlate P-gp function or expression with *in vitro* sensitivity to the anthracylines, previous treatment and primary/secondary disease. It was possible however, to identify individual patients whose blast cells exhibited P-gp expression and function, who were deemed resistant to anthracyclines in the MTT assay and indeed showed a modulatory effect. Furthermore, it was possible to evaluate which modulator would have the greatest effect. However it must be noted that patients whose cells were found sensitive to the anthracyclines, *in vitro,* sometimes showed similar modulatory effects teamed with positive P-gp expression and function.

5. DISCUSSION

The continued search for increased response rates in AML to cytotoxic agents has led to the extensive characterisation of phenotypes that confer resistance by a variety of mechanisms. Overcoming this resistance become paramount in recent studies. Our study enabled us to utilise two separate methodologies that examined both the mechanisms and expression of resistance.

We observed raised drug accumulation in the assessment of P-gp function at 80nM with GF120918, however we found no increase in sensitivity to the anthracyclines at 100nM using the MTT assay. Perhaps this could be overcome by using concentrations comparable to those of PSC833 and CsA.

This study, as with others,[6] established a correlation between expression and function of Pgp. However we were unable to correlate these observations, with *in vitro* resistance to the anthracyclines in the group of patients we examined. Whilst this may appear a paradoxical result, we were able, in individual patients, to observe cells with positive P-gp expression and function coupled with *in vitro* resistance to the anthracylines, it was further possible to identify which modulator had the greatest effect. However since we noticed that some patients sensitive, *in vitro*, to the anthracyclines could also show strong modulatory effects coupled with expression and function of P-gp we believe that, in future studies, if such patients were identified as positive for expression and function P-gp using only flow cytometry methodology the assumption could be made that they were resistant to the anthracyclines and thus treated unnecessarily with modulators, whereas in fact there is the possibility that these patients could be sensitive.

This has led us to the conclusion that both flow cytometry and the MTT assay should play an active joint role in future studies of MDR

ACKNOWLEDGMENTS

Alena W. Elgie was supported by the Kent Leukaemia and Cancer Equipment Fund and she acknowledges their valued support in this project.

REFERENCES

1. Tsuruo T. Mechanisms of multidrug resistance and implications for therapy. Japanese Journal of Cancer Research, (1988) 79, 285–296.
2. Campos L. Guyotat D. Archimbaud E. et al. Clinical significance of multidrug resistance P-Glycoprotein expression on acute nonlymphoblastic leukemia cells at diagnosis. Blood (1992).79, 473–476.
3. List A. Spier C. Cline A. et al. Expression of the multidrug resistance gene product (P-glycoprotein) in myelodysplasia is associated with a stem cell phenotype. Br J Haematology (1991) 78, 28–34.
4. Xu-Rong Jiang. Stephen M Kelsey. Yu-Ling Wu. Adrian C Newland. Circumvention of P-glycoprotein-mediated drug resistance in human leukaemic cells by non-immunosuppressive cyclosporin D analogue, SDZ PSC833. Br J Haematology, (1995) 90, 375–383.
5. Hyafil F. Vergely C. Du Vignaud P. Grand-Perret T. *In vitro* and *in vivo* reversal of multidrug resistance by GF120918, an acridonecarboxamide derivative. Cancer Research, (1993) 53, 4595–4602.
6. Ivy SP. Olshefski RS. Taylor BJ. Patel KM. Reaman GH. Correlation of P-glycoprotein expression and function in childhood acute leukemia: A children's cancer group study. Blood,(1996) 88. 309–318.

QUININE IMPROVES RESULTS OF INTENSIVE CHEMOTHERAPY (IC) IN MYELODYSPLASTIC SYNDROMES (MDS) EXPRESSING P-GLYCOPROTEIN (PGP)

Updated Results of a Randomized Study

E. Wattel, E. Solary, B. Hecquet, D. Caillot, N. Ifrah, A. Brion, N. Milpied, M. Janvier, A. Guerci, H. Rochant, C. Cordonnier, F. Dreyfus, A. Veil, L. Hoang-Ngoc, A. M. Stoppa, N. Gratecos, A. Sadoun, H. Tilly, P. Brice, B. Lioure, B. Desablens, B. Pignon, J. P. Abgrall, M. Leporrier, B. Dupriez, D. Guyotat, P. Lepelley, and P. Fenaux[*]

Groupe Français des Myélodysplasies (GFM) and Groupe GOELAMS

Keywords: myelodysplastic syndromes, intensive chemotherapy, drug resistance, mdr, quinine.

ABSTRACT

We designed a randomized trial of IC with or without quinine, an agent capable of reverting the multidrug resistance (mdr) phenotype, in patients aged ≤ 65 years with high risk MDS. Patients were randomized to receive Mitoxantrone $12mg/m^2/d$ d_{2-5} + AraC $1g/m^2/12h$ d_{1-5}, with (Q^+) or without (Q^-) quinine (30mg/kg/day). 131 patients were included. PGP expression analysis was successfully made in 91 patients and 42 patients (46%) had positive PGP expression. In PGP positive cases, 13 of the 25 (52%) patients who received quinine achieved CR, as compared to 3 of the 17 (18%) patients treated with chemotherapy alone (p=0.02). In PGP negative cases, the CR rate was 35% and 49%, respectively in patients who received quinine or chemotherapy alone (difference not significant). In the 42 PGP

---

[*] Correspondence and reprint requests: Pr. P. Fenaux, Service des Maladies du Sang, CHU, 1 place de Verdun, 59037 Lille France. Fax: 33(0)3 20 44 40 94; Tel: 33 (0)3 20 44 43 48.

Drug Resistance in Leukemia and Lymphoma III, edited by Kaspers *et al.*
Kluwer Academic / Plenum Publishers, New York, 1999.

positive patients, median Kaplan-Meier (KM) survival was 13 months in patients allocated to the quinine group, and 8 months in patients treated with chemotherapy alone (p=0.01). In PGP negative patients, median KM survival was 14 months in patients allocated to the quinine group, and 14 months in patients treated with chemotherapy alone. Side effects of quinine mainly included vertigo and tinnitus that generally disappeared with dose reduction. Mucositis was significantly more frequently observed in the quinine group. No life threatening cardiac toxicity was observed. In conclusion, results of this randomized study show that quinine increases the CR rate and survival in PGP positive MDS cases treated with IC. The fact that quinine had no effect on the response rate and survival of PGP negative MDS suggests a specific effect on PGP mediated drug resistance rather than, for instance, a simple effect on the metabolism of Mitoxantrone and/or AraC.

INTRODUCTION

Intensive anthracycline AraC chemotherapy, in MDS and AML following MDS, gives lower complete remission (CR) rates and shorter CR duration than in de novo AML (1–14). Reasons for the lower response rates to chemotherapy in MDS are unknown but could include a higher incidence of expression of the multidrug resistance (mdr) gene in MDS than in de novo AML, as mdr gene expression is generally associated with poorer results of intensive chemotherapy in AML and MDS (15).

The decreased intracellular accumulation of a variety of cytotoxic agents, characteristic of the mdr phenotype, can be reversed *in vitro* by a number of non cytotoxic agents but the *in vivo* use of most of these agents is precluded by serum protein binding or clinical toxicity (16–23). Intravenous infusion of conventional doses of quinine allows the achievement of sufficient serum concentration to reverse the anthracycline resistance in mdr models, and can be safely administered in combination to mitoxantrone and AraC (24–26). In the preliminary results of a recent randomized trial, the French Groupe Ouest Est des Leucémies Aiguës Myéloïdes (Goelams) showed that the addition of quinine to mitoxantrone-AraC chemotherapy could improve the CR rates in AML, particularly in AML post MDS (27). Differences were not significant, including in AML post MDS, but the number of patients in this subgroup was relatively small, and PGP expression had been studied in only a limited number of centers. Thus the Goelams group and the Groupe Français des Myélodysplasies (French MDS group: GFM) performed a similar randomized study of mitoxantrone-AraC chemotherapy and quinine in MDS and AML post MDS. Randomization was stopped after the second interim analysis, as the CR rate in cases that expressed PGP was significantly superior with the addition of quinine.

PATIENTS AND METHODS

Eligibility Criteria

Inclusion criteria were (1) MDS, according to FAB criteria, (2) age ≤ 65 years (3) marrow blasts ≥ 5%, ie refractory anemia with excess blasts (RAEB), RAEB in transformation (RAEB-T) chronic myelomonocytic leukemia (CMML) or MDS having progressed to AML (AML post MDS) (4) patient diagnosed in a center where PGP expression was assessable or adequate material sent to a referral center (5) written informed consent of the patient.

Protocol Design

Patients allocated to chemotherapy alone (control group) received an induction course of mitoxantrone (MXN) 12mg/m^2/d d$_{2-5}$ and AraC 1g/m^2/12h d$_{1-5}$. Patient allocated to the quinine group received the same MXN-AraC regimen with quinine formiate at a dosage of 30 mg/kg/d started 24 hours before the first dose of MXN and administered in continuous IV infusion until 24 hours after the end of the last MXN infusion. Toxicity was assessed according to the WHO grading system.

PGP Expression

In AML post MDS, PGP expression was determined by flow cytometry using MRK16 antibody, a monoclonal antibody which recognizes an extracellular determinant of P-glycoprotein, in a previously described indirect immunofluorescent assay (25). Briefly, cells were fixed in 1% paraformaldehyde for 30mn at 4°C and incubated in human AB serum before a 30mn incubation with MRK16 antibody (2 µg/ml), then with fluorescein-conjugated F(ab')$_2$ fragments of goat antimouse IgG (37.5 µg/ml; Silenius laboratories). The percentage of positive cells was determined by flow cytometry using a Becton-Dickinson FACScan flow cytometer. A non relevant IgG2a was used with the same goat antimouse second step reagent to calibrate the assay on the FACScan and determine the positivity for individual cells. P-glycoprotein-positive K562/ADM cells were used as positive control. MRK 16 staining was measured by the Kolmogorov-Smirnov (KS) statistic to compare MRK16-stained cells with the control, as previously described (28).

In non transformed MDS patients, PGP expression was assessed by immunocytochemistry on marrow slides with JSB1 MoAb using the alkaline phosphatase-antialkaline phosphatase (APAAP) technique or the avidin-biotin-peroxydase technique, as previously described (15). A sample was considered positive when at least 5% of blasts were stained with JSB1 in the absence of control staining.

Endpoints

The complete remission (CR) rate, in cases with PGP expression, was the major endpoint. CR criteria included: (i) marrow blasts <5%; (ii) neutrophils >1500/mm^3, platelets > 100000/mm^3, Hemoglobin>10g without transfusion requirement; (iii) normalization of the karyotype if initially abnormal (at least 10 mitoses examined); (iiii) disappearance of major myelodysplastic features in the bone marrow (with the exception of mild dysplasia, as seen after chemotherapy). Partial remission (PR) criteria included: <5% marrow blasts and persistence of cytopenia(s) but with an increase in neutrophils by at least 1000/mm^3, of platelets by at least 50,000/mm^3, of hemoglobin by at least 2g/dl, or disappearance of cytopenias but persistance of either major myelodysplastic features or cytogenetic abnormalities. Death in aplasia was defined by death during the period of aplasia following chemotherapy administration. Failure corresponded to all other situations.

The CR duration and survival in with PGP positive cases; the CR rate, CR duration and survival in the overall population and in PGP negative patients were considered as secondary endpoints.

Statistical Analysis

Prognostic factors were assessed using the appropriate regression models, either logistic regression or Cox model. These factors, derived from previous studies (11, 29) were age, sex, FAB classification, WBC count, hemoglobin level, platelet count, absolute number of circulating blasts, percentage of bone marrow blasts, cytogenetic abnormalities and time from diagnosis to treatment.

RESULTS

Initial Characteristics of the Patients

Table 1 summarizes initial characteristics of the 131 patients. No significant differences in pretreatment characteristics were found between the 2 groups.

PGP expression analysis was successfully made in 91 patients. Forty-two patients (46%) had positive PGP expression and 49 (54%) were PGP negative. In the remaining 40 patients (30%) PGP expression could not be evaluated, mainly due to the absence or poor quality of cellular samples, and rarely to laboratory technical problems.

In the 91 patients where PGP expression was successfully assessed and in the 42 PGP positive patients, no significant difference in pretreatment characteristics was observed between patients allocated to receive or not quinine (Tables 2 and 3). Of note was the presence, in the whole 131 patients and in the 91 patients where PGP was successfully assessed, of a trend for more cases of MDS-AML in the group that did not receive quinine (Table 1 and 2), as those patients appear to respond less favorably to chemotherapy than patients still in MDS phase (11). However, this difference was not significant. Furthermore, it was not found in PGP positive patients (Table 3).

Table 1. Initial characteristics of the 131 patients

	Quinine group (n=62)	Chemotherapy alone (n=69)	p value
Mean age (range)	50 (19-66)	52 (18-68)	ns
M/F	36/26	40/29	
Mean time (range) from diagnostic to treatment (months)	10.5 (3-61)	14.5 (3-135)	ns
FAB at the time of treatment			ns
MDS-AML	30	49	
RAEB	9	8	
RAEB-T	22	11	
CMML	1	1	
Karyotype (99 patients)			ns
Normal	19	21	
Isolated -7	7	5	
Isolated del 5q	3	1	
+ 8	1	1	
Other single abn	9	12	
Complex abn	9	11	

Table 2. Initial characteristics of the 91 patients in whom PGP expression was succesfully assessed

	Quinine (n=42)	Chemotherapy alone (n=49)	p value
Mean age (range)	50 (19-66)	51 (18-68)	ns
M/F	24/18	28/21	
Mean time (range) from diagnosis to treatment (months)	8 (3-53)	16 (3-135)	ns
FAB at the time of treatment			ns
MDS-AML	19	35	
RAEB	6	5	
RAEB-T	16	8	
CMML	1	1	
Karyotype (70 patients)			ns
Normal	14	15	
Isolated -7	4	3	
Isolated del 5q	3	1	
+ 8	0	0	
Other single abn	7	8	
Complex abn	5	10	

Response to Treatment (Table 4)

Of the 131 patients, 57 (44%) achieved CR, 22 (17%) PR, 30 (23%) had resistant disease and 22 (16%) died during aplasia. Of the 91 patients in whom PGP expression was successfully assessed, 37 (41%) achieved CR, 20 (22%) PR, 19 (21%) had resistant disease and 15 (16%) died during aplasia. The CR rate was 38% in PGP positive cases and 43% in PGP negative cases (difference not significant).

Table 3. Initial characteristics of the 42 PGP positive patients

	Quinine (n=25)	Chemotherapy alone (n=17)	p value
Mean age (range)	52 (19-66)	54 (27-66)	ns
M/F	19/6	16/1	ns
Mean time (range) from diagnosis to treatment (months)	9 (3-53)	12 (3-50)	ns
FAB at the time of treatment			ns
MDS-AML	11	10	
RAEB	5	2	
RAEB-T	9	4	
CMML	0	1	
Karyotype (34 patients)			ns
Normal	9	6	
Isolated -7	2	1	
Isolated del 5q	2	0	
+ 8	1	1	
Other single abn	4	4	
Complex abn	3	2	

Table 4. Response to treatment and evolution

	Quinine	Chemotherapy alone	p value
Whole study population (131 patients)			
n	62	69	
CR (%)	29 (47)	28 (41)	ns
Median CR duration (months)	16	14	ns
Median survival (months)	13	11	ns
PGP positive cases (42 patients)			
n	25	17	
CR (%)	13 (52)	3 (18)	0.02
CR duration (months)	Median: 14	4, 6, 14	
Median survival (months)	13	8	0.01
PGP negative cases (49 patients)			
n	17	32	
CR (%)	6 (35)	15 (49)	ns
Median CR duration (months)	9	14	ns
Median survival (months)	14	14	ns

Of the 62 patients allocated to the quinine group, 29 (47%) achieved CR, as compared to 28 of the 69 (41%) patients treated with chemotherapy alone (difference not significant). Similarly, there was no significant difference in the incidence of death during aplasia between the 2 groups: 13% in the quinine arm versus 20% in the control arm.

In PGP positive cases, 13 of the 25 (52%) patients who received quinine achieved CR, as compared to 3 of the 17 (18%) patients treated with chemotherapy alone (p=0.02, Mantel-Haenszel test). On the other hand, in PGP negative cases, the CR rate was 35% and 49%, respectively in patients who received quinine or chemotherapy alone (difference not significant).

CR Duration and Survival

Median follow up of the 131 patients was 9 months. Median Kaplan-Meier estimate of overall survival was 12 months. Of the 57 patients who achieved CR, 34 received consolidation CT, 20 were autografted (using bone marrow or peripheral stem cells harvested after CR achievement) and 3 were allografted in first CR. Allografted patients were censored at the time of transplantation. Thirty-six patients relapsed after 2 to 37 months and 21 were still in CR after 7 to 59 months, with a median CR duration of 14 months. Median Kaplan-Meier estimate of survival was 13 months in the 62 patients allocated to the quinine group and 11 months in the 69 patients allocated to the control group (difference not significant, Figure 1).

In the 42 PGP positive patients, median Kaplan-Meier estimate of survival was 13 months in patients allocated to the quinine group, and 8 months in patients treated with chemotherapy alone (p=0.01, Figure 2). In PGP negative patients, median Kaplan-Meier estimate of survival was 14 months in patients allocated to the quinine group, and 14 months in patients treated with chemotherapy alone (difference not significant, Figure 3).

Toxicity of the Regimen

Toxicity of quinine was observed in 17 of 62 quinine-treated patients (27%) and included tinnitus (13/62, 21%), vertigo (8/62, 13%), bradycardia (1/62: 2%), QT interval increase on ECG (4/62: 6%), and mild hearing loss (6/62, 10%).

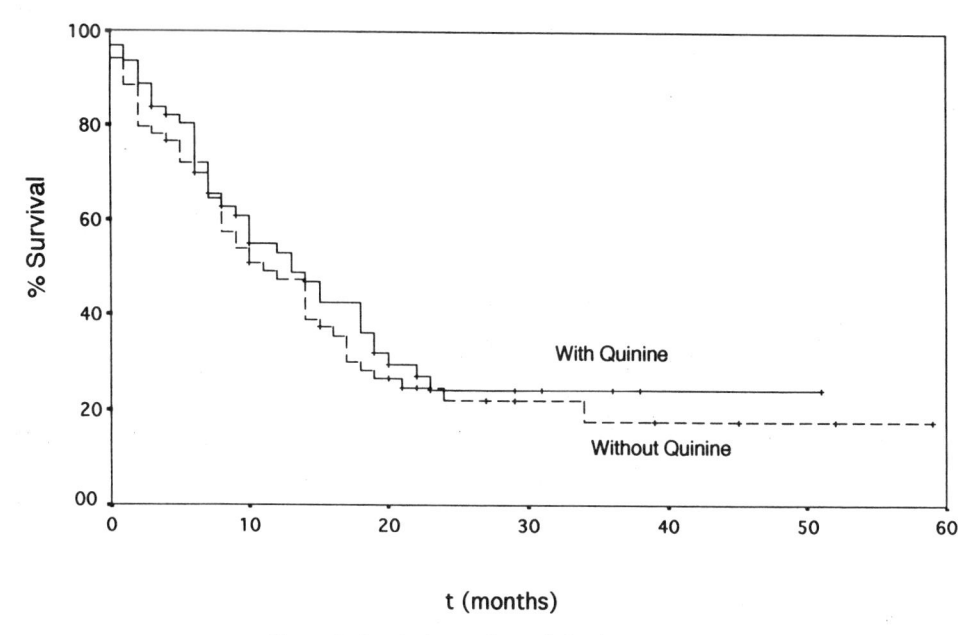

Figure 1. Survival according to induction treatment.

In 15 patients, quinine-induced side effects decreased or disappeared after unique 20% quinine dose-decrease. In 2 patients, quinine infusion had to be stopped after 2 days due to excessive QT increase (1 case) or hearing loss (1 case).

Hematologic toxicity is detailed in Table 5. In patients who achieved CR, mean duration neutropenia and time to discharge from hospital were longer in patients allocated to

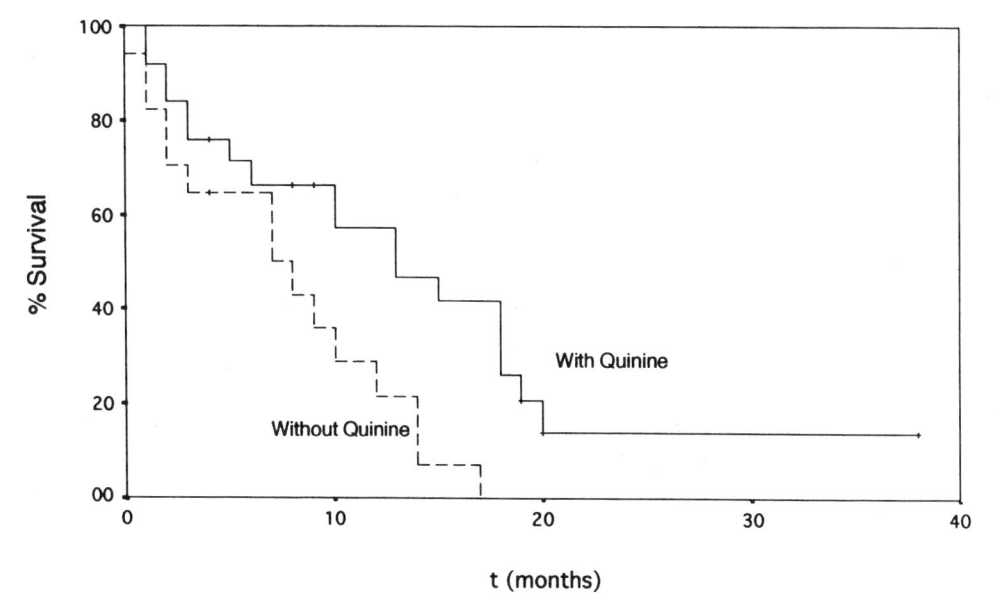

Figure 2. Survival of the PGP positive patients according to induction treatment.

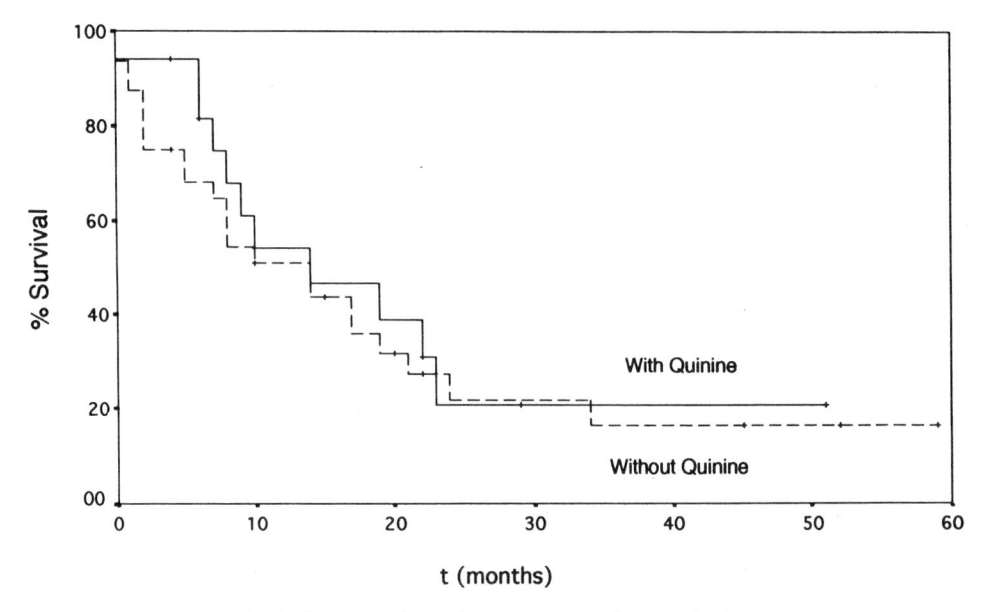

Figure 3. Survival of the PGP negative patients according to induction treatment.

the quinine arm. However, this difference was not significant. There was a significantly prolonged duration of hospitalization in patients treated with quinine

Non hematologic toxicity is detailed in Table 6. There was no significant difference in the incidence of > WHO grade 2 diarrhea, vomitis, nausea, liver and heart toxicity between the 2 arms. Mucositis was significantly more frequently observed in the quinine group (Table 6).

DISCUSSION

Forty six percent of the 91 patients tested were found to express PGP. MDR 1 expression is observed in 40 to 70% of patients with de novo untreated MDS, i.e., more often than in de novo untreated AML in most reported series (19, 30–40). PGP expression is especially frequent in MDS-AML and high risk MDS (i.e., RAEB, RAEB-T and CMML). We had previously found a significant higher CR rate in PGP positive MDS patients treated with intensive anthracycline-AraC regimen when compared to PGP negative cases (15). These results prompted us to combine chemotherapy to quinine in a randomized trial.

We found no significant difference in CR rate, CR duration and survival between chemotherapy alone and chemotherapy combined to quinine in the overall patient population.

Table 5. Hematologic toxicity according to induction treatment in patients who achieved CR

	Quinine (n = 29)	Chemotherapy alone (n = 28)	p value
Mean duration of leukopenia (days)	26 ± 9	23± 12	0.1
Mean duration of neutropenia (days)	28 ± 8	24 ±5	0.07
Mean duration of thrombocytopenia (days)	27 ± 12	25 ± 6	0.3
Mean time to discharge from hospital (days)	36 ± 9	31 ± 7	0.02

Table 6. Nonhematologic toxicity (WHO Grade 2) according to induction treatment

	Quinine (62 patients)	Chemotherapy alone (69)	p value
Mucositis (%)	18 (29)	10 (14)	0.04
Nausea (%)	17 (28)	14 (21)	ns
Diarrhea (%)	19 (31)	16 (23)	ns
Liver (%)	11 (17)	12 (17)	ns
Vomiting (%)	19 (31)	16 (23)	ns
Hearth (%)	2 (3)	1 (1)	ns

However, in PGP positive cases, a significantly higher CR rate, more prolonged CR duration and better survival were observed in patients treated with quinine when compared to patients treated with chemotherapy alone. A possible explanation to those results could be an effect of quinine on the metabolism of Mitoxantrone and/or AraC. Indeed, several drugs currently investigated as mdr reversing agents, including PSC833, can modify the metabolism of antineoplastic agents, including anthracyclines and epipodophyllotoxins (41, 42). This effect can result pharmacologically in an increase in drug concentration and possibly in higher efficacy (and also toxicity). However, in the present study, quinine had no effect on the response rate, CR duration and survival in PGP negative MDS. Furthermore, in previous studies of the Goelams group, serum levels of quinine achieved by continuous infusion of this drug were sufficient to circumvent the mdr phenotype of a mdr positive cell line (25–27). These findings strongly suggest a specific effect of quinine on PGP mediated drug resistance rather than a simple effect on drug metabolism.

To our knowledge, this study is the first to demonstrate some benefit of the addition of a drug reversing agent to antineoplastic drugs in a randomized trial. Quinine, like verapamil (Dalton *et al.*, 1995) and cyclosporine A (43), belongs to the first generation of resistance modifiers. Several phase I/II trials with verapamil and cyclosporine A agents in relapsing AML (44), multiple myeloma (43) and non-Hodgkin's lymphoma (19, 45) have suggested that these drugs could yield some benefit in combination with anthracyclines, vinca alkaloids or epipodophyllotoxins. However, those studies were not randomized.

The favorable effect of quinine on PGP mediated drug resistance obtained in the present study could be due to a better efficacy of quinine, as compared to many of the other potential reversing agents tested so far. Apart from our group, quinine has not been assessed clinically as a reversing agent by other groups, to our knowledge. On the other hand, quinine -and possibly other reversing agents-could have a greater reversing effect on PGP positive blasts from MDS patients than on PGP positive tumor cells from other neoplasms. In the case of AML, preliminary results from the Goelams group already suggested a greater effect of quinine on the drug sensitivity of blasts from AML occuring after MDS and myeloproliferative disorders, than on blasts from de novo AML cases (27).

Second generation resistance modifiers such as PSC833 (41), dexverapamil (46) or Cinchonine (47) have been designed in order to increase specificity for PGP expression and to decrease toxicity. In vitro studies have shown that those drugs allowed sufficient modulation of P-glycoprotein under serum conditions at concentrations achievable *in vivo* and clinical studies with those drugs are underway (39). Because our results suggest that reversing agents may be clinically useful in MDS, it will be important to test those drugs in this group of disorders and to compare their clinical usefulness with that of quinine.

Side effects of quinine mainly included tinnitus and vertigo. They generally disappeared with 20% dose reduction. No life threatening cardiac toxicity was observed. There was a trend for more prolonged duration of neutropenia and a significantly prolonged duration of hospitalization in patients treated with quinine. In addition, quinine induced a significant increase in the incidence of mucositis.

In addition to PGP, other molecules, including multidrug resistance-associated protein (MRP) (48) and lung resistance protein (LRP) (29) interfere with the transport of cytotoxic drugs. LRP expression, in particular, is observed in about 40% of MDS and is only partially correlated with PGP expression (39, 49). Little is known about MRP expression in MDS. Finally, in addition to alteration of drug transport, drug resistance may arise from alterations at any other step in the cell-killing pathways including drug metabolism (50), drug target and DNA repair mechanisms (51) and in the ability of cells to recognize a toxic insult and engage apoptosis. Some of these mechanisms have prognostic implication in AML and/or MDS treated with intensive chemotherapy (52, 54) and may provide important targets in the modulation of drug resistance.

ACKNOWLEGMENTS

Supported by the Programme Hospitalier de Recherche Clinique (Centre Hospitalier Universitaire of Lille).

REFERENCES

1. Martiat P., Ferrant A., Michaux J.L., Sokal G. (1988) ; Intensive chemotherapy for acute non-lymphoblastic leukemia after primary myelodysplastic syndrome. *Hematol Oncol*, **6** : 299–305.
2. Michels SD., Mc Kenna RW., Arthur DC., Brunning RD. (1985) Therapy related acute myeloid leukemia and myelodysplastic syndrome : a clinical and morphologic study of 65 cases. *Blood*, **65** : 1364–1372.
3. Hoyle C.F., De Bastos M., Wheatley K., Sherrington P.D., Fischer P.J., Rees J.K.H., Gray R., Hayhoe F.G.J. (1989) AML associated with previous cytotoxic therapy, MDS or myeloproliferative disorders: results from the MRC's 9th AML trial. *Br J Haematol*, **72** : 45–53.
4. De Witte T., Muus P., De Pauw B., Haanen C. (1990) Intensive antileukemic treatment of patients younger than 65 years with myelodysplastic syndromes and secondary acute myelogenous leukemia. *Cancer*, **66**, 831–837.
5. Fenaux P., Morel P., Rose C., Lai J.L., Jouet J.P., Bauters F. (1991). Prognostic factors in adult de novo myelodysplastic syndromes treated by intensive chemotherapy. *Br J Haematol*, **77**, 497–501.
6. De Witte T., Suciu S., Peetermans M., Fenaux P., Strijckmans P., Hayat M., Jaksic J., Selleslag D., Zittoun R., Dardenne M., Solbu G., Zwierzina H., Muus P. (1995) A pilot study of intensive chemotherapy for bad prognosis myelodysplasia (MDS) and secondary acute myeloid leukemia (sAML) following MDS of more than 6 months duration. A study by the Leukemia Cooperative Group of the European Organisation for Research and Treatment in Cancer (EORTC-LCG). *Leukemia*, **9**, 1805–1811.
7. Berstein S., Brunetto V., Davey F., Mayer RJ., Wurster-Hill D., Schiffer C., Bloomfield C. (1993) Intensive chemotherapy for patients with myelodysplastic syndromes. *Blood*, **82**, (suppl 1), 1960.
8. Ruutu T., Hänninen A., Järventie G., Koistinen P., Koivunen E., Kätkä K., Nousiainen T., Pelliniemi T.T., Remes K., Timonen T., Volin L., Elonen E. (1994) Intensive treatment of poor prognosis myelodysplastic syndromes (MDS) and acute myeloid leukemia subsequent to MDS with idarubicin and cytarabine (abstract). *Br J Haematol*, **87** (suppl. 1) : 19.
9. Aul C., Runde V., Germing U., Burk M., Heyll A., Hildebrandt B., Willers R. (1995) Remission rates, survival and prognostic factors in 94 patients with advanced MDS treated with intensive chemotherapy. *Ann Hematol*, **70** (suppl 2), A138.
10. Aul C., Runde V., Gattermann N., Germing U., Schneider W., (1994) Treatment of advanced primary myelodysplastic syndromes with AML-type chemotherapy: results in 76 patients. *Leuk Res*, **18**, suppl : 22 (abstr).
11. Hiddemann W., Büchner T., Wörmann B., Koch P., Aul C., Balleisen L., Bennet J. (1995) Intensive therapy of high risk myelodysplastic syndromes with sequential intermediate dose cytosine arabinoside and mitoxantrone with or without GM-CSF (abstract). *Ann Hematol*, **70** (suppl II) : A109.

12. Gore S.D., Burke P.J. (1995) Long-term survival of subsets of patients with advanced myelodysplastic syndromes (MDS) treated with intensive chemotherapy (abstract). *Blood,* **86** (suppl 1) : 339a.
13. Wattel E., de Botton S., Laï J.L., Preudhomme C., Lepelley P., Bauters F., Fenaux P. (1997). Long term follow up of de novo myelodysplastic syndromes treated with intensive chemotherapy: incidence of long survivors and outcome of partial responders. *Br J Haematol,* **98,** 983–991.
14. Gardin C., Chaibi P., de Revel T., Rousselot P., Turlure P., Micléa J.M., Nédellec G., Dombret H. (1997) Intensive chemotherapy with idarubicin, cytosine arabinoside, and granulocyte colony-stimulating factor (G-CSF) in patients with secondary and therapy-related acute myelogenous leukemia. *Leukemia,* **11** : 16–21.
15. Lepelley P., Soenen V., Preudhomme C., Lai J.L., Cosson A., Fenaux P. (1994). Expression of the multidrug resistance P-glycoprotein and its relationship to hematological characteristics and response to treatment in myelodysplastic syndromes. *Leukemia,* **8,** 998–1004.
16. Bennis S., Ichas F., Robert J. (1995). Differential effects of verapamil and quinine on the reversal of doxorubicin resistance in a human leukemia cell line. *Int J Cancer,* **62,** 283–90.
17. Dorr R.T., Liddil J.D. (1991). Modulation of mitomycin C-induced multidrug resistance in vitro. *Cancer Chemother Pharmacol,* **27,** 290–4.
18. Genne P., Duchamp O., Solary E., Pinard D., Belon J.P., Dimanche-Boitrel M.T., Chauffert B. (1994). Comparative effects of quinine and cinchonine in reversing multidrug resistance on human leukemic cell line K562/ADM. *Leukemia,* **8,** 160–4.
19. Malayeri R., Filipits M., Suchomel R.W., Z˙chbauer S., Lechner K., Pirker R. (1996). Multidrug resistance in leukemias and its reversal. *Leuk Lymphoma,* **23,** 451–8.
20. Solary E., Velay I., Chauffert B., Caillot D., Bidan J.M., Dumas M., Casasnovas O., Guy H. (1990). Quinine circumvents the doxorubicin resistance of a multidrug resistant human leukemic cell-line, K562/DXR. *Nouv Rev Fr Hematol,* **32,** 361–3.
21. Sonneveld P. (1996). Reversal of multidrug resistance in acute myeloid leukaemia and other haematological malignancies. *Eur J Cancer,* **6,** 1062–1069.
22. Wigler P.W., Patterson F.K. (1994). Reversal agent inhibition of the multidrug resistance pump in human leukemic lymphoblasts. *Biochim Biophys Acta,* **1189,** 1–6.
23. Pajeva I.K., Wiese M., Cordes H.P., Seydel J.K. (1996). Membrane interactions of some catamphiphilic drugs and relation to their multidrug-resistance-reversing ability. *J Cancer Res Clin Oncol,* **122,** 27–40.
24. Solary E., Bidan J.M., Calvo F., Chauffert B., Caillot D., Mugneret F., Gauville C., Tsuruo T., Carli P.M., Guy H. (1991a). P-glycoprotein expression and in vitro reversion of doxorubicin resistance by verapamil in clinical specimens from acute leukaemia and myeloma. *Leukemia,* **5,** 592–7.
25. Solary E., Velay I., Chauffert B., Bidan J.M., Caillot D., Dumas M., Guy H. (1991b). Sufficient levels of quinine in the serum circumvent the multidrug resistance of the human leukemic cell line K562/ ADM. *Cancer,* **68,** 1714–9.
26. Solary E., Caillot D., Chauffert B., Casasnovas R.O., Dumas M., Maynadie M., Guy H. (1992). Feasibility of using quinine, a potential multidrug resistance- reversing agent, in combination with mitoxantrone and cytarabine for the treatment of acute leukemia. *J Clin Oncol,* **10,** 1730–6.
27. Solary E., Witz B., Caillot D., Moreau P., Desablens B., Cahn J.Y., Sadoun A., Pignon B., Berthou C., Maloisel F., Guyotat D., Casassus, P, Ifrah N., Lamy Y., Audhuy B., Colombat P., Harousseau J.L. (1996). Combination of quinine as a potential reversing agent with mitoxantrone and cytarabine for the treatment of acute leukemias: a randomized multicenter study. *Blood,* **88,** 1198–1205.
28. Leith C.P., Chen I.M., Kopecky K.J., Appelbaum F.R., Head D.R., Godwin J.E., Weick J.K., Willman C.L. (1995). Correlation of multidrug resistance (MDR1) protein expression with functional dye/drug efflux in acute myeloid leukemia by multiparameter flow cytometry: identification of discordant MDR-/efflux+ and MDR1+/efflux- cases. *Blood,* **86,** 2329–2342.
29. Morel P., Hebbar M., Lai J.L., Duhamel A., Preudhomme C., Wattel E., Bauters F., Fenaux P. (1993). Cytogenetic analysis has strong independent prognostic value in de novo myelodysplastic syndromes and can be incorporated in a new scoring system: a report on 408 cases. *Leukemia,* **7,** 1315–23.
30. Kuwazuru Y., Yoshimura A., Hanada S., Utsunomiya A., Makino T., Ishibashi K., Kodama M., Iwahashi M., Arima T., Akiyama S. (1990). Expression of the multidrug transporter, P-glycoprotein, in acute leukemia cells and correlation to clinical drug resistance. *Cancer,* **66,** 868–73.
31. Wood P., Burgess R., MacGregor A., Yin J.A. (1994). P-glycoprotein expression on acute myeloid leukaemia blast cells at diagnosis predicts response to chemotherapy and survival. *Br J Haematol,* **87,** 509–14.
32. Sato H., Preisler H., Day R., Raza A., Larson R., Browman G., Goldberg J., Vogler R., Grunwald H., Gottlieb A., *et al.* (1990). MDR1 transcript levels as an indication of resistant disease in acute myelogenous leukaemia. *Br J Haematol,* **75,** 340–5.

33. Campos L., Guyotat D., Archimbaud E., Calmard-Oriol P., Tsuruo T., Troncy J., Treille D., Fiere D. (1992). Clinical significance of multidrug resistance P-glycoprotein expression on acute nonlymphoblastic leukemia cells at diagnosis. *Blood*, **79**, 473–476.
34. Marie J.P., Legrand O., Russo D., Zhou D., Suberville A.M., Zittoun R. (1992). Multidrug resistance (MDR) gene expression in acute non lymphoblastic leukemia: sequential analysis. *Leuk Lymphoma*, **8**, 261–265.
35. Hegewisch-Becker S., Hossfeld D.K. (1996). The MDR phenotype in hematologic malignancies: prognostic relevance and future perspectives. *Ann Hematol*, **72**, 105–117.
36. Guerci A., Merlin J.L., Missoum N., Feldmann L., Marchal S., Witz F., Rose C., Guerci O. (1995). Predictive value for treatment outcome in acute myeloid leukemia of cellular daunorubicin accumulation and P-glycoprotein expression simultaneously determined by flow cytometry. *Blood*, **85**, 2147–2153.
37. Pirker R., Wallner J., Geissler K., Linkesch W., Haas O.A., Bettelheim P., Hopfner M., Scherrer R., Valent P., Havelec L., *et al.* (1991). MDR1 gene expression and treatment outcome in acute myeloid leukemia [see comments]. *J Natl Cancer Inst*, **83**, 708–712.
38. Zöchbauer S., Gsur A., Brunner R., Kyrle P.A., Lechner K., Pirker R. (1994). P-glycoprotein expression as unfavorable prognostic factor in acute myeloid leukemia. *Leukemia*, **8**, 974–977.
39. List A.F. (1996). Role of multidrug resistance and its pharmacological modulation in acute myeloid leukemia. *Leukemia*, **10**, 937–42.
40. McKenna S.L., Padua R.A. (1997). Multidrug resistance in leukaemia. *Br J Haematol*, **96**, 659–74.
41. Gonzalez O., Colombo T., De Fusco M., Imperatori L., Zucchetti M., D'Incalci M. (1995). Changes in doxorubicin distribution and toxicity in mice pretreated with the cyclosporin analogue SDZ PSC 833. *Cancer Chemother Pharmacol*, **36**, 335–40.
42. Sonneveld P., Marie J.P., Huisman C., Vekhoff A., Schoester M., Faussat A.M., van Kapel J., Groenewegen A., Charnick S., Zittoun R., L'wenberg, B (1996). Reversal of multidrug resistance by SDZ PSC 833, combined with VAD (vincristine, doxorubicin, dexamethasone) in refractory multiple myeloma. A phase I study. *Leukemia*, **10**, 1741–50.
43. Weber D., Dimopoulos M., Sinicrope F., Alexanian R. (1995). VAD-cyclosporine therapy for VAD-resistant multiple myeloma. *Leuk Lymphoma*, **19**, 159–63.
44. List A.F., Spier C., Greer J., Wolff S., Hutter J., Dorr R., Salmon S., Futscher B., Baier M., Dalton W. (1993). Phase I/II trial of cyclosporine as a chemotherapy-resistance modifier in acute leukemia [see comments]. *J Clin Oncol*, **11**, 1652–60.
45. Miller T.P., Grogan T.M., Dalton W.S., Spier C.M., Scheper R.J., Salmon S.E. (1991). P-glycoprotein expression in malignant lymphoma and reversal of clinical drug resistance with chemotherapy plus high-dose verapamil. *J Clin Oncol*, **9**, 17–24.
46. Wilson W.H., Bates S.E., Fojo A., Bryant G., Zhan Z., Regis J., Wittes R.E., Jaffe E.S., Steinberg S.M., Herdt J., et a. (1995). Controlled trial of dexverapamil, a modulator of multidrug resistance, in lymphomas refractory to EPOCH chemotherapy. *J Clin Oncol*, **13**, 1995–2004.
47. Genne P., Dimanche-Boitrel M.T., Mauvernay R.Y., Gutierrez G., Duchamp O., Petit J.M., Martin F., Chauffert B. (1992). Cinchonine, a potent efflux inhibitor to circumvent anthracycline resistance in vivo. *Cancer Res*, **52**, 2797–2801.
48. Beck J., Niethammer D., Gekeler V. (1996). MDR1, MRP, topoisomerase IIalpha/beta, and cyclin A gene expression in acute and chronic leukemias. *Leukemia*, **10**, S39-S45.
49. Lepelley P., Grardel N., Preudhomme C., Wattel E., Cosson A., Fenaux P. (1998). Expression of LRP and its correlation with other drug resistance proteins and outcome in myelodysplastic syndromes (MDS). *Leuk Lymphoma*, **29**, 547–551.
50. Holmes J., Wareing C., Jacobs A., Hayes J.D., Padua R.A., Wolf C.R. (1990). Glutathione-s-transferase pi expression in leukaemia: a comparative analysis with mdr-1 data. *Br J Cancer*, **62**, 209–12.
51. Gieseler F., Glasmacher A., K‰mpfe D., Wandt H., Nuessler V., Valsamas S., Kunze J., Wilms K. (1996). Topoisomerase II activities in AML and their correlation with cellular sensitivity to anthracyclines and epipodophyllotoxines. *Leukemia*, **10**, 1177–80.
52. Campos, L., Rouault, J.P., Sabido, O., Oriol, P., Roubi, N., Vasselon, C., Archimbaud, E., Magaud, J.P. & Guyotat, D. (1993). High expression of bcl-2 protein in acute myeloid leukemia cells is associated with poor response to chemotherapy. *Blood*, **81**, 3091–6.
54. Wattel, E., Preudhomme, C., Hecquet, B., Vanrumbeke, M., Quesnel, B., Dervite, I., Morel, P. & Fenaux, P. (1994). p53 mutations are associated with resistance to chemotherapy and short survival in hematologic malignancies. *Blood*, **84**, 3148–3157.

6

TREATMENT OF POOR PROGNOSIS AML PATIENTS USING PSC833 (VALSPODAR) PLUS MITOXANTRONE, ETOPOSIDE, AND CYTARABINE (PSC-MEC)

R. Advani, G. Visani, D. Milligan, H. Saba, M. Tallman, J. M. Rowe,
P. H. Wiernik, J. Ramek, K. Dugan, B. Lum, J. Villena, E. Davis, E. Paietta,
M. Litchman, A. Covelli, B. Sikic, and P. Greenberg

Stanford Medical Center, Stanford, California
Policlinico S. Orsola, Bologna
Heartlands Hospital, Birmingham
Moffit Cancer Center, Tampa, Florida
Northwestern Medical Center, Chicago, Illinois
Rochester Medical Center, New York
Albert Einstein Medical Center, Bronx, New York
Novartis Pharmaceuticals E. Hanover, New Jersey
Novartis Pharma AG, Switzerland

Keywords: Refractory/relapsing AML, multidrug resistance, P-glycoprotein, clinical trials.

1. ABSTRACT

The failure of convenional chemotherapy in relapsed or refractory and other poor risk AML patients has been linked to expression of the multidrug resistance gene (*mdr1*) product P-glycoprotein (P-gp). PSC 833 is a non-competitive inhibitor of P-gp and has been shown *in vitro* and *in vivo* to restore sensitivity of resistant tumor cells to anticancer drugs (ACDs). Induction chemotherapy consisting of cytarabine (C) in combination with PSC 833 and escalating doses of mitoxantrone (M) and etoposide (E) over 5 or 6 days were tested in two phase I/II studies in poor prognosis AML. Overall, 59 patients were evaluated: their age ranged between 18 and 70 years. Fourteen patients had primary refractory disease, 25 had relapsed within 9 months from first complete remission (CR), 5 were in second relapse, 10 had secondary AML, and 4 had relapsed post-bone marrow transplantation. PSC 833 was given as a constant i.v. infusion at a rate of 10 mg/kg/24h for 5 or 6 days, depending on the duration of chemotherapy. In both studies a loading dose of 2 mg/kg of PSC 833 was given on day 1. In the 5-day regimen, the final study doses of the cytotoxic agents were C 1 g/m^2/d, M 4.0 mg/m^2/d, and E 40 mg/m^2/d. In the 6-day regimen, the final study doses of the cytotoxic agents were C 1 g/m^2/d, M 4.5 mg/m^2/d and E 30 mg/m^2/d. The combined efficacy results of both studies indicate that PSC-MEC is active in all treatment indications, complete remission being achieved in 2/5 (40%) second relapses, 8/25 (32%) early relapses, 3/10 (30%) secondary AML, 3/15 (20%) refractory patients and 1/4 (25%) post-BMT relapses. Based on historical controls, this observed overall CR rate (29%) is higher than expected in this high risk patient population. Our data indicate that, in refractory/relapsed AML patients, PSC-MEC regimens had encouraging antileukemic effects, is well tolerated, and has led to Phase III trials in this setting.

2. INTRODUCTION

Standard induction therapy produces CR in 52% to 72% of patients with *de novo* AML;[1-8] the rate of remission depends on a variety of factors, such as age of the patient, history of MDS, and cytogenetic and immunophenotypic profile.[9,10] Overall median remission duration is 8 to 12 months, median survival is 9 to 16 months. About 40% of patients who received intensification with high dose cytarabine in either induction or consolidation therapy were disease-free at 4 years.[8,11,12] However, the benefits of intensive therapy have been confined to younger patients (i.e. < 55-year old): only 20% of *de novo* AML patients without a transplant or intensive post remission therapy are long-term survivors.

After relapse from the initial remission, a significant proportion of patients is unable to achieve a second CR: combination regimens incorporating high dose cytarabine in relapsed or refractory AML report complete response rates of 22–70% with durations averaging 3–6 months.[13-17] This broad range relates to the selection of subjects: the most prominent prognostic factors are duration of first remission and age.[18-24] Patients who fail to achieve CR after receiving two adequate attempts at induction are considered to have primary refractory disease. The prognosis for such patients is exceptionally grim, and response to salvage regimens is rare[24]. With the exception of occasional younger patients salvaged by bone marrow transplantation, patients treated with chemotherapy for relapsed or refractory AML are assumed to have minimal chances of long-term disease-free survival.

3. MULTIDRUG RESISTANCE

Failure of conventional chemotherapy in relapsed or refractory AML has been linked to expression of the multidrug resistance gene-1 (*mdr-1*),[25-27] that encodes a 170-kd transmembrane glycoprotein known as P-glycoprotein (P-gp).[28,29] P-gp functions as an adenosine triphosphate (ATP)-dependent efflux pump, and is capable of extruding a wide variety of structurally unrelated drugs taken up by cells through passive diffusion, including the anthracyclines and vinca alkaloids that are frequently used for treating AML.[30] Expression of P-gp results in decreased intracellular accumulation of and resistance to multiple chemotherapeutic agents, a phenomenon which has been termed multidrug resistance (MDR).[31]

transplantation. PSC 833 was given as a constant i.v. infusion at a rate of 10 mg/kg/24h for 5 or 6 days, depending on the duration of chemotherapy. In both studies a loading dose of 2 mg/kg of PSC 833 was given on day 1. In the 5-day regimen, the final study doses of the cytotoxic agents were C 1 g/m^2/d, M 4.0 mg/m^2/d, and E 40 mg/m^2/d. In the 6-day regimen, the final study doses of the cytotoxic agents were C 1 g/m^2/d, M 4.5 mg/m^2/d and E 30 mg/m^2/d. The combined efficacy results of both studies indicate that PSC-MEC is active in all treatment indications, complete remission being achieved in 2/5 (40%) second relapses, 8/25 (32%) early relapses, 3/10 (30%) secondary AML, 3/15 (20%) refractory patients and 1/4 (25%) post-BMT relapses. Based on historical controls, this observed overall CR rate (29%) is higher than expected in this high risk patient population. Our data indicate that, in refractory/relapsed AML patients, PSC-MEC regimens had encouraging antileukemic effects, is well tolerated, and has led to Phase III trials in this setting.

2. INTRODUCTION

Standard induction therapy produces CR in 52% to 72% of patients with *de novo* AML;[1-8] the rate of remission depends on a variety of factors, such as age of the patient, history of MDS, and cytogenetic and immunophenotypic profile.[9,10] Overall median remission duration is 8 to 12 months, median survival is 9 to 16 months. About 40% of patients who received intensification with high dose cytarabine in either induction or consolidation therapy were disease-free at 4 years.[8,11,12] However, the benefits of intensive therapy have been confined to younger patients (i.e. < 55-year old): only 20% of *de novo* AML patients without a transplant or intensive post remission therapy are long-term survivors.

After relapse from the initial remission, a significant proportion of patients is unable to achieve a second CR: combination regimens incorporating high dose cytarabine in relapsed or refractory AML report complete response rates of 22–70% with durations averaging 3–6 months.[13-17] This broad range relates to the selection of subjects: the most prominent prognostic factors are duration of first remission and age.[18-24] Patients who fail to achieve CR after receiving two adequate attempts at induction are considered to have primary refractory disease. The prognosis for such patients is exceptionally grim, and response to salvage regimens is rare[24]. With the exception of occasional younger patients salvaged by bone marrow transplantation, patients treated with chemotherapy for relapsed or refractory AML are assumed to have minimal chances of long-term disease-free survival.

3. MULTIDRUG RESISTANCE

Failure of conventional chemotherapy in relapsed or refractory AML has been linked to expression of the multidrug resistance gene-1 (*mdr-1*),[25-27] that encodes a 170-kd transmembrane glycoprotein known as P-glycoprotein (P-gp).[28,29] P-gp functions as an adenosine triphosphate (ATP)-dependent efflux pump, and is capable of extruding a wide variety of structurally unrelated drugs taken up by cells through passive diffusion, including the anthracyclines and vinca alkaloids that are frequently used for treating AML.[30] Expression of P-gp results in decreased intracellular accumulation of and resistance to multiple chemotherapeutic agents, a phenomenon which has been termed multidrug resistance (MDR).[31]

TREATMENT OF POOR PROGNOSIS AML PATIENTS USING PSC833 (VALSPODAR) PLUS MITOXANTRONE, ETOPOSIDE, AND CYTARABINE (PSC-MEC)

R. Advani, G. Visani, D. Milligan, H. Saba, M. Tallman, J. M. Rowe,
P. H. Wiernik, J. Ramek, K. Dugan, B. Lum, J. Villena, E. Davis, E. Paietta,
M. Litchman, A. Covelli, B. Sikic, and P. Greenberg

Stanford Medical Center, Stanford, California
Policlinico S. Orsola, Bologna
Heartlands Hospital, Birmingham
Moffit Cancer Center, Tampa, Florida
Northwestern Medical Center, Chicago, Illinois
Rochester Medical Center, New York
Albert Einstein Medical Center, Bronx, New York
Novartis Pharmaceuticals E. Hanover, New Jersey
Novartis Pharma AG, Switzerland

Keywords: Refractory/relapsing AML, multidrug resistance, P-glycoprotein, clinical trials.

1. ABSTRACT

The failure of convenional chemotherapy in relapsed or refractory and other poor risk AML patients has been linked to expression of the multidrug resistance gene (*mdr1*) product P-glycoprotein (P-gp). PSC 833 is a non-competitive inhibitor of P-gp and has been shown *in vitro* and *in vivo* to restore sensitivity of resistant tumor cells to anticancer drugs (ACDs). Induction chemotherapy consisting of cytarabine (C) in combination with PSC 833 and escalating doses of mitoxantrone (M) and etoposide (E) over 5 or 6 days were tested in two phase I/II studies in poor prognosis AML. Overall, 59 patients were evaluated: their age ranged between 18 and 70 years. Fourteen patients had primary refractory disease, 25 had relapsed within 9 months from first complete remission (CR), 5 were in second relapse, 10 had secondary AML, and 4 had relapsed post-bone marrow

Since 1989 several studies have reported a frequency of the *mdr-1* phenotype in about 30 to 50% of AML patients, depending on the technique and the threshold used,[32-35] with higher percentage (50–80%) in AML patients relapsing after or refractory to chemotherapy.[21,36,37] Sixty-five percent of AML subjects primarily resistant to induction treatment or relapsing early (<6 months) overexpress P-gp as opposed to only 37% of subjects, relapsing later than 6 months.[38]

The correlation between *mdr-1* gene expression and treatment outcome is well-documented in AML.[39] Many studies have reported a relationship between the absence of remission and the overexpression of P-gp,[40-50] or the overexpression of P-gp and refractory disease.[36,51] In a study on a small number of patients, the predictive value of P-gp expression at primary diagnosis or at early relapse is 94% and 66.6% for response and 90% and 94.1% for nonresponse, respectively.[38]

4. MODULATION OF MDR

A large number of compounds have been investigated for their ability to reverse the P-gp mediated MDR.[52] Examples include verapamil, amiodarone, quinacrine, phenothiazines, neuroleptics, quinidine, and cyclosporin A.[53,54] A recent preliminary report of a randomized study using quinine as a resistance modulating agent (RMA) plus intensive chemotherapy for AML post-MDS and high risk MDS patients indicated that quinine increased the CR rate and disease-free survival in P-gp positive patients but not in those who were P-gp negative.[55] In addition, a trial with Cyclosporin A, one of the most potent RMAs tested in clinical trials to date,[56,57] in 42 subjects with poor risk AML has been recently reported.[57] Overall 63% of subjects achieved a complete remission. Interestingly, 9 of 11 (82%) subjects relapsing within 1 year from the first complete remission achieved a second CR.

However, most of these agents produced severe toxic effects such as blocking of ion channels, modulation of other physiological pathways,[55,58] or, in the case of cyclosporines, immunosuppression and nephrotoxicity.[59]

4.1. PSC 833

PSC 833 (valspodar) is an analogue of cyclosporine D, but, unlike cyclosporine A, is not immunosuppressive or nephrotoxic.[60-62] PSC 833 has been shown to be approximately five-fold to 30-fold more potent than cyclosporine A and almost 100-fold more potent than verapamil. It can reverse MDR in vitro at concentrations of 0.5 to 2.0 µmol/L.[61] The increased potency of PSC 833 over agents such as verapamil and cyclosporine A is due, in part, to the fact that PSC 833 is a high affinity, noncompetitive inhibitor of P-gp, and is not appreciably transported by P-gp.[63] In contrast, verapamil and cyclosporine A are both substrates for P-gp and appear to exert their modulatory effects by competitive inhibition.[64,65] Data from phase I/II trials indicate that PSC 833 is well tolerated and that levels that reverse MDR in vitro (1000 to 2000 ng/mL) can be readily achieved *in vivo* with both the oral[66] and the parenteral formulation.[67-70] The dose limiting toxicity of PSC 833 is cerebellar ataxia, which is short-lasting and fully reversible. At the recommended dose of 10mg/kg/day PSC 833 continuous i.v. infusion, less than 3% of patients experience grade 3 ataxia. As with the oral formulation, intravenous PSC 833 does cause reversible changes in liver transaminases and bilirubin.

Because P-gp has a physiologic role in normal tissues responsible for the transport and excretion of cytotoxic drugs, treatment with P-gp inhibitors delays the elimination of anticancer drugs, and can thereby cause increased toxicity associated with those drugs. In phase 1 studies the dose-normalized AUC increased by 61–74% for doxorubicin and by 84% (mean values) for etoposide, when these drugs were given in combination with PSC 833.[67,71] The mean decreases in clearance were 29–33%, and 40%, respectively.

4.2. PSC-MEC Phase I Studies

Mitoxantrone and etoposide, with or without intermediate-dose cytarabine, have proven to be an effective regimen in refractory or relapsed AML with acceptable toxicity. Ho et al.[72] investigated the efficacy and tolerance of a combination of mitoxantrone and etoposide in refractory and poor risk AML. Of the 41 refractory or early-relapsed subjects who were evaluable for response and toxicity 16 (39%) attained complete remission (CR). Spadea et al.[73] used a combination of mitoxantrone, etoposide and intermediate dose cytarabine in subjects with poor risk AML. Thirty-eight patients were either resistant to one induction cycle or had relapsed within 6 months from CR: 16 of them (42.4%) achieved CR. In another trial using a similar drug-combination but different schedule and dosing, Archimbaud et al.[74] observed a 44% CR rate in 70 early relapsing or refractory patients, with only 3% surviving free of disease longer than 2 years.

Two phase I/II trials with PSC 833 in combination with mitoxantrone (M), etoposide (E), and intermediate-dose cytarabine (C) (PSC-MEC) over 5[70] or 6[69] days, respectively, in patients with poor risk AML have been completed. These were dose-finding studies designed to assess the safety of the regimen and the pharmacokinetic interactions of PSC 833 with the two cytotoxic drugs of the combination, i.e. mitoxantrone and etoposide, that are P-gp-substrates. Poor risk patients were defined as patients who were refractory to front-line induction therapy, relapsed within 6 to 9 months from the first complete remission, were in second relapse, or had secondary AML.

In all patients, PSC 833 was given as a constant i.v. infusion at a rate of 10 mg/kg/24h for 5 or 6 days, depending on the duration of chemotherapy. In both studies, the i.v. infusion of PSC 833 was started concomitantly with a 2 mg/kg loading dose given i.v. over 2 hours. The final doses of the PSC-MEC regimens in these two trials are shown in Table 1.

It is worth noting that the doses of cytotoxic agents are quite consistent among the two trials: in the 6-day regimen, the decrease in the mitoxantrone dose (4.5 mg/m^2 vs. 4.0 mg/m^2) was compensated by the increase in etoposide dose (30 mg/m^2 vs. 40 mg/m^2).

In the study by Visani et al, twenty-two patients with poor prognosis AML, i.e. refractory to first-line induction or relapsing within 9 months of attaining CR, were enrolled. The median age of these patients is 42 years (range 18–69 years). Eight patients had primary refractory disease, 7 each had relapsed within 6 or 7–9 months after CR, respectively. Six patients had secondary leukemia.

Mitoxantrone was dose-escalated from 3.0 mg/m^2/d in cohort I (n=10) to 4.5 mg/m^2/d in cohort II (n=6): in both cohorts PSC 833 i.v. infusion was given at 10

Table 1. Final dose of cytotoxic drugs on the 5- and 6 day PSC-MEC regimens

Study	Cytarabine	Mitoxantrone	Etoposide
Visani et al[69]	1 g/m^2/d × 6	4.5 mg/m^2/d × 6	30 mg/m^2/d × 6
Advani et al[70]	1 g/m^2/d × 5	4.0 mg/m^2/d × 5	40 mg/m^2/d × 5

mg/kg/24h over 7 days. Dose-limiting toxicities (DLT) observed in cohort I and II were three episodes of prolonged grade 4 hyperbilirubinemia and one grade 4 mucositis. Since the long duration of grade 4 bilirubinemia was felt to be secondary to the 7-day infusion of PSC 833, this was shortened by 24 hours in the final cohort. The only DLT observed in this cohort was a single episode of grade 4 aplasia. Pharmacokinetics of PSC 833 was evaluated in all the patients, and blood levels of PSC 833 after the loading dose ranged from 1200 to 6000 ng/mL (1.0–6.0 µM).

Overall, 6 patients (27%) achieved CR, and 18 failed chemotherapy. Causes for failures included: 10 refractory leukemia, 2 marrow regeneration failures, 2 early deaths, and 2 not assessable.

Similar results were found in a phase I/II US trial that further supports dose modification of mitoxantrone and etoposide when used with PSC 833. In this phase II multicentre study, 37 patients with relapsed or refractory AML or secondary AML were accrued. Indications for treatment included early relapse (< 6 mo.) (n = 11), ≥ 2 relapses (n = 5), secondary/post-MDS AML (n = 10), primary refractory AML (n = 7) and relapse post-BMT (n = 4). The first 6 pts were treated with M 5 mg/m^2/d, E 50 mg/m^2/d, C 1 mg/m^2/d (ie, with ~50% lower M and E doses than standard). Due to excess toxicity the next 31 pts received 20% lower M & E doses, with markedly reduced toxicities and good drug tolerance. Marrow hypoplasia was achieved in 33/35 evaluated pts. Blood PSC 833 levels (10 pts) ranged from 1000–3000 ng/ml (1–3 µM), levels capable of in vitro MDR-1 modulation. Pharmacokinetic (PK) analyses during 31 PSC-MEC courses for E in 27 pts showed a 1.7-fold increase in area under the curve (AUC) (P = 0.0009) and a 46% decrease in clearance (P = 0.001) compared to historical controls without PSC. The mean T 1/2 for M in 28 pts during 30 PSC-MEC courses, was 3.6 hr (95% CI 3.3–4.0), which is longer than that previously reported in the absence of PSC (mean 2.0 hr; 95% CI 1.4–2.7; P < 0.05). Twelve pts achieved CR (32%), 4 PR, and 21 failed therapy. Nine of 12 CRs received consolidative therapy including four BMTs. Median remission duration of pts achieving CR was 5.5 mo (range, 0.7–13.3 mo.). Survival of CR + PR pts was 8.3 mo. (range, 4.8–17.5+ mo).

5. CONCLUSIONS

Several strategies to overcome drug resistance during chemotherapy have been evaluated. These include the combination of "non-cross-resistant" chemotherapy, utilization of extremely high doses of chemotherapy in conjunction with hematopoietic stem cells, and/or co-administration of agents that block specific mechanisms of drug resistance.

Evidence from many of these studies also suggests that clinical resistance is multifactorial. In addition to the "classic" pattern of MDR mediated by P-gp, at least two alternative mechanism of MDR have recently been identified. The MDR-associated protein (MRP) transports drugs that are glutathione-S conjugates and, like P-gp, confers resistance through drug efflux.[75-77] The lung-resistance protein (LRP) is a nuclear major vault protein homolog that may function to disrupt the transport of drugs from the cytoplasm to the nucleus.[78] Preliminary studies indicate that both MRP and LRP are expressed at high levels in normal hematopoietic cells and in leukemic cells, where their expression may be associated with MDR.[79,80] At least one report has shown that MRP gene expression is upregulated in patients with relapsing AML,[81] but further studies are needed to establish the prognostic significance of this gene in drug-resistant malignancies. In a study by List et

Table 2. Probability of achieving second CR according to response to the previous treatment.

Prognostic group	Frequency of second CR
First salvage therapy	
1st CR ≥ 2 years	73%
1st CR ≥ 1 year, < 2 years	47%
1st CR ≥ 0 year, < 1 years	14%
Second salvage therapy	0%
Total patient number	206

From: Estey E, Thall P, and David C. Cancer Chemother Pharmacol 40(Suppl):S9-S12, 1997.

al.,[79] immunocytochemical staining for LRP was detected in 33% of patients with relapsing AML. In this study LRP overexpresion was predictive for a poor response to therapy.

On the other hand, studies to date clearly suggest that *mdr1* expression is important in determining therapeutic outcome in patients with relapsed or refractory acute leukemia. Reversing resistance due to P-gp may benefit patients by improving therapeutic response to established cytotoxic regimens. PSC 833 appears to interact specifically with P-gp, while not binding to cyclophilin, the latter accounting for the immunosuppressive effects of Cyclosporine A.

Results from completed phase I/II trials in poor risk AML patients are encouraging if compared to remission rates of between 15 and 52% for early relapsed subjects in other studies with intermediate or high dose cytarabine containing regimens.[74,82] The chance of attaining complete remission after salvage therapy for refractory or relapsed AML patients is primarily dependent on the duration of their first remission (see Table 2)

Based on historical controls, the expected complete remission rate for the patients accrued on the two PSC-MEC studies was between 10% and 19%. The efficacy results of both studies combined are shown in Table 3 by pre-treatment disease status: the observed complete remission rate is twice as high as expected in this population.

Another recent preliminary investigation using PSC 833 plus chemotherapy for relapsed/refractory AML have shown similar encouraging results as these studies.[83] In contrast, a recent study not showing benefit from PSC 833 plus chemotherapy had a different experimental design and marked regimen-related toxicity, which may have contributed to the relatively poor outcome of those patients.[84]

Phase I/II studies with PSC-MEC indicated that intravenous administration of PSC 833 is well tolerated. Hyperbilirubinemia was only observed at higher doses or over prolonged administration of PSC 833 in some cohorts. Ataxia was not reported in these studies. Since PSC 833 affects the elimination of many P-gp substrate anti-cancer drugs, the

Table 3. Combined results from PSC+MEC phase I/II studies [69,70]

Treatment indication	Total N.	CR N.	CR %
Refractory	15	3	20
Relapsed < 9 mos	25	8	32
Second relapse	5	2	40
Secondary AML	10	3	30
Post-BMT relapse	4	1	25
Total	59	17	29

use of PSC 833 in combination with cytotoxic agents requires appropriate dose reductions to yield effective treatment with acceptable toxicities. Based on the clinical experience with PSC 833, it is now possible to predict what the PK effects will be and to institute appropriate dose reductions in the scheduled chemotherapy regimen.

Modulating clinical MDR in selected hemopoietic malignancies appears a promising approach: phase III randomized trials, which have started, are needed to determine if this new therapeutic strategy is ultimately beneficial to patients.

REFERENCES

1. Rai, KR, HollandJF, Glidwell OJ, et al: Treatment of acute myeloid leukemia: A study by Cancer and Leukemia Group B. Blood 58:1203–1212, 1981.
2. Yates J, Glidwell O, Wiernik P, et al: Cytosine arabinoside with daunorubicin or adraimycin for therapy of acute myeloid leukemia: a CALGB study. Blood 60:453–462, 1982.
3. Omura GA, Vogler WR, Lefabte J, et al: Treatment of acute myelogenous leukemia: Influence of three induction regimens and maintenance with chemotherapy or BCG immunotherapy. Cancer 49:1530–1536, 1982.
4. Sauter C, Berchtold W, Foopp M, et al: Acute myelogenous leukemia: Maintenance chemotherapy after early consolidation treatment does not prolong survival. Lancet 1:379–382, 1984.
5. Vogler WR, Winton EE, Gordon DS, et al: A randomized comparison of post remission therapy in acute myelogenous leukemia: A Southwestern Cancer Study Group trial. Blood 63: 1039–1045, 1984.
6. Priesler H, David RB, Kirshner J, et al: Comparison of 3 remission induction regimens and two post-induction regimens for the treatment of acute non-lymphocytic leukemia. Blood 69:1441–1448, 1987.
7. Bishop JF, Lowenthal RM, Joshua D, et al: Etoposide in acute non-lymphocytic leukemia. Blood 75:1–6, 1990.
8. Mayer RJ, Davis RB, Schiffer CA, et al: Intensive post-remission chemotherapy in adults with acute myeloid leukemia. N Engl J Med 3331:896–903, 1994.
9. Stone and Mayer: . Hematol Clin North Am, 7:47, 1993.
10. Keating MJ, Estey E, Katarjian H: Acute Leukemia. In: DeVita VT Jr, Hellman S, and Rosemberg SA eds. *Cancer: Principles & Practice of Oncology*. JB Lippincott, Philadelphia, 1993, p.1938–1964.
11. Bishop JS, Matthews JP, Young GA, et al: A randomized trial of high-dose cytarabine in induction in acute myeloid leukemia. Blood 87:1710, 1996.
12. Weick JK, Kopecky TJ, Appelbaum FR, et al: A randomized investigation of high-dose versus standard-dose cytosine arabinoside with daunorubicin in patients with previously untreated acute myeloid leukemia: A Southwest Oncology Group study. Blood 88:2841, 1996.
13. McCalley DL. Treatment of adult acute leukaemia. Clinical Pharmacy 1992; 11:767–796.
14. Estey E, Plunkett W, Keating M et al. Variables predicting response to high dose cytosine arabinoside therapy in patients with refractory acute leukaemia. Leukaemia 1987; 1(8):580–583.
15. Willemze R, Ribbe WE, Zwaan FE. Experience with intermediate and high dose cytosine arabinoside in relapsed and refractory acute leukaemia. Neth J Med 1983; 26:215–219.
16. Hiddemann W, Aul C, Maschmeyer G et al. High-dose versus intermediate dose cytosine arabinoside combined with mitoxantrone for treatment of relapsed and refractory acute myeloid leukaemia: results of an age adjusted randomized comparison. Leukaemia and Lymphoma; 10 Suppl:133–137.
17. Herzig RH, Wolff SN, Lazarus HM et al. High dose cytosine arabinoside therapy for refractory leukaemia. Blood 1983; 62: 361–9.
18. Hiddemann W, Büchner T. Treatment strategies in acute myeloid leukaemia (AML). Blut 1990; 60:163–171.
19. Keating MJ, Kantarjian H, Smith TL et al. Response to induction therapy and survival after relapse in acute myelogenous leukaemia. J Clin Oncol 1989; 7:1071–1080.
20. Rees JKH, Swirsky D, Gray RG, et al: Principal results of the Medical Research Council's 8th acute myeloid leukemia trial. Lancet 2:1236, 1986.
21. Keating MJ, Kantarjian H, Smith TL, et al: Response to salvage therapy and survival after relapse in acute myelogenous leukaemia. J Clin Oncol 7:1071, 1989.
22. Hiddemann W, Martin WR, Sauerland CM, et al: Definition of refractoriness against conventional chemotherapy in acute myeloid leukemia: a proposal based on the results of retreatment by thioguanine, cytosine

arabinoside, and daunorubicin (TAB 9) in 150 patients with relapse after standardized first line therapy. Leukemia 4:184, 1990.
23. Estey E, Thall P, and David C: Design and analysis of salvage therapy in acute myelogenous leukemia. Cancer Chemother Pharmacol 40(Suppl):S9-S12, 1997.
24. Bolwell BJ, Cassileth PA, Gale RP: High dose cytarabine:a review. Leukemia 2:253, 1998.
25. Fojo AT, Whang-Peng J, Gottesmann MM. Amplification of DNA sequences in human multidrug-resistance KB carcinoma cells. Proc Natl Acad Sci USA 82:7661–7665, 1985.
26. Gros P, Neriah BY, Croop JM, et al. Isolation and expression of a complementary DNA that confers multidrug resistance. Nature 323:728–731, 1986.
27. Goldstein LJ, Galski H, Fojo A, et al. Expression of a multidrug resistance gene in human cancers. J Natl Cancer Inst 2:116–124, 1989.
28. Juliano RL, Ling V. A surface glycoprotein modulating drug permeability in Chinese hamster ovary cell mutants. Biochem Biophys Acta 455:152–162, 1976
29. Kartner N, Riordan JR, Ling V. Cell surface P-glycoprotein associated with multidrug resistance in mammalian cell lines. Science 2211285–1288, 1983.
30. Gottesman MM, Pastan I. Biochemistry of multidrug resistance mediated by the multidrug transporter. Ann Rev Biochem 62:385–427, 1993.
31. Biedler JL, Riehm H. Cellular resistance to actinomycin D in Chinese Hamster cells *in vitro*: cross-resistance, radioautographic and cytogenetic studies. Cancer Res 30:1174–1184, 1970.
32. Pastan P, Schouten H. Multidrug resistance mediated by P-glycoprotein in haematological malignancies. Neth J Med 42:218–231, 1993.
33. Licht T, Pastan I, Gottesman M, et al. P-glycoprotein mediated multidrug resistance in normal and neoplastic haemopoietic cells. Annals Hematol 69:159–171, 1994.
34. Nooter K, Sonneveld P. Clinical relevance of P-glycoprotein expression in haematological malignancies. Leuk Res 18:23–243, 1994.
35. Marie JP. P-glycoprotein in adult hematological malignancies. Hematol Oncol Clin N Am 9:239–250, 1995.
36. Zhou D, Marie JP, Suberville A, Zittoun R. Relevance of MDR-1 gene expression in acute myeloid leukemia and comparison of different diagnostic methods. Leukemia 6:879–885, 1992.
37. List AF, Spier CM, Cline A et al. Expression of the multidrug resistance gene product (P-glycoprotein) in myelodysplasia is associated with a stem cell phenotype. Br J Haematol 1991; 78:28–34.
38. Nuessler V, Pelka-Fleischer R, Zweirzina H et al. P-glycoprotein expression in patients with acute leukaemia—clinical relevance Leukemia 10:523–531 1996.
39. Holmes J, West R. The effect of MDR1 gene expression on outcome in acute myeloid leukaemia. Brj Cancer 69:382–384, 1994.
40. Te Boekhorst P, de Leeuww K, Schoester M, et al. Predominance of functional multidrug resistance (MDR-1) phenotype in CD34[+] myeloid leukemia cells. Blood 79:3157–3162, 1993.
41. Campos L, Guyotat D, Archimbaud E, et al. Clinical significance of multidrug resistance P-glycoprotein expression on acute nonlymphoblastic leukemia cells at diagnosis. Blood 79:473–476, 1992.
42. Lamy T, Goasguen D, Mordeletb E, et al. P-glycoprotein (P-170) and CD34 expression in adult acute leukemia (AML). Leukemia 8:1879–1883, 1994.
43. Wood P, Burgess R, McGregor A, Liu Yin J. P-glycoprotein expression on acute myeloid leukaemia blasts cells at diagnosis predicts response to chemotherapy and survival. Br J Haematol 87:509–514, 1994.
44. Kuwazuru Y, Yoshimura A, Hanada S, et al. Expression of the multidrug transporter P-glycoprotein in acute leukemia cells and correlation to clinical drug resistance. Cancer 66:868–873, 1990
45. Marie JP, Zittoun R, Sikic B. Multidrug resistance gene (*mdr*) expression in adult acute leukemias: correlation with treatment outcome and *in vitro* drug sensitivity. Blood 78:586–592, 1991.
46. Pirker R, Wallner J, Geissler K, et al. MDR-1 gene expression and treatment outcome in acute myeloid leukemia. J Natl Cancer Inst 83:708–712, 1991.
47. Michieli M, M. Damiani D, Geromin A, et al. Overexpression of multidrug resistance-associated p-170 glycoprotein in acute non-lymphocytic leukemia. Eur J Haematol 48:87–92, 1992.
48. Tirikainen M, Elonen E, Ruutu T, Jansson S, Krusius T. Clinical significance of P-glycoprotein expression in acute leukemia as analysed by immunocytochemistry. Eur J Haematol 50:279–285, 1993.
49. Zoechbauerm S, Gsur A, Brunner R, Kyrle P, Lechner K, Pirker R. P-glycoprotein expression as unfavorable prognostic factor in acute myeloid leukemia. Leukemia 8:975–977, 1994.
50. Basara N, Radosevic-Radojkovic N, Colovic M, Boskovic D, Rolovic Z. *In vitro* drug sensitivity of leukemic progenitors and P-glycoprotein expression in adult myeloid leukemia: correlation with induction treatment outcome. Eur J Haematol 55:83–87, 1995.

51. Zhou D, Zittoun R, Marie JP. Expression of multidrug resistance-associated protein (MRP) and multidrug resistance (MDR1) genes in acute myeloid leukemia. Leukemia 9:1661–1666, 1995.
52. Lum Bl, Fisher GA, Brophy NA, et al. Clinical trials of modulation of multidrug resistance. Pharmacokinetic and pharmacodynamic considerations. Cancer 72:3502–3514, 1993.
53. Ford J and Hait W. Pharmacology of drugs that alter multidrug resistance in cancer. PharmacolRev 42:156–199,1993.
54. Fisher GA, Lum BL, Hausdorff J, et al. Pharmacological considerations in the modulation of multidrug resistance. Eur J Cancer 32A:1082–1088, 1996.
55. Solary E, Witz B, Caillot D, et al. Combination of quinine as a potential reversing agent with mitoxantrone and cytarabine for the treatment of acute leukemias: a randomized multicenter study. Blood 88:1198–1205, 1996.
56. Sonneveld P, Nooter K. Reversal of drug-resistance by cyclosporin-A in a patient with acute myelocytic leukaemia. Brit J Haem 1990; 75:208–211.
57. List AF, Spier C, Greer J, et al. Phase I/II trial of cyclosporin as a chemotherapy-resistance modifier in acute leukemia. J Clin Oncol 1993;11:1652–1660.
58. Fisher GA and Sikic BI. Clinical studies with modulators of multidrug resistance. Hematol Oncol Clin North AM 9:363–382, 1995.
59. Yahanda AM, Adler KM, Fisher GA, et al. Phase I trial of etoposide with cyclosporine as a modulator of multidrug resistance. J Clin Oncol 10:1624–1634, 1992.
60. Twentyman PR. Modification of cytotoxic drug resistance by non-immunosuppressive cyclosporins. Br J Cancer 57:254–258, 1988.
61. Boesch D, Muller K, Poutier-Manzanedo A, Loor F. Restoration of daunomycin retention in multidrug resistant P388 cells by submicromolar concentrations of SDZ PSC 833. Exp Cell Res 196:26–32, 1991.
62. Twentyman PR and Bleehen NM. Resistance modification by PSC-833, a novel non-immunosuppressive cyclosporin. Eur J Cancer 27:1639–1542, 1991.
63. Archinal Mattheis A, Rzepka RW, Wtanabe T, et al. Analysis of the interactions of SDZ PSC 833 ([3'keto-BMT1]-Val2]cyclosporine), a multiresistance modulator, with P-glycoprotein. Oncol Res 7:603–610, 1995.
64. Foxwell BM, Mackie A, Ling V, et al. Identification of the mutlidrug resistance-related P-glycoprotein as a cyclosporine binding protein. Mol Pharmacol 36:534–546, 1989.
65. Twentyman PR. Cyclosporins as drug resistance modifiers. Bochem Pharmacol 43:109–117, 1992.
66. Sonneveld P, Marie JP, Huisman C, et al. Reversal of multidrug resistance by PSC 833 combined with VAD in refractory multiple myeloma: a phase I study. Leukemia 10:1741–1750, 1996.
67. Boote DJ, Dennis IF, Twentyman PR, et al. Phase I study of etoposide with SDZ PSC 833 as a modulator of multidrug resistance in patients with cancer. J Clin Oncol 14:610–618, 1996.
68. Sonneveld P, Lowenberg B, Vossebled P, et al. Dose finding study of PSC 833, a novel MDR reversing agent, with daunorubicin and Ara-C in uneated eldelry patients with acute myelod leukemia (AML). Blood 90(Suppl 1) Abstract 2517, 1997.
69. Visani G, Milligan D, Leoni F, et al. A phase I dose-finding study of PSC 833, a novel MDR reversing agent, with mitoxantrone, etoposide and cytarabine (PSC-MEC) in poor prognosis acute leukemia (AML). Blood 90(Suppl 1) Abstract 2518, 1997.
70. Advani R, Saba H, Tallman M, et al. Treatment of poor prognosis AML patients with PSC 833 plus mitoxantrone, etoposide and cytarabine (PSC-MEC). Blood 90(Suppl 1) Abstract 2260, 1997.
71. Sikic b. Pharmacologic approaches to reversing multidrug resistance. Seminars in Hematol 34(Suppl 5):40–47, 1997.
72. Ho AD, Lipp T, Ehninger G et al. Combination of mitoxantrone and etoposide in refractory acute myelogenous leukaemia - an active and well-tolerated regimen. J Clin Oncol. 1988; 6:213–217.
73. Spadea A, Petti MC, Fazi P et al. Mitoxantrone, etoposide and intermediate-dose cytarabine (MEC): an effective regimen for poor risk acute myeloid leukaemia. Leukaemia 1993; 7 (No. 4):549–552.
74. Archimbaud E, Thomas X, Leblond V, et al. Timed sequential chemotherapy for previously treated acute myeloid leukaemia:long-term follow-up of etoposide, mitoxantrone, and cytarabine - 86 trial. J Clin Oncol 1995; 13:11–18.
75. Cole SP. Bhradwaj G, Gerlach JH, et al. Overexpression of a transporter gene in a multidrug-resistant human lung cancer cell line. Science 258:1650–1654, 1992.
76. Muller M, Meijer C, Zaman GJ, et al. Overexpression of the gene encoding the multidrug resistance-associated protein results in increased ATP-dependent glutathione S-conjugate transport. Proc Natl Acad Sci USA 91:13033–13037, 1994.
77. Eijdems EW, Zaman GJ, de Haas M, et al. Altered MRP is associted with multidrug resistance and reduced drug accumulation in human SW-1573 cells. Br J Cancer 72:298–306, 1995.

78. Scheffer GL. Wijngaard PL, Flens MJ, et al. The drug resistance-related protein LRP is the human major vault protein. Nat Med 1:578–582, 1995
79. List AF, Spier CS, Grogan TM, et al. Overexpression of the major vault transporter protein lung-resistance protein predicts treatment outcome in acute myeloid leukemia. Blood 87:2464–2469, 1996
80. Ross DD, Doyle LA, Schiffer CA, et al. Expression of multidrug resistance-associated protein (MRP) mRNA in blast cells from acute myeloid leukemia (AML) patients. Leukemia 10:48–55, 1996.
81. Schenider E, cowan KH, Bader H, et al. Increased expression of the multidrug resistance-associated protein gene in relapsed leukemia. Blood 85:186–190, 1995.
82. Harousseau JL, Reiffers J, Hurteloup P et al. Treatment of relapsed acute myeloid leukaemia with idarubicin and intermediate-dose cytarabine. J Clin Oncol 1989; 7(1):45–49.
83. List A, Karanes C, Dorr R, et al. Modulation of anthracycline resistance in poor-risk acute myeloid leukemia (AML) with SDZ PSC 833: results of a phase I/II multicenter study. Blood 88(Suppl 1) Abstract 1156, 1996.
84. Kornblau SM, Estey E, Madden T, et al. Phase I study of mitoxantrone plus etoposide with multidrug resistance blockade by SDZ PSC 833 in relapsed or refractory acute myelogenous leukemia. J Clin Oncol 15:1796–1802, 1997

ASSESSMENT OF P-GLYCOPROTEIN EXPRESSION BY IMMUNOCYTOCHEMISTRY AND FLOW CYTOMETRY USING TWO DIFFERENT MONOCLONAL ANTIBODIES COUPLED WITH FUNCTIONAL EFFLUX ANALYSIS IN 34 PATIENTS WITH ACUTE MYELOID LEUKEMIA

S. Poulain,[1] P. Lepelley,[1] N. Cambier,[2] A. Cosson,[1] P. Fenaux,[2] and E. Wattel[2]

[1]Laboratoire d'Hématologie A
[2]Service des Maladies du Sang
Chu, Lille, France

Keywords: P-glycoprotein, immunocytochemistry, flow cytometry, rhodamine-123, acute myeloid leukemia.

1. ABSTRACT

Drug resistance often results in failure of anticancer chemotherapy in leukemias. A large number of studies have been published on the effect of P-glycoprotein (Pgp) expression on prognosis in AML. However, a consensus has been difficult to reach, due to the variable results obtained by different laboratories. Pgp expression was investigated here in bone marrow samples from 34 patients with AML including 19 newly diagnosed cases and 15 relapsing patients. Pgp expression was performed by immunocytochemistry (ICC) using the aviding-biotin-peroxydase technique with JSB1 and UIC2 MoAbs. Flow cytometry (FCM) analysis of Pgp expression was performed using UCI2 MoAbs in an indirect immunofluorescent assay without cell permeabilization. Rhodamine 123 (Rh 123) uptake was measured in the presence or absence of verapamil. Result was discordant in only 1/20 samples studied with both JSB1 and UIC2 by ICC. Results of Pgp expression were consistent on FCM and ICC in 23 of the 28 (82%) samples tested. Overall, Pgp expression was observed by ICC or FCM in 23 (67%) patients, including 11 (58%) newly diagnosed patients and 12 (80%) patients in relapse. Functional Rh123 efflux (Rh123+) was observed in 20 cases (59%) : 10 de novo AML (53%) vs 10 AML in relapse (67%). The functional efflux was correlated with Pgp expression in 25 of the 34 cases analyzed (p=0.013). 3 (9%) and 6 (18%) samples were Pgp−/Rh123+ and Pgp+/Rh123− respectively. Nine of the 14 pts (64%) treated with intensive anthracyclin-Ara C chemotherapy achieved complete remission, including 5/5 (100%) Pgp− cases vs 4/9 (44%) Pgp+ cases (p=0.04) and 4/6 (67%) Rh 123− vs 4/7 (57%) Rh123+ cases (p=0.5). In conclusion, assessment of Pgp expression by ICC and FMC using 2 different MoAbs coupled with functional efflux analysis confirms that Pgp expression is correlated with disease stage and response to treatment in AML. Discordant Pgp/Rh123 cases suggest a non functional Pgp or another alteration of drug transport.

2. INTRODUCTION

Multidrug resistance may be related to the overexpression of multidrug resistance gene (MDR1), which encodes a 170 Kd glycoprotein (Pgp), an energy dependant membrane protein which functions as a transmembrane drug efflux pump (1). Pgp has a broad substrate specificity and can export a wide range of structurally unrelated drugs, including vinca-alkaloids, anthracyclines and etoposide. Several authors have report Pgp expression as predictive of lower remission rates and survival in acute leukemia (2,3,4). The presence of Pgp can be mesured at the level of gene expression, amount of protein or functional activity. To date, a number of different methods as western blot, immunocytochemistry (ICC) and flow cytometry (FCM) have been used to detect protein expression. Many monoclonal antibodies (MoAbs) have been proposed: MRK16, UIC2, C219, JSB1…(5,6,7). The results are often not reliable because of the different methods used, and the definition of Pgp overexpression fluctuates in most publications.When comparative studies were made, concordances between methods was found in 70–80% of the cases (8). This issues were recently discussed at an international workshop, where standardisation of detection methods was suggested (9). The best assay is not yet determined and a combinaison of FCM and immunocytochemical tests is required to evalue the MDR phenotype.

The aim of our study was to compare three different methods of MDR assessment in acute myeloid leukemia (AML), each of them detecting Pgp expression at a different level: immunocytochemistry, using two different monoclonal antibodies JSB1 and UIC2 directed respectively against internal and external Pgp epitopes, flow cytometry with an indirect immunofluorescent assay using UIC2 without cell permeabilisation and the fluorescent dye rhodamine (Rh123) efflux, measured in the presence or absence of verapamil.

3. MATERIALS AND METHODS

3.1. Patients

Thirty four patients with acute myeloid leukemia including 19 patients at diagnosis and 15 patients in relapse were studied. Median age was 46 years (5 to 80). FAB classification of AML revealed: 5 M0, 9 M1, 11 M2, 7 M4, 2 M5. Fourteen patients were treated by conventional intensive combination chemotherapy including cytosine arabinoside (Ara C) and anthracycline and were evaluable for response.

3.2. Immunocytochemistry

Pgp expression was determined on bone marrow smears obtained by aspiration and frozen at −20°C until use. The immunocytochemical reaction was performed using the avidin-biotin-peroxydase (ABC) technique and JSB1 (Novocastra, New Castle, UK), or UIC2 (Immunotech, Marseille, France) as monoclonal antibodies according to our previous report (10). Controls were performed with a non reactive MoAb (Mouse IgG2a and IgG1). Slides were fixed for 10 min in cold acetone, washed on buffered saline prior to labelling, and incubated with blocking horse normal serum. Endogenous peroxydase was blocked with H2O2 azide mixture (Dako reagent).Slides were incubated sequentially with 1/10 diluted JSB1 or 1/5 diluted UIC2 overnight at +4°C, then with biotin-labeled horse anti-mouse immunoglobulin for 60 min (Vector, Burlingame, CA, USA) and finally with peroxidase-conjugated avidin-biotin complex for 60 min. All incubations were carried out in a humid chamber. The reaction was developed using 0.05% diaminobenzidine and 0.01% H2O2 and slides were counterstained with Giemsa. Positive cells appeared with brownish granules. Staining intensity was reported as negative (−), intermediate (+) and high (++).

3.3. Flow Cytometry

Bone marrow mononuclear cells (MNC) were separated by density gradient centrifugation using Ficoll-Hypaque (density 1.077) and washed in RPMI + 10% foetal calf serum (FCS). Cells were cryopreserved in 90% FCS and 10% dimethyl sulfoxide and stored in liquid nitrogen. Cryopreserved AML blasts were thawed in prewarmed media and pre-incubated for 1 hour at 37°C for the functional assay. The viability of the leukemic blasts was determined using trypan blue exclusion. Sample with more than 20 % of stained cells were excluded from study.

Pgp detection was performed by indirect immunofluorescence. Briefly, 5×10^5 cells were incubated with UIC2 at 4°C for one hour. Appropriate isotypic controls at the same protein concentration was substituted in the control tube. Cells were washed in PBS+ 1% bovine serum albumine and another incubation was performed for 30 min in dark with the FITC antimouse antibody. After washing, cells were resuspended in PBS and were analysed on flow cytometer (FASCan, Becton Dickinson San Jose, California) using LysisII software.

UIC2 staining was mesured by the Kolmogorov-Smirnov (KS) statistic to compare UIC2 stained cells with the control. Positive MDR1 expression was defined by a D value ≥ 0.15 and/or by a mean fluorescence intensity (MFI) ratio between UIC2 and control staining ≥ 1.5.

For functional assay, cells were stained with 200 ng/ml Rh 123 for 45min at room temperature and after washing, were incubated in dye free medium for 2 hours at 37°C with or without verapamil (10 μmol). One aliquot was placed at 4°C for measurement of baseline Rh123 accumulation. After efflux, the cells were washed, pelleted and resuspended in fresh 4°C media for immediate flow cytometric analysis. In preliminary tests, no significant difference in the ability of leukemic blasts to exclude the fluorescent dye was observed between fresh and cryopreserved cells. Propidium iodide at a concentration of 5μg/ml was added immediately before analysis to allow exclusion of dead cells. Gating was electively directed on morphological cytometric blast cell characteristics, according to the side scatter and forward scatter parameters. In cases with <80% blasts, mononuclear cells were labelled with CD34-phycoerythrine MoAbs after Rh 123 test, and the efflux was evaluated on CD 34 positive cells.The Rh 123 test was analysed as positive if the mean fluorescence intensity ratio between efflux and accumulation (E/A) was < 0.8. The reversal power of verapamil was analysed by the (Verapamil- efllux)/ Efflux x 100 ratio.

Adriamycine resistant and sensitive K 562 cell lines were used as positive and negative controls, respectively.

4. RESULTS

4.1. Immunocytochemistry

Of the 33 smears staining with JSB1, 20 (61%) gave a positive result (Table 1).They corresponded to 10/18 newly diagnosed AML (55%) and 10/14 AML in relapse (71%). Staining was frequently weak but the percentage of positive cells exceeded 20% in all cases. Twenty samples were studied with both UIC2 and JSB1 by ICC and discordants results were obtained in only one case (p<0.001).

4.2. Flow Cytometry

Pgp expression. Seventeen of the 29 samples (57%) tested were found positive after FCM analysis (FCM+, Table 1). The D value ranged from 0.15 to 0.44. The results obtained by D value were correlated with MFI data. Results of PgP expression were consistent on ICC and FCM in 23 of the 28 samples tested (82%). Three samples were ICC+/FCM− (pts 3, 4, 11) and 2 were ICC−/FCM+ (pts 17, 32). Overall, Pgp expression was observed by ICC or FCM in 23 patients (67%) including 11 (58 %) newly diagnosed and 12 (80%) in relapse.

Efflux of Rh 123. Rh 123 efflux was observed in 20 of the 34 cases analysed (59 %) corresponding to 10 (53%) de novo AML versus 10 (67%) AML in relapse. The mean E/A ratio was 0.43 (range 0.18 to 0.68). The efflux was completely (17 cases) or partially (3 cases) blocked in the presence of verapamil .

The functional efflux (Rh123 +) was correlated with Pgp expression in 25 of the 34 cases analysed by both methods (p= 0.013). Three (9%) and 6 (18%) samples were Pgp−/Rh 123+ (pts 9, 18, 30) and Pgp+/Rh123 − (pts 3, 5, 8, 15, 32, 34) respectively. These discordances were not explained by the FAB type or the disease stage.

All the effluxing specimens were CD 34+. We found a statistically significant correlation between Rh 123 efflux and the CD 34 expression (p= 0,006).

No significant correlation was noted between the MDR1 phenotype and FAB typing, or other hematologic characteristics.

Fourteen patients, including 13 cases evaluated for functional efflux, received intensive anthracycline-Ara-C chemotherapy and 9 (64 %) achieved complete remission, including 5/5 (100 %) Pgp-negative patients vs 4/9 (44 %) Pgp-positive patients (p=0.04) and 4/6 (67 %) Rh123− patients vs 4/7 (57 %) Rh123+ patients (p=0.5) (Fisher's test).

5. DISCUSSION

As new therapeutics are designed to circumvent multidrug resistance in AML, accurate identification of patients who could benefit from such resistance modifiers is essen-

Table 1. P-glycoprotein expression and Rhodamine efflux in the 34 patients with AML

Patient n°	FAB	CD34 expression	Immunocytochemistry JSB1*	UIC2*	Flow cytometry D value	Rh123 test (E/A)**	Conclusion
			Patients at diagnosis				
1	M0	+	–	ND	0.02	0.83	Pgp–/Efflux–
2	M0	+	++ (70%)	ND	ND	0.38	Pgp+/Efflux–
3	M0	+	++ (100%)	++ (100%)	0.02	0.88	Pgp+/Efflux–
4	M1	+	+ (34%)	++ (90%)	0.11	0.45	Pgp+/Efflux+
5	M1	ND	+ (56%)	ND	0.28	0.82	Pgp+/Efflux–
6	M1	ND	ND	ND	0.11	0.85	Pgp–/Efflux–
7	M1	–	–	–	0.14	0.81	Pgp–/Efflux–
8	M1	–	+ (100%)	ND	0.32	0.93	Pgp+/Efflux–
9	M1	+	–	–	ND	0.55	Pgp–/Efflux+
10	M1	+	+ (32%)	+ (67%)	0.17	0.33	Pgp+/Efflux+
11	M2	+	+ (59%)	+ (62%)	0.1	0.29	Pgp+/Efflux+
12	M2	–	–	–	ND	0.85	Pgp–/Efflux–
13	M2	+	–	–	0.08	0.8	Pgp–/Efflux–
14	M2	+	+ (96%)	+ (24%)	0.33	0.66	Pgp+/Efflux+
15	M4	–	+ (100%)	ND	0.23	0.86	Pgp+/Efflux–
16	M4	+	–	–	0.1	0.8	Pgp–/Efflux–
17	M4	+	–	ND	0.28	0.18	Pgp+/Efflux+
18	M4	+	–	–	0.12	0.54	Pgp–/Efflux+
19	M5	+	++ (100%)	+ (16%)	0.37	0.26	Pgp+/Efflux+
			Patients at relapse				
20	M0	+	+ (55%)	+ (79%)	0.38	0.36	Pgp+/Efflux+
21	M0	+	–	–	0.06	0.9	Pgp–/Efflux–
22	M1	+	–	–	0.02	0.92	Pgp–/Efflux–
23	M1	+	+ (96%)	ND	0.19	0.43	Pgp+/Efflux+
24	M2	ND	+ (60%)	ND	ND	0.52	Pgp+/Efflux+
25	M2	ND	+ (21%)	ND	0.44	0.25	Pgp+/Efflux+
26	M2	+	+ (27%)	+ (57%)	0.15	0.4	Pgp+/Efflux+
27	M2	+	+ (55%)	ND	ND	0.48	Pgp+/Efflux+
28	M2	+	+ (48%)	ND	0.38	0.29	Pgp+/Efflux+
29	M2	+	+ (56%)	ND	0.18	0.3	Pgp+/Efflux+
30	M2	+	–	–	0.1	0.68	Pgp–/Efflux+
31	M4	+	+ (22%)	+ (92%)	0.4	0.32	Pgp+/Efflux+
32	M4	–	–	+ (100%)	0.28	0.9	Pgp+/Efflux–
33	M4	+	ND	+ (29%)	0.2	0.68	Pgp+/Efflux+
34	M5	–	+ (100%)	ND	0.17	0.85	Pgp+/Efflux–

* P-glycoprotein expression scored as : (–) negative, (+) intermediate, (++) high ; ( ) : percentage of positive cells
**E/A : mean fluorescence intensity between efflux and accumulation ND : Not done

tial. The aim of our study was to contribute to the standardization of Pgp detection methods in leukemias and to explore the relation between expression and function. Only one discordant result was observed when a sample from the same patients were studied by both UIC2 and JSB1 by ICC. The main advantage of this assey is that the morphology remains intact and that Pgp staining can be evaluated in individual cells. The drawback of the method is that it depends on to personal interpretation. In addition, analysis is often restricted to several hundred of cells. However in myelodysplaticsyndroms, where percentage of blasts is low, this technique remains very useful.

By flow cytometric detection, we observed in most cases a relatively low level of UIC2 staining, resulting in an overlap of the fluorescence distribution of control and test specimen. UIC2 staining was measured by the Kolmogorov-Smirnov statistic.This method appears to be very useful in flow cytometric when weak staining is present, especially in clinical specimens. Like other authors, we found low levels of Pgp expression in leukemic samples, when compared to resistant cell lines.

Results of Pgp expression were consistent on FCM and ICC in 23 of the 28 samples tested. Three samples were ICC+/FCM– and 2 were ICC–/FCM+. These discrepancies can be explained by the presence of masking epitopes or by a very low density of Pgp antigen.

Measurement of the efflux function by the Rh 123, a mitochondrial dye, is rapid and easy to perform (11). The use of a viability marker constitutes an important criterion of specificity. CD34 expression was found to correlate with the efflux activity. This indicates that functional activity is predominantly observed in immature CD34+ AML and may contribute to chemoresistance in poorly differentiated myeloid leukemia (12).

Our results showed that Rh 123 efflux is strongly related to the presence of Pgp ($p = 0.013$). Discordants results betweeen function and expression were detected in nine cases. The efflux assay also identified several atypical cases in which functional efflux, partially or completely blocked by verapamil was found in the absence of detectable MDR1 expression. The identification of Pgp–/Efflux + AML (9%) suggests that other non MDR1 mediated efflux may operate in these cases (13). One alternative drug transporter protein is multidrug resistance-associated protein (MRP) (14,15). Increased expression of MRP has been demonstrated in many Pgp negative resistant cell lines with decreased drug accumulation.While MRP expression has been detected in leukemic cells, its role in treatment failure remains controversial (16).

We found 6 (18%) Pgp+/Efflux– cases. Some evidence exists for the presence of non functional MDR1 protein in normal blood cells as mature monocytes which express a very low level of Pgp expression without detectable functional efflux (17). This lack of activity may correspond to a low level of expression (18). Alternatively, protein modification in localization or structure may have the same consequence (19).

In conclusion, assessment of Pgp expression by ICC and FCM using 2 different monoclonal antibodies coupled with functional efflux analysis confirms that Pgp expression is correlated with disease stage and response to treatment in AML. Eighteen percent of the Pgp+ AML are Rh123– suggesting a non functional Pgp in these cases. Conversely, 9 % of the Rh123+ AML are Pgp–, suggesting another alteration of drug transport in these patients.

REFERENCES

1. Gottesman M.M., Pastan I. Biochemistry of multidrug resistance mediated by the multidrug transporter. Ann. Rev. Biochem., 1993, 62, 385–427.
2. Guerci A., Merlin J.L., Missoum N., Feldmann L., Marchal S., Witz F., Rose C., Guerci O. Predictive value for treatment outcome in acute myeloid leukemia of cellular daunorubicin accumulation and P-glyprotein expression simultaneously detemined by flow cytometry. Blood, 1995, 85, 2147–2153.
3. Nüssler V., Pelka-Fleischer R., Zwierzina H., Nerl C., Beckert B., Gieseler F., Diem H., Ledderose G., Gullis E., Sauer H., Wilmanns W. P-glycoprotein expression in patients with acute leukemia-clinical relevance. Leukemia, 1996, 10, 523–531.
4. Leith C.P., Kopecky K.J., Godwin J., Mc Connell T., Slovak M.L., Chen I.M., Head D.R., Appelbaum F.R, Willman C.L. Acute myeloid leukemia in the elderly : assessment of multidrug resistance (MDR1) and cy-

togenetics distinguishes biological subgroups with remarkably distinct responses to standart chemotherapy: A Southwest Oncology Group study. Blood, 1997, 9, 3323–3329.
5. Mechetner E.B., Roninson I. Efficient inhibition of glycoprotein-mediated multidrug resistance with a monoclonal antibody. Proc. Natl. Acad., Sc. USA, 1992, 89, 5824–5828.
6. Miwa H., Kita K., Nishii K., Morita N., Takahura N., Ohishi K., Mahmud N., Kageyama S., Fukumoto M., Shirakawa S. Expression of MDR1 gene in acute leukemia cells: association with CD7+ acute myeloblastic leukemia/acute lymphoblastic leukemia. Blood, 1993, 82, 3445–3451.
7. Lehne G., de Angelis P., Clausen O.P.F., Egeland T., Tsuruo T., Rugstad H.E.Binding diversity of antibodies against external and internal epitopes of the multidrug resistance gene product P-glycoprotein. Cytometry, 1995, 20, 228–237.
8. Marie J.P., Huet A.M, Faussat A.M., Perrot J.Y., Chevillard S., Barbu V., Bayle C., Boutorrat J., Calvo F., campos-Guyotat L., Colosetti P., Cazin J.L., Cremoux P., Delvincourt C., Demur C., Drenou B., Fenneteau O., Feuillard J., Garnier-Suillerot A., Genne P., Gorisse M.C., Gosselin P., Jouault H., Lacave R., Le Calvez G., LegliseM.C., Leonce S., Manfait M., Maynadie M., Merle-Beral H., Merlin J.L., Mousseau M., Morjani H., Pio F., Pinguet F., Poncelet P., Racadot E., Raphael M., Richard B., Rossi J.F., Schlegel N., Viehl P., Zhou D.C., Robert J. Multicentric evaluation of the MDR phenotype in leukemia. Leukemia, 1997, 11, 1086–1094.
9. Beck W.T., Grognan T.M., Willman C.L., Cordon-Cardo, Parham D.M., Kuttesch J.F., Andreeff M., Bates S.E., Berard C.W., Boyett J.M., Brophy N.A., Broxtermann J.H., Chan H.L.S., Dalton W.S., Dietel M., Fojo A.T., Gascoyne R.D., Head D., Houghton P.J., Srivastava D.K., Lehnert M., Leith C.L., Paietta E., Pavelic Z.P., Rimsza L., Roninson I.B., Sikic B.I., Twentyman P.R., Warnke R., Weinstein R. Methods to detect P-glycoprotein-associated multidrug resistance in patients tumors: consensus recommendations. Cancer Res., 1996, 56, 3010–3020.
10. Lepelley P., Soenen V., Preudhomme C., Lai J.L., Cosson A., Fenaux P. Expression of the multidrug resistance P-glycoprotein and its relationship to hematological characteristics and response to treatment in myelodysplastic syndromes. Leukemia, 1994, 8, 998–1004.
11. Ludescher C., Thaler J., Drach D., Drach J., Spitaler M., Gaattringer C., Huber H., Hoffman J. Detection of activity of P-glycoprotein in human tumour samples using rhodamine 123. Br. J. Haematol., 1992, 82, 161–168.
12. te Boekhorst P.A.W., de Leeuw K., Shoester M., Wittebol S., Nooter K., Hagemeijer A., Löwenberg B., Sonneveld P. Preominance of functional Multidrug Resistance (MDR1) phenotype in CD34+ acute myeloid leukemia cells. Blood, 1993, 82, 3157–3162.
13. Leith C.P., Chen I.M., Kopecky K.J., Appelbaum F.R., Head D.R., Godwin J.E., Weick J.K., Willman C.L. Correlation of multidrug resistance (MDR1) protein expression with functional dye/drug efflux in acute myeloid leukemia by multiparameter flow cytometry: indentification of discordant MDR1/Efflux+ and MDR1+/Efflux– cases. Blood,1995, 86, 2329–2342.
14. Cole S.P.C., Bhardwaj G., Gerlach J.H., Mackie J.E., Grant C.E., Almquist K., Stewart A., Kurz E., Duncan A., Deeley R. Overexpression of a transporter gene in a multidrug-resistant human lung cancer cell line. Science, 1992, 258, 1650–1654.
15. Cole S.P.C., Defley R.G. Multidrug resistance associated with overexpression of MRP Cancer Treat. Res., 1996, 87, 39–62.
16. Hart S.M., Ganesshagru K., Hoffbrand A.V., Prentice H.G., Mehta A.B. Expression of the multidrug resistance-associated protein (MRP) in acute leukaemia. Leukemia, 1994, 8, 2163–2168.
17. Klimecki W.T., Futscher B.W., Grogan T.M., Dalton W.S. P-glycoprotein expression and function in circulating blood cells from normal volunteers. Blood, 1994, 83, 2451–2458.
18. Bailly D., Muller C., Jaffrezou J.P., Demur C., Cassar G., Bordier C., Laurent G. Lack of correlation between expression and function of P-glycoprotein in acute myeloid leukemia cell lines. Leukemia, 1995, 9, 799–807.
19. Cumber P.M., Jacobs A., Hoy T., Whittaker J.A., Tsuruo T., Padua R.A. Increased drug accumulation ex vivo with cyclosporin in chronic lymphatic leukemia and its relationship to epitope masking of P-glycoprotein. Leukemia, 1991, 5, 1050–1053.

8

PRELIMINARY IMMUNOCYTOCHEMICAL STUDIES OF MDR-1 AND MDR-3 Pgp EXPRESSION IN B-CELL LEUKAEMIAS

Annemarie Larkin,[1*] Elizabeth Moran,[1] Denis Alexander,[2] and Martin Clynes[2]

[1]National Cell and Tissue Culture Centre
Bioresearch Ireland, Dublin City University
Glasnevin, Dublin 9, Ireland
[2]Department of Haematology
Belfast City Hospital
Belfast BT9 7AB, Northern Ireland

Keywords: MDR-1, MDR-3, P-glycoprotein, B-cell leukaemia, immunocytochemistry.

ABSTRACT

P-glycoproteins (Pgps) belong to the family of ATP binding cassette (ABC) transporter proteins. In humans two Pgp genes have been identified; *mdr-1* and *mdr-3*. Classical Multiple Drug Resistance (MDR) is associated with over expression of the *mdr-1* gene product, P-170. No role for *mdr-3* in MDR has yet been proven. However there is evidence that *mdr-3* overexpression may be associated with drug resistance in certain B-cell lymphocytic leukaemias. In an immunocytochemical study we have looked at a selection of B-cell leukaemias for *mdr-1* and *mdr-3* encoded Pgp expression using monoclonal antibodies specific for the *mdr-1* and *mdr-3* encoded gene products. In B-CLL patients a differential pattern of MDR-3 positive staining was observed; suggesting that MDR-3 positivity may be associated with a more malignant phenotype in B-CLL. This pattern was not observed with MDR-1 positivity. We also observed MDR-3 positivity in an AML stage M5a patient which is the first report of MDR-3 Pgp expression being detected in AML; suggesting that MDR-3 Pgp expression may be limited to particular subtypes of this dis-

---

*Correspondence to: AM Larkin, National Cell and Tissue Culture Centre, Bioresearch Ireland, Dublin City University, Glasnevin, Dublin 9, Ireland.

ease. Results from B-NHL cases were inconclusive with varying expression of MDR-1 and MDR-3 Pgps observed. Work is currently underway to further explain the significance of these findings.

INTRODUCTION

P-glycoproteins (Pgps) belong to the family of ATP binding cassette (ABC) transporter proteins.[1] In humans there are two Pgp genes *mdr-1* and *mdr-3* which show 80% homology.[2–3]

Overexpression of the *mdr-1* gene product is associated with Classical Multiple Drug Resistance (MDR) in cultured cell lines and in certain tumours.[4–5]

There have been several published studies of *mdr-1*/ Pgp detection in various haematological malignancies. Reports of these studies vary considerably, probably due to the lack of standarisation of detection systems, however *mdr-1*/ Pgp overexpression is thought to be implicated as a cause of clinical resistance in Acute Myleoid Leukaemia (AML) and Multiple Myeloma (MM) and possibly in late stages of Acute Lymphocytic Leukaemia (ALL) and non-Hodgkins Lymphoma (NHL). In other haematological neoplasms a prognostic role for *mdr-1*/ Pgp has not been established.

Although a role in drug resistance for *mdr-3* has not been proven, studies involving *mdr-3* transformed yeast systems[6] and earlier work on haematological malignancies providing strong evidence that *mdr-3* may encode a functional drug pump in certain B-cell leukaemias, supports such a role for this gene.[7–8] Arai et al. have recently demonstrated that *mdr-3* Pgp has functional drug efflux capacity in acute lymphocytic leukaemia bloods.[9]

mdr-1 expression has been shown to occur in all types of leukaemias except B-cell pro-lymphocytic leukaemia (B-PLL), high levels of *mdr-3* gene expression have been observed in PLL patients with no detectable *mdr-1* expression.[7–8] From these initial studies it appeared that *mdr-3* expression is limited to leukaemias of B-cell origin, in addition this expression appears to be further restricted to certain developmental stages of B-cells.

Chronic Lymphocytic Leukaemia (CLL) has a highly variable clinical course and presents great difficulty in prognosis and therapy. Previous studies have shown that in general B-CLL cases express *mdr-1* and *mdr-3*.[8,10-12] *mdr-1*/ Pgp overexpression appears to be intrinsic rather than acquired in this disease. Higher *mdr-3* expression levels were associated with prior treatment and also with advanced disease. These correlations were not observed with *mdr-1* expression levels.[8,11] However a later study found no evidence that overexpression of *mdr-3* was related to rhodamine efflux in B-CLL, but did find once again a tendency toward higher *mdr-3* expression in patients with advanced disease.[10]

There appears to be a high correlation between *mdr-1*/ Pgp overexpression and clinical drug resistance in AML.[13] To date *mdr-3* expression has not been detected in myeloid leukaemias.[7,8,10] *mdr-1*/ Pgp has been more frequently detected in French American British classification (FAB), classes M4, M5a and M5b and less frequently in FAB, M3;[14] this pro-lymphocytic M3 subclass, is highly sensitive to chemotherapy.

Most of the work on *mdr-1*/ Pgp in NHL has been performed on frozen lymph node sections. In general samples from treated patients appear to express more *mdr-1*/ Pgp than untreated patients. There appears to be no difference in *mdr-1*/ Pgp expression between high and low grade lymphomas and between B and T sub types.[12] As to whether absence of *mdr-1*/ Pgp is an indicator of better clinical response; three studies have showed a correlation.[15-17] A larger study did not prove such a correlation.[18] There have been no published reports of *mdr-3*/ Pgp expression being investigated. To investigate whether *mdr-3* plays a role in the clinical resistance of B-NHL, we have examined a selection of B-NHL malignancies for *mdr-3* and *mdr-1* encoded protein levels. Also we have looked at a small number of B-CLL cases, to define further the exact significance of *mdr-3* expression in this disease and to ascertain whether this gene does indeed represent an independent marker of more agressive disease. In this preliminary immunocytochemical study we have also investigated *mdr-3* and *mdr-1* Pgp levels in three FAB subclasses of AML.

METHODS

mdr-1 encoded Pgp was detected using the MDR-1 specific monoclonal antibody, BRI MAb 6/1C.[19] *mdr-3* encoded Pgp was detected using a new MDR-3 specific MAb developed in our laboratory, BRI MAb 6/1G (manuscript in preparation).

Haematological Samples

Cytospin preparations of peripheral blood, bone marrow and pleural fluid were kindly provided by the Department of Haematology, Belfast City Hospital, Belfast, Northeren Ireland.

Immunocytochemical Studies

All immunocytochemical studies were performed according to the method of Hsu *et al.*,[20] using an avidin-biotin horseradish peroxidase (HRP) conjugated kit (ABC) plus an appropriate secondary antibody from Dako, UK.

Briefly, cytospin preparations were fixed for 2 mins in ice cold acetone and allowed to air dry for at least 15 mins prior to immunostaining. Endogenous peroxidase activity was quenched by placing cytospins in 0.6% (vol/vol) H_2O_2/ methanol. All slides were blocked for non-specific staining with 20% (vol/vol) normal rabbit serum for 20 mins. Primary antibodies were applied to each sample (BRI Anti-MDR-3 MAb, 6/1G diluted 1:2 to 1:10 in TBS/0.05% (vol/vol) Tween 20, the MDR-1 specific antibody 6/1C used as neat supernatant or as ascitic fluid diluted 1:40 in TBS/0.05% (vol/vol) Tween 20) for 2 hrs. This was followed by a 30 min incubation with biotinylated rabbit anti-mouse IgG (1/300 dilution in TBS/ 0.05% (vol/vol) Tween 20). Finally ABC (HRP conjugated) was applied for 25 mins and the peroxidase substrate 3'-3 diaminobenzidine tetrahydrochloride (DAB, Dako) was then applied for 5–7 mins. All incubations were carried out at room temperature and slides were washed after each incubation in 3 changes of TBS/0.05% (vol/vol) Tween 20 over 15 mins.Cells were lightly stained with haematoxylin, differentiated in 1% (vol/vol) acid alcohol and 'blued' in Scott's tap water. Following dehydration in graded alcohols slides were cleared in xylene and mounted in DPX (BDH, UK). Negative control slides in which primary antibody was replaced by control mouse immunoglobulins (Vector Labs) (used within the manufacturers recommended concentration range) were included in all experiments.

RESULTS

B-CLL

Two cases of B-CLL showed MDR-1 positivity in normal and malignant cell types. A differential pattern of MDR-3 positive staining was observed with the larger malignant cells (more pleiomorphic, possibly associated with higher grade/ more malignant phenotype) showing more intense MDR-3 positivity than smaller malignant cells. Both of these patients had recieved prior treatment.

AML

Of three AML cases included in this study a specimen from a patient presenting with AML, French American British (FAB) classification, M0 was negative for *MDR-1* and *MDR-3* protein expression. An AML, FAB M1 sample showed *MDR-1* Pgp positivity but did not show any MDR-3 positivity. The third sample, FAB M5a exhibited weak MDR-1 positivity in monoblasts with very intense MDR-3 positivity (which was very granular in nature) also observed in these monoblasts. None of these patients had received prior treatment.

B-NHL

Peripheral blood from one B-NHL patient (diagnosis not further classified) was negative for both *MDR-1* and *MDR-3* Pgp expression. One case of mantle cell lymphoma showed MDR-3 positivity and was negative for MDR-1; a second case however showed a reversal of these results. A small number of follicle centre lymphomas gave conflicting results in this study although in two cases there appears to be co-expression of *MDR-1* and *MDR-3* Pgps. One case of follicle centre lymphoma (atypical CD5 +ve type) showed weak positivity for MDR-1 and did not show any MDR-3 positivity prior to treatment. At 16 days post treatment MDR-1 expression was increased significantly; intense MDR-3 specific staining was also observed. Further post treatment samples from this patient are being investigated.

DISCUSSION

B-CLL has been previously shown to express both the *mdr-1* and the *mdr-3* genes.[8,10-12] We found MDR-1 and MDR-3 Pgp expression in two post treatment samples of B-CLL. A differential pattern of MDR-3 positive staining was observed with intense MDR-3 positivity, possibly indicating a more malignant phenotype in both cases. This differential staining pattern was not observed with MDR-1 positivity. These observations are in agreement with previous work which suggests that *mdr-1* does not appear to play a significant role in CLL, however as we have already mentioned *mdr-3* may play an important role in B-CLL. *mdr-3* expression and not *mdr-1* expression was significantly higher in patients with advanced B-CLL than those with early stage disease in a study carried out by Sonneveld et al.[11] Ludscher et al.[10] also found a tendancy toward higher *mdr-3* expression in patients with advanced stages of CLL. Our observations and these earlier studies suggest that *mdr-3*/ Pgp overexpression may represent a marker of a more malignant phenotype/ more aggressive disease in B-CLL. As the number of cases in our study was small, we are currently examining more B-CLL cases for MDR-3 and MDR-1 Pgp levels.

To date *mdr-3* expression has not been reported in AML. The *mdr-1* gene product has been shown to be frequently expressed in AML at diagnosis (i.e. prior to treatment) and at relapse. A recent review on AML by Marie et al.[13] has reported a high correlation between *mdr-1*/ Pgp overexpression and clinical drug resistance. In our study two untreated cases of AML (FAB, M0 and M1) showed MDR-1 positivity and were both negative for MDR-3 Pgp. A FAB, M5a untreated patient showed weak MDR-1 positivity but showed intense MDR-3 positivity. Since AML stage M5a has an undifferentiated monoblastic lineage; the possibility exists that *mdr-3* is not expressed in certain sub types: M0, M1, M2 and M3 all of which have myeloblastic/ myelocytic morphology. It is intended to examine MDR-3 reactivity in a wider range of AML subtypes to further investigate these observations. *mdr-3* expression may be restricted to the M5a and M5b subtypes which have a monocytic morphology. It has already been suggested that *mdr-3* expression may be restricted to certain B-cell developmental stages; no *mdr-3* expression has been found in MM which presents with end stage B-cells.[8] Analysis of *mdr-3* expression in a selection of B-cell leukaemias revealed that expression of this gene is associated with the differentiation/ maturation stages of the B-cell neoplasm.[12]

The B-NHL cases studied (mantle cell, follicle centre and unclassified B-NHL) showed varying levels of MDR-3 and MDR-1 Pgp expression. Interestingly in one B-NHL we examined the malignant cells comprised of lymphoplasmacytoid cells which are late stage B-cells; this sample was negative for both MDR-1 and MDR-3 Pgps. A high level of MDR-3 positivity appeared to develop following treatment in one case of follicle centre lymphoma (atypical, CD5+ve). Further post treatment samples are currently being investigated for MDR-3 and MDR-1 Pgp expression levels.

A more extensive study is planned to investigate whether expression is significantly related to treatment/ outcome in various B-NHL neoplasms (including mantle cell and follicle centre lymphomas) and also to assess the significance of the MDR-1/ MDR-3 expression levels observed in other B-cell malignancies examined in this preliminary study.

REFERENCES

1. Schinkel AH, Roelofs MEM, Borst P. Characterisation of the human MDR-3 P-glycoprotein and its recognition by P-glycoprotein-specific monoclonal antibodies. *Ca Res*, **51(10)**, 2628–2635 (1991).
2. Roninson IB, Chin JE, Choi K et al.. Isolation of human mdr DNA sequences amplifed in multidrug resistant KB carcinomas cells. *Proc. Natl. Acad. Sci. USA*, **83**, 4538 (1986).
3. Van Der Bliek AM, Baas F, Ten Houte-De-Lange T, Kooiman PM, Van Der Velde-Koerts T, Borst P. The human *mdr-3* gene encodes a novel p-glycoprotein homologue and gives rise to alternatively spliced mRNAs in liver. *EMBO J*, **6**, 3325 (1987).
4. Roninson IB. The role of *mdr-1* (P-glycoprotein) gene in multidrug resistance in vitro and in vivo. *Biochem Pharacol*, **43**, 95–102 (1992).
5. Clynes M. Cellular models for multidrug resistance in cancer. *In Vitro Cell Dev Biol*, **29A**, 171–179 (1993).
6. Kino K, Taguchi Y, Yamada K, Komano T, Ueda K. Aureobasidin A an antifungal cyclic depsipeptide antibiotic, is a substrate for both human MDR-1 and MDR-2/ P-glycoproteins. *FEBS Lett*, **399**, 29–32 (1996).
7. Nooter K, Sonnevald P, Janssen A, Oostrum R, Boersma T, Herweijer H, Valerio D, Hagemeijer A, Baas F. Expression of the *mdr-3* gene in prolymphocytic leukemia: association with cyclosporin-A induced increase in drug accumulation. *Int J Ca.*, **45**, 626–631(1989).
8. Herweijer H, Sonneveld P, Baas F, Nooter K. Expression of *mdr-1* and *mdr-3* Multidrug-resistance Genes in Human Acute and Chronic Leukemias and association with stimulation of drug accumulation by cyclosporine. *J Natl Ca Inst.*, **82(13)**,1133–1140 (1990).
9. Arai Y, Masuda M, Sugawara I, Arai T, Motoji T, Tsuruo T, Oshimi K, Mizoguchi H. Expression of the MDR-1 and MDR-3 gene products in acute and chronic leukemias. *Leuk Res*, **21**, 313–319 (1997).
10. Sonneveld P, Nooter K, Burghouts JTM, Herweijer H, Adriaansen HJ, van Dongen JJM. High Expression of the *mdr-3* Multiple Resistance Gene in Advanced Stage Chronic Lymphocytic Leukemia. *Blood*, **79(6)**, 1496–1500 (1992).
11. Nooter K, Sonneveld P. Multidrug resistance (MDR) genes in haematological malignancies. *Cytotechnology.*, **12**, 213–230 (1993).
12. Ludescher C, Hilbe W, Eisterer W, Preuss E, Huber C, Gotwald M, Hofmann, Thaler J. Activity of P-glycoprotein in B-cell Chronic Lymphocytic leukaemia determined by a flow cytometric assay. *J. Natl. Cancer. Inst.*, **85 (21)**, 1751–1758 (1993).
13. Marie JP, Zhou DC, Gurbuxani S, Legrand O, Zittoun R. Mdr-1/ P-glycoprotein in Haematological Neoplasms. *Eur J Ca.*, **32A(6)**, 1034–1038 (1996).

14. Nussler V, Pelka-Fleischer R, Zwierzina H, Nerl C, Beckert B, Gieseler F, Diem H, Ledderose, Gullis E, Sauer H, Wilmanns W. P-glycoprotein expression in patients with acute leukemias - clinical relevance. *Leukemia* **10**, Suppl 3, S23-S31 (1996).
15. Pileri SA, Sabattini, Falani B, Tazzari PL, Gherlinzoni F, Michieli MG, Damiani D, Zucchini L, Gobbi M, Tsuro T, Baccarani M. Immunohistochemical detection of the multidrug transport protein P170 in human normal tissues and malignant lymphomas. *Histopathology,* **19**,131–140 (1991).
16. Cheng A, Su I, Chen Y, Lee T, Wang C. Expression of p-glycoprotein and glutathione-S transferase in recurrent lymphomas: the possible role of Epstein-Barr virus, immunophenotypes, and other predisposing factors. *J Clin Oncol*, **11**,109–115 (1993).
17. Rodriguez C, Commes T, Robert J, Rossi J. Expression of p-glycoprotein and anionic glutathione s transferase genes in non-Hodgkins's lymphoma. *Leuk Res,* **17**, 149–156 (1993).
18. Niehans G, Jaszcz W, Brunetto V, *et al.* Immunohistochemical identification of p-glycoprotein in previously untreated, diffuse large cell and immunoblastic lymphomas. *Ca Res*, **52**, 3668–3657 (1992).
19. Moran E, Larkin AM, Doherty G, Kelehan P, Kennedy SM, Clynes M. A new mdr-1 encoded P-170 specific monoclonal antibody: (6/1C) on paraffin wax embedded tissue without pre treatment of sections. *J Clin Pathol.*, **50(6)**, 465–471 (1997).
20. Hsu SM, Raine L, Fanger H. Use of avidin-biotin-peroxidase complex (ABC) in immunoperoxidase techniques. *J Histchem Cytochem.,* **29**, 577–580 (1981).

A MUTATION IN THE PROMOTER OF THE MULTIDRUG RESISTANCE GENE (*MDR*1) IN HUMAN HEMATOLOGICAL MALIGNANCIES MAY CONTRIBUTE TO THE PATHOGENESIS OF RESISTANT DISEASE

Deborah Rund, Idit Azar, and Olga Shperling

Hematology Department
Hadassah University Hospital
Ein Kerem, POB 12000
Jerusalem, Israel 91120

1. ABSTRACT

The overexpression of the multidrug resistance gene *MDR*1 has been found to be associated with therapy-resistance in hematological malignancies. Yet the cellular mechanisms underlying this increased expression are completely unknown. Point mutations in the *MDR*1 promoter have been found in osteogenic sarcoma (Stein et al., Eur J of Cancer, 30A: 1541–1545, 1994). We therefore analyzed DNA from hematological malignancies for *MDR*1 promoter point mutations. Two pairs of overlapping PCR primers were designed which did not amplify the *MDR*3 gene. Amplified DNA was screened using single strand conformation polymorphism (SSCP). 139 patients and 93 normal controls were studied. Fifteen patients (11%) were found to have abnormal bands on the SSCP analysis. Of these, 9 had acute myeloid leukemia (AML), 4 chronic lymphocytic leukemia (CLL), 1 acute lymphocytic leukemia (ALL), and 1 nonHodgkin's lymphoma (NHL). Sequence analysis revealed that all patients were heterozygous for a point mutation in the promoter (T-C transition at +8). Four normals (4%) were found to be heterozygous for the mutation. Confirmation of the mutation was performed by oligonucleotide probe hybridization. All but two of the AML patients have died due to chemoresistant disease (one is lost to followup). Of the CLL patients, one is alive with progressive disease, and the others have died. Further studies will assess the effect of this mutation on *MDR*1 gene transcription.

Drug Resistance in Leukemia and Lymphoma III, edited by Kaspers *et al.*
Kluwer Academic / Plenum Publishers, New York, 1999.

2. INTRODUCTION

The human multidrug resistance gene *MDR1*[1] encodes a 170 kd transmembrane glycoprotein (P-glycoprotein, abbreviated P-gp), which confers energy-dependent resistance to a number of naturally occuring, structurally unrelated types of chemotherapeutic agents. This gene is variably expressed in normal tissues of the body, including high level tissue-specific expression in certain organs. In other tissues, such as mature bone marrow, expression is very low. The gene has been under study for over a decade. The human gene *MDR1* and the two murine homologues *mdr1* and *mdr3* are highly conserved in mammalian species[1] and their protein structure bears striking similarity to many polypepetides involved in cellular export or import in prokaryotes. This suggests an important physiological role for P-gp, but the precise cellular function of P-gp is still under debate.

Despite the great interest in P-gp, the regulatory mechanisms controlling murine and human *MDR1* gene expression in normal tissues, as well as malignancies, are not well understood. Recently, many studies have concentrated on *MDR1* activity in hematopoietic tissues. Many of these types of studies have been performed in malignant cell lines. However, it is quite likely that the regulation of these genes in malignant cells is quite different from that occurring in normal tissues or even in actual human maligancies.[2] There is a much lower level of expression of these genes at physiological levels (both in normal tissues or in human malignant cells) than are expressed in transformed cell lines.[2] This suggests that studies performed exclusively on highly drug-resistant cell lines may not shed light on drug resistance mechnisms which are active in vivo.[2]

Point mutations in a gene may affect the coding region or the noncoding regions. Promoter regions are particularly susceptible to mutations, as they contain CpG islands which are hotspots for mutation generation.[3] The occurence of these mutations is thought to be an endogenous process.[3] Mutations affecting the promoter region may either decrease or increase gene activity. In non-malignant tissues, promoter mutations have been found to be a common mechanism causing changes in "developmentally programmed expression". This has been studied extensively for the promoter of the human γ-globin gene, for which "genetically-programmed" downregulation of expression occurs as a normal part of erythroid cell ontogeny. Point mutations in the promoter, located at the binding sites of transacting factors crucial for regulated gene expression, lead to persistent elevations in fetal hemoglobin, even when present in the heterozygous state.

Recently, two different, recurrent point mutations were discovered in the promoter region of the *MDR1* gene in 7 out of 9 untreated human osteosarcomas, versus none of 8 malignant fibrous histiosarcomas.[4] The investigators screened for point mutations in a region of the *MDR1* promoter known to contain drug-responsive elements, which result in increased expression upon exposure to chemotherapeutic drugs.[4] The mutations identified were not found to increase basal promoter activity when put into plasmid constructs used in *cat* assays. However, they did result in increased *cat* expression upon exposure of transfected cells to *MDR1*-sensitive drugs.[4] The level of *cat* expression was modestly increased, as would be expected to result from mutations of this type.

We routinely test all patients with acute leukemia, and many with other hematological malignancies, for *MDR1* phenotype using rhodamine 123 dye exclusion.[5,6] Rhodamine 123 dye exclusion is a functional assay[5] which is known to be able to determine even low, physiologically significant levels of P-glycoprotein activity.[7]

We screened for mutations in the *MDR1* gene promoter in hematological malignancies with the goal of identifying cis-acting sequences which may be important for *MDR1* regulation in hematopoietic tissue. The patients who were examined had been previously evaluated for *MDR*1 activity using rhodamine 123 efflux. Screening for mutations was performed in patients who were rhodamine efflux-positive as well as those who were rhodamine efflux negative, for comparative purposes.

3. MATERIALS AND METHODS

Peripheral blood mononuclear cells were separated over Ficoll gradients. Cells were then stained with rhodamine 123 using the method outlined by Chaudhary.[5] We used 150 ng/ml of rhodamine 123 for staining, for 15 minutes at 37°C with an efflux time of 2 hours. 10 µM verapamil was used as an *MDR*1 inhibitor. Cells were counterstained with propidium iodide immediately prior to analysis to identify dead cells (if any were present), which were removed from the analysis by gating. We defined a positive result as one in which the Kolmogorov-Smirnov (abbreviated K-S) D value[8] was equal to or greater than 0.15.[9–11] Cell lines which were high level positive (P388^R) and *MDR*1 negative (P388^S, K562) as well as cells which were low level positive (NIH3T3 cells[6]) were used for calibration.

Normal DNA samples were obtained from the National Laboratory for the Genetics of Israeli Populations, Sackler School of Medicine of Tel Aviv University, Tel Aviv, Israel.

DNA was isolated from patient samples using standard Proteinase K digestion followed by phenol-chloroform extraction.[12]

PCR analysis was performed as previously described.[12] Two primer sets were designed which did not cross-react with *MDR*3, which spanned the region from –238 to +170. SSCP analysis was performed using standard techniques.[13,14] Sequencing of PCR fragments was performed using the Thermo Sequenase Terminator kit. Confirmation of the mutation was made using sequence analysis of the opposite strand, followed by dot blot analysis using ^{32}P-labelled oligonucleotide probes.[12]

4. RESULTS

DNA from rhodamine efflux-positive as well as rhodamine efflux-negative patients was screened for the presence of point mutations using the SSCP technique. A total of 139 patients were examined, in addition to 93 normal controls. Table 1 lists the distribution of their diagnoses.

A number of patients were found to have aberant bands on single strand conformation polymorphism (SSCP) analysis (not shown). Sequence analysis was performed of

Table 1.

Diagnosis	# Tested	Positive (%)
AML (primary)	50	6 (12%)
AML (secondary)	22	1 (4.5%)
CLL	32	4 (12.5%)
NHL	20	1 (5%)
ALL	9	1 (11%)
MDS	6	0
normals	93	4 (4%)

both strands. The sequence analysis revealed that the patients were heterozygous for a T to C transition at +8 relative to the transcription start site. Dot blot hybridization with radioactive oligonucleotide probes complemetary to the mutant and wild type sequences confirmed this finding. The mutation was also found in oral mucous membrane epithelial cells (not shown) obtained by saline mouthwash, indicating that it is constitutional.

The rhodamine efflux status of the patients who were positive for the point mutation was examined. Of primary AML patients, 75% of those with the mutation were positive for rhodamine 123 efflux, compared to 50% of patients in our population who did not carry the mutation.

The clinical status of the AML patients who were positive for the promoter mutation was examined. The age at diagnosis was lower for primary AML patients carrying the mutation than it was for those without the mutation (32.8 years, compared to 42 years for those without mutation, p<0.001). Of the 8 patients with 1° AML who carried the point mutation, 5 relapsed (71%) at an average of 33.5 weeks and survived an average of 54.8 weeks. 2 are alive (one, who had acute promyelocytic leukemia, survives over 150 weeks; one, a child, >200 weeks). One, who could not be located, was lost to followup at 93 weeks. This data is similar to that of the patients at our institution who were rhodamine efflux-positive, regardless of whether or not they carried the mutation.

All of the CLL patients who carried the point mutation were rhodamine efflux positive. However, they were all male, and over 90% of male CLL patients in our cohort are rhodamine efflux-positive irrespective of whether or not they carry the mutation.

The clinical status of the patients with CLL was examined. Of 4 patients, 2 had somewhat early onset disease (ages 51 and 53).

One of these had progressive CLL over 3 years (to Stage IV), following which he developed metastatic Mertle Cell tumor and died. The other rapidly developed progressive disease (Stage IV within a year of diagnosis) and died of sepsis after chemotherapy.

5. DISCUSSION

Both the murine and human *MDR*1 genes have been studied to ellucidate their cis-acting regulatory mechanisms. The promoter was sequenced.[15] This promoter lacks a CAAT or TATA box, but has SP1 and AP1 binding sites. Recent studies[16] have shown that certain specific nucleotide sequences are important in controlling the level of *MDR*1 expression. Both positive and negative regulatory mechanisms seem to be operating. Binding sites for nuclear proteins have been identified by footprinting, methylation interference assays and gel retardation assays. One of the sites for nuclear protein binding which is conserved across species between rodent and human is an SP1 binding site.[17] Of note is that an initiator sequence was identified which is required for proper transcription initiation, at nt -6 to +11.[18]

We have identified a point mutation which is present at high frequency in human hematopoietic malignancies. It was present in AML and CLL at 3 times the frequency that it was found in normal DNA samples. While we do not yet have the data demonstrating what the precise effect of the mutation is on *MDR*1 gene expression, we hypothesize that it has a positive effect on *MDR*1 transcription. Since the mutation is located one base pair downstream from the initiator sequence, in the 5' untranslated region, we suggest that it may influence the rate of RNA transcription. Further studies are underway in our laboratory to investigate this possibility.

ACKNOWLEDGMENTS

This work was supported by the Israel Cancer Research Fund. We thank Dr. Dvora Filon for assistance with some of the experiments.

REFERENCES

1. Pastan I, Gottesman M: Multidrug resistance. Ann Rev Med 1991;42:277–286
2. Simon S, Schindler M: Cell biological mechanisms of multidrug resistance in tumors. Proc Natl Acad Sci USA 91:3497–3504, 1994
3. Jones P: DNA methylation errors and cancer. Cancer Research 1996;56:2463–2467
4. Stein U, Walther W, Wunderlich V: Point mutations in the mdr1 promoter of human osteosarcomas are associated with *in vitro* responsiveness to multidrug resistance relevant drugs. Euro J Cancer 1994;30A:1541–1545
5. Chaudhary P, Roninson I: Expression and activity of P-glycoprotein, a multidrug efflux pump, in human hematopoietic stem cells. Cell 1991;66:85–94
6. Broxterman H, Lankelman J, Pinedo H, Eekman C, Wahrer D, Ossenkoppele G, Schuurhuis G: Theoretical and practical considerations for the measurement of P-glycoprotein function in acute meyloid leukemia. Leukemia 1997;11:1110–1118
7. Webb M, Raphael C, Asbahr H, Erber W, Meyer B: The detection of rhodamine 123 drug efflux at low levels of drug resistance. Br J Haematol 1996;93:650–655
8. Young I: Proof without prejudice: use of Kolgomorov-Smirnov test for the analysis of histograms from flow systems and other sources. J. Histochem Cytochem 1977;25:935–941
9. Beck W, Grogan T, Williams C, Cordon-Cardo C, Parham D, Kuttesch J, Andreef M, Bates S, Berard C, Boyett J, Brophy N, Broxterman H, Chan H, Dalton W, Dietel M, Fojo A, Gascoyne R, Head D, Houghton P, Srivastava D, Lehnert M, Leith C, Paietta E, Pavelic Z, Rimsza L, Roninson I, Sikic B, Twentyman P, Warnke R, Weinstein R: Methods to detect P-glycoprotein-associated resistance in patients' tumors: consensus recommendations. Cancer Research 1996;56:3010–3020
10. Ivy S, Olshevski R, Taylor B, Patel K, Reaman G: Correlation of P-glycoprotein expression and function in childhood acute leukemia,. Blood 1996;88:309–318
11. Pall G, Spitaler M, Gofman J, Thaler J, Ludescher C: Multidrug resistance in leukemia: a comparison of different diagnostic methods. Leukemia 1997;11:1067–1072
12. Rund D, Cohen T, Filon D, Dowling CE, Warren TC, Barak I, Rachmilewitz EA, Kazazian HH, Oppenheim A: Evolution of a genetic disease in an ethnic isolate: beta-thalassemia in the Jews of Kurdistan. Proc Natl Acad Sci USA 1991;88:310–314
13. Hayashi K: PCR-SSCP: a simple and sensitive method for detection of mutations in the genomic DNA. PCR Method Applications 1991;1:34–38
14. Glavac D, Dean M: Optimization of the single-strand conformation polymorphism (SSCP) technique for detection of point mutations. Human Mutation 1993;2:404–414
15. Ueda K, Pastan I, Gottesman M: Isolation and sequence of the promoter region of the human multi-drug resistance (P-glycoprotein) gene. J Biol Chem 1987;262:17432–17436
16. Cornwell M, Smith D: SP1 activates the *MDR*1 promoter through one of two distinct G-rich regions that modulate promoter activity. J Biol Chem 1993;26:19505–19511
17. Cohen D, Yu L, Rzepka R, Horwitz S: Identification of two nuclear protein binding sites and their role in the regulation of the murine multidrug resistance *mdr*1a promoter. DNA and Cell Biology 1994;13:641 649
18. van Groenigen M, Valentijn L, Baas F: Identification of a functional initiator sequence in the human *MDR*1 promoter. Biochimica Biophysica Acta 1993;1172:138–146

10

REPRODUCIBLE FLOW CYTOMETRIC METHODOLOGY FOR MEASURING MULTIDRUG RESISTANCE IN LEUKAEMIC BLASTS

M. Pallis,[1] J. Turzanski,[1] S. Langabeer,[2] and N. H. Russell[1]

[1]Nottingham City Hospital and University of Nottingham
Nottingham, United Kingdom
[2]UCL Hospitals
London, United Kingdom

Keywords: MDR, daunorubicin, standardised flow cytometry, AML.

1. ABSTRACT

In order to bring MDR analysis into a clinical setting, reproducible assays with clear cut off points to define MDR positivity must be used. Sensitivity can also be increased by combining the results of more than one assay. We have used a combination of flow cytometric assays to define MDR positive and negative blasts in 47 AML patients entered into MRC trials. Our primary test is a standardised and reproducible assay for anthracycline accumulation in which we use carboxylate microspheres to bind the fluorescent drug daunorubicin (dnr). Cells and beads are incubated concurrently with dnr. Cellular dnr accumulation is quantified as a cell: bead fluorescence ratio. Confirmatory assays for MDR comprise the cyclosporin modulation assay for rhodamine 123 uptake and also measurement of lung resistance protein and multidrug resistance associated protein (with LRP-56 and MRPr1 respectively).

27/47 (57%) samples had both low dnr accumulation and at least one positive confirmatory test (a modulated functional assay and/or protein overexpression) and were categorised as "confirmed MDR". 15/47 patients (32%) were MDR negative in all 4 assays. 5/47 (11%) patients had unconfirmed low dnr accumulation. None of the patients in this cohort had high dnr accumulation alongside overexpressed LRP or MRP or functional P-glycoprotein. We believe that this approach to MDR analysis enhances the value of the highly reproducible functional assays. The use of a primary and confirmatory tests is also likely to improve specificity.

2. INTRODUCTION

2.1. Multidrug Resistance in AML

In AML, as in other malignancies, two membrane pumps—P-glycoprotein (P-gp) and multidrug-resistance associated protein (MRP), as well as the major vault protein LRP have been associated with multidrug resistance.[1-6] The expression of these three proteins is heterogeneous: blast populations may be negative for all three; P-gp is expressed in 19–75% of samples and is more prevalent in the elderly;[3,4,7] LRP is expressed in normal haemopoietic cells and is overexpressed in about 35% blasts.[5,8] MRP overexpression has not yet been adequately defined, although high message levels have been found to correspond to low daunorubicin accumulation.[6] More than one mechanism of multidrug resistance may be expressed in the same blast population.[8]

2.2. MDR Measurement in a Clinical Setting: The Need for Reliable Tests

Our growing understanding of the role of MDR in chemoresistance has given rise to at least two trends in the approach to induction chemotherapy in AML. The first is to inhibit P-glycoprotein-mediated MDR through the addition of resistance modulators such as cyclosporin A or PSC 833, which increase the cellular retention of MDR drugs.[9] The second approach is to use an induction regime such as FLAG, which avoids MDR drugs altogether.[10] Both approaches need multicentre trials to validate their use. Such trials also demand that the patients' initial MDR status should be known, so that the association between therapy and outcome for MDR positive patients can be compared and contrasted with their MDR negative counterparts.

2.3. Assays for MDR

The measurement of MDR proteins and message has proved to be a considerable technical challenge, and multicentre studies have demonstrated lack of agreement between laboratories, with nonetheless a consensus opinion that flow cytometry is a promising way forward.[11] As well as being useful for measuring proteins, flow cytometry can be used for measuring *functional* multidrug resistance. The functional assay system is based on the fact that certain fluorescent, lipophilic and cationic drugs (e.g. daunorubicin) or probes (e.g. rhodamine 123) accumulate inside drug-sensitive cells, but are expelled by MDR cells.[12,13] Broxterman has described a reproducible assay in which cells and fluorescent probes are incubated with and without the P-glycoprotein-specific resistance modifier SDZ PSC 833.[14] Results are expressed as the ratio of cell fluorescence intensity with modifier to cell fluorescence intensity without modifier. From a technical viewpoint, the advantage of using a fluorescence ratio in flow cytometric assays is that the ratio corrects for variables such as flow cytometer type and performance, batch variation in probes and cellular characteristics.

However, a thorough MDR investigation of the patient presenting with AML would need to incorporate an assay for MDR mechanisms which do not respond to modifiers such as that involving LRP. Recognising the need for a reproducible assay of probe accumulation which does not depend on resistance modifiers, we developed a procedure for standardising the measurement of total daunorubicin accumulation in leukaemic cells.[15] We used commercially available microbeads to bind daunorubicin and we constructed a cell-to-bead fluorescence ratio, a novel parameter for recording cellular daunorubicin accumulation reproducibly. We have used this standardised assay as our primary test for MDR, which was measured in leukaemic blasts from patients entered into MRC trials. We have also measured the cyclosporin and PSC 833 modulation ratios as well as LRP and MRP in these samples.

3. MATERIALS AND METHODS

3.1. Patients and Sampling

On initial diagnosis, blood or marrow from patients with AML entered into MRC AML 11 and AML 12 trials were sent to University College London for cryopreservation. Samples were selected for MDR analysis on the basis that they had not been in transit for more than 48 hrs before cryopreservation and that there were initially at least 5×10^7 blast cells in a vial. Selected samples were sent on dry ice to Nottingham City Hospital for analysis.

3.2. Sample Pre-Incubation

Thawed leukemic blasts were suspended in RPMI 1640 with 20% FCS and 1% each of L-glutamine and hepes buffer (both from Sigma) and rested at 37°C in a 5% CO_2 atmosphere for 90 minutes. We found that dead cells have a tendency to clump during this thawing/resting procedure and clumps were removed before proceeding further. Cell viability was measured after 90 minutes, and samples with < 85% viability were excluded from further analysis.

3.3. The Daunorubicin Cell: Bead Fluorescence Ratio

Bead ratio was determined as described.[15] Briefly, rested leukaemic blast cells were resuspended in culture medium (as above, except with 10% FCS) at 10^6/ml and incubated with 2×10^{-6} M daunorubicin at 37°C for 75 min and then pelleted at 4°C, rinsed in 3ml of cold PBS with 1% BSA and 0.1% sodium azide (PBSAA buffer) and resuspended in propidium iodide, 50 µg/ml in PBSAA. 5 µl Polysciences 10 µm carboxylate microspheres (Catalogue no. 18133, Park Scientific, Northampton, UK) suspended in 1 ml of PBSAA were incubated with the same concentration of daunorubicin alongside the cells, and were also rinsed and analysed alongside the cells. Daunorubicin was initially purchased from Sigma, and latterly the clinical preparation Cerubidin (Rhone Polenc Rorer) was substituted. A preliminary study using U937 cells confirmed that the cell: bead ratios were consistent between preparations.

3.4. Cyclosporin and PSC 833 Modulation of Rhodamine 123 Fluorescence

Rested leukaemic blast cells were resuspended at 10^6/ml and incubated with 200ng/ml rhodamine 123 (Sigma) with and without 2×10^{-6} PSC833 or 5µg/ml cyclosporin A at 37°C for 75 min and then pelleted at 4°C. Cells were then rinsed in 3ml of cold PBS with 1% BSA and 0.1% sodium azide (PBSAA buffer) and resuspended in propidium iodide, 50 µg/ml in PBSAA.

3.5. LRP and MRP

Unconjugated antibodies MRP-r1 and LRP56 (both from Monosan, Uden, Netherlands) were used according to manufacturers' instructions, with the minor modification that a blocking step in 20% normal rabbit serum was used prior to second layer labelling.

3.6. Flow Cytometry

For flow cytometric analysis a Becton Dickinson FACScan was used with a logarithmic amplifier and Cellquest software. Figure 1 shows Facsplots generated for one patient. In functional assays linearised geometric mean probe fluorescence of the cells incubated at 4^0C was subtracted from test fluorescence at 37^0C before calculating the ratios. Antibody binding was measured (i) using the Kolmogoroff Smirnoff D value calculated by the Cellquest program and (ii) for quantitative analysis, the channel number corresponding to

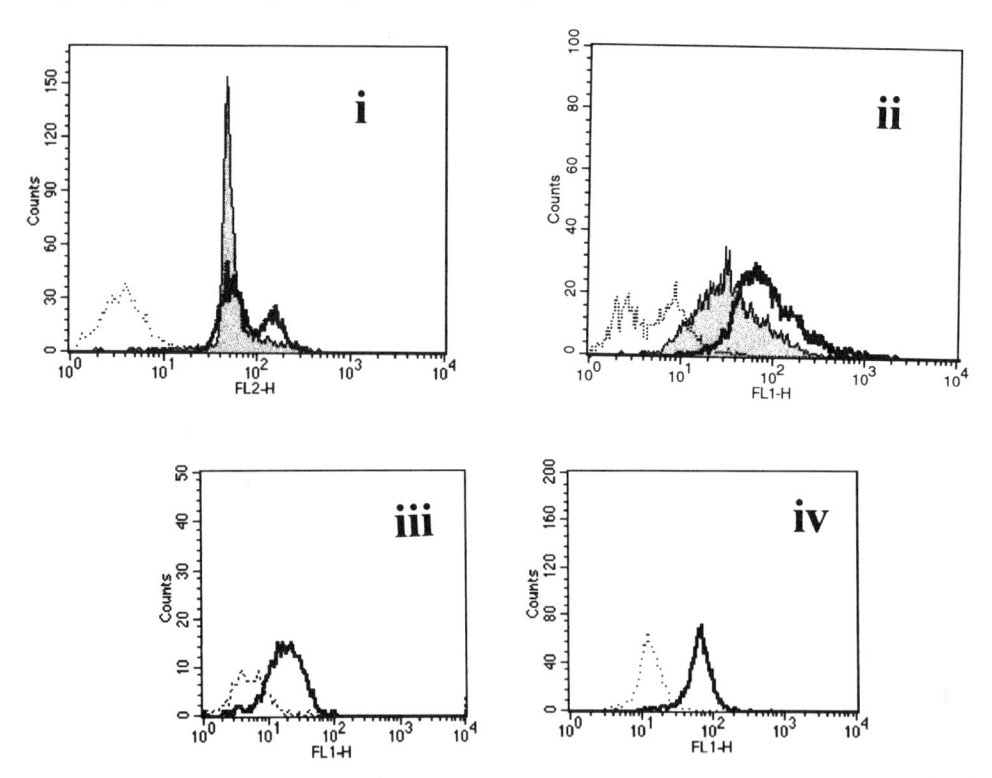

Figure 1. FACScan plots for MDR determinants in an AML patient who was MDR positive in all 4 tests. (i) Histogram showing cellular daunorubicin fluorescence after incubation at 37^0C (solid line), after incubation at 4^0C (dotted line) and bead fluorescence (shaded peak). The dnr cell:bead ratio was 1.4. An FL1/FL2 dotplot was initially constructed (not shown) to allow clear discrimination of propidium iodide negative events, which were gated for subsequent analysis. (ii) Histogram showing rhodamine 123 fluorescence with (solid line) or without (shaded peak) cyclosporin. (Propidium iodide positive events have been gated out.) Fluorescence after incubation at 4^0C is shown as a dotted line. The logarithmic scale belies the magnitude of the increase in fluorescence caused by cyclosporin, which in this example is 2.3-fold. (iii, iv) LRP and MRP expression (solid lines) respectively. Isotype control fluorescence is shown by dotted peaks. Overexpression is defined in section 4.3.

the 90th percentile fluorescence on test and control histograms was determined using Dako Flowmate software as a sensitive measure of increased fluorescence which may be occurring on a subset of cells.

4. RESULTS

4.1. The Daunorubicin Cell: Bead Fluorescence Ratio (dnr Ratio)

Preliminary studies, published elsewhere, confirmed that there is reproducible binding of daunorubicin to carboxylate microspheres under the standardised conditions described in Section 3.3, with a CV of 5.47% over a 3 month period.[15] Importantly, as shown in Figure 2, we noted that when our flow cytometer was serviced and recalibrated, the sensitivity increased, such that the apparent fluorescence after instrument service was 54% higher than before service. This illustrates the importance of standardising fluorescence in long-term studies, even on a single instrument. We previously demonstrated the reproducibility of the cell:bead ratio: repeat assays on 20 patients up to eight months after the first series of assays correlated with an R value of 0.86.[15]

The dnr ratios for the patient cohort in this study ranged between 0.59 and 3.56 (median 1.69). There was no clear cut off point between high and low fluorescence (Figure 3).

4.2. Measurement of P-Glycoprotein

P-glycoprotein was measured functionally using cyclosporin and PSC833 modulation assays. On examination of the scatterplots of these variables plotted against the dnr ratios, the cyclosporin modulation assay was selected as a confirmatory test for MDR on the grounds that samples with a high dnr ratio (>2.1:1) had modulation ratios very near unity. The cut off point, which was set at 1.06 to allow a little variation about the mean, was thus consistent with low dnr accumulation. 19/47 patients had an elevated rhodamine 123 accumulation in the presence of cyclosporin A. The ratio for PSC 833 modulated increases in rhodamine 123 uptake was greater than unity in 45/47 patients, and it was not

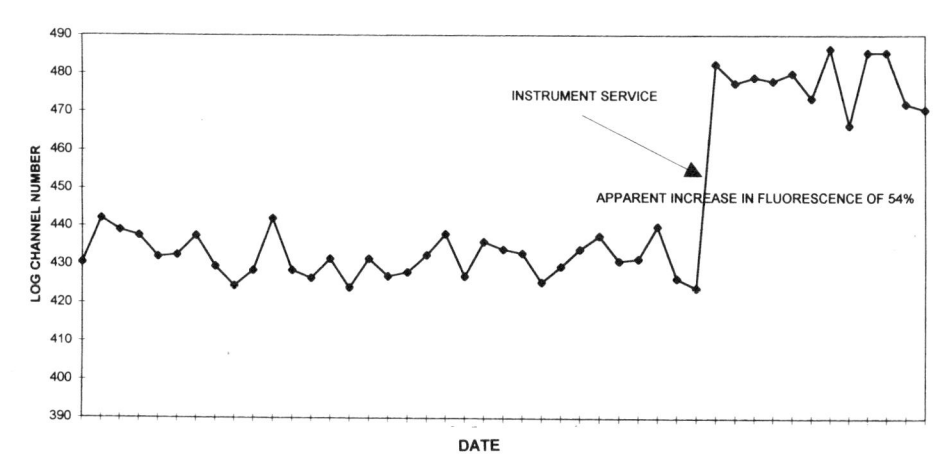

Figure 2. Serial measurements of bead: daunorubicin fluorescence before and after instrument calibration. This figure illustrates the fact that routine servicing of a flow cytometer may increase sensitivity, and thus the fluorescence will appear to increase.

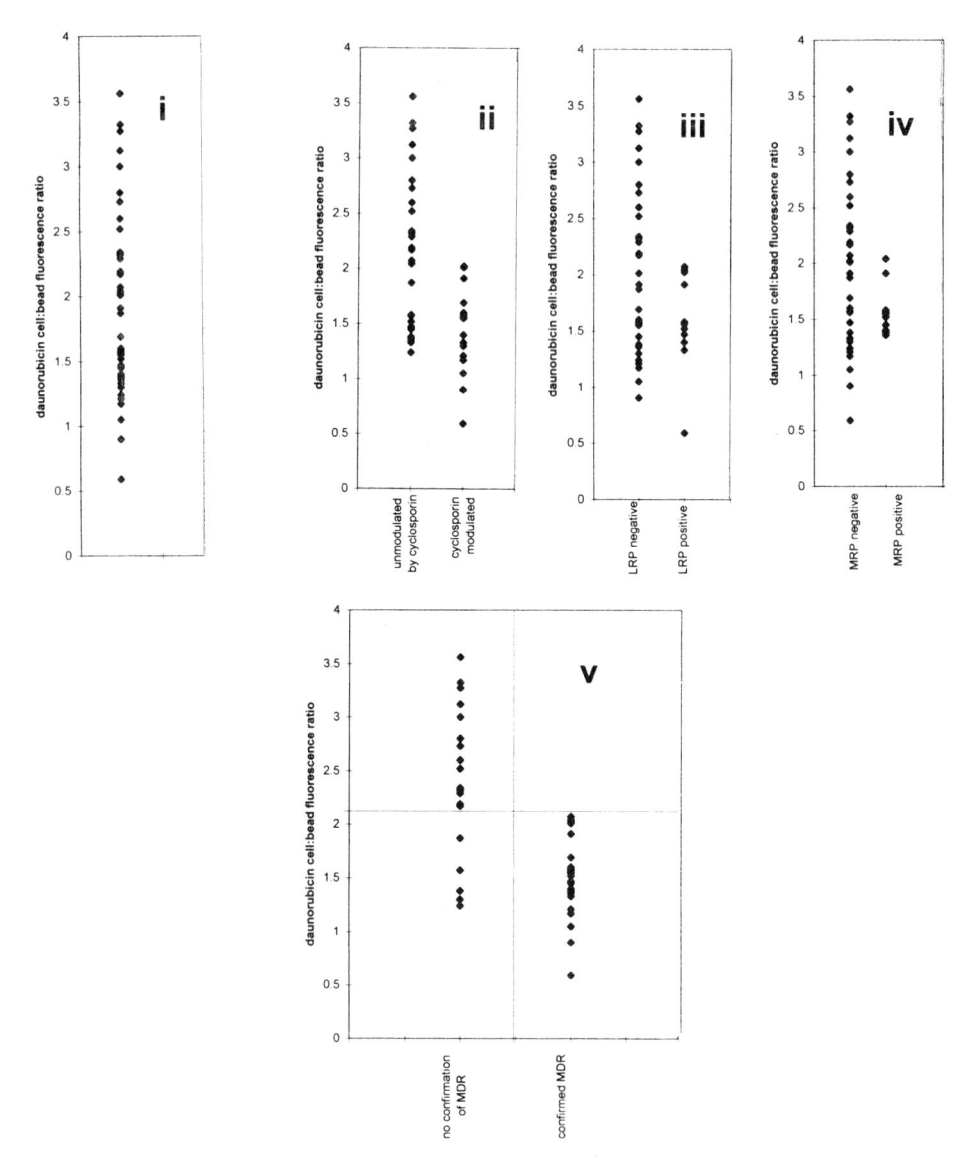

Figure 3. (i) dnr ratios in 47 AML patients, showing the lack of a clear cut-off point between high and low accumulators. (ii) dnr ratios sorted by positive (n=19) and negative (n=28) cyclosporin modulation of rhodamine 123. (iii) dnr ratios sorted by overexpressed (n=12) and normal (n=35) LRP. (iv) dnr ratios sorted by overexpressed (n=11) and normal (n=36) MRP. (v) dnr ratios sorted by positive (n=27) and negative (n=20) confirmatory tests.

clear from examining the scatterplot (Figure 4) where the cut off point between positive and negative modulation should be drawn.

4.3. Measurement of MRP and LRP

We compared two methods of quantifying protein expression. Firstly, we used the Kolmogoroff/Smirnoff statistic calculated by the Cellquest software to ascribe the quantitative D value to the difference between test and control distributions. Secondly we used

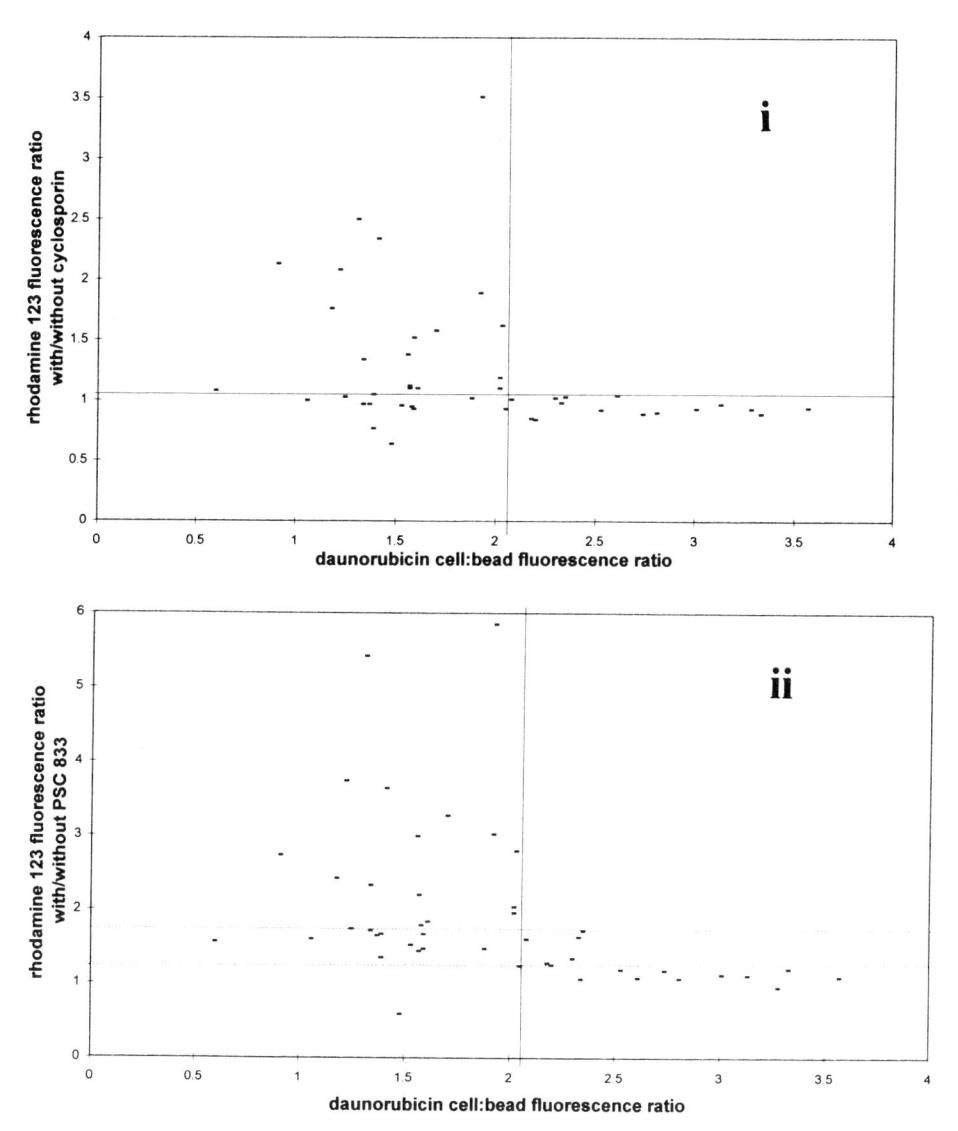

Figure 4. Scatterplots of the dnr ratio (x axis) plotted against (i) the cyclosporin modulation ratio, (ii) the PSC 833 modulation ratio. The intercepts draw attention to the ease of dichotomising cells which were either sensitive to cyclosporin and low accumulators of daunorubicin OR cyclosporin insensitive and high daunorubicin accumulators. PSC 833 values were not so amenable to dichotomisation.

Dako Flowmate software to calculate 90th centile fluorescence, in order to explore a measure which may be sensitive to changes occuring in a subset of cells. We divided the 90th centile test antibody fluorescence by control antibody fluorescence. As exemplified in Figure 5, the D value is sensitive to an increase in the fluorescence of the entire population, whereas 90th centile fluorescence is sensitive to an increase in subset fluorescence. The association of daunorubicin accumulation with LRP is dependent on the parameter used to measure LRP (Figure 5, iii and iv); the correlation coefficient between the two ways of measuring LRP was only 0.6.

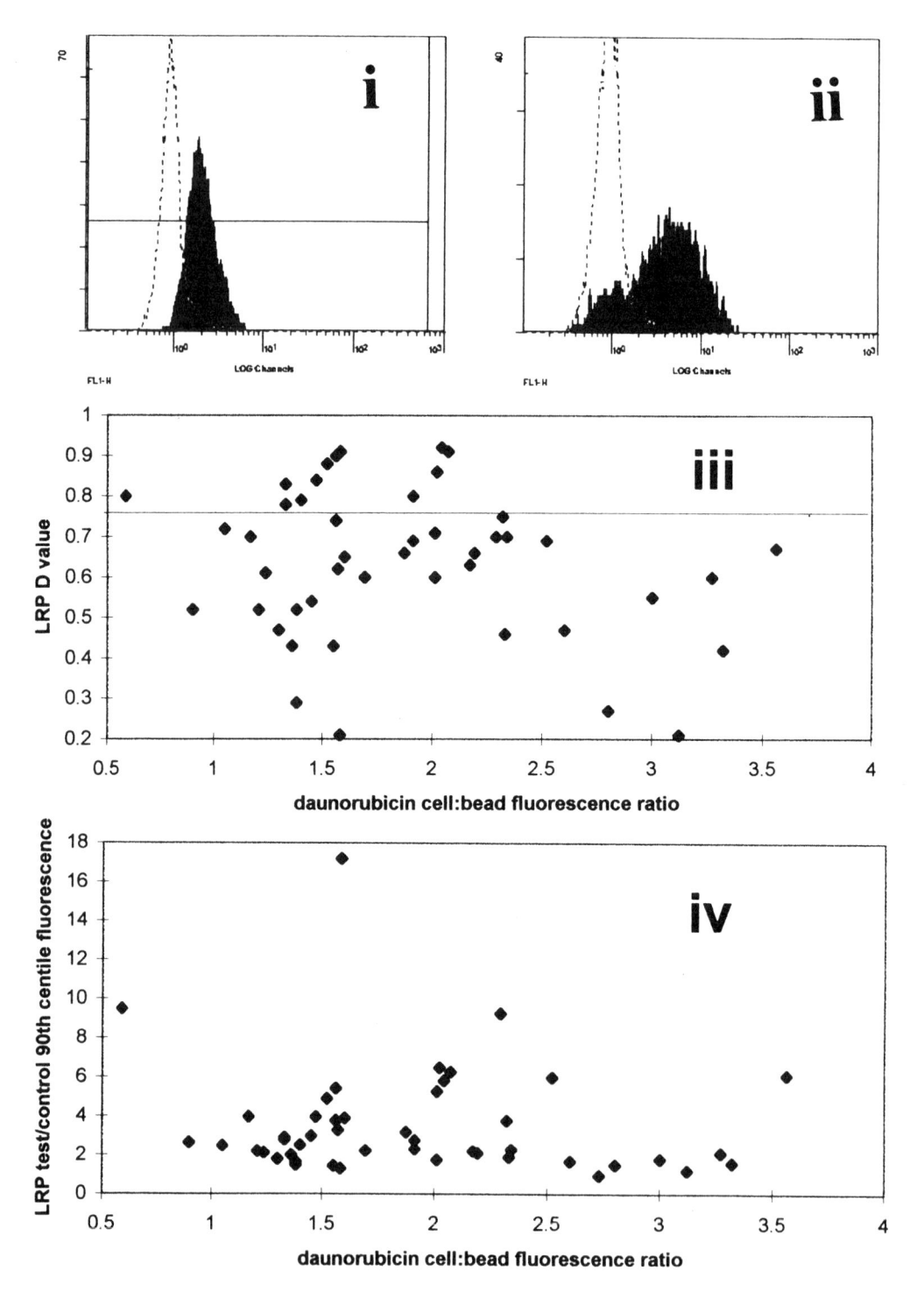

Figure 5. LRP expression (i) in a sample with relatively high, homogenous expression, (ii) in a sample with high expression on a subset. The D value for sample (i) was greater than for sample (ii) but the situation was reversed for the parameter test/blank 90th centile fluorescence. (iii) Scatterplot of the dnr ratio plotted against LRP D values, illustrating that none of the samples with D values greater than 0.75 had a high dnr ratio (iv) Scatterplot of the dnr ratio plotted against 90th centile values.

On the basis of the scatterplot illustrated in Figure 5 (iii), in which the patients with the highest D values had dnr ratios of < 2.1:1, the D value with a cut off point of 0.75 was chosen to represent LRP protein overexpression. LRP was overexpressed in 12 patients. MRP was more homogenously expressed than LRP, and thus the D values accorded well with 90th centile fluorescence (Figure 6). On the basis of the scatterplots, a D value of >0.85 was chosen to define MRP overexpression. Of the 11 samples overexpressing MRP, 2 also had cyclosporin modulation of rhodamine 123, 3 had elevated LRP and 3 showed evidence of all 3 mechanisms. A further 2 patients had elevated LRP with cyclosporin modulation but not MRP.

4.4. Distribution of Results According to Both the dnr Ratio and Confirmatory Tests

As illustrated in Figure 2, with a cut off point of 2.1 for the dnr ratio, 1.06 for the cyclosporin ratio, 0.75 for LRP overexpression and 0.85 for MRP overexpression, 27/47 samples had confirmed MDR. 15 samples had a high dnr ratio and no other evidence of MDR. 5 samples had a low dnr ratio with no positive confirmatory test.

5. DISCUSSION

Low cellular daunorubicin accumulation in AML is characteristic of P-gp, LRP and MRP positive blast cells.[6,8,14,16] Due to its fluorescent properties and clinical role, dnr is hypothetically an ideal substrate for the flow cytometric assay of MDR. However, before assays for dnr accumulation in leukaemia could merit clinical application, two issues needed to be resolved: firstly, was the range of values for daunorubicin accumulation sufficiently broad for clear discrimination between low and high accumulators and secondly could cellular dnr fluorescence be standardised? We have shown that there is no clear cut off point between high and low accumulation of daunorubicin, but we have also established that when other assays are used as confirmatory tests for MDR, the discrimination between confirmed MDR samples and MDR negative samples is clarified. Furthermore, using carboxylate beads which function as an internal standard for cellular daunorubicin fluorescence, we have established that fluorescence can be standardised, and moreover that it *needs* to be standardised, since changes in the sensitivity of fluorescence detection, such as occur when an instrument undergoes routine servicing, can cause major inconsistencies in measurement.

The large majority of samples in this study either had confirmed MDR or were MDR negative. No samples with high values for LRP, MRP or functional P-gp were high daunorubicin accumulators. There were however 5 samples which were low accumulators of dnr in the absence of a confirmatory test for MDR. There could be a physiological explanation for this, e.g., an undescribed MDR mechanism. However technical failure is also a possibility, and the most likely reason for this is poor sample quality. In multicentre clinical trials, the handling of samples before they reach the laboratory is difficult to control and the possiblity that low daunorubicin accumulation by these 5 samples was due to *in vitro* sublethal damage should not be excluded. In this context it makes sense for an approach such as ours in which more than one test is used to confirm MDR.

P-glycoprotein has been evaluated using functional rather than antibody data. The decision not to use antibody data was based partly on reports of good inter-centre reproducibility using a functional assay,[14] but not using antibody.[17] Also there is evidence that

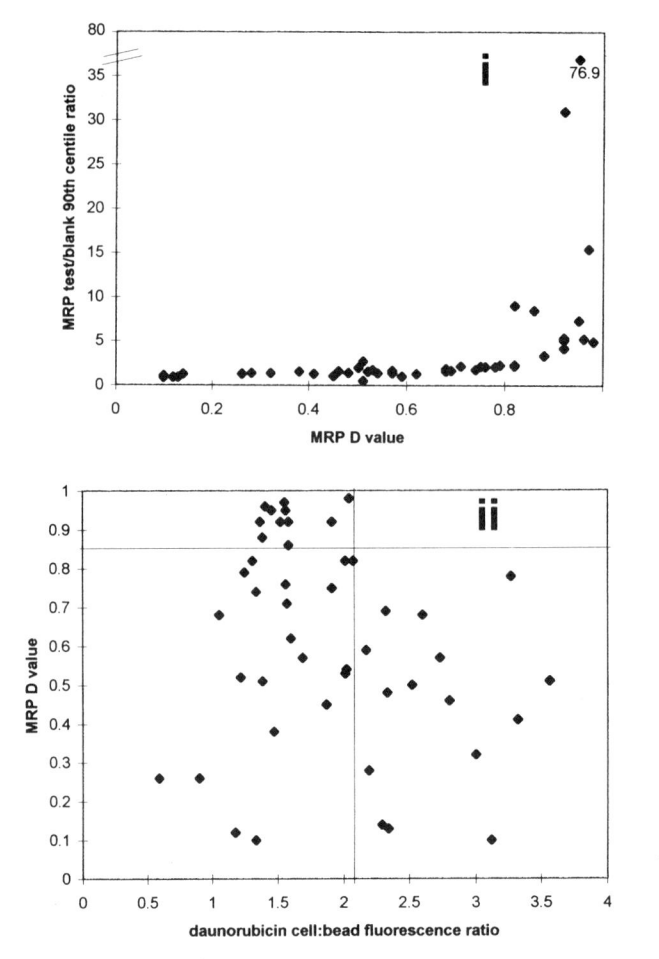

Figure 6. (i) Scatterplot of D values and 90th centile test/control fluorescence for MRP. (ii) Scatterplot of the dnr ratio plotted against MRP D values, illustrating that the samples with D values greater than 0.85 all had a low dnr ratio.

patients whose MDR drug uptake can be modulated by cyclosporin or PSC 833 in vitro are not always identifiable by their P-glycoprotein expression.[8,18,19]

It has been argued that a positive/negative dichotomy should be avoided in MDR analysis, for example the Memphis workshop concluded that dichotomisation "compromised the reliability of conclusions,"[11] and the study of P-glycoprotein by Perrot and colleagues showed wide discrepancies in flow cytometric data interpretation.[17] However, if the effect of MDR on treatment outcome is to be analysed, it is essential to provide a dichotomous analysis. An advantage to the approach described in this paper is that all the measurements were initially made on a continuous scale—based on mean fluorescence for the functional studies and D values for the proteins—and that cut off points were set only after examining daunorubicin accumulation in association with other variables.

In this study we noted that high protein levels can occur either as the entire blast population overexpresses a protein or as a subpopulation overexpresses a protein. Both parameters identified the same MRPhigh cases. In contrast, LRP is often expressed on a subset of blasts. Identification of the LRPhigh subset may be important for predicting overall survival of leukaemia patients, and failure to identify this subset may help account for the current discrepancies in the literature over the value of LRP in predicting outcome.

In conclusion, the flow cytometric measurement of daunorubicin accumulation is a clinically appropriate assay for MDR in AML and can be measured reproducibly using a standardised assay. The use of confirmatory assays for MDR allows results to be dichotomised and improves the specificity of the laboratory findings.

REFERENCES

1. Izquierdo MA, Scheffer GL, Flens MJ, Schroieijers AB, van der Valk P, Scheper RJ. Major vault protein LRP-mediated multidrug resistance. Eur J Cancer 1996;32A:979–984.
2. Loe DW, Deeley RG, Cole SPC. Biology of the multidrug resistance-associated protein, MRP. Eur J Cancer 1996;32A:945–957.
3. Marie J-P. P-glycoprotein in adult hematological malignancies. Hematology/Oncology Clinics of N America 1995;9:239–249.
4. Sonneveld P. Multidrug resistance in acute myeloid leukaemia. Balliere's Clinical Haematology 1996;9:185–203.
5. List AF, Spier CS, Grogan TM, Johnson C, Roe DJ, Greer JP, Wolff SN, Broxterman HJ, Scheffer GL, Scheper RJ, Dalton WS. Overexpression of the major vault transporter protein lung-resistance protein predicts treatment outcome in acute myeloid-leukemia. Blood 1996;87(6):2464–2469.
6. Xu D, Knaust E, Pisa P, Palucka K, Lundenberg J, Arestrom I, Peterson C, Gruber A. Levels of mdr1 and mrp mRNA in leukaemic cell populations from patients with acute myelocytic leukaemia are heterogenous and inversely correlated to cellular daunorubicin accumulation. Br J Haematol 1996;92:847–854.
7. Leith CP, Kopecky KJ, Godwin J, McConnell T, Slovak ML, Chen IM, Head DR, Appelbaum FR, Willman CL. Acute myeloid leukemia in the elderly: Assessment of multidrug resistance (MDR1) and cytogenetics distinguishes biologic subgroups with remarkably distinct responses to standard chemotherapy. A southwest oncology group study. Blood 1997;89(9):3323–3329.
8. Michieli M, Damiani D, Ermacora A, Raspadori D, Michelutti A, Grimaz S, Fanin R, Russo D, Lauria F, Masolini P, Baccarani M. P-glycoprotein (pgp) and lung resistance-related protein (LRP) expression and function in leukaemic blast cells. Br J Haematol 1997;96:356–365.
9. Sonneveld P. Reversal of multidrug-resistance in acute myeloid-leukemia and other hematological malignancies. European Journal Of Cancer 1996;32A(6):1062–1069.
10. Estey E, Thall PF, Andreeff M, Beran M, Kantarjian H, O'Brien S, Escudier S, Robertson LE, Koller CA, Kornblau S, Pierce S, Freireich EJ, Deisseroth A, Keating M. Use of Granulocyte Colony-Stimulating Factor Before, During and After Fludarabine Plus Cytarabine Induction Therapy of Newly Diagnosed Acute Myelogenous Leukemia or Myelodysplastic Syndromes: Comparison with Fludarabine plus Cytarabine Without Granulocyte Colony-Stimulating Factor. J Clin Oncol 1994;12:671–678.
11. Beck WT, Grogan TM, Willman CL, Cordoncardo C, Parham DM, Kuttesch JF, Andreeff M, Bates SE, Berard CW, Boyett JM, Brophy NA, Broxterman HJ, Chan HSL, Dalton WS, Dietel M, Fojo AT, Gascoyne RD, Head D, Houghton PJ, Srivastava DK, Lehnert M, Leith CP, Paietta E, Pavelic ZP, Rimsza L, Roninson IB, Sikic BI, Twentyman PR, Warnke R, Weinstein R. Methods to detect p-glycoprotein-associated multidrug-resistance in patients' tumors — consensus recommendations. Cancer Research 1996;56(13):3010–3020.
12. Sonneveld P, van den Engh GJ. Differences in uptake of adriamycin and daunomycin by normal BM cells and acute leukemia cells determined by flow cytometry. Leukemia Research 1981;5:251–257.
13. Broxterman HJ, Lankelma J, Pinedo HM. How to probe clinical tumor samples for p-glycoprotein and multidrug resistance-associated protein. European Journal Of Cancer 1996;32A(6):1024–1033.
14. Broxterman HJ, Sonneveld P, Feller N, Ossenkoppele G, Wahrer DCR, Eekman CA, Schoester M, Lankelma J, Pinedo HM, Lowenberg B, Schuurhuis GJ. Quality Control of multidrug resistance assays in adult acute leukaemia: correlation between assays for P-glycoprotein expression and activity. Blood 1996;87:4809–4816.
15. Pallis M, Russell NH. Functional multidrug resistance in acute myeloblastic leukaemia: a standardized flow cytometric assay for intracellular daunorubicin accumulation. British Journal Of Haematology 1998;100(1):194–197.
16. te Boekhorst PAW, Lowenberg B, Vankapel J, Nooter K, Sonneveld P. Multidrug-resistant cells with high proliferative capacity determine response to therapy in acute myeloid-leukemia. Leukemia 1995;9(6):1025–1031.

17. Perrot JY, Faussat AM, Zhou DC, Zittoun R, Robert J, Marie JP. Evaluation multicentrique du phenotype MDR dans les leucemies: analyse intermediare de l'experience francaise. Bulletin Du Cancer 1996;83(8):634–640.
18. Leith CP, Chen IM, Kopecky KJ, Appelbaum FR, Head DR, Godwin JE, Weick JK, Willman CL. Correlation of multidrug resistance (MDR-1) protein expression with functional dye/drug efflux in acute myeloid leukemia by multiparameter flow cytometry: identification of discordant MDR-/efflux+ and MDR1+/efflux- cases. Blood 1995;86:2329–2342.
19. Sincock PM, Ashman LK. Expression of c-kit and functional drug efflux are correlated in de novo acute myeloid leukaemia. Leukemia 1997;11:1850–1857.

11

NATURAL FLUORESCENCE IMAGING OF LEUKEMIC CELLS FOR STUDYING UPTAKE AND RETENTION OF ANTHRACYCLINES

M. Monici,[1,4] F. Fusi,[2,4] P. Mazzinghi,[1] A. Degli Innocenti o Nocentini,[3]
I. Landini,[3] I. Banchelli,[3] B. Bartolozzi,[3] V. Santini,[3] and P. A. Bernabei[3]

[1]Istituto di Elettronica Quantistica-CNR, Florence, Italy
[2]Dip. di Fisiopatologia Clinica, University of Florence, Italy
[3]Div. di Ematologia, Policlinico di Careggi, University of Florence, Italy
[4]Sezione A, INFM, Florence, Italy

INTRODUCTION

Cells exposed to light of appropriate wavelength show fluorescence emission in the UV-visible spectral range. This phenomenon, called natural fluorescence (NF), is related to cell compounds, i.e. proteins (1), nicotinic coenzymes (2), flavins (3), etc., engaged in structural and metabolic processes. Thus a correlation does exist between NF emission and morpho-functional state of cells.

Recently, we developed a NF-based microscopic method that allows to perform single-cell microspectrofluorometry and fluorescence imaging (4). It was applied to the study of normal peripheral blood cells and leukemic cell lines (5), identifying both the nature of the single cell observed and its functional state.

The multispectral fluorescence imaging technique (MFI) is efficient in detecting both cell natural fluorescence (NF), even if its intensity is very low, and emission of exogenous fluorochromes interacting with cells.

In this paper, the application of MFI to the study of leukemic cell-drug interaction is described. In particular, pharmacodynamics of anthracyclines is considered.

Multispectral imaging, combining spectral and spatial resolution, gives information on fluorochrome localization, intensity and range of emission.

Two aspects of cell-drug interaction can be analysed: 1) drug effect on cell morphology and metabolism, by monitoring NF changes; 2) drug intracellular localization, when the drug is a fluorescent molecule, and this is the case of many antiblastic agents.

The example is reported of a study carried out on cells treated with the antiblastic drug doxorubicin.

MATERIALS AND METHODS

The apparatus for image acquisition consists of an inverted epifluorescence microscope (Nikon Diaphot) equipped with an oil-immersion CF-UV fluor objective 100x (N.A. 1.30). A high pressure mercury lamp (Osram HBO 100W) or an Argon laser are used as excitation sources. A set of filters selects the excitation wavelength, including interference filters and an infrared cut-off filter (Schott KG1). The fluorescence is analysed by a digital CCD camera (Compuscope CCD 800, 768 × 512 pixels) with lumogen coating for improved UV-violet sensitivity. The CCD detector is cooled to -20°C by a thermoelectric Peltier cooler, integrated in the camera, to achieve a dark current < 0.1 el./pixel/sec. The images are directly digitised, with 14 bit dynamics, in the CCD controller, and transmitted to the storage computer on a digital interface. A motorised filter wheel, which can hold up to 8 different interference filters, allows multispectral acquisition under software control by the host PC.

The image can be alternatively routed to a multichannel spectral analyser (Hamamatsu, PMA 11) for the acquisition of the full spectral features of selected spots of the sample, with a resolution of 1.5 nm.

The images shown here were obtained using filters peaked at 450, 550, 600 and 658 nm, with 50 nm bandpass. Each 14 bit monochrome image was then linearly compressed to 8 bit, to match the dynamics of the output devices, and combined together in a single RGB image. This procedure does not produce photometrically corrected images, but improves the discrimination of cell structures by the use of a multispectral approach, simply combining three wavelength bands in a single RGB image. No other image enhancement procedures were used at this stage, even the background subtraction was found unnecessary.

HL60 leukemic cells were cultured in RPMI 1640 medium, with FCS 10% and splitted twice weekly.

Cells, adherent to polylysine coated slides were setted in a flow, thermostatic microchamber and treated with doxorubicin [10^{-6} M] for 30 and 60min.

Before single-cell analysis, cells were washed thrice and suspended in PBS with albumin 1% in order to avoid NF of the media.

RESULTS AND DISCUSSION

Imaging and spectral analysis allow to study, on single cell-basis, both the uptake and retention of the drug employed.

Figure 1a shows the excitation-emission spectra of doxorubicin dissolved in Ham's modified F12 medium. In Figure 1b the emission spectra recorded from treated and untreated HL60 cells can be observed. The comparison among the spectra reported in Figures 1a and 1b clearly demonstrates that the yellow-red component in treated cell fluorescence emission is due to the drug.

The interaction between doxorubicin and leukemic cells has been investigated utilizing MFI technique with two different excitation conditions: the 365 nm wavelength, particularly suitable to excite NF of cells (Figure 2a), and the 436 wavelength, quite near to the optimum for drug fluorescence excitation (Figure 2b).

Drug fluorescence is evident at 365 nm excitation also. This is due to its higher fluorescence quantum yield in comparison with that of natural fluorochromes. Moreover,

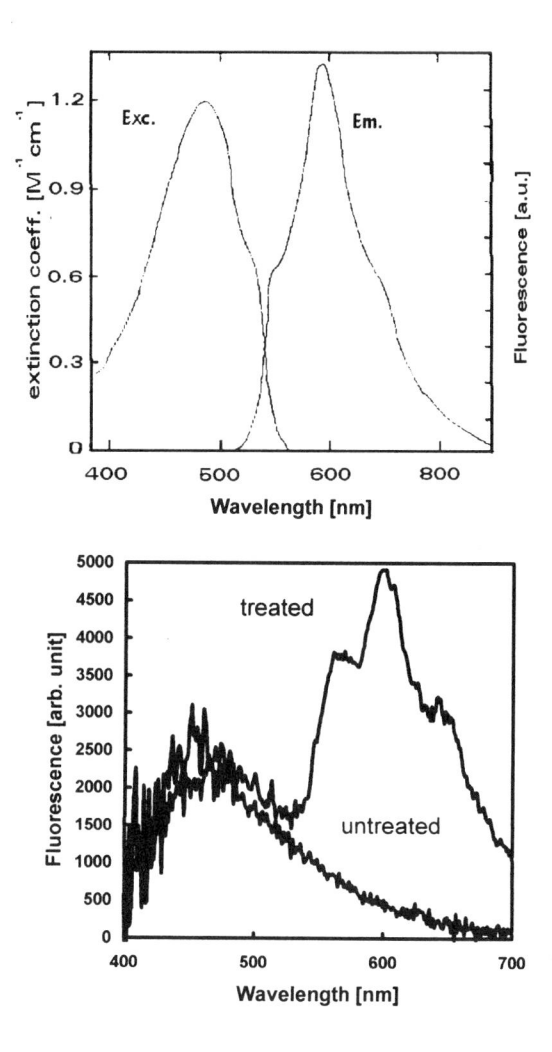

Figure 1. (Top) Excitation and emission spectra of doxorubicin. (Bottom) Emission spectra recorded from HL60 cells treated and untreated with doxorubicin.

changes in the excitation-emission spectra of doxorubicin are possible, owing to drug metabolisation and binding with cell structures.

In Figure 2a, the intense red fluorescence at nuclear level indicates a great concentration of the drug in this area. In the cytoplasm, the faint yellow-red fluorescence of the drug is almost completely hidden by the blue-green NF of cell components. This indicate that drug concentration in cytoplasm is low. NF of treated cells seems to be more intense and to have a different evolution time in comparison with that observed in untreated cells.

In Figure 2b, where cell NF is practically absent, drug intracellular distribution is even more evident. Doxorubicin is highly concentrated in the nucleus (red fluorescence). Drug concentration rapidly decreases in cytoplasm (yellow-green fluorescence).

CONCLUSIONS

The results show that cell-drug interaction produces deep changes in cell NF. The contribute of the different fluorophores (cellular compounds and drug) to the emission and

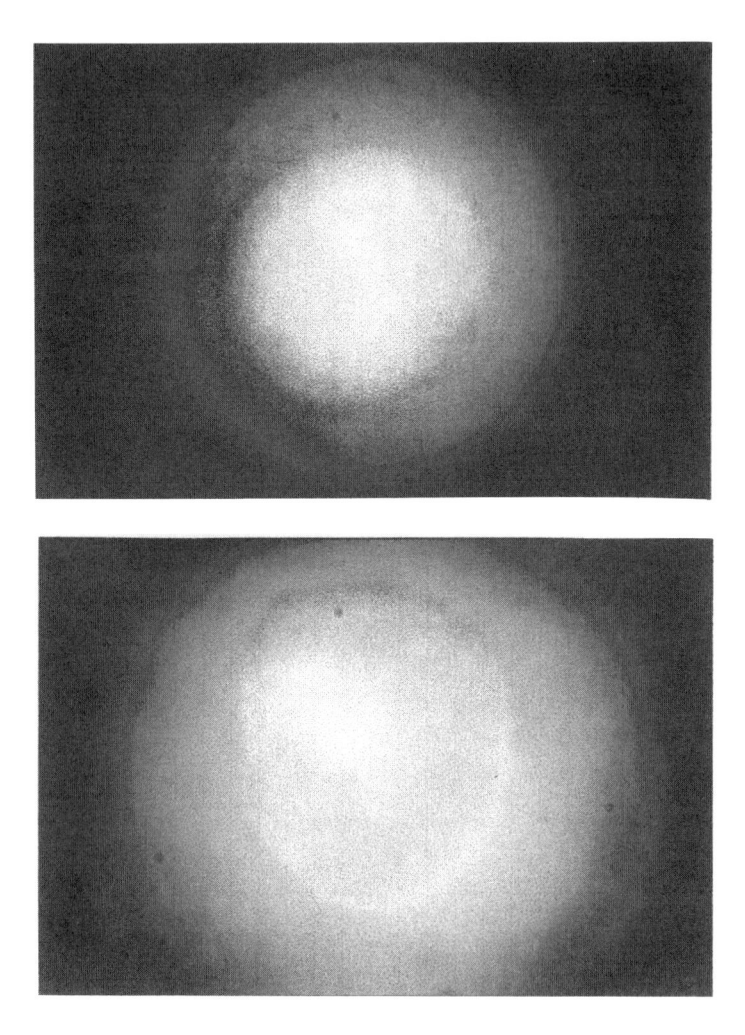

Figure 2A. Multispectral NF images of HL60 cells treated with doxorubicin for excitation wavelength at 365 nm: 30 min. (top) and 60 min. (bottom) of incubation time respectively.

Natural Fluorescence Imaging of Leukemic Cells 93

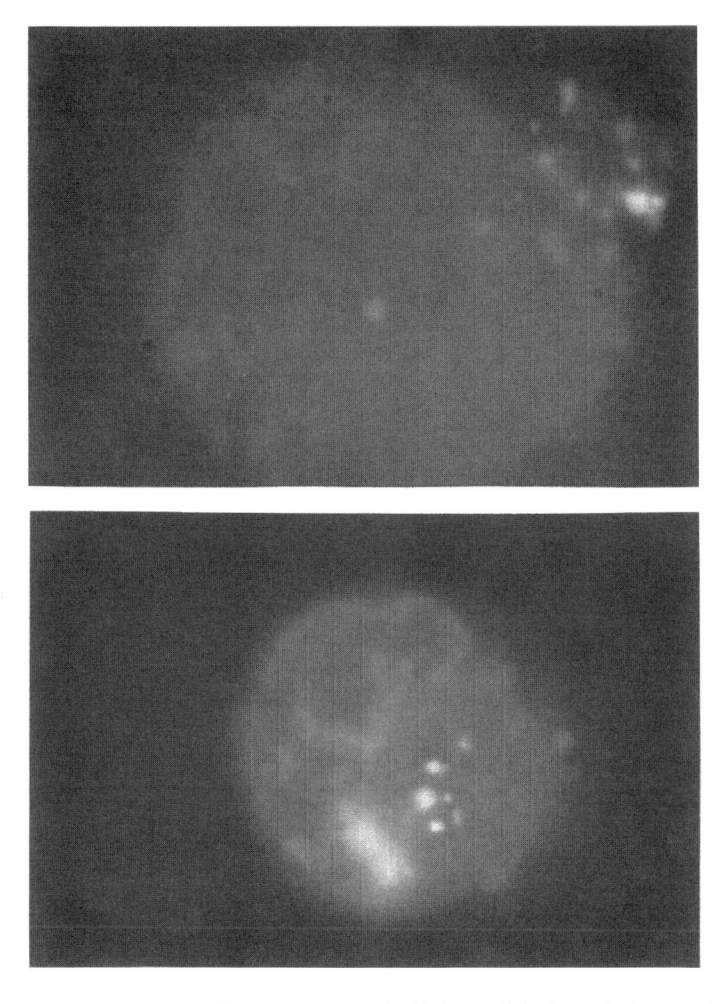

Figure 2B. Multispectral NF images of HL60 cells treated with doxorubicin for excitation wavelength at 436 nm: 30 min. (top) and 60 min. (bottom) of incubation time respectively.

their localisation can be revealed. Information about the functional state of cells can be deduced. In conclusion the MFI technique could be a promising tool to study cell-drug interaction in order to evaluate uptake, retention, localisation of the drug and its effect on cell metabolism.

REFERENCES

1. Weynrib I. and Steiner R.F., The luminescence of aromatic aminoacids, in Excited states of proteins and nucleic acids, R. F. Steiner and I. Weynrib eds., pp. 227–318, MacMillan Press, London and Basingstoke, UK, 1971.
2. Kohen E., Hirschberg J.C., Kohen C., Wouters A., Pearson A., Salmon J.M. and Thorell B., Multichannel microspectrofluorometry for topographic and spectral analysis of NAD(P)H fluorescence in single living cells. Biochim. Biophys. Acta, 396: 149–154, 19775.

3. Benson C., Meyer R. A., Zaruba M.E. and McKhann G. M., Cellular autofluorescence - Is it due to flavins?, J. Histochem. Cytochem., 27: 44–48, 1979.
4. Monici, G. Agati, P. Mazzinghi, R. Pratesi, F. Fusi, P. A. Bernabei, I. Landini, P. Rossi Ferrini. Image analysis of cell natural fluorescence. Diagnostic applications in haematology. In: In: Biomedical Systems and Technologies, SPIE Vol. 2928, N. I. Croitoru, M. Frenz, T. A. King, R. Pratesi, A. M. Verga Scheggi, S. Seeger, O. S. Wolfbeis Eds., 180–187, Vienna, 1996.
5. Monici, P. A. Bernabei, F. Fusi, P. Rossi Ferrini, I. Landini e P. Mazzinghi. Natural fluorescence imaging for the discrimination of normal peripheral blood cells and leukemic ones. British J. of Haematology, 93(supplement 2): 344, 1996.

ARTIFICIAL NEURAL NETWORKS AS VERSATILE TOOLS FOR PREDICTION OF MDR-MODULATORY ACTIVITY

C. Tmej,[1] P. Chiba,[2] K. -J. Schaper,[3] G. Ecker,[1] and W. Fleischhacker[1]

[1]Institute of Pharmaceutical Chemistry
[2]Institute of Medical Chemistry
University of Vienna
Waehringer Strasse 10, A-1090 Wien, Austria
[3]Medical and Pharmaceutical Chemistry
Borstel Research Center
Parkallee 1-40, D-23845 Borstel, Germany

Keywords: Modulators of Multidrug resistance, propafenone, structure-activity relationship, artificial neural networks, Free-Wilson analysis.

1. ABSTRACT

Following our ongoing studies on structure-activity relationship studies of propafenone-type modulators of multidrug resistance, we performed both a Free-Wilson analysis and a combined Hansch/Free-Wilson analysis on a set of 48 compounds using artificial neural networks (ANN). In comparison to classical multiple linear regression (MLR) analysis, the ANN showed equal or even slightly better predictive power in leave one out cross validation procedures and was remarkably superior when performing a leave 8 out cross validation. Additionally, it was possible to train a network using only 14 compounds and to properly predict the MDR-modulating activity of the remaining 34 compounds. In this case, the MLR analysis completely failed due to insufficient number of cases.

Attempts to extract informations on which input descriptors are important using a genetic input selection algorithm failed. Best results were obtained using those descriptors which showed highest statistical significance in MLR analyses.

Drug Resistance in Leukemia and Lymphoma III, edited by Kaspers *et al.*
Kluwer Academic / Plenum Publishers, New York, 1999.

2. INTRODUCTION

Development of multiple drug resistance (MDR) has been suspected as a major cause of treatment failure in cancer therapy. One of the most important and best understood resistance mechanisms is overexpression of membrane bound transport proteins like P-glycoprotein (PGP) or multidrug resistance related proteins (MRPs).[1] Several studies have reported evidence for a correlation of PGP expression with unfavourable response to chemotherapy in acute myeloid leukemia.[2] Additionally, clinical studies have shown that inhibition of the multidrug transporter P-glycoprotein may reverse resistance in leukemias, lymphomas and multiple myeloma.[3] Thus, in contrast to the treatment of solid tumors, the concept of coadministration of low molecular weight MDR modulators has proven beneficial effects in hematological malignancies.[4] Nevertheless, dose limiting side effects are common, which emphasizes efforts on the design of new, highly active and highly specific MDR modulators.

In our ongoing studies on structure-activity relationships of propafenone-type MDR modulators,[5] we extended our investigations on the use of artificial neural networks (ANN). Neural computing has shown major advantages in the analysis of data sets with complex non-linear relationships.[6] Thus, after a proper "learning procedure", ANNs are able to "recognize" existing patterns and relationships. Additionally, a trained network can be used to predict all kind of properties, as has recently been demonstrated for the prediction of molecular lipophilicity (logP values) based only on connection matrices of investigated molecules.[7] In this paper we investigated the training of an ANN to predict MDR modulating activity of propafenone-type modulators of multidrug resistance and compared the results with those obtained recently by multiple linear regression analysis.[8] As independent data input we used a combination of indicator variables based on a Free-Wilson type matrix and physicochemical parameters like lipophilicity values (logP) and molar refractivity (MR).

3. MATERIALS AND METHODS

3.1. Chemistry and Free-Wilson Data Matrix

Table 1 and Figure 1 show the chemical structure of compounds **1–48** used in the present study. All derivatives were synthesized in analogy to previously reported procedures.[8] Descriptors X_1-X_{19} describe the structural difference to propafenone (**1**), which was used as reference molecule. All compounds exhibit an aryloxypropanolamine backbone and differ in the substituents on the central aromatic ring system (R2, descriptors X_8-X_{19}) and on the nitrogen atom (R1, descriptors X_1-X_7). Numbers in Table 1 are compound numbers: analog **9** contains the X_1 substituent in R1 position (NH-n-Pr replaced by 1-piperidyl) as well as the X_8 substituent in R2 position (ortho-COC_2H_4Ph replaced by ortho-$CH(OH)C_2H_4Ph$).

3.2. Calculation of Physicochemical Properties

The logP values were calculated according to the method of Ghose and Crippen[9] using the software package MOLGEN.[10] As previously demonstrated on a series of propafenone analogs, the calculated values are in excellent agreement with those obtained experimentally using two different HPLC methods.[11] The molecules were generated using

Table 1. Chemical structure and X-descriptor characteristics of compounds 1–48

Descr.[a]	—	X_1	X_2	X_3	X_4	X_5	X_6	X_7
—	1[b]	2	3	4	5	6	7	8
X_8		9	10	11	12			
X_9		13	14	15	16			17
X_{10}			18				19	
X_{11}		20		21	22		23	24
X_{12}		25			26		27	
X_{13}			28				29	
X_{14}		30	31	32	33			
X_{15}	34	35				36		
X_{16}	37	38		39		40		
X_{17}		41	42		43			
X_{18}		44	45					
X_{19}		46	47		48			

[a] the descriptors X_1 to X_7 in the first row indicate substituents in R1 position of Figure 1, whereas the descriptors X_8 to X_{19} in the first column indicate substituents in R2 position;
[b] numbers in the table are compound numbers: **1** is the parent molecule propafenone with no structural modification; analog **9** contains the X_1 substituent in R1 position (NH-n-Pr replaced by 1-piperidyl) as well as the X_8 substituent in R2 position (*ortho*-COC$_2$H$_4$Ph replaced by *ortho*-CH(OH)C$_2$H$_4$Ph), etc.

the builder function and were energetically minimized with the optimization tool. Both conformationally independent logP and MR values were calculated and the difference to the parent compound propafenone (1) was used as Hansch-type descriptor. For the determination of the logP contribution of substituents on the nitrogen atom ($\Delta logP_N$) the difference of logP values of the corresponding phenylpropiophenone derivative and propafenone was calculated. The logP increment of the acyl substituent on the central aromatic moiety ($\Delta logP_{AC}$) was obtained *via* subtraction of the logP value of the corresponding phenyloxypropanolamine from that of propafenone. In this case, additionally the indicator variables M and P were used to indicate whether the acyl moiety is shifted from the ortho to the meta (M) or para position (P) to the propoxy group.

3.3. Cell Lines

The CCRF-CEM T lymphoblast cell line, as well as the resistant line were obtained as described previously.[12] Cells were kept in RPMI1640 medium supplemented with 10% fetal calf serum under standard culture conditions. The resistant CCRF vcr1000 cell line was kept in medium containing 1000 ng/mL vincristine. The selecting agent was washed out at least 1 week prior to the experiments. The cell line used in our studies was selected in the presence of increasing doses of vincristine without prior mutagenization. This cell line has been chosen because of distinct PGP-expression. In addition, no significant contribution of other factors to MDR was observed.

3.4. MDR-Modulating Activity

The daunomycin efflux assay was used to measure the inhibition of PGP-mediated transmembrane transport. Briefly, cells were pelleted, the supernatant was removed by aspi-

X_1	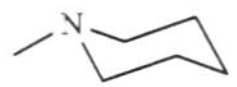
X_2	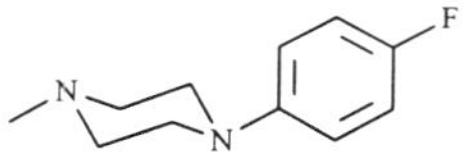
X_3	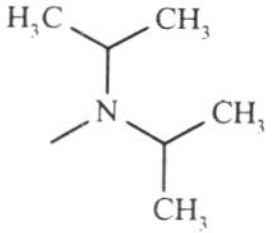
X_4	
X_5	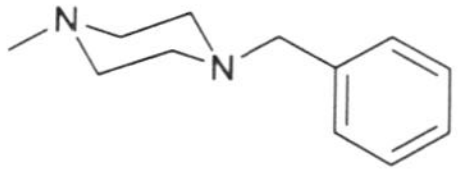
X_6	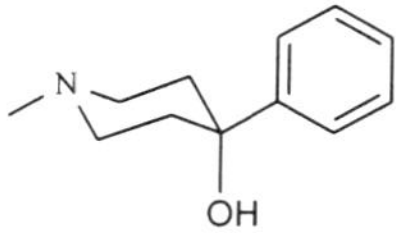
X_7	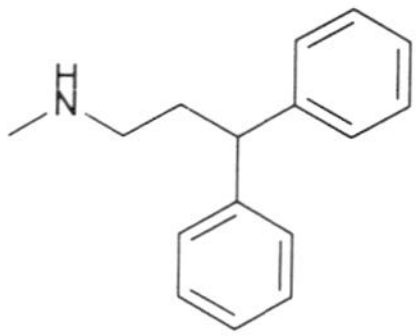

X_8	(ortho) $CH(OH)C_2H_4Ph$
X_9	(ortho) $CH(OCH_3)C_2H_4Ph$
X_{10}	(ortho) $COCH_3$
X_{11}	(ortho) COC_2H_4Naphth
X_{12}	(ortho) COC_2H_5
X_{13}	(ortho) COPh
X_{14}	(ortho → para) COC_2H_4Ph
X_{15}	5-OH
X_{16}	5-OCH_2Ph
X_{17}	(ortho → para) $COCH_3$
X_{18}	(ortho → meta) COC_2H_4Ph
X_{19}	(ortho → meta) $COCH_3$

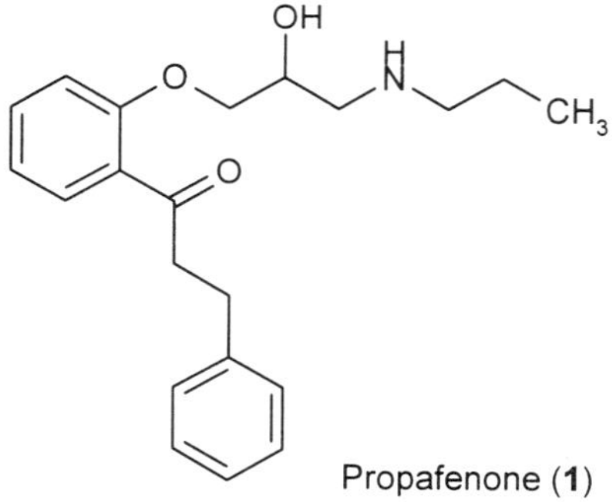

Propafenone (**1**)

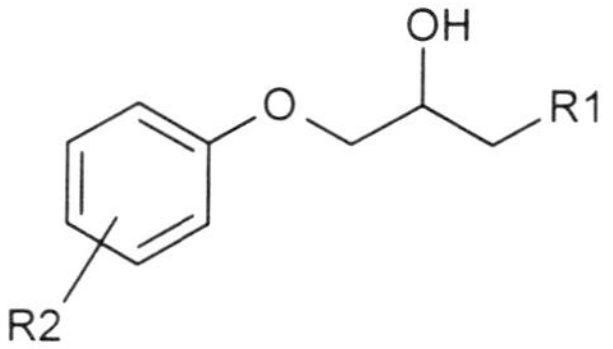

R1: X_1-X_7

R2: X_8-X_{19}

Figure 1. All X-descriptors state the difference to the lead compound propafenone; X_{17}–X_{19} indicate a shift of the acyl group to the para or meta position, whereas X_{15} and X_{16} indicate the presence of OH or OCH_2Ph in para position to the propoxy group (i.e. no change of ortho-COC_2H_4Ph).

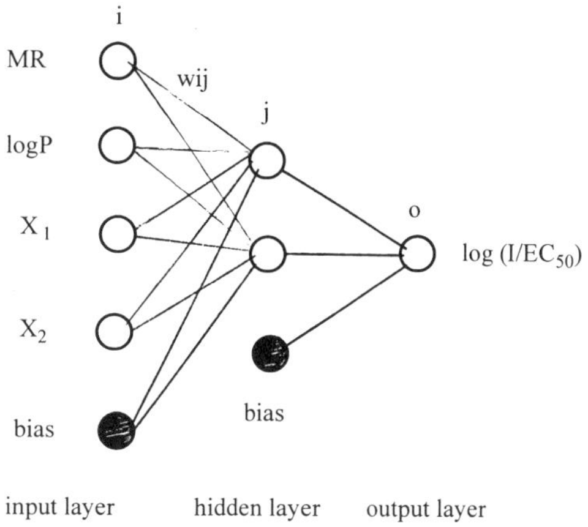

Figure 2. The variables x_i, which are used as data input into the input neurons are combined with adjustable weights $w_{i,j}$ and summed up in the units of the hidden layer. This value is further transformed in the hidden layer neuron via a sigmoidal function. The result is "sent" to the output neuron (combined with the corresponding weight).

ration and the cells were resuspended at a density of 1 × 10⁶/mL in RPMI1640 medium containing daunomycin (Sigma Chem. Comp., St. Louis, MO) at a final concentration of 3.0 µM. Cell suspensions were incubated at 37°C for 30 min. Tubes were chilled on ice and pelleted at 500 g in an Eppendorf 5403 centrifuge (Eppendorf, Germany). Supernatants were removed and the cell pellet was resuspended in medium which was prewarmed to 37°C and contained either no modulator or chemosensitizer at various concentrations dependent on solubility and expected potency of the modifier. Eight concentrations (serial dilution 1:2.5) were tested for each modulator. After 1, 2, 3 and 4 min, aliquots of the incubation mixture were transferred to tubes containing an equal volume of ice cold stop solution (RPMI1640 medium containing verapamil at a final concentration of 10 µg/mL). Zero time-points were done by immediately pipetting daunomycin preloaded cells into ice cold stop solution. Non PGP expressing parental CCRF-CEM cells were used as controls for simple plasma membrane diffusion, whereby initial daunomycin fluorescence levels were adjusted to be equal to initial levels observed in resistant cells. Samples drawn at the respective time points were kept in an ice water bath and measured within one hour on a Becton Dickinson FACSCALIBUR flow cytometer (Becton Dickinson, Vienna, Austria). Viable cells were gated on the basis of forward and side scatter. The excitation wavelength was 488 nm and the emission was measured in the FL3 channel (650–780 nm). 5000 gated events were accumulated for the determination of mean fluorescence values. Time points were fitted by an exponential curve and the first order rate constant (V_{max}/K_m) was determined as the slope of the curve at the zero time point. A correction for simple diffusion was achieved by subtracting the efflux rates observed in the parental line. EC_{50} values of modifiers were calculated from dose response curves of (V_{max}/K_m) vs. modifier concentration. The EC_{50} values of the compounds ranged from 0.07 µM for **7** to 302.05 µM for **43**.

3.5. Artificial Neural Networks

The powerful TRAJAN software package[13] was used in our study. Generally, a feed-forward, fully connected three layer perceptron was used. The basic configuration of this most commonly used type of artificial neural network is shown in Figure 2.

Starting with a set of n input neurons in the first layer the components x_i are combined with adjustable weights $w_{i,j}$ and summed up (linear Post Synaptic Potential function) in the units of the hidden layer. This multidimensional vector is further "squashed" into the output neuron via a sigmoidal function. The backpropagation algorithm as the best known training algorithm for supervised ANN learning[14] repeats this process thus adjusting the weights after each epoch until the overall Root Mean Square (RMS) error between actual and target output is minimized. Generally, we started the training procedure with randomly selected weights and used an RMS error lower than 0.01 as stopping condition for network training. The momentum factor, which causes the algorithm to pick up speed, was set to 0.6. The learning rate, which determines the size of changes applied to the weights after each epoch, was set to 0.3.

3.5.1. Network Design. One of the most common problems in neural computing is a so called overtraining of the network. This often occurs, when the ratio of number of cases to number of adjustable weights (often refered to as ρ) is smaller than 1.[15] In this case, the network simply "memorizes" the data, which results on the one hand in a perfect description of the data set, but on the other hand in a very poor predictive ability. With a unique Automatic Network Design Algorithm Trajan offers the possibility to favour small networks, thus preventing overlearning. Using this algorithm, a large number of different networks has been analyzed by checking the performance against a verification pattern. The automatic network design usually was run overnight, and the Unit Penalty was set to 0.001, thus favouring smaller networks. The number of iterations was set to 100.

3.5.2. Genetic Input Selection. One of the biggest disadvantages of the use of neural computing in medicinal chemistry is the fact, that it is nearly impossible to extract information on how learning and prediction works.[16] Thus, a well trained network is able to predict the pharmacological activity of the compounds, but it is very difficult to get information on how input variables influence activity. Nevertheless, exactly this information is needed to proceed in a drug development process. One possibility to overcome this problem is to use a genetic input selection (GIS) algorithm. Genetic algorithms are a powerful tool to find minima on complex hypersurfaces in a very short time.[17] Thus, we used the GIS algorithm incorporated in the TRAJAN software package to reduce the number of input neurons to the absolutely necessary minimum to achieve proper predictions. This procedure on the one hand leads to a further improvement of ρ and on the other hand should indicate, which input variables are necessary for prediction of MDR-modulating activity. Generally, the Unit Penalty was set to 0.001. The Smoothing Factor was set to 0.3, the Mutation Rate to 1 and the Cross Over rate to 0.3.

3.6. Statistical Validation of Predictive Ability

As mentioned above, the most important feature for the quality of a created ANN is the predictive ability. Besides a high correlation coefficient (r) for a plot of fited vs. observed activities, a high cross validated r^2 (now often denoted as predictive power Q^2) is the best proof for high predictive ability.[18] In a leave n out cross validation procedure, a set of n compounds is removed from the data set, the network is trained with the remaining (a-n) compounds and the activity of the discarded test compounds is predicted on basis of the relationship found. This procedure is repeated a/n times and a correlation is derived between the predicted and the observed outputs. Q^2 is calculated as $Q^2 = (SD-PRESS)/SD$; $SD = \Sigma(i_{actual} - Mean)^2$, and $PRESS = \Sigma(i_{predicted} - i_{actual})^2$. In this study, we used both leave 1 out (L1O) and leave 8 out (L8O) cross validation to estimate the predictive ability of our networks and to compare the results with those previously obtained in multiple linear regression analysis.[8] Additionally, we selected 14 compounds (structurally as diverse as possible) as training set and used the remaining 34 derivatives as test set.

4. RESULTS AND DISCUSSION

4.1. Non-Linear Free-Wilson Analysis

In the present study the Fujita-Ban modification[19] of the Free-Wilson method was used. Indicator variables X_1-X_{19} were used as input variables and the $\log(1/EC_{50})$ values were compared with results obtained at the output neuron. Using the automatic network designer for evaluation of the optimal network architecture, a 19:5:1 configuration was suggested. Systematic investigations using a leave one out crossvalidation procedure confirmed this architecture as giving the best predictive ability (Table 2, Figure 3). Although the predictive power Q^2 is lower than that obtained in multiple linear regression (MLR) analysis ($Q^2_{L1O} = 0.66$), the value of $Q^2_{L1O} = 0.56$ shows that it is possible to train an ANN for prediction of MDR-modulatory activity of compounds using only indicator variables for description of the chemical structure of the compounds.

To further test the reliability of this approach, we performed a leave 8 out cross validation. Thus, the set of 48 compounds was divided into 6 groups, each containing 8 compounds. The network was trained with 40 compounds and the activity of the remaining 8 derivatives was predicted. This procedure was repeated 6 times. The plot of predicted vs. observed $\log(1/EC_{50})$ values for all 48 compounds showed an r value of 0.93 and Q^2_{L8O} was 0.79 (Figure 4).

In contrast, MLR analysis using the same procedure showed remarkably lower predictivity ($Q^2_{L8O} = 0.43$). Furthermore, using only 14 compounds for training of the network, the remaining 34 derivatives were predicted with a r of 0.82 ($Q^2 = 0.32$). In this case, the MLR procedure completely failed due to an insufficient number of cases (14 cases vs. 20 adjustable coefficients!). This clearly shows the advantage of ANNs to extract relevant information from a small data set and to use this information for prediction.

Genetic input selection did not improve predictivity ($Q^2_{L1O} = 0.57$), but selected 12 out of 19 structural features as being important for PGP inhibitory activity of propafenone type modulators (Table 3, Row 1). Interestingly, the 12 descriptors selected are completely different to those obtained in the MLR-analysis as contributing statistically significant to MDR-modulating activity (10 out of 19, Table 3, Row 2). Thus, using this set of descriptors as input, we obtained a network with remarkably higher Q^2_{L1O} value (0.64). This indicates, that in our case the genetic algorithm did not lead to a proper minimum. Furthermore, most

Table 2. Predictive ability of various networks with different architecture

	19:1:1[a]	19:2:1	19:3:1	19:4:1	19:5:1	19:6:1
Training[b]						
r	0.925	0.999	0.996	0.997	0.997	0.999
r^2	0.856	0.998	0.992	0.993	0.993	0.998
s	0.335	0.040	0.081	0.072	0.072	0.042
Prediction[c]						
r	0.710	0.690	0.665	0.730	0.825	0.775
r^2	0.505	0.476	0.443	0.530	0.681	0.601
s	0.621	0.640	0.660	0.605	0.499	0.557
Q^2	0.330	0.350	0.090	0.290	0.563	0.370

[a] Network architecture: 19 input neurons, 1 hidden layer neuron, 1 output neuron.
[b] Statistics of plot calculated vs. observed $\log(1/EC_{50})$ values.
[c] Statistics of plot predicted vs. observed $\log(1/EC_{50})$ values, obtained by a leave 1 out cross validation.

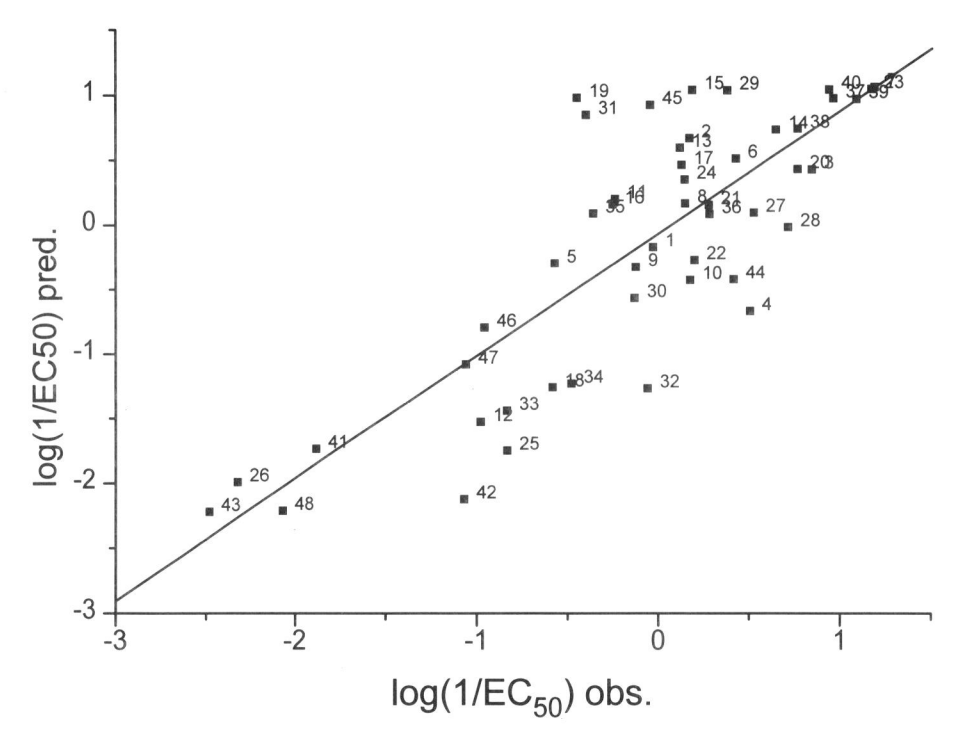

Figure 3. Plot of predicted vs. observed MDR modulating activity (expressed as log(1/EC$_{50}$) values) of compounds **1–48**. The predicted values were obtained by a leave one out cross validation using an ANN (19:5:1) and descriptors X$_1$-X$_{19}$ as input variables; r = 0.825, s = 0.499, Q^2 = 0.563.

of the descriptors indeed seem to additively contribute to MDR modulating activity. With the exception of X$_4$ and X$_6$, all descriptors describe variations on the central aromatic ring, which further strengthens the importance of the ortho-phenone moiety.

4.2. Combined Hansch/Free-Wilson Analysis

We previously could demonstrate, that high lipophilicity of the compounds is a major prerequisite for high MDR-modulating activity.[20] Additionally, hydrogen bond donor strength[21] and charge of several substructures[22] was also shown to be of some importance. Thus, we extended the Free-Wilson data set and added several physicochemical parameters like overall logP, partial lipophilicity of the substituent on the central aromatic ring

Table 3. Descriptors classified as important by a genetic input selection algorithm

	Descriptors
Row 1	X$_4$, X$_6$, X$_8$, X$_{10}$, X$_{12}$, X$_{14}$-X$_{17}$, X$_{19}$
Row 2	X$_2$-X$_7$, X$_9$, X$_{11}$-X$_{13}$, X$_{16}$, X$_{17}$
Row 3	logP, ΔlogP$_{AC}$, ΔlogP$_N$, MR, P, X$_3$-X$_6$, X$_9$, X$_{11}$, X$_{13}$, X$_{16}$, X$_{17}$
Row 4	logP, ΔlogP$_{AC}$, ΔlogP$_N$, MR, M, P, X$_6$-X$_9$, X$_{15}$, X$_{16}$
Row 5	MR, P, X$_2$, X$_4$, X$_5$, X$_7$, X$_8$

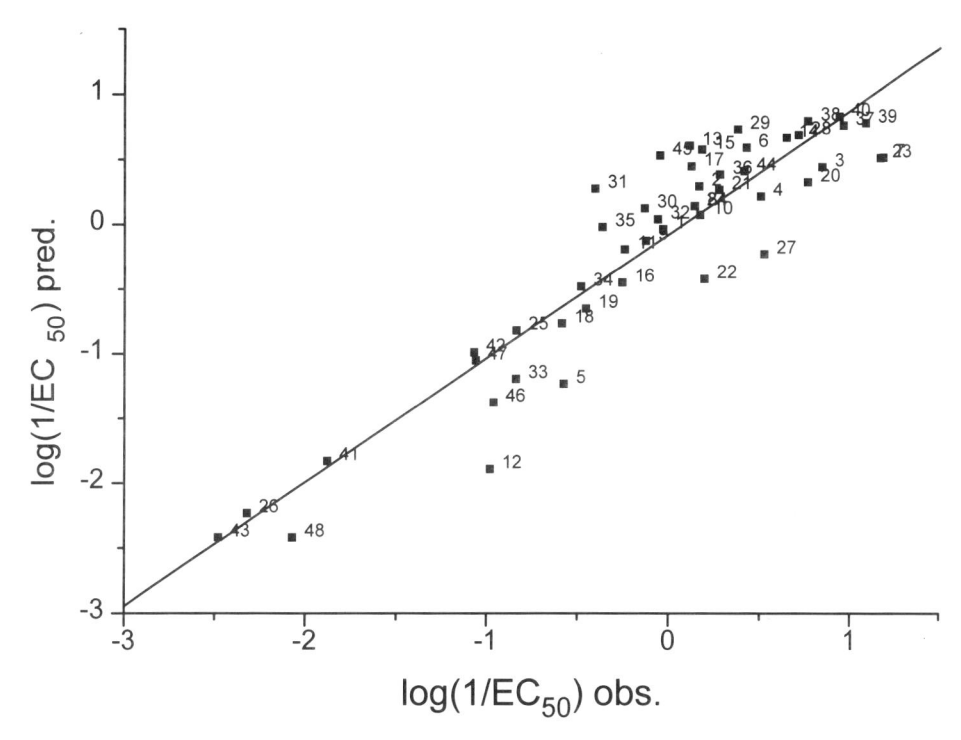

Figure 4. Plot of predicted vs. observed MDR modulating activity (expressed as log(1/EC$_{50}$) values) of compounds **1–48**. The predicted values were obtained by a leave 8 out cross validation using an ANN (19:5:1) and descriptors X$_1$-X$_{19}$ as input variables; r = 0.930, s = 0.350, Q^2 = 0.794.

(ΔlogP$_{AC}$) and on the Nitrogen atom (ΔlogP$_N$) and molar refractivity (MR), which accounts for both steric and electronic interaction forces. Additionally, we included the indicator variables M and P, which denote the information whether the acyl moiety on the central aromatic ring is shifted from ortho-position (to the ether oxygen) to meta- or para-position.

Using all 25 descriptors as input variables, a 25:5:1 network was trained and a leave one out cross validation was performed. Taking into account the unfavourable low ρ value (0.37), the predictive power Q^2 was remarkably high (Q$^2_{L1O}$ = 0.71). In this case, the genetic input selection led to a dramatic loss of predictivity, with 14 descriptors remaining in the input matrix (Table 3, Row 3; Q$^2_{L1O}$ = 0.41). To test, whether predictiveness increases with increasing ρ, we reduced the input matrix according to the following assumptions:

With the exception of X$_6$ and X$_7$, all variations on the nitrogen atom mainly contribute to activity via their lipophilicity value, as could be shown previously. Thus, X$_1$ - X$_5$ were replaced by ΔlogP$_N$.

Furthermore, descriptors X$_{10}$ - X$_{14}$ and X$_{17}$ - X$_{19}$ were replaced by their corresponding ΔlogP$_{AC}$ values and the information of the substitution pattern on the central aromatic ring (M, P).

This reduced the number of input neurons to 12 (Table 3, Row 4) and increased ρ to 3.8 due to a 12:1:1 architecture of the network. Indeed, predictivity was enhanced to Q$^2_{L1O}$ = 0.77.

In analogy to the Free-Wilson approach, we further reduced the X-descriptors according to the results of the MLR analysis (Table 3, Row 5). In this case, only 7 input

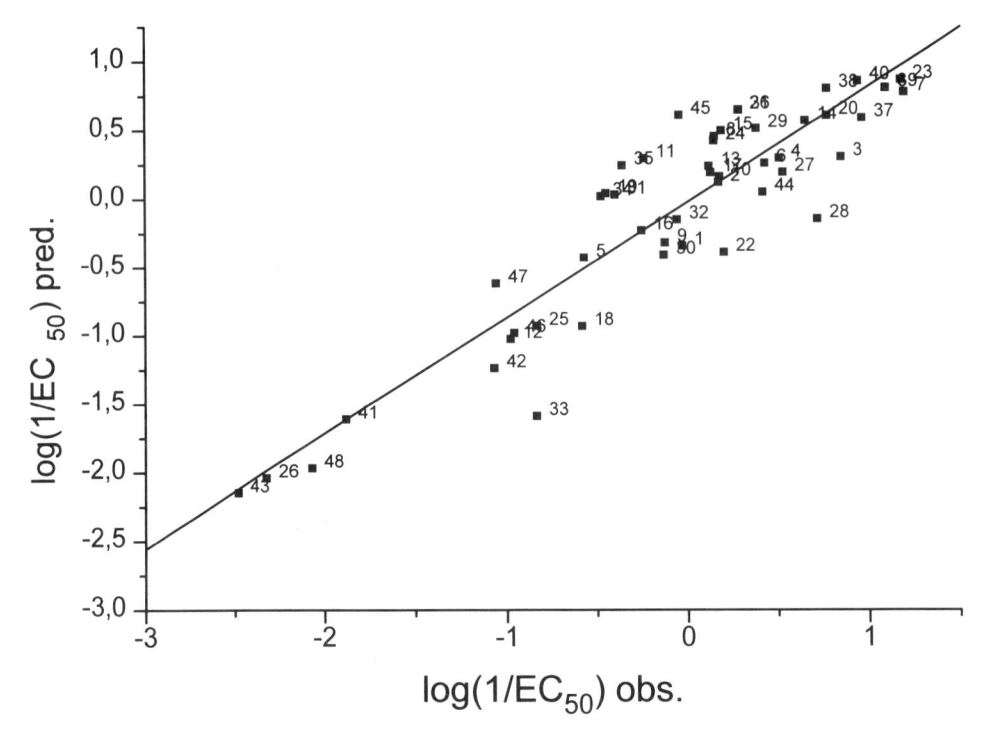

Figure 5. Plot of predicted vs. observed MDR modulating activity (expressed as log(1/EC$_{50}$) values) of compounds **1–48**. The predicted values were obtained by a leave 1 out cross validation using an ANN (7:4:1) and descriptors MR, P, X$_2$, X$_4$, X$_5$, X$_7$ and X$_8$ as input variables; r = 0.920, s = 0.320, Q^2 = 0.850.

variables were used to describe all compounds. The automatic network design showed a 7:4:1 architecture as optimum. Although ρ decreased to 1.5, a remarkable improvement in predictivity was achieved (Figure 5; Q$^2_{L1O}$ = 0.85). This value is even slightly superior to that obtained in MLR-analysis.

In summary, artificial neural networks were used to perform both a Free-Wilson analysis and a combined Hansch/Free-Wilson analysis on a set of 48 propafenone-type modulators of multidrug resistance. In both cases, in comparison to classical multiple linear regression analysis, the ANN showed equal or slightly better predictive power in leave one out cross validation procedures and was remarkably superior when performing a leave 8 out cross validation. Additionally, it was possible to train a network using only 14 compounds and to properly predict the MDR-modulating activity of the remaining 34 compounds. In this case, the MLR analysis failed completely due to an insufficient number of cases.

Nevertheless, attempts to extract informations on which input descriptors are important using a genetic input selection algorithm failed. Best results were obtained using those descriptors which showed highest statistical significance in MLR analyses. Thus, it was possible to train an artificial neural network for prediction of MDR-modulating activity of propafenone-type modulators, but it was not yet possible to conclusively extract information on which descriptors are important for this recognition/prediction process.

Extending our studies on different classes of modulators will show, whether artificial neural networks generally are a new tool in the prediction of MDR modulating activity and whether it will be possible to extract information important for design of highly active inhibitors of P-glycoprotein.

ACKNOWLEDGMENT

We gratefully acknowledge the financial support provided by the Austrian Science Fund (grant # P11760-MOB).

REFERENCES

1. Kane, S.E. Multidrug resistance of cancer cells. Adv. Drug Res. 1996, 28, 182–238.
2. Broxterman, H.L., Schuurhuis, G.J. Transport proteins in drug resistance: detection and prognostic significance in acute myeloid leukemia. J. Intern. Med. Suppl. 1997, 740, 147–151.
3. Sonneveld, P., Lokhorst, H.M., Vossebeld, P. Drug resistance in multiple myeloma. Semin. Hematol 1997, 34, 34–39.
4. Raderer, M., Scheithauer, W. Clinical trials of agents that reverse multidrug resistance. Cancer 1993, 72, 3553–3563.
5. Ecker, G., Chiba, P. Structure-activity-relationship studies on modulators of the multidrug transporter P-glycoprotein - an overview. Wien. Klin. Wochenschr. 1995, 107, 681–686.
6. Andrea, T.A., Kalayeh, H. Applications of neural networks in quantitative structure-activity relationships of dihydrofolate reductase inhibitors. J. Med. Chem. 1991, 34, 2824–2836.
7. Schaper, K.J., Samitier, M.L.R. Calculation of Octanol/Water Partition Coefficients (logP) using artificial neural networks and connection matices. Quant. Struct. Act. Relat. 1997, 16, 224–230.
8. Tmej, C., Chiba, P., Huber, M., Richter, E., Hitzler, M., Schaper, K.J., Ecker, G. A combined Hansch/Free-Wilson approach as predictive tool in QSAR studies on propafenone-type modulators of multidrug resistance. Archiv. der Pharmazie 1998, 331, 233–240.
9. Ghose, A.K., Pritchett, A., Crippen, G.M. Atomic physicochemical parameters for three dimensional structure directed quantitative structure-activity relationships III: Modeling hydrophobic interactions. J. Comput. Chem. 1988, 9, 80–90
10. Baricic, P., Mackov, M.; distributed by Hudecek, M., P. Horova 18, 841 07 Bratislava, Slowakia
11. Prets, S., Jungreithmair, A., Chiba, P., Ecker, G. Comparison of different methods for estimation of lipophilicity of propafenone-type modulators of multidrug resistance. Sci. Pharm. 1996, 64, 627–636.
12. Gekeler, V., Frese, G., Noller, A., Handgretinger, R., Wilisch, A., Schmidt, H., Muller, C., Dopfer, R., Klingebiel, T., Diddens, H., Probst, H., Niethammer, D. Mdr1/P-glycoprotein, topoisomerase and glutathione-S-transferase gene expression in primary and relapsed state adult and childhood leukemias. Br. J. Cancer 1992, 66, 507–517.
13. TRAJAN V 3.0, Trajan Software Ltd., Trajan House, Durham, England.
14. Karna, K.N., Breen, D.M. An artificial neural networks tutorial: Part1 - basics. Neural Networks 1989, 1, 4–22.
15. So, S.-S., Richards, G. Application of neural networks: Quantitative structure-activity relationships of the derivatives of 2,4-diamino-5-(substituted-benzyl)pyrimidines as DHFR inhibitors. J. Med. Chem. 1992, 35, 3201–3207.
16. Aoyama, T., Ichikawa, H. Obtaining the correlation indices between drug activity and strucutral parameters using a neural network. Chem. Pharm. Bull. 1991, 39, 372–378.
17. Holland, J.H. Adaption in natural and artificial systems; The Univeristy of Michigan Press, An Arbor, MI, 1975
18. Cramer, R.D. III, Patterson, D.E., Bunce, J.D. Comparative molecular field analysis (CoMFA). 1. Effect of shape on binding of steroids to carrier proteins. J. Am. Chem. Soc. 1988, 110, 5959–5967.
19. Fujita, T., Ban, T. Structure-activity study of phenylethylamines as substrates of biosynthetic enzymes of sympathetic transmitters. J. Med. Chem. 1971, 14, 148–152.
20. Ecker, G., Chiba, P., Hitzler, M., Schmid, D., Visser, K., Cordes, H.P., Csöllei, J., Seydel, J.K., Schaper, K.-J. Structure-activity relationship studies on benzofurane analogs of propafenone-type modulators of tumor cell multidrug resistance. J. Med. Chem. 1996, 39, 4767–4774.
21. Chiba, P., Ecker, G., Schmid, D., Drach, J., Tell, B., Goldenberg, S., Gekeler, V. Structural requirements for activity of propafenone type modulators in PGP-mediated multidrug resistance. Mol. Pharmacol. 1996, 49, 1122–1130.
22. Chiba, P., Holzer, W., Landau, M., Bechmann, G., Lorenz, K., Plagens, B., Hitzler, M., Richter, E., Ecker, G. Substituted 4-acylpyrazoles and -pyrazolones: Synthesis and MDR-modulating activity. J. Medicinal Chem. 1998, 41, 4001–4011.

DISCORDANCE OF P-GLYCOPROTEIN EXPRESSION AND FUNCTION IN ACUTE LEUKEMIA

Barbara De Moerloose,[1*] Catharina Dhooge,[1] and Jan Philippé[2]

[1]Department of Pediatrics
[2]Clinical Chemistry, Microbiology, and Immunology
University Hospital Gent
De Pintelaan 185, B-9000 Gent, Belgium

Keywords: MDR, P-glycoprotein, leukemia, flow cytometry.

1. ABSTRACT

Since March 1996, 93 consecutive samples of 45 adults and 41 children, suffering from acute leukemia, were evaluated prospectively for P-glycoprotein (P-gp) expression and function by flow cytometry. P-gp antigen expression was determined with the monoclonal antibodies 4E3 and MRK16. Transport function was assessed by measuring the modulating effect of verapamil on the intracellular retention of Rhodamine 123.

P-gp positivity at relapse was not significantly more frequent than at initial diagnosis in our study group, neither with the immunologic assay, nor with the functional test. There was no correlation between the results of the immunologic and the functional test. Discordant test results were observed in 11/41 children (12/44 samples) and 14/45 adults (15/49 samples), independent of the type of leukemia. 2/12 and 2/15 samples scored positive with one of the monoclonal antibodies and were functionally inactive. In 10/12 and 13/15 samples however, an efflux pump was active and dependent of verapamil, but without detectable antigen. The functional flow cytometric assay allows evaluation of non-P-gp efflux pumps and, therefore, is more clinically relevant since it may better identify patients who would benefit from the use of P-gp inhibitors.

---

[*] Research assistant of the Fund for Scientific Research (FWO), Flanders.

2. INTRODUCTION

One of the best studied mechanisms that cause multidrug resistance (MDR) is the expression of the P-glycoprotein (P-gp), a 170-kD calcium-dependent efflux pump with ATPase activity, located in the plasma cell membrane.[1] P-gp expression is claimed to be an independent parameter of poor response to chemotherapy and bad oucome in AML of the adult by several authors.[2,3,4,5,6] Some studies however have shown that patients with clinically resistant AML do not always have evidence of P-gp overexpression.[7,8,9] The role of P-gp in other hematological malignancies remains even more controversial[10,11,12] and recent clinical trials with P-gp reversing agents have yielded disappointing results.[13]

Levels at which drug resistance becomes clinically relevant are unknown, but probably low.[14] Therefore, accurate measurement of low levels of P-gp in clinical samples remains an elusive goal. Flow cytometry seems to be clearly superior to immunocytochemistry and rt-PCR in distinguishing specimens with low or intermediate levels of P-gp expression;[15] the Rhodamine 123 efflux test equally detects low levels of drug resistance[16]. Moreover, functional assays could help to evaluate effects of chemotherapy combined with chemosensitizers in leukemic blasts and they give an accurate identification of patients that may benefit from therapies containing such P-gp inhibitors.

Comparison of P-gp antigen expression and transport function was examined recently in adult AML[9,17,18] and in childhood leukemia[19,20] and yielded different results. Adult ALL patients were not evaluated. Using flow cytometric immunologic and functional assays, we examined P-gp in 45 adults and 41 children with acute leukemia. Seven patients were examined at both initial diagnosis and relapse, or at two different relapse episodes.

3. MATERIALS AND METHODS

3.1. Patients

From march 1996 to march 1998, 93 bone marrow and blood samples of 11 adults with ALL, 34 adults with AML, 34 children with ALL and 7 children with AML were evaluated consecutively at the time of diagnosis. No cryopreserved material was used. 68 samples were collected at initial diagnosis and 25 at relapse. All patients were classified according to the FAB classification and immunophenotyping was performed in 76 cases. Serial samples were obtained in seven patients.

Patient characteristics are listed in Table 1 and 5.

3.2. Flow Cytometry

Mononuclear cells were isolated by gradient centrifugation on Ficoll-hypaque. Samples of the human myeloid leukemia cell line K562 and its P-gp expressing resistant clone K562/VLB were included in each experiment as negative and positive control respectively.

3.2.1. Determination of P-gp Expression. Cells (5.10^5) were incubated for 30 minutes with a matched-isotype control antibody (IgG2$_a$, Dako Corporation, Glostrup, Denmark) and with the monoclonal antibodies 4E3 (7.5 µg/ml, Dako Corporation, Carpinteria, USA) or MRK16 (5 µg/ml, Kamiya Biomedical Company, Thousand Oaks, USA) which recognize different external epitopes of P-gp. Cells were washed twice in PBS/BSA/NaN$_3$ and incubated for 20 minutes with fluorescein isothiocyanate-labeled or phycoerythrin-la-

Table 1. Patient characteristics*

	de novo ALL (33)	relapse ALL (15)	de novo AML (35)	relapse AML (10)
Gender				
Ratio M/F	18/15	6/9	26/9	4/6
Age				
< 1year	1			2
1<<2 year	1		2	
2<<10 year	15	5	4	
10<<60 year	13	9	14	4
>60 year	3	1	15	4
FAB classif				
M0			4	1
M1			6	2
M2			14	4
M4			5	0
M5			5	3
RAEB-t			1	0
SecondaryLineage	1		9	
B	26	11		
T	2	1		
Biphenotypic	4	3		
Undifferent.	1			
Cytogenetics				
Favorable	2	0	3	2
Unfavorable	4	3	10	3
Others	19	11	16	4
Not available	7	1	7	

*Eleven adults and 34 children are suffering from ALL; 34 adults and 7 children from AML. Five patients were examined at both initial diagnosis and at relapse, 2 patients at different relapse episodes. Favorable cytogenetic results are t(8;21) and inv(16) in AML and hyperdiploidy in ALL. Unfavorable cytogenetic parameters are -7, del7q, -5, del5q, +13, 11q23 and complex abnormalities for AML; t(9;22), t(4;11) and 11q23 for ALL.

beled goat F(ab')$_2$ anti-mouse IgG (Caltag Laboratories, Burlingame, UK). Cells were stained with an immunologic marker (if immunophenotyping results were available) to identify the cell population of interest.

Fluorescence was analyzed on a FACSort flow cytometer (Becton Dickinson). At least 10.000 events were counted.

Kolmogorov-Smirnov (KS) statistics were performed on the resulting fluorescence histograms of the isotypic and the specific antibody. A sample was considered positive if the KS D-value was > 0.15 and if the mean fluorescence of the cells was at least 10% brighter after staining with the specific antibody, compared to the isotypic matched control antibody (mean fluorescence index (MFI) > 1.10).

3.2.2. Functional Assay. Functional analysis of P-gp was carried out by studying the accumulation and retention pattern of 200 ng/ml Rhodamine 123 (Rho 123) in the absence and presence of verapamil (Isoptine, Knoll, Belgium), as described by others[23] Briefly, 10^5 cells were incubated for 1 hour at 37°C with 200 ng/ml Rho 123 in the absence or presence of 10 µM verapamil. The intracellular Rho 123 accumulation was measured. Cells were washed twice with cold (4°C) HBSS without fenol red and resuspended in HBSS without fenol red. Cells were incubated for 1 hour at 37°C with or without 10 µM verapamil and the remaining intracellular Rho 123 retention after the efflux period was measured. Results were expressed as ratios which are calculated after the accumulation or efflux period of 1 hour each, by division of the median intracellular Rho 123 fluorescence in the presence of verapamil by the median Rho 123 fluorescence in the absence of verapamil. The functional assay is considered positive if the cells exhibit Rho 123 efflux and if the intracellular Rho 123 fluorescence enhances in the presence of verapamil by at least 10 % (Retention ratio >1.10). The reversing effect of verapamil (%) was calculated by dividing the median fluorescence shift (rho 123 retention in the presence of verapamil - rho 123 retention in the absence of verapamil) by the median rho 123 retention in the presence of verapamil.

3.3. Statistical Analysis

The correlation between P-gp expression as determined by 4E3 or MRK16, and between P-gp expression and function, was estimated by the Pearson correlation test (r = correlation coefficient).

4. RESULTS

4.1. Comparison of the Antigenic Determinations and the Functional Assay

Correlation of the MFI of the samples after incubation with 4E3 or MRK16 revealed a correlation coefficient of 0.51 for the overall population; 0.37 for the children with AML, 0.50 for the children with ALL, 0.98 for the adults with ALL and 0.57 for the adults with AML (Figure 1).

After comparison of the results of the antigenic determination and the functional assay, 4 different immunologic/functional (I/F) phenotypes are being observed, as demonstrated in Figure 2. The typical MDR1 phenotype (=I+/F+) was found in 9 children and 11 adults (Table 2 and 3). Discrepant test results were found in 12/44 samples of children and 15/49 samples of adults, independent of the type of leukemia. The majority of discordant samples has the I-/F+ phenotype (10/12 children and 13/15 adults). 2/12 children and 2/15

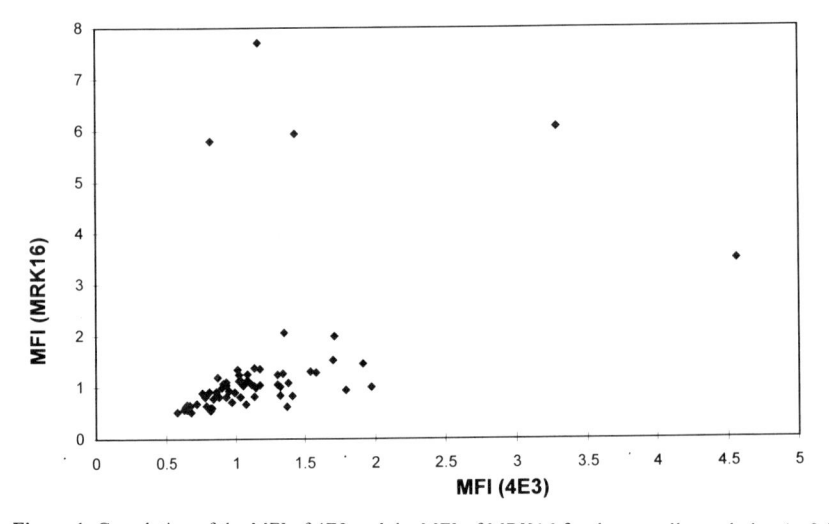

Figure 1. Correlation of the MFI of 4E3 and the MFI of MRK16 for the overall population (r=0.51).

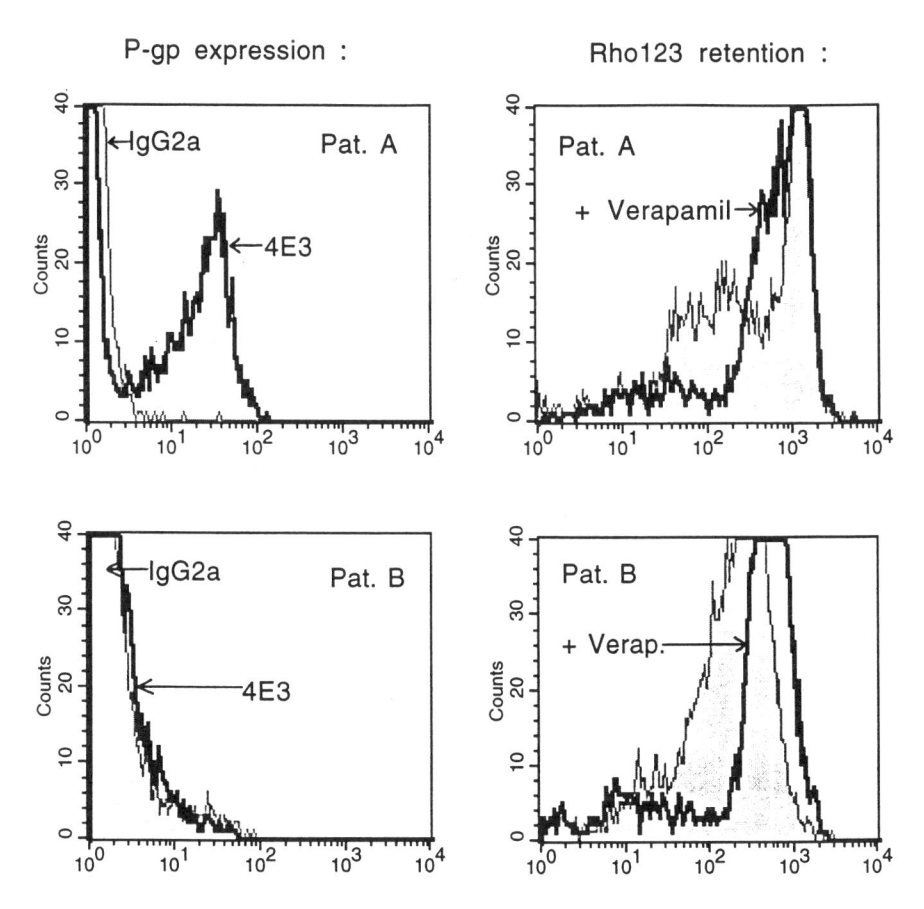

Figure 2. Illustration of 4 different phenotypes. The comparison of the flow cytometric immunologic and functional assays reveals four different results. The histograms on the left represent the results of the immunologic assay : the gray line is the fluorescence of the cells after staining with the isotypic matched control antibody; the black line after staining with the monoclonal antibody 4E3. The immunologic assay is positive when the cellular fluorescence after staining with 4E3 enhances in comparison with the isotypic antibody. The histograms on the right show the intracellular rho 123 retention in the absence of verapamil (gray line) and in the presence of verapamil (black line). Positive cells have a brighter intracellular rho 123 fluorescence in the presence of verapamil than in the absence of verapamil. Patient A is a double positive patient; patient B shows a discordant phenotype with a negative immunologic but positive functional test; patient C is positive for the immunologic assay and negative for the functional test and patient D is double negative.

adults had the I+/F- phenotype; the immunologic assay in this group of patients was twice positive for both MRK16 and 4E3, and twice positive for 4E3 but negative for MRK16.

On the contrary, all 3 patients who scored positive for MRK16 and negative for 4E3, had a double positive (I+/F+) phenotype.

After statistical analysis of MFI and retention ratio, we found a very poor correlation for the overall population (r=0.01; Figure 3). Correlation of the MFI and the reversing effect of verapamil also results in a poor correlation (r=0.04 for the children and r=0.15 for the adults; Figure 4.1 and 4.2 respectively).

In 8 adults and 4 children a Rho 123 efflux was observed which was not influenced by the presence of verapamil.

P-gp expression :   Rho123 retention :

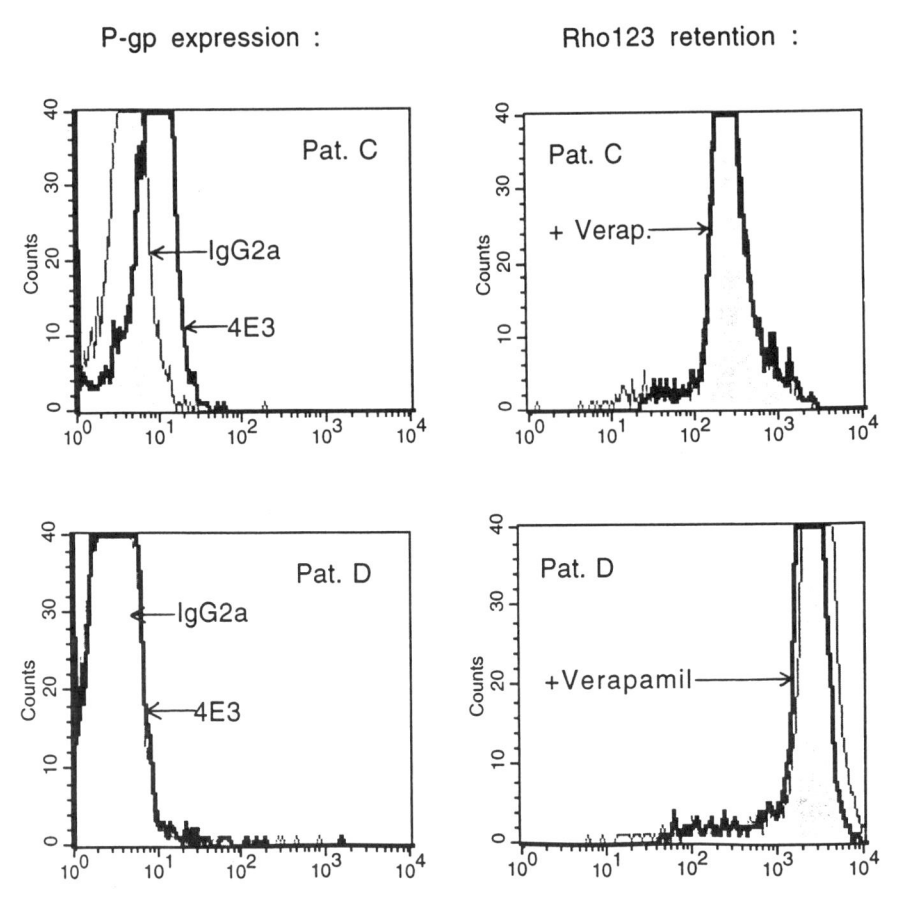

Figure 2. (*Continued*)

In 9 adults with AML, the cells had a bright fluorescence after staining with the isotypic matched control antibody ($IgG2_a$) : 4 of these patients had the I-/F- phenotype, 4 had the I-/F+ phenotype and 1 had the I+/F+ phenotype. These phenotypes did not change after incubation of the cells with human AB serum, prior to incubation with 4E3, MRK16 or $IgG2_a$ (data not shown).

4.2. P-gp Expression and Function in AML and ALL

In AML samples, no difference in P-gp levels was found between presentation (35 samples) and relapse (10 samples) using the functional assay (60%, Table 4). The immunologic assay on the contrary showed an increase in P-gp positivity between initial diagnosis (34%) and relapse (50%) but the number of relapsed patients is small. P-gp positivity, at initial diagnosis or at relapse, was larger using the functional assay compared to the immunologic assay (60% versus 34% and 60% versus 50%).

In ALL samples, P-gp positivity was larger using the functional assay compared to the immunologic assay as well (33% versus 15% at initial diagnosis and 27% versus 13% at relapse). P-gp positivity in ALL was not more frequent at relapse compared to the initial

Table 2. Results of the immunologic (I) and functional (F) flow cytometric assays in 44 samples of 41 children suffering from AML or ALL

Diagnosis	Number	I+/F+	I+/F-	I-/F+	I-/F-
AML					
de novo					
M0	1			1	
M2	1	1			
M4	1	1			
M5	2		1		1
RAEBt	1	1			
relapse					
M5	2	1		1	
ALL					
de novo					
B-lineage	20	4		3	13
Biphenotypic	3			2	1
relapse					
B-lineage	10		1	3	6
T-lineage	1				1
Biphenotypic	2	1			1

diagnosis, by neither of the 2 assays (15% and 33% compared to 13% and 27% respectively, Table 4).

P-gp expression was found in AML in 34% of the cases at initial diagnosis and in 50% at relapse, compared to only 15% and 13% in ALL at initial diagnosis or at relapse respectively. A positive functional assay was also more frequently found in AML compared to ALL.

Table 3. Results of the immunologic (I) and functional (F) flow cytometric assays in 49 samples of 45 adults suffering from AML or ALL

Diagnosis	Number	I+/F+	I+/F-	I-/F+	I-/F-
AML					
de novo					
M0	3	2	1		
M1	6	1		3	2
M2	13	4		6	3
M4	4			2	2
M5	3				3
relapse					
M0	1				1
M1	2	1			1
M2	4	2		1	1
M5	1		1		
ALL					
de novo					
B-lineage	6				6
T-lineage	2			1	1
Biphenotypic	1				1
Undiff.	1	1			
relapse					
B-lineage	2				2

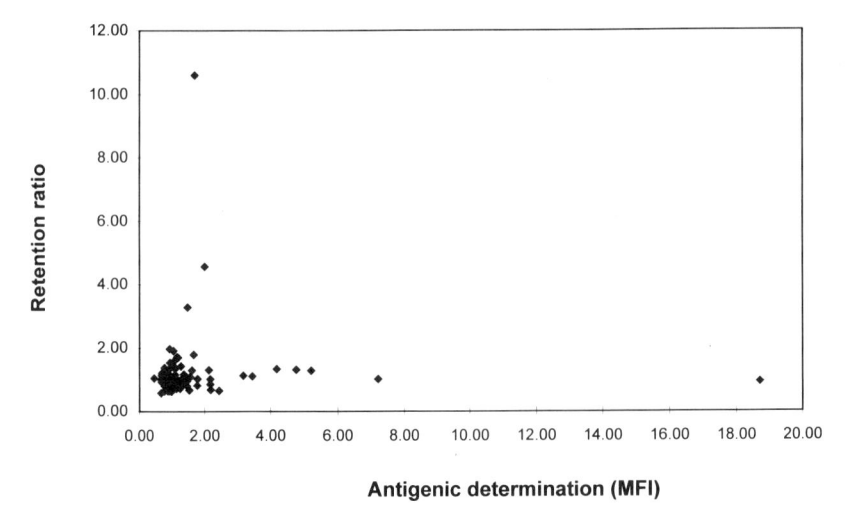

Figure 3. Correlation of antigenic determination (MFI) and Rho 123 retention ratio in the overall population.

4.3. Sequential Analysis

Sequential analysis was performed in 7 patients (Table 5). Two patients experienced two relapse episodes, five others were evaluated at initial diagnosis and at a subsequent relapse. In one patient (PDS C) P-gp was detected with 4E3 and MRK16 at the first relapse, but not at the second relapse. There was no enhancement of P-gp positivity in the other patients, except for one (V P). This man scored positive for the immunologic assay; Rho 123 efflux was present but not influenced by the presence of verapamil.

5. DISCUSSION

During the past two years, we evaluated 45 adults and 41 children suffering from ALL or AML, by means of two flow cytometric assays. We preferred the functional assay using the fluorescent dye Rho 123 as P-gp substrate and verapamil as P-gp inhibitor. Rho 123 is a more sensitive way to measure P-gp function than a similar assay with daunorubicin[9,21] and it is proven to detect low levels of drug resistance.[16] We used two antibodies recognizing separate external epitopes (4E3 and MRK16) because occasional false positive[15] or false negative results, for example because of epitope masking,[22] have been reported. We correlated these two test in order to detect drug efflux in the absence of P-gp expression, which might be an indication of other mechanisms of drug resistance.[24]

Both methods showed a wide range of values for P-gp expression or function between individual patients. P-gp expression was much lower in the patient samples compared to the cell line K562/VLB and we found lower levels of P-gp positivity using the immunologic assay compared to the functional test, which is in accordance with findings of other authors.[20]

P-gp expression and pumping activity in ALL was less frequent compared to AML (Table 4), which is also reported previously.[23] There was a slight increase in P-gp expression at relapse in the adults with AML, compared to the initial diagnosis, but no increase in P-gp function; there was also no increase in the children and the adult ALL patients

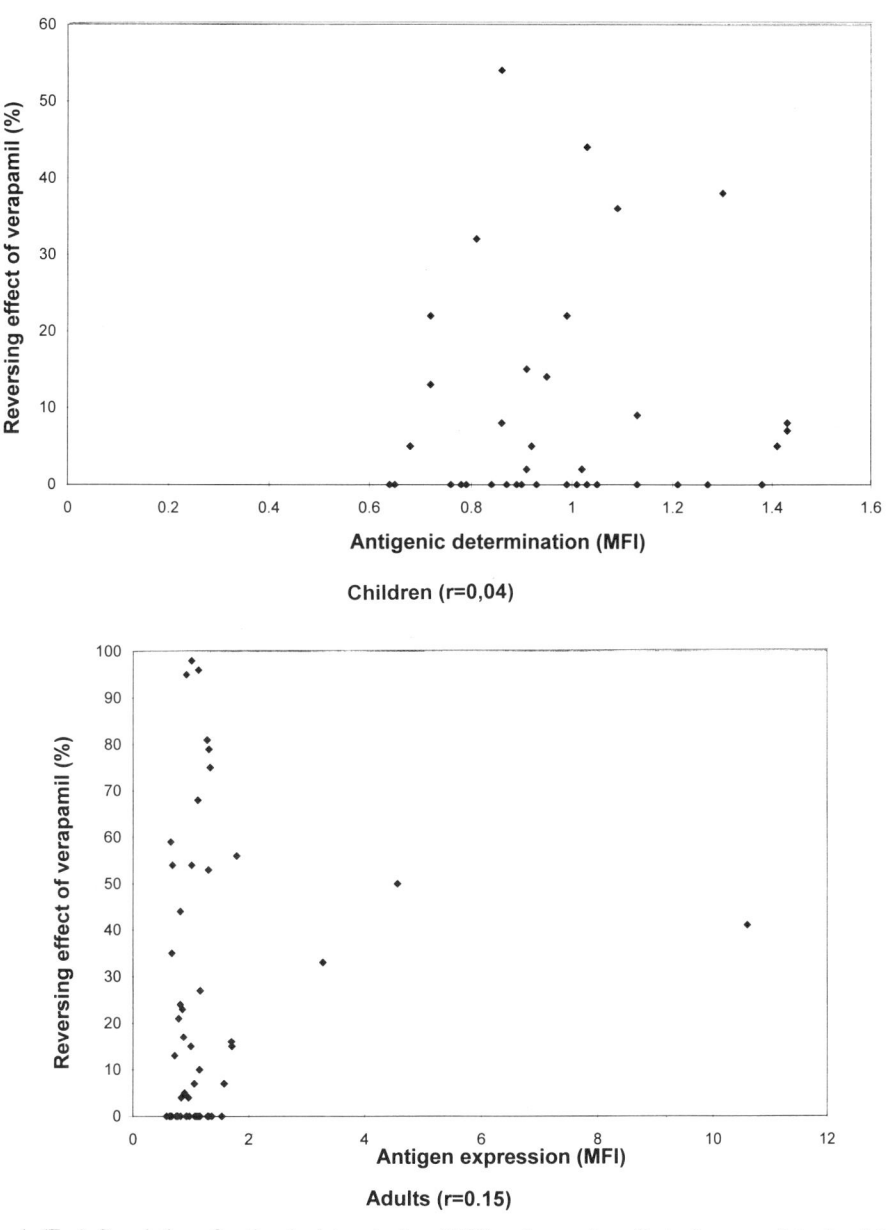

Figure 4. (Top) Correlation of antigenic determination (MFI) and reversing effect of verapamil in the children (r=0.04). (Bottom) Correlation of antigenic determination (MFI) and reversing effect of verapamil in the adults (r=0.15).

with the immunologic, nor with the functional assay. Ivy et al.[19] and Tafuri et al.,[20] who examined childhood leukemias, found significant increases of P-gp function at relapse; they observed no increase of P-gp expression using the monoclonal antibodies at relapse.

The best correlation (r = 0.98) between 4E3 and MRK16 was found in the adult population, suffering from ALL, the weakest correlation (r = 0.36) amongst the children with AML.

Table 4. P-gp positivity according to the immunologic and functional assay in ALL and AML at initial diagnosis and at relapse for the overall population

	De novo ALL (33)	Relapse ALL (15)	De novo AML(35)	Relapse AML (10)
Immunologic	5 (15%)	2 (13%)	12 (34%)	5 (50%)
Functional	11 (33%)	4 (27%)	21 (60%)	6 (60%)

There was no correlation between the retention ratio and the antigenic determination using 4E3 and MRK16 in our setting (r = 0.01), nor between the reversing effect of verapamil and the antigenic determination (r = 0.04 for the children and r = 0.15 for the adults). On the contrary, Ivy et al.[19] examined childhood leukemic samples with Rho 123 efflux and the monoclonal antibody MRK™16 and found an excellent correlation (r = 0.82). Tafuri et al.[20] also used rho 123 and the monoclonal antibodies 4E3 and MRK16 in childhood leukemia (merely childhood ALL) and found a good correlation (r = 0.6). Bailly et al.[17] however, reported a lack of correlation between P-gp expression, evaluated by the monoclonal antibodies MRK16 and UIC2, and Rho 123 kinetics in AML cell lines. Xie et al.[18] also found no correlation (r = 0.11) between antigen expression (using MRK16) and daunorubicin accumulation despite additional refinements such as neuraminidase pretreatment and antigen quantification. A poor correlation (r=0.06) between P-gp function, meas-

Table 5. Phenotypes of 7 patients who were analysed both at initial diagnosis and subsequently at relapse (5) or at 2 different relapse episodes (2)

Initials	Age	Sex	Diagnosis	Cytogenetics	Phenotype	CR	Outcome
PDS C	<1y	F	AML M5 Relapse 1	11q23	I+/F+	yes	Relapse 2 after BMT
			AML M5 Relapse 2	11q23	I-/F+		Dead
DC B	10y	F	ALL Biphen. after CML	t(9;22)	I-/F+	no	Relapse after BMT
	11y		ALL Biphen. Relapse	t(9;22)	I+/F+		Dead
M N	17y	F	B ALL Relapse 1	46,XX	I-/F+	yes	Relapse after BMT
			B ALL Relapse 2	46,XX	I-/F-		Dead
B R	71y	F	B ALL	46,XX	I-/F-	yes	Relapse
	72y		B ALL Relapse	t(9;22)	I-/F-	yes	Alive
V P	75y	M	Secondary AML M5	48,XY,+8	I-/F- +efflux	no	Relapse
			AML M5 Relapse		I+/F- +efflux		Dead
O T	33y	M	AML M2	inv(16)	I-/F+	yes	Relapse
	34y		AML M2 Relapse		I-/F+	yes	Alive
VC B	28y	M	AML M1	-7,11q23	I-/F- +efflux	yes	Early relapse, Relapse after BMT
	29y		AML M0 Relapse 2		I-/F- + efflux		Dead

ured by daunorubicin uptake, and P-gp determination by the monoclonal antibody 4E3 was reported previously.[25]

We found discrepant test results in 12/44 samples of children and 15/49 samples of adults. These discrepancies were independent of the type of leukemia (Table 2–3). The majority of discordant samples has the I-/F+ phenotype (10/12 children and 13/15 adults). 2/12 children and 2/15 adults had the I+/F- phenotype.

Discrepant test results are reported by several authors.[6,9,18-20] Ivy et al.[19] found a positive functional test in 5/103 children without detectable antigen. Leith et al.[9] reported 10/60 adults suffering from AML with the I-/F+ phenotype, and 6/60 cases with an I+/F- phenotype.

The I+/F- phenotype may be caused by aspecific cross-reactions of the monoclonal antibodies or by non-functional P-gp. Posttranslational modifications, e.g., mediated by protein kinase C, may alter the state of activity of P-gp, as described in tissue cultures.[23]

Functional efflux, detected without P-gp antigen expression, probably indicates that alternate non-P-gp mediated efflux mechanisms are present. The use of fluorescent dyes for the evaluation of P-gp activity should always consider possible other efflux pumps such as MRP.[23,24] We found amongst the patients without P-gp expression, Rho 123 efflux, not inhibited by verapamil, in 12; and efflux, inhibited by verapamil, in 22.

The I-/F+ phenotype may also be caused by insufficient staining with the monoclonal antibodies. In three patients, we detected weak P-gp expression after subsequent testing and only in dual-parameter flow cytometry.

Functional assays seem to be more sensitive than antigenic determination of P-gp and they evaluate the presence of other efflux pumps. They offer opportunities to evaluate in vitro which leukemia patients will profite from chemotherapy combined with chemosensitizers.

ACKNOWLEDGMENTS

This work was supported by an FWO grant "Kom op".

REFERENCES

1. Kartner L., Riordan J.R. and Ling V. Cell surface P-glycoprotein associated with multidrug resistance in mammalian cell lines. Science 1983,221,1285–1288.
2. Leith C.P., Kopecky K.J., Godwin J.,McConnell T., Slovak M.L., Chen I-M., Head D.R., Appelbaum F.R. and Willman C.L. Acute myeloid leukemia in the elderly : Assessment of multidrug resistance (MDR1) and cytogenetics distinguishes biologic subgroups with remarkably distict responses to standard chemotherapy. A Southwest Oncology Group study. Blood 1997,89,3323–3329.
3. Del Poeta G., Venditti A., Aronica G., Stasi R., Cox M.C., Buccisano F., Bruno A., Tamburini A., Suppo G., Simone M.D., Epiceno A.M., Del Moro B., Masi M., Papa G. and Amadori S. P-glycoprotein expression in de novo acute myeloid leukemia. Leukemia and Lymphoma 1997,27,257–274.
4. Van de Heuvel-Eibrinck M.M., van der Holt B., te Boekhorst P.A.W., Pieters R., Schoester M., Löwenberg B. and Sonneveld P. MDR1 expression as an independent prognostic factor for response and survival in de novo acute myeloid leukaemia. Br. J. Haem. 1997,99,76–83.
5. Wood P., Burgess R., MacGregor A. and Liu Yin J.A. P-glycoprotein expression on acute myeloid leukaemia blast cells at diagnosis predicts response to chemotherapy and survival. Br. J. Haem.1994,87,509–514.
6. Guerci A., Merlin J.L., Missoum N., Feldmann L., Marchal S., Witz F., Rose C. and Guerci O. Predictive value for treatment outcome in acute myeloid leukemia of cellular daunorubicin accumulation and P-glycoprotein expression simultaneously determined by flow cytometry. Blood 1995,85,2147–2153.

7. Zhou D-C, Zittoun R, Marie J-P. Expression of the multidrug-resistance associated protein (MRP) and multidrug resistance (MDR1) genes in acute myeloid leukemia. Leukemia 1995,9,1661–1667.
8. Hart S.M., Ganeshaguru K., Scheper R.J., Prentice H.G., Hoffbrand A.V. and Mehta A.B. Expression of the human major vault protein LRP in acute myeloid leukemia. Exp. Hem. 1997,25,1227–1232.
9. Leith C. P., Chen I-M., Kopecky K.J., Appelbaum F.R., Head D.R., Godwin J.E., Weick J.K. and Willman C.L. Correlation of multidrug resistance (MDR1) protein expression with functional dye/drug efflux in acute myeloid leukemia by multiparameter flow cytometry : Identification of discordant MDR$^-$/Efflux$^+$ and MDR$^+$/Efflux$^-$ cases. Blood 1995,86,2329–2342.
10. Wattel E., Lepelley P., Merlat A., Sartiaux C., Bauters F., Jouet J.P. and Fenaux P. Expression of the multidrug resistance P glycoprotein in newly diagnosed adult acute lymphoblastic leukemia : absence of correlation with response to treatment. Leukemia 1995,9,1870–1874.
11. Sievers E.L., Smith F.O., Woods W.G., Lee J.W., Bleyer W.A., Willman C.L. and Bernstein I.D. Cell surface expression of the multidrug resistance P-glycoprotein (P-170) as detected by monoclonal antibody MRK-16 in pediatric acute myeloid leukemia fails to define a poor prognostic group: a report from the Childrens Cancer Group. Leukemia 1995,9,2042–2048.
12. Pearson L., Leith C.P., Duncan M.H., Chen I-M., McConnell T., Trinkaus K., Foucar K. and Willman C.L. Multidrug resistance-1 (MDR1) expression and functional dye/drug efflux is highly correlated with the t(8;21) chromosomal translocation in pediatric acute myeloid leukemia. Leukemia 1996,10,1274–1282.
13. Fisher G.A. and Sikic B.I. Clinical studies with modulators of multidrug resistance. Hematol. Oncol. Clin. N. Am. 1995,9,363–382.
14. Musto P., Melillo L., Lombardi G., Matera R., Di Giorgio G. and Carotenuto M. High risk of early resistant relapse for leukaemic patients with presence of multidrug resistance associated P-glycoprotein positive cells in complete remission. Br. J. Haem. 1991,77,50–53.
15. Beck W.T., Grogan T.M., Willman C.L., Cordon-Cardo C., Parham D.M., Kuttesch J.F., Andreeff M., Bates S.E., Berard C.W., Boyett J.M., Brophy N.A., Broxterman H.J., Chan H.S.L., Dalton W.S., Dietel M., Fojo A.T., Gascoyne R.D., Head D., Houghton P.J., Srivastava D.K., Lehnert M., Leith C.P., Paietta E., Pavelic Z.P., Rimsza L., Roninson I.B., Sikic B.I., Twentyman P.R., Warnke R. and Weinstein R. Methods to detect P-glycoprotein-associated Multidrug Resistance in patients' tumors : Consensus recommendations. Cancer Research 1996,56,3010–3020.
16. Webb M., Raphael C.L., Asbahr H., Erber W.N. and Meyer B.F. The detection of rhodamine 123 efflux at low levels of drug resistance. Br. J. of Haematology 1996,93,650–655.
17. Bailly J.D., Muller C., Jaffrezou J.P., Demur C., Gassar G., Bordier C. and Laurent G. Lack of correlation between expression and function of P-glycoprotein in AML cell lines. Leukemia 1995,9,799–804.
18. Xie X-Y, Robb D. Chow S. and Hedley D.W. Discordant P-glycoprotein antigen expression and transport function in acute myeloid leukemia. Leukemia 1995,9,1882–1887
19. Ivy S.P., Olshefski R.S., Taylor B.J., Patel K.M., Reaman G.H. Correlation of P-glycoprotein expression and function in childhood acute leukemia : a children's cancer group study. Blood 1996,88,309–318.
20. Tafuri A., Sommaggio A., Burba L., Albergoni M.P., Petrucci M.T., Mascolo M.G., Testi A.M., Basso G. Prognostic value of rhodamine-efflux and MDR-1/P-170 expression in childhood acute leukemia. Leuk. Res. 1995,19,927–931.
21. Lamy T., Drenou B., Grulois I., Fardel O., Jacquelinet C., Goasguen J., Dauriac C., Amiot L., Bernard M., Fauchet R.and Le Prise P.-Y. Multi-drug resistance (MDR) activity in acute leukemia determined by rhodamine 123 efflux assay. Leukemia 1995,9,1549–1555.
22. Cumber P.M., Jacobs A., Hoy T., Fisher J., Whittaker J.A., Tsuruo T. and Padua R.A. Expression of the multiple drug resistance gene (mdr-1) and epitope masking in chronic lymphatic leukaemia. Br. J. Haem. 1990,76,226–230.
23. Ludescher C., Eisterer W., Hilbe W., Gotwald M., Hofmann J., Zabernigg A., Cianfriglia M. and Thaler J. Low frequency of activity of P-glycoprotein (P-170) in acute lymphoblastic leukemia compared to acute myeloid leukemia. Leukemia 1995,9,350–356.
24. Feller N., Kuiper C.M., Lankelma J., Ruhdal J.K., Scheper R.J., Pinedo H.M. and Broxterman H.J. Functional detection of MDR1/P170 and MRP/P190-mediated multidrug resistance in tumour cells by flow cytometry. Br. J. Cancer 1995,72,543–549.
25. Chin-Yee I., Keeney M., Rudzitis L., Alshammari S. and Lohmann R.C. Poor correlation between P glycoprotein measured by drug (daunorubicin) uptake assay and monoclonal antibody 4E3. (Abstract) Blood 1994,84,S2594

14

MULTIDRUG RESISTANCE RELATED PROTEINS IN PRIMARY CUTANEOUS LYMPHOMAS

Christian W. van Haselen,[1,*] Marcel J. Flens,[2] Rik J. Scheper,[2] Paul van der Valk,[2] George L. Scheffer,[2] Johan Toonstra,[1] and Willem A. van Vloten[1]

[1]Department of Dermatology
University Hospital Utrecht
[2]Department of Pathology
University Hospital Vrije
Universiteit Amsterdam, The Netherlands

Keywords: cutaneous lymphomas, P-glycoprotein, multidrug resistance protein, lung resistance protein.

1. ABSTRACT

1.1. Background

In patients with primary cutaneous B-cell lymphomas (CBCL) and primary cutaneous T-cell lymphomas (CTCL), extracutaneous sites may become involved and then polychemotherapy is indicated. Multi-agent chemotherapy may induce long lasting complete remissions in CBCL's. Most CTCL's, especially mycosis fungoides (MF), and CD30 negative primary cutaneous large T-cell lymphoma (PCLTCL) respond poorly or partially to Multi-agent Chemotherapy.

---

[*] Correspondence to: C.W. van Haselen, Department of Dermatology, University Hospital Utrecht, P.O. Box 85500 3508 GA Utrecht, The Netherlands. Phone: 31 30 2507443; Fax: 31 30 2505404

Drug Resistance in Leukemia and Lymphoma III, edited by Kaspers *et al.*
Kluwer Academic / Plenum Publishers, New York, 1999.

1.2. Purpose

We have studied whether cutanous lymphomas express the following multidrug resistance (MDR) related proteins: multidrug resistance protein (MRP), lung resistance protein (LRP) and P-glycoprotein (Pgp).

1.3. Methods

From the files of the Dutch Cutaneous Lymphoma Working Group we selected pretreatment punch biopsy specimens of the skin from 14 patients with MF, 10 patients with a PCLTCL and 8 patients with a CBCL. In several patients with a clinical relapse of their disease after multi-agent chemotherapy, punch biopsy specimens of cutaneous lesions were available (6 MF, 3 PCLTCL, 1 CBCL). Benign dermatoses with a dense lymphoid infiltrate were included as a control. Immunohistochemistry was done on formalin fixed, paraffin-embedded punch biopsy specimens with monoclonal antibodies MRPr1 (anti-MRP); LRP-56 (anti-LRP); C219 (anti-Pgp). Staining was performed by the biotin-streptavidin immunoperoxidase method.

1.4. Results

MRPr1 staining was found in the cytoplasm of ≥ 5%-50% of lymphoid cells in 13 out of 14 cases of MF and in 6 out of 10 patients with a PCLTCL. In 2 out of 8 cases of CBCL ≥ 5%-50% positive tumorcells were found. Strong staining (≥50% of the cells positive) was found in 10 out of the total of 24 CTCL cases. LRP56 staining of lymphoid cells was found in 1 out of 14 cases of MF and in 1 out of 10 cases of PCLTCL and in 1 out of 8 cases of CBCL. C219 expression was found in 4 out of 10 cases of PCLTCL and in 2 out of 8 cases of CBCL. After chemotherapy both a higher staining intensity and a higher number of positive cells were found with MRPr1 especially in patients with MF.

1.5. Conclusion

The present study shows that lymphoid cells in both primary cutaneous lymphomas and benign skin disorders may express MDR related proteins and that the expression profile of these proteins is roughly related to the tumor cell phenotype. However, the functional role of these proteins in clinical drug resistance in primary cutaneous lymphomas has to be proven.

2. INTRODUCTION

By definition primary cutaneous lymphomas represent a subgroup of non-Hodgkin's lymphomas that clinically present in the skin. Extracutaneous involvement may occur later in the disease course. Primary cutaneous lymphomas show considerable variation in clinical presentation, histology, immunophenotype and prognosis.[1]

We will summarize the clinicopathological features of the studied cutaneous lymphomas and focus on their clinical chemosensitivity.

2.1. Mycosis Fungoides

Mycosis fungoides (MF), an epidermotropic cutaneous T-cell lymphoma (CTCL), has an indolent clinical course with slow progression over years or sometimes decades

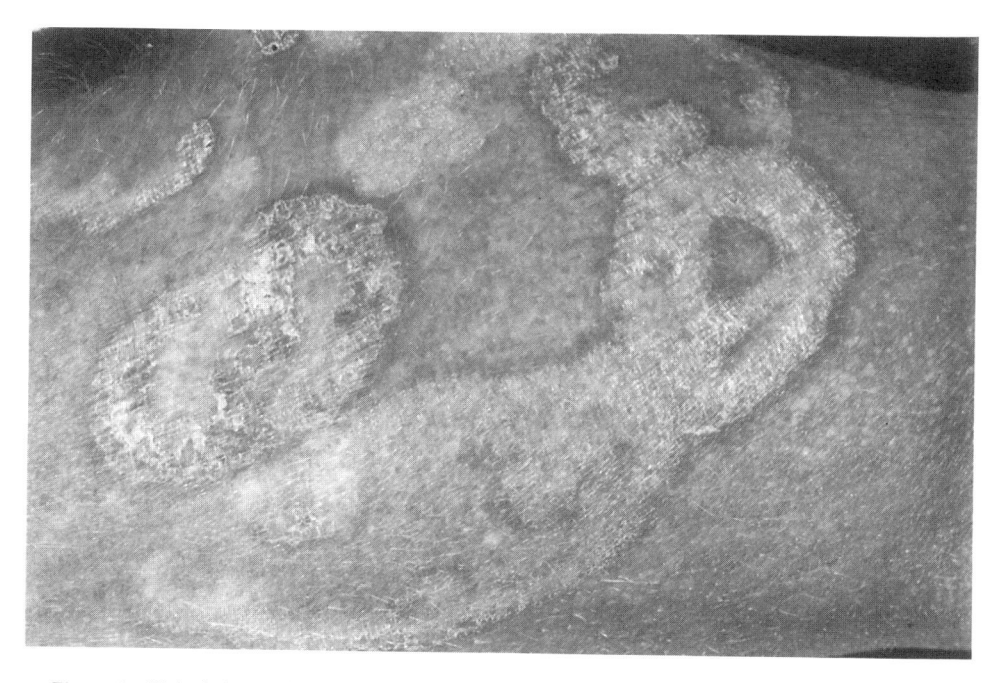

Figure 1. Clinical picture of mycosis fungoides with annular, red scaling plaques on the right upper leg.

from patches to plaques and eventually tumors (Figure 1). MF cells in early disease seem to proliferate only in the skin. However, the multiplicity of lesions in patients with MF indicates that these cells circulate through the peripheral blood, although they are difficult to detect by T-cell receptor rearrangement analysis. In patients with MF stage Ia, b (only cutaneous manifestations), treatment with multi-agent chemotherapy as compared to skin-targeted therapies does not contribute to a better survival.[2] In the event that extracutaneous sites become involved, multi-agent chemotherapy is indicated. However both cutaneous MF lesions and extracutaneous MF involvement are or become often refractory to treatment and may even progress during therapy.

2.2. Primary Cutaneous Large Cell Lymphomas

Most primary cutaneous T-cell lymphomas other than MF and Sézary syndrome belong to the gruop of primary cutaneous large T-cell lymphomas (PCLTCL). These lymphomas often present with (ulcerated) nodules or tumors (Figure 2). Previous studies demonstrated that in the PCLTCL group expression of the CD30 antigen on the majority of tumor cells is the most important prognostic parameter. Thus, whereas CD30+ PCLTCL have an excellent prognosis (limited disease, good response to therapy, 4-year survival >90%) the prognosis of CD30- PCLTCL is often poor (early dissemination to extracutaneous sites, frequent relapses during or after therapy, 4-year survival <25%).[1]

2.3. Cutaneous B-Cell Lymphoma

Patients present with nonscaling, solitary or grouped papules, plaques and/or tumors, which may be surrounded by (annular) erythemas (Figure 3). If left untreated, the skin lesions gradually increase in size over years. However, extracutaneous involvement is un-

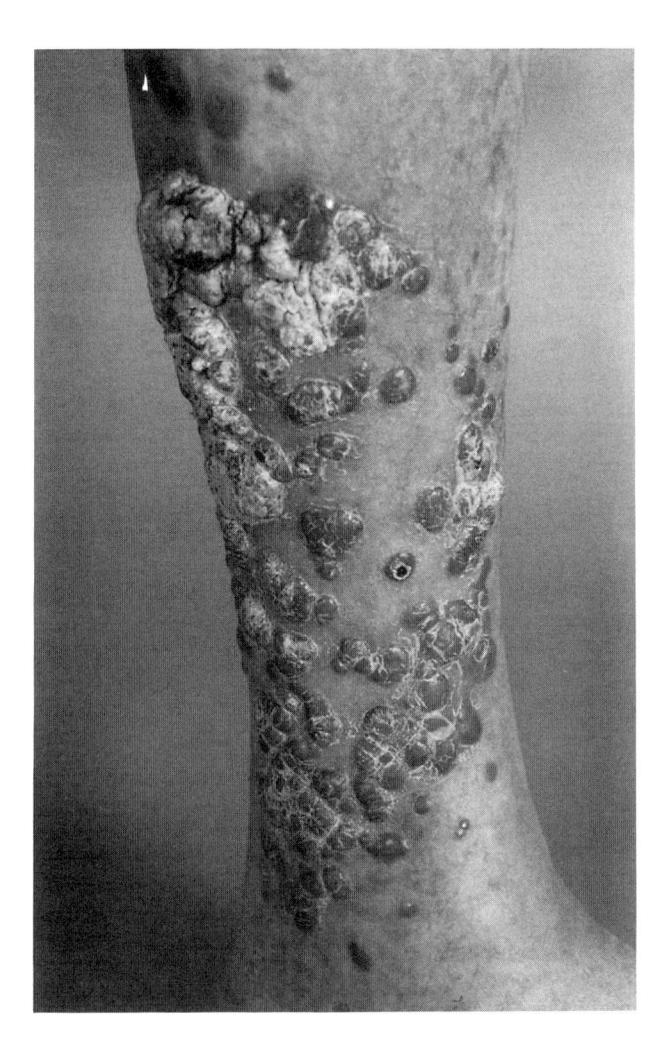

Figure 2. CD30- primary cutaneous T-cell lymphoma with multiple scaling nodules and tumors confluencing to hyperkeratotic plaques on the lower left leg.

common. The preferred mode of treatment is radiotherapy when the disease is localized to a small skin area. In the case that chemotherapy is indicated, (more skin sites are involved or the disease is disseminated to extracutaneous structures) often complete remission can be achieved[1].

2.4. Multidrug Resistance

Failure of multi-agent chemotherapy to induce a remission in cutaneous lymphomas may be due to pharmacokinetic mechanisms (low drug concentration at the level of the tumor cells).[3] However, in general multidrug resistance (MDR) is thought to result from processes at the cellular level.[4,5] Intrinsic drug resistance of tumor cells may be due to cell growth kinetics; in low grade tumors (lymphomas) a subpopulation of the tumor cells that is responsible for persistence and regrowth of the tumor, is in the G0-phase of the cell cycle, whereas rapidly proliferating cells are more vulnerable to the toxic effects of chemotherapy. Mechanisms involved in blocking the apoptotic pathway may also contribute to drugresistance.[6] In this study we focussed on the expression of multidrug resistance pro-

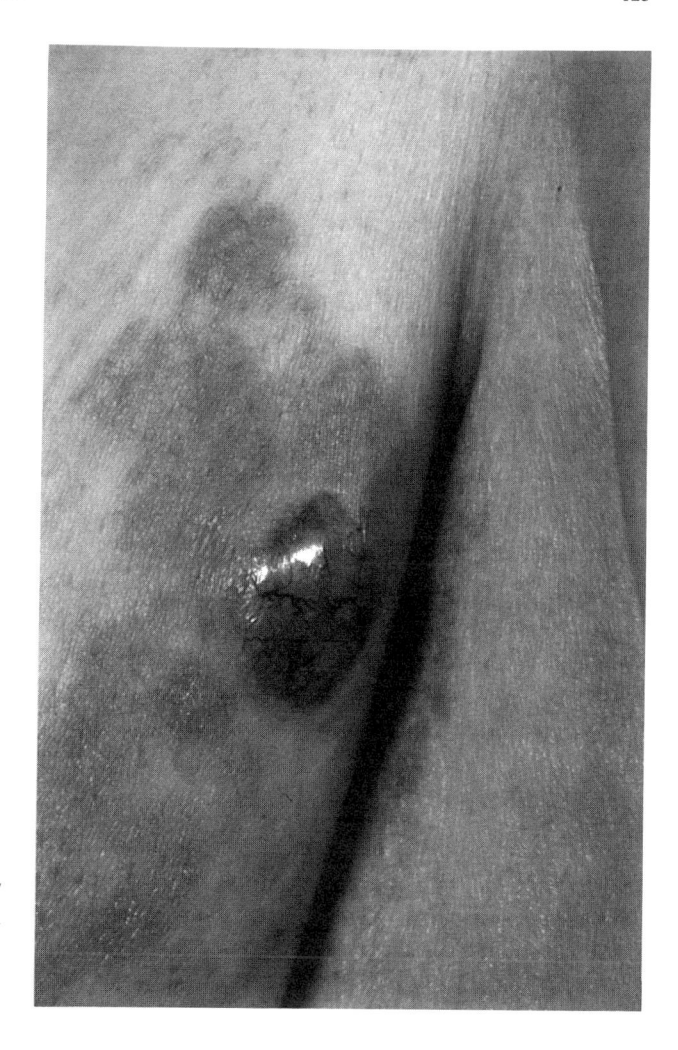

Figure 3. Cutaneous centroblastic/centrocytic B-cell lymphoma with a tumor with teleangiectasias on a non-infiltrated, sharply demarcated, irregular base on the right arm.

tein (MRP), lung resistance protein (LRP) and P-glycoprotein (Pgp), proteins associated with mechanisms that are capable to keep the cellular concentration of the drugs los (efflux of drugs, diminished drup uptake and sequestration). They have been grouped as MDR related proteins.[7]

P-glycoprotein (Pgp), a drug efflux protein, is capable to keep the cellular concentration of the drug low[8]. Expression of Pgp can be found on a subpopulation of normal hematopoietic stem cells and in many other cells of the body such as macrophages, stromal cells, lymphocytes, CD8+ T-cells and natural killer cells and also in hematological malignancies.[8]

MRP is also a drug efflux pump which was detected in a broad range of human tissues and in distinct tumor types.[9–12] However, in refractory lymphomas MRP expression was detected in the minority of the cases.[13]

LRP was first identified in a lung cancer cell line. LRP is like Pgp and MRP distributed in a range of normal human tissues. LRP is also expressed in many human cancer cell lines, significantly related with resistance to a variety of drugs. LRP is the major component of large cellular organelles called "vaults". The exact function of vaults is sofar unclear. LRP overexpression at diagnosis was found to be a strong and independent marker for (poor) respons to chemotherapy and unfavourable outcome in acute myeloid leukaemias and cisplatin-treated ovarium carcinomas.[14,15]

In this pilot study we investigated whether the clinical differences in therapy response of the selected primary cutaneous lymphomas are associated with a specific expression profile of the proteins MRP, LRP and Pgp.

3. PATIENTS AND METHODS

3.1. Patients

Thirty-two patients with a primary cutaneous lymphoma were selected from the files of the Dutch Cutaneous Lymphoma Working Group. The diagnosis was made according to the criteria of the European Organization for Research and Treatment of Cancer (EORTC) classification for primary cutaneous lymphomas.[1] The main clinicopathological data of the selected patients are summarized in Table 1.

Eight patients with untreated early mycosis fungoides (MF) (plaque/patch stage) and 6 patients treated with psoalen and ultraviolet A radiation with progressive disease into the tumor stage, were selected.

We compared plaques and tumors from one patient when available. Furthermore we compared tumorcells of MF patients with the CD4+/8- phenotype to those with the CD4-/8- phenotype.

In 6 selected MF cases we compared staining before and during therapy. In these cases punch biopsy specimens were taken from lesional skin both before and after 3 or 4 courses of polychemotherapy in patients with progressive disease.

In the group of 10 patients with a primary cutaneous large T-cell lymphoma (PCLTCL) we compared 3 CD30 positive to 7 CD30 negative lymphomas. Post treatment

Table 1. Summary of pretreatment staining results with Pgp, MRP and LRP for CD4+ vs CD4- MF, plaque vs tumor MF, CD30+ vs CD30- PCLTCL, and CBCL

	no/weak (<5%)			Positive (≥5%-50%)			Strong positive (≥50%)		
	Pgp	MRP	LRP	Pgp	MRP	LRP	Pgp	MRP	LRP
MF									
CD4+(n=10)	ND	1	9	ND	5	1	ND	4	0
CD4- (n=4)	ND	0	4	ND	1	0	ND	3	0
MF									
PL (n=8)	ND	1	8	ND	5	0	ND	2	0
TU (n=6)	ND	0	5	ND	1	1	ND	5	0
MF									
total (n=14)	ND	1	13	ND	6	1	ND	7	0
PCLTCL									
CD30- (n=7)	4	3	6	3	2	0	0	2	0
CD30+ (n=3)	2	1	3	1	1	1	0	1	0
PCLTCL									
total (n=10)	6	4	9	4	3	1	0	3	0
CBCL									
total (n=8)	6	6	7	2	2	1	0	0	0

ND = not done MF = mycosis fungoides PL = plaque TU = tumor PCLTCL = primary cutaneous large T-cell lymphoma CBCL = cutaneous B-cell lymphoma.

punch biopsy specimens from three patients who received multi-agent chemotherapy and had progressive disease during the disease course, were included.

Furthermore a group of patients with a primary cutaneous centroblastic/centrocytic B-cell lymphoma (CBCL) was selected. In one patient a post treatment punch biopsy specimen was available.

Patients with benign dermatoses (actinic reticuloid, lichen planus, pseudo T-cell lymphoma, pseudo B-cell lymphoma and eczema were included as controls).

3.2. Immunohistochemistry

Four micrometer sections of formaldehyde-fixed and paraffin-embedded tumor specimens were mounted on poly L-lysine-coated slides and dried overnight (37°C). Sections were then dewaxed and dehydrated. Endogenous peroxidase was blocked by incubation with 0.3% H_2O_2 in methanol. Antigen retrieval was done by heating in the microwave (3x5 min) (C219). For MRPr1 and LRP-56 an antigen retrieval was not done.

Non-specific binding sites were blocked by incubation with normal rabbit or normal goat serum (1:50 Dako, Kopenhagen, Denmark) followed by monoclonal antibodies MRPr1 (dil 1:50, rat IgG 2a), LRP-56 (dil 1:50, mouse IgG 2b) and C219 (dil 1:40, mouse Ig, Centocor). All dilutions were made in phosphate buffered saline and 1% bovine serum albumin.

Biotinylated rabbit anti-mouse immunoglobuline (1:150 Dako) and streptavidin-biotin horse-radish peroxidase complex (1:500 Zymed lab Inc, San Francisco, CA)) were employed as second and third steps. Bound peroxidase was developed with 4 mg (w/v) 3,3' diamino-benzidine-tetra hydrochloride and 0,02% H_2O_2 in phosphate buffered saline (Sigma, St. Louis, MO). The slides were counterstained with hematoxyllin and mounted. Epidermal staning was used as an internal positive control. Omission of the first antibody was used as a negative control. All incubations were performed at room temperature.

Immunostaining for MRPr1, LRP-56 and C219 was semi-quantitatively expressed as follows: no, weak (<5% positive tumor cells), positive (≥5%-50% positive tumor cells) and strongly positive staining (≥50% positive tumor cells). Immunostaining score was performed in the most representative part of the infiltrate, i.e. the most dense part with the fewest admixture with reactive cells. All slides were scored by two observers. No major discrepancies (>1 category) occurred, and smaller discrepancies in scoring results were resolved after parallel examination of the slides.

4. RESULTS

The pretreatment staining results for MRP, LRP and Pgp in primary cutaneous lymphomas are shown in Table 1.

4.1. MRP

MRPr1 was localized intracytoplasmatic in a granular fashion in keratinocytes and adnexal structures (internal positive control).

In most cases the tumor cells including T and B-cells showed often moderate to very strong granular, intracytoplasmatic staining in varying percentages of tumor cells. The staining intensity was related to the percentage of positive cells (so where ≥ 50% of the cells stained, the cells stained (very) strong). Interestingly the infiltrate cells showed a

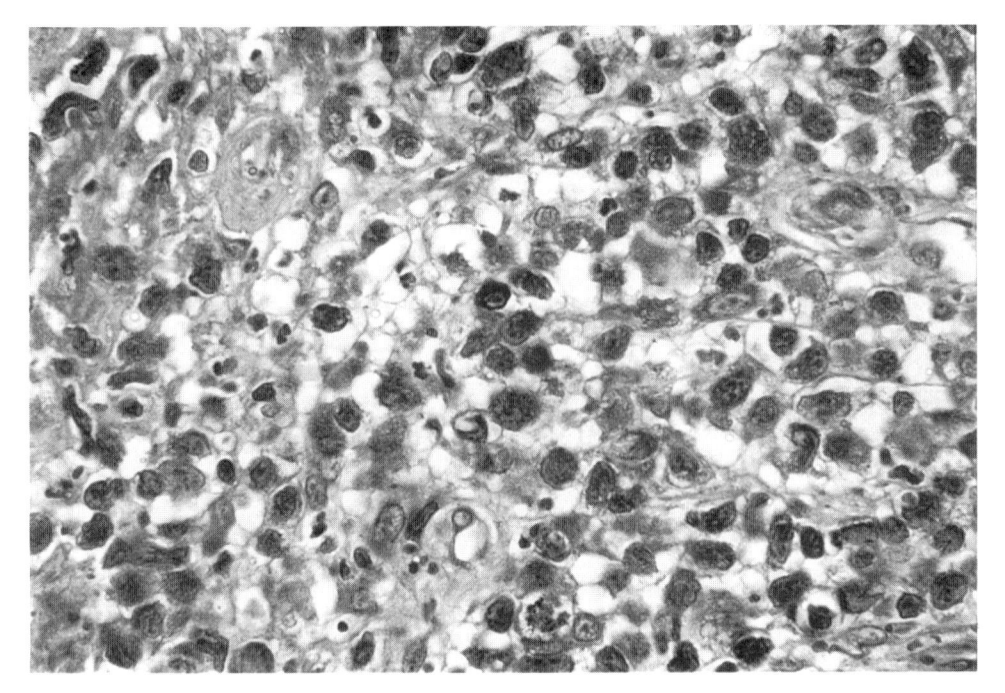

Figure 4. Tumor stage MF. Very strong immunostaining of virtually all tumor cells with MRPr1. (Original magnification x 600, hematoxyllin counterstaining).

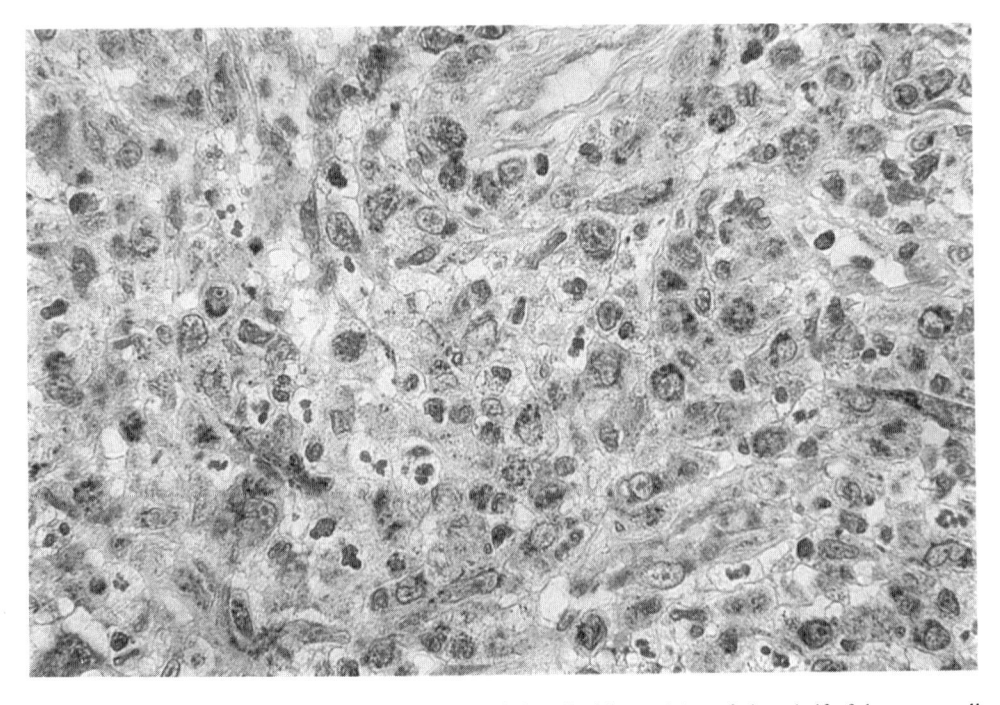

Figure 5. CD30+ PCLTCL, anaplastic subtype. Tumor lesion. Positive staining of about half of the tumor cells with MRPr1 (x600).

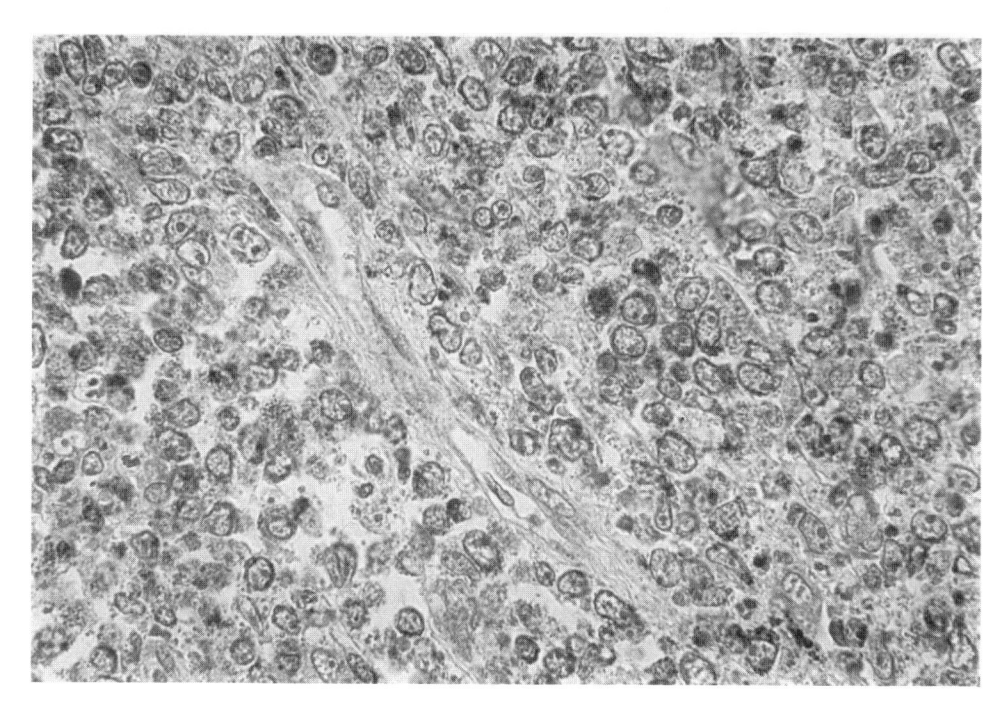

Figure 6. Malignant B-cell lymphoma (centrocytic/centroblastic subtype). Nodular lesion. MRPr1 immunostaining shows about 30% positive cells (x600).

varying staining intensity. For instance larger tumor cells and blast forms showed stronger staining than smaller tumor cells. Furthermore, T-cell lymphomas showed stronger staining intensity and number of positive cells than B-cell lymphomas. Reactive, non-malignant cells in the infiltrate were weakly MRP positive in both types of lymphomas and also in benign dermatoses.

With MRPr1 6 out of 14 MF cases were positive. Three out of 10 cases of PCLTCL were positive (no clear difference between the CD30+ and CD30- group). Two out of 8 cases of CBCL were positive.

Strong positive staining; ($\geq$ 50% of the tumor cells stain (very) strong), was found in 7 out of 14 cases of MF, 3 out of 10 cases of PCLTCL and in none of the cases of CBCL.

Within the MF group strong positive MRPr1 staining was found in 5 out of 6 cases of tumor stage MF in both the plaque and the tumor in the same patient. Two out of 8 cases of plaque stage MF were scored "strong positive". Furthermore CD4-, 8- cases of MF were strong positive in 3 out of 4 cases as compared to 4 out of 10 cases with CD4+, 8- MF. In the group of CTCL a slight increase in staining intensity was found in pre-treatment punch biopsy specimens as compared to punch biopsy specimens from lesional skin after polychemotherapy: A slight increase from "positive" to "strong positive" after multi-agent chemotherapy was found in 3 out of 6 cases of MF and in 1 out of 3 cases of PCLTCL (after radiotherapy). About the same staining score was found in 2 out of 6 cases of MF, in 1 out of 3 cases of PCLTCL and the only case of CBCL remained negative after multi-agent chemotherapy. Decrease in staining after chemotherapy was also seen in one case of MF and in one case of PCLTCL. In this latter case the punch biopsy specimen was taken from a patient with a good response to therapy.

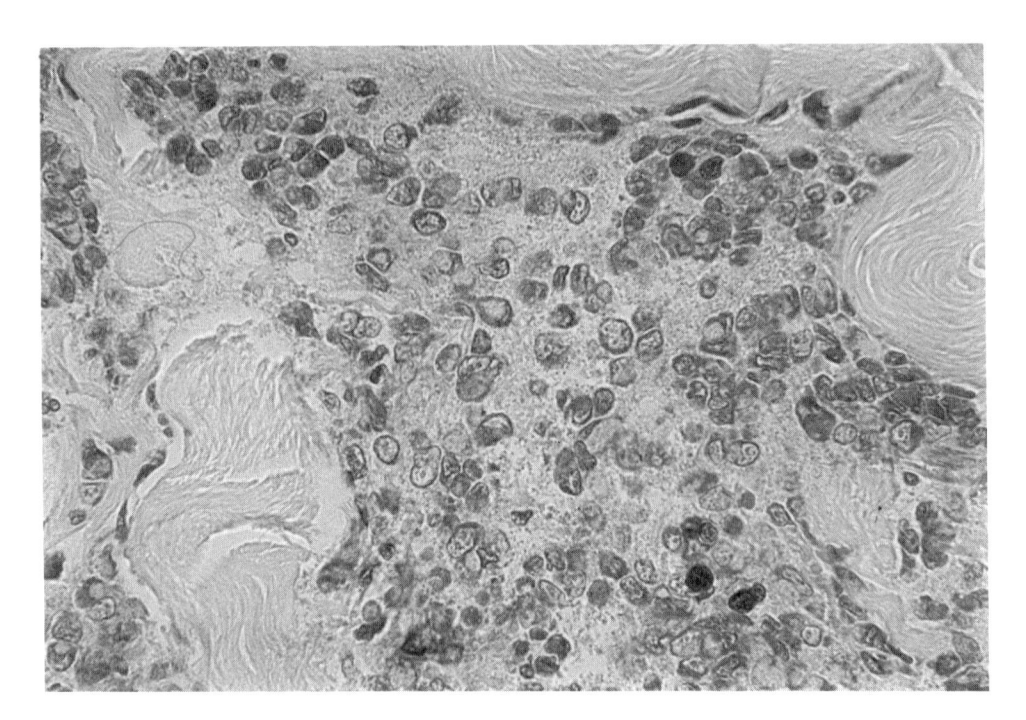

Figure 7. LRP56 immunostaining in tumorstage mycosis fungoides. About 30% of the tumor cells is positive (x600).

4.2. LRP

LRP56 positive staining of the keratinocyte cytoplasm in a granular fashion, was seen.

Tumor cells (i.e., cells with cerebriform nuclei; blast forms and large anaplastic cells) were positive (cytoplasmatic staining) in only one CD4+/8- case of tumor stage MF and in one case of CD30+ PCLTCL. In one case of CBCL both centroblasts and centrocytes were positive. We found no differences in pre- and posttreatment punch biopsy specimens. (The same negative staining score in all 6 cases of MF, in 2 cases of PCLTCL and in the only case of CBCL; except for one case with negative staining after multi-agent chemotherapy induced clinical remission).

4.3. Pgp

Weak cytoplasmatic staining of keratinocytes was found in all cases tested (C219 MoAb). In a case of PCLTCL 30+ strong staining cells were found that were identified as eosinophils. The specificity of this staining could not be identified. Weak cytoplasmatic staining of about 20% of the tumor cells was found in 1 out of 6 patients with MF (other 8 cases not done).

Three out of 7 CD30- and 1 out of 3 CD30+ PCLTCL cases stained positive. No strong positive cases were found. Two out of 8 cases of CBCL were positive for Pgp.

No changes in staining score were found in MF cases before and after treatment. Also staining of tumor cells in cases of PCLTCL after multi-agent chemotherapy remained about the same. One case of CBCL remained negative after three unsuccesful courses of multi-agent chemotherapeutic treatment.

We found no associations between the expression of the three different MDR related proteins.

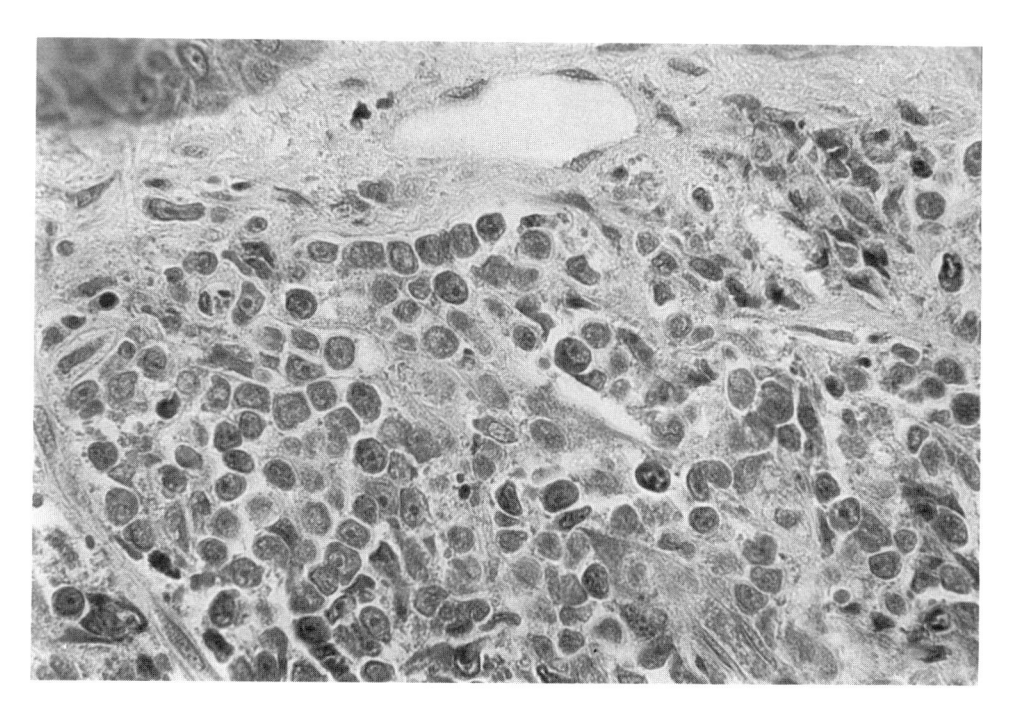

Figure 8. CD30- PCLTCL, immunoblastic subtype. Tumor lesion. Immunostaining with C219 shows about 30% positive cells (x600).

5. DISCUSSION

During the past decade, several different parameters have been found to be of prognostic value in patients with primary cutaneous lymphomas.[1] For clinicans who have a major interest in predicting the patient's response to treatment, the detection of chemotherapy resistant cells at diagnosis may have diagnostic and prognostic implications and may even influence choice of therapy.[16]

It is tempting to evaluate the expression of MDR related proteins in primary cutaneous lymphomas with a divers clinical behaviour and as a most conspicious feature, a diversity in response to chemotherapy.[1] In extracutaneous non Hodgkin's lymphomas the MDR phenotype has been described.[13] However, it is difficult to elaborate the contribution to clinical drug resistance in refractory lymphomas.[13] Multi-agent chemotherapy may induce long lasting remissions in CBCL. However, patients with MF and CD30- PCLTCL have a poor prognosis in the case that extracutaneous sites are involved because they respond poorly or partially to multi-agent chemotherapy. In contrast to CD30- PCLTCL, CD30+ PCLTCL have an excellent prognosis with a good response to therapy.[1]

5.1. MRP

MRP expression in primary cutaneous lymphomas has not yet been investigated. In this study we found that MRP expression in MF was common. A staining percentage of 5–50% tumor cells was found in 6 out of 14 patients and strong positive staining (≥50% tumor cells positive) was seen in 7 out of 14 patients with a tendency of stronger staining of MF cells in tumor stage MF in both plaque and tumor lesions. Also the CD4-/8- phenotype was associated with stronger staining as compared to the CD4+/8- phenotype. In MF loss of CD antigens is an indication for tumor progression.[1] Therefore these findings suggest that disease progression in MF as reflected by the formation of tumors and loss of the CD4 marker may be associated with increased MRP expression.

In half of the MF cases a slight increase in MRP expression in posttreatment punch biopsies of therapy resistant lesions was found. This finding corresponds with a study of Zhan et al., who quantified MRP expression in relapsed and refractory lymphoma.[13] Elevated MRP expression in a subgroup of MF patients might indicate a selection of chemoresistant subclones although we cannot prove whether this reflects a pure MRP mediated selection or whether this selection is the result of other mechanisms[6] with only a secondary contribution of MRP or, as a third possibility, is related aspecifically with disease progression.[1]

MRP expression in PCLTCL was in general less strong as compared to MF cases. As a most conspicuous finding we did not find differences between the CD30+ and CD30- patients.

Upregulation of MRP expression was found in only one case of PCLTCL in a punch biopsy of lesional skin after relapse following radiotherapy. This finding indicates a nonspecific upregulation, probably related to tumor progression.

MRP expression in CBCL was less frequently found and the staining intensity was much weaker as compared to the group of CTCL.

5.2. LRP

LRP expression was uncommon in cases of MF and PCLTCL, so LRP expression in MF seems not contributing to drug resistance in the majority of the cases. Overexpression in a MF-patient after multi-agent chemotherapy and LRP expression in a CD30- PCLTCL before multi-agent chemotherapy with decreased staining intensity in a regressing lesion after succesfull multi-agent chemotherapy indicates that LRP expression might play a role in a subgroup of CTCL although the same reserves as mentioned for MRP are applicable.

LRP expression was found in none of the patients with a cutaneous B-cell lymphoma.

5.3. Pgp

Cytoplasmatic Pgp expression was found in only 1 out of 6 cases of MF. However, there was no increase after therapy. Weak cytoplasmatic Pgp expression was found in small percentages in PCLTCL and in analogy with MRP and LRP expression not related to the expression of the CD30 antigen.

Like in MF cases Pgp expression seems not relevant for PCLTCL and cutaneous B-cell lymphomas (weak cytoplasmatic staining in a minority of the cases).

In conclusion it is indicated that lymphoid cells in CBCL and CTCL may have an intrinsic drug resistance as indicated by the expression of one or more MDR related proteins. Especially MRP expression reflected by MRPr1 staining, might play a role in CTCL (increased expression after multi-agent chemotherapy and in progressive disease in MF, stronger expression in the CTCL group as compared to the CBCL group). LRP expression may be important in a subgroup of CTCL. The value of Pgp expression in this group is not clear. Understanding of the phenomenon of drugresistance in primary cutaneous lymphomas is warranted, several different mechanisms may be involved in MDR in some of these lymphomas. However, these study illustrates the complexity of the MDR phenotype.

REFERENCES

1. Willemze R, Kerl H. Sterry W, Berti E, Cerroni L, Chimenti S, Diaz-Peréz JL, Geerts ML, Goos M, Knobler R, Ralfkiaer E, Santucci M, Smith N, Wechsler J, Van Vloten WA, Meijer CJLM. EORTC classification for primary cutaneous lymphomas: A proposal from the cutaneous lymphomas study group of the European Organization for Research and Treatment of Cancer. *Blood* 1997; 90: 354–71.
2. Kay FJ, Bunn PA, Steinberg SM. A randomized trial comparing combination electron beam radiation and chemotherapy with topical therapy in the initial treatment of mycosis fungoides. *N Engl J Med* 1989; 321, 1784.
3. Pui C, Relling MV, Mason E, Rivera GK, Crist WM, Evans WE. Pharmacokinetic resistance in childhood leukaemia. *In: drug resistance in leukaemia and lymphoma II*. Eds. R. Pieters, GJL Kaspers and AJP Veerman. Harwood Academic Publishers 1997 The Netherlands pp 1–7.
4. Rossi JF. Biological and clinical aspects of chemoresistance. Part 2: leukaemias. *Retinoids today and tomorrow* 1996; 45: 28–31.
5. Yuen AR, Sikic BI. Multidrug resistance in lymphomas. *J Clin Oncol* 1994; 12: 2453–2459.
6. Landowski TH, Gleason-Guzman MC, Dalton WS. Selection for drug resistance results in resistance to fas-mediated apoptosis. *Blood* 1997; 89: 1854–61.
7. den Boer ML, Zwaan MC, Pieters R, Kazemier KM, Rottier MMA, Flens MJ, Scheper RJ and Veerman AJ. Optimal immunocytochemical and flow cytometric detection of Pgp, MRP and LRP in childhood acute lymphoblastic leukemia. *Leukemia* 1997; 11: 1078–85.
8. Marie JP. P-glycoprotein in adult hematologic malignancies. *Hematology/oncology clinics of North-America* 1995; 9: 239–48.
9. Legrand O, Perrot JY, Tang R, Simonin G, Gurbuxani S, Zittoun R, Marie JP. Expression of the multidrug resistance-associated protein (MRP) MRNA and protein in normal peripheral blood and bone marrow haemopoietic cells. *Br J Haematol* 1996; 94: 23–33.
10. Flens MJ, Izquierdo MA, Scheffer GL, Fritz JM, Meijer CJLM, Scheper RJ and Zaman GJR. Immunochemical detection of the multidrug resistance-associated protein MRP in human multidrug-resistant tumor cells by monoclonal antibodies. *Cancer Res* 1994; 54: 4557–63.
11. Nooter K, Westerman MA, Flens MJ, Zaman GJR, Scheper RJ, van Wingerden KE, Burger H, Oostrum R, Boersma T, Sonneveld P, Gratema JW, Kok T, Eggermont AMM, Bosman FT and Stoter G. Expression of the multidrug resistance-associated protein (MRP) gene in human cancers. *Clin Cancer Res 1995*; 147: 1545–52.
12. Flens MF, Zaman GJR, van der Valk P, Izquierdo MA, Schroeijers AB, Scheffer GL, van der Groep P, de Haas M, Meijer CJLM and Scheper RJ. Tissue distribution of the multidrug resistance protein. *Am J Pathol* 1996; 148: 1237–47.
13. Zhan Z, Sandor VA, Gamelin E, Regis J, Dickstein B, Wilson W, Fojo AT, Bates SE. Expression of the multidrug resistance-associated protein gene in refractory lymphoma: Quantitation by a validated polymerase chain reaction assay. *Blood* 1997; 89: 3795–3800.
14. Izquierdo MA, Scheffer GL, Flens MF, Schroeijers AB, van der Valk P and Scheper RJ. Major vault protein LRP-related multidrug resistance. *Eur J Cancer* 1996; 32A: 979–84.
15. Izquierdo MA, Scheffer GL, Flens MJ, Giaccone G, Broxterman HJ, Meijer CJLM, van der Valk P and Scheper RJ. Broad distribution of the multidrug resistance-related vault lung resistance protein in normal human tissues and tumors. *Am J Pathol* 1996; 148: 877–87.
16. Wilson WH, Bates SE, Fojo A, Bryant G et al. Controlled trial of dexverapamil, a modulator of multidrug resistance, in lymphomas refractory to EPOCH chemotherapy. *J Clin Oncol* 1995; 13: 1995–2004.

THE LUNG RESISTANCE PROTEIN (LRP) PREDICTS POOR OUTCOME IN ACUTE MYELOID LEUKEMIA

Robert Pirker, Gudrun Pohl, Thomas Stranzl, Ralf W. Suchomel, Rik J. Scheper,[*] Ulrich Jäger, Klaus Geissler, Klaus Lechner, and Martin Filipits

Divisions of Oncology and Hematology
Department of Internal Medicine I
University of Vienna Medical School
Währinger Gürtel 18, A-1090 Vienna, Austria

Keywords: lung resistance protein, LRP, drug resistance, acute myeloid leukemia, prognosis.

1. ABSTRACT

To determine the clinical significance of the lung resistance protein (LRP) in acute myeloid leukemia (AML), we have studied LRP expression of leukemic blasts and its association with clinical outcome in patients with de novo AML. LRP expression of leukemic blasts was determined by immunocytochemistry by means of monoclonal antibody LRP-56. LRP expression at diagnosis was detected in 31 out of 86 (36%) patients and correlated with white blood cell count (p = 0.01). The complete remission rate of induction chemotherapy was 72% for all treated patients (n = 82). The complete remission rate was 81% for patients without LRP expression but only 55% for patients with LRP expression (p = 0.01). Overall survival and disease-free survival were estimated according to Kaplan-Meier in 82 and 59 patients, respectively. At a median follow-up of 16 months, median overall survival was 17 months for LRP-negative patients but only 8 months for LRP-positive patients (p = 0.006). Disease-free survival was 9 months for LRP-negative patients and 6 months for LRP-positive patients (p = 0.078). Thus LRP predicts for poor outcome indicating that the LRP gene is a clinically relevant drug resistance gene in AML.

---

[*] Department of Pathology, Free University Hospital, 1007 MB Amsterdam, The Netherlands.

2. INTRODUCTION

Drug resistance remains a major problem in the treatment of acute myeloid leukemia (AML). Potential resistance mechanisms are those involved in the multidrug resistance (MDR) phenotype.[1,2] They include the MDR1 gene[1] and the multidrug resistance protein (MRP) gene.[3] Expression of MDR1 RNA as well as P-gp have been shown to be associated with worse outcome in AML.[4-7] MRP expression did not predict for clinical outcome in the initial analysis of our study.[8] However, an update of this study showed a trend toward shorter survival for patients with intermediate or high MRP levels as compared to patients with low levels.[9] In the subgroup of patients with inversion in chromosome 16, patients with a deletion of the MRP gene had a longer overall and disease-free survival.[10] Whether MRP gene deletion is the reason for the good prognosis of patients with inversion in chromosome 16 remains unclear, because lack of MDR1 RNA/P-gp expression might also explain the good prognosis of patients with this AML subtype.[11]

Recently, the lung resistance protein (LRP) was detected in MDR cell lines and its gene has been cloned.[12,13] The LRP gene is homologous to the major vault protein of the rat. Vaults are ribonucleoprotein particles which are located in the cytoplasm and probably involved in transport processes.[14,15] LRP is thus believed to contribute to the drug resistance of these cell lines, probably via affecting drug transport. LRP overexpression is associated with resistance to doxorubicin, vincristine, carboplatin, cisplatin and melphalan.[16] LRP is overexpressed in normal colon tissue, normal lung tissue, renal proximal tubules, adrenal cortex and macrophages,[17] but its physiological function remains to be evaluated. To determine whether LRP is a clinically relevant drug resistance gene in AML, we have studied LRP expression of leukemic cells and its relationship to clinical outcome in previously untreated patients with de novo AML. Here we summarize the results of this study which has been published in more detail elsewhere.[18]

3. PATIENTS AND METHODS

3.1. Patients

Eighty-six patients (37 females, 49 males) with de novo AML were studied (Table 1). Eighty-two patients received standard induction chemotherapy protocols, whereas 4 patients did not receive chemotherapy (Table 1). Treatment consisted of daunorubicin 45 mg/m^2 daily on days 1–3 and cytarabine 200 mg/m^2 daily on days 1–7 (DA protocol) in 21 patients and additional etoposide 100 mg/m^2 daily on days 1–5 (DAE protocol) in 50 patients. Three patients were treated with idarubicin plus cytarabine (IA protocol). Six patients with FAB subtype M3 received all-trans retinoic acid (ATRA) prior to chemotherapy. Two patients received intermediate-dose cytarabine followed by DAE as second induction chemotherapy cycle. Response to induction chemotherapy was assessed according to standard criteria. Fifty-six out of 59 patients in complete remission received consolidation therapy. Seventeen patients underwent bone marrow transplantation.

3.2. Immunocytochemistry

Mononuclear cells were isolated from either peripheral blood (n = 37), bone marrow (n = 36) aspirates or both sources (n = 13) by Ficoll-Paque (Pharmacia) gradient centrifu-

Table 1. Characteristics of patients

	All patients	LRP-negative patients	(%)	LRP-positive patients	(%)	P
No. of patients	86	55	(100)	31	(100)	
Age (years)						
Median	56	54		61		0.1†*
Range	15-88	15-88		18-82		
Patients 50 years	52	31	(56)	21	(68)	0.3‡
Sex (F/M)	37/49	22/33		15/16		
White blood cell count						
Median	21750	14380		52300		0.01†
Range	400-280700	400-250000		740-280700		
FAB subtype						
M0	5	2	(4)	3	(10)	0.2*
M1	16	9	(17)	7	(23)	
M2	22	17	(31)	5	(16)	
M3	9	8	(15)	1	(3)	
M4	16	9	(16)	7	(23)	
M4Eo	5	3	(5)	2	(6)	
M5	10	4	(7)	6	(19)	
M6	3	3	(5)	0	(0)	
Lactate dehydrogenase (U/l)						
Median	463	433		583		0.1†
Range	104-3800	104-2460		194-3800		
Karyotype (n=79)						
Good prognosis#	20	16	(29)	4	(13)	0.3*
Intermediate prognosis	29	19	(35)	10	(32)	
Poor prognosis	30	17	(31)	13	(42)	
Induction therapy						
DA	21	14	(25)	7	(23)	0.4*
DAE	50	31	(56)	19	(62)	
IA	3	1	(2)	2	(6)	
ATRA + DA or DAE	6	6	(11)	0	(0)	
Intermed.-dose cytarabine + DAE	2	1	(2)	1	(3)	
None	4	2	(4)	2	(6)	
Bone marrow transplantation	17	13	(24)	4	(13)	

†Kruskal-Wallis test
‡Chi-square test
§Fisher's exact test
*Exact chi-square test
¶Protocols and karyotype classification are described in 'Patients and Methods'
#Good prognosis versus all other karyotypes: p=0.1

gation. Smears were prepared and stored at -20°C until use. Cells were fixed in cold acetone and incubated in 3% H_2O_2 in order to block endogenous peroxidase activity. Immunocytochemistry was performed with the monoclonal antibody LRP-56 as described.[18] Antibody binding was detected by the avidin-biotin-peroxidase method. The slides were counterstained with Mayer's Hämalaun and mounted with Aquatex (Merck). All washes were performed in phosphate-buffered saline.

The small-cell lung cancer cell line SW1573 and its drug-resistant variant SW1573/2R120 were used as negative and positive controls for LRP expression, respectively.[12,13] In addition, experiments without the monoclonal antibody LRP-56 were used as negative controls.

3.3. Survival Analysis

Survival durations were estimated according to Kaplan-Meier.[19] Overall survival was measured from the time of diagnosis until the time of either death or last control. Disease-free survival was measured from the time of complete remission until the time of relapse or death. Patients who underwent bone marrow transplantation were censored at the time of transplantation.

3.4. Statistical Analysis

Frequencies were tested by chi-square analysis or Fisher's exact test. In addition, Kruskal-Wallis tests were performed. Comparisons of survival curves were done with the log-rank test.

4. RESULTS

LRP expression was immunocytochemically determined by means of the monoclonal antibody LRP-56 and samples were scored LRP-positive if ≥5% of the blasts were stained. LRP was positive in 31 out of 86 (36%) patients (Table 1). In those 13 cases where samples from both sources were studied, no differences between peripheral and bone marrow blasts were observed (data not shown).

LRP expression correlated with white blood cell count (p=0.01) but was independent of age, percentage of patients older than 50 years, sex and serum lactate dehydrogenase levels (Table 1). Interestingly, 8/9 (89%) patients with promyelocytic leukemia (FAB M3) did not express LRP but this was not significantly different from other FAB subtypes (p=0.1). Patients with inv16, t(8;21) or t(15;17) were categorized as good prognosis patients and they showed a trend (p=0.1) toward negative LRP (Table 1).

Eighty-two patients received standard induction chemotherapy. The treatment protocols were not different between LRP-negative and LRP-positive patients (Table 1). The complete remission rate of induction chemotherapy was 72% for all treated patients. Resistant disease (after at least two treatment cycles) and early death (within four weeks after begin of treatment) occurred in 11% and 12% of the patients, respectively. Four (5%) patients were not evaluable because they received only one treatment cycle which did not result in complete remission. The complete remission rate was 81% for patients without LRP expression but only 55% for patients with LRP expression (p=0.01) (Table 2). Resistant disease was seen in 4 (8%) LRP-negative and in 5 (17%) LRP-positive patients. Early death occurred in 5 (9%) negative and 5 (17%) positive patients (Table 2).

Overall survival and disease-free survival were estimated according to Kaplan-Meier in 82 and 59 patients, respectively. Relapses and deaths occurred in 41 and 54 patients, respectively. At a median follow-up of 16 months, median overall survival was 17 months for LRP-negative patients but only 8 months for LRP-positive patients (p=0.006) (Figure 1). Median disease-free survival was 9 months for LRP-negative and 6 months for LRP-positive patients (p=0.078) (Figure 2).

Table 2. LRP and outcome of induction chemotherapy

	No. of patients	Complete remission	Resistant disease	Early death	Not evaluable
Total	82	59 (72%)	9 (11%)	10 (12%)	4 (5%)
LRP⁻ patients	53	43 (81%)	4 (8%)	5 (9%)	1 (2%)
LRP⁺ patients	29	16 (55%)	5 (17%)	5 (17%)	3 (11%)

LRP expression of leukemic cells was compared with outcome of induction chemotherapy.
Induction chemotherapy protocols are described in 'Patients and Methods'.
Statistical analysis (chi-square test) for complete remission: p=0.01

5. DISCUSSION

In the present study, LRP expression of leukemic cells was observed in 36% of AML patients at diagnosis and did predict for both poor response to induction chemotherapy and shorter survival. The association of LRP expression with poor outcome stresses the clinical relevance of LRP and also suggests that drug resistance in AML is multifactorial, involving at least P-gp and LRP.

Similar percentages of LRP expression were reported by others.[17,20] The association of LRP expression with shorter survival is consistent with the findings by List et al. who reported a trend of LRP expression toward worse outcome on a heterogenous study population that included patients with de novo, secondary or relapsed AML.[20]

Although an association of LRP expression with high WBC was seen (Table 1), the poor outcome of LRP-positive patients cannot be explained by their higher WBC because in our study WBC had no impact on clinical outcome (data not shown). Lack of LRP expression in most FAB M3 patients (Table 1) might contribute to the good response to anthracyclines as well as good prognosis of this AML subtype.[21]

In conclusion, the LRP gene appears to be another clinically relevant drug resistance gene in AML. This will have to be considered in the planning of strategies to overcome drug resistance in this disease and warrants the development of modifiers not only of P-gp function[22,23] but also of LRP function.

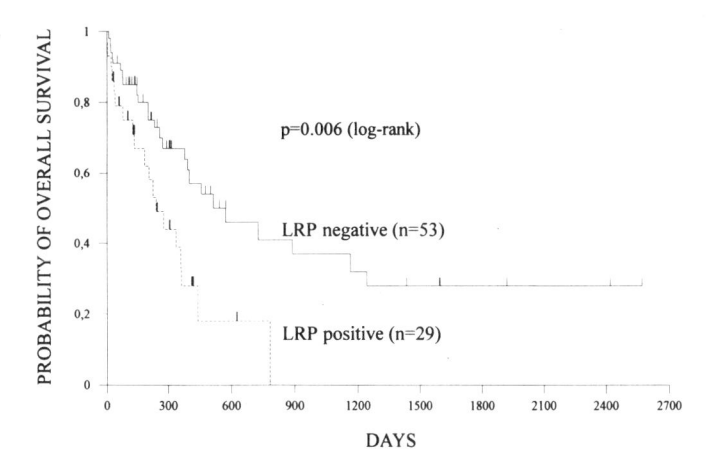

Figure 1. LRP and overall survival. Overall survival was estimated according to Kaplan-Meier in 82 patients. Survival data based on LRP expression are shown.

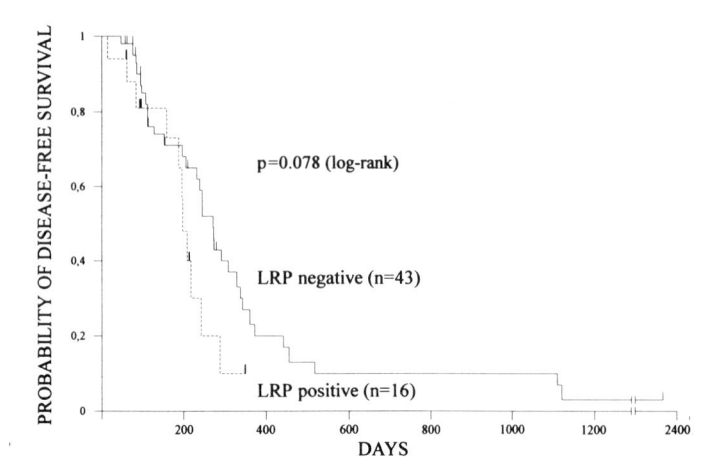

Figure 2. LRP and disease-free survival. Disease-free survival based on LRP expression was estimated according to Kaplan-Meier in 59 patients.

ACKNOWLEDGMENT

This study was supported by the 'Fonds zur Förderung der wissenschaftlichen Forschung' (project number P12264-MED).

REFERENCES

1. Pastan I, Gottesman M. Multiple-drug resistance in human cancer. N Engl J Med 1987, 316, 1388–1393
2. Filipits M, Suchomel RW, Zöchbauer S, Malayeri R, Pirker R. Clinical relevance of drug resistance genes in malignant diseases. Leukemia 1996, 10 (Suppl. 3), 10–17
3. Cole SPC, Bhardwaj G, Gerlach JH, Mackie JE, Grant CE, Almquist KC, Stewart AJ, Kurz EU, Duncan AMV, Deeley RG. Overexpression of a transporter gene in a multidrug-resistant human lung cancer cell line. Science 1992, 258, 1650–1654
4. Pirker R, Wallner J, Geissler K, Linkesch W, Haas OA, Bettelheim P, Hopfner M, Scherrer R, Valent P, Havelec L, Ludwig H, Lechner K. MDR1 gene expression and treatment outcome in acute myeloid leukemia. J Natl Cancer Inst 1991, 83, 708–712
5. Marie J-P, Zittoun R, Sikic BI. Multidrug resistance (mdr1) gene expression in adult acute leukemias: correlations with treatment outcome and in vitro drug sensitivity. Blood 1991, 78, 586–592
6. Campos L, Guyotat D, Archimbaud E, Calmard-Oriol P, Tsuruo T, Troncy J, Treille D, Fiere D. Clinical significance of multidrug resistance P-glycoprotein expression on acute nonlymphoblastic leukemia cells at diagnosis. Blood 1992, 79, 473–476
7. Zöchbauer S, Gsur A, Brunner R, Kyrle PA, Lechner K, Pirker R. P-glycoprotein expression as unfavorable prognostic factor in acute myeloid leukemia. Leukemia 1994, 8, 974–977
8. Filipits M, Suchomel RW, Zöchbauer S, Brunner R, Lechner K, Pirker R: Multidrug resistance-associated protein (MRP) in acute myeloid leukemia: no impact on treatment outcome. Clin Cancer Res 1997, 3, 1419–1425
9. Filipits M, Stranzl T, Pohl G, Suchomel RW, Zöchbauer S, Brunner R, Lechner K, Pirker R. MRP expression in acute myeloid leukemia: an update. This volume (Chapter 16)
10. Kuss BJ, Deeley RG, Cole SPC, Willman CL, Kopecky KJ, Wolman SR, Eyre HJ, Lane SA, Nancarrow JK, Whitmore SA, Callen DF. Deletion of gene for multidrug resistance in acute myeloid leukaemia with inversion in chromosome 16: prognostic implications. Lancet 1994, 343, 1531–1534
11. Zöchbauer S, Haas OA, Schwarzinger I, Lechner K, Pirker R. Multidrug resistance in acute myeloid leukaemia with inversion in chromosome 16 or FAB M4Eo subtype. Lancet 1994, 344, 894

12. Scheper RJ, Broxterman HJ, Scheffer GL, Kaaijk P, Dalton WS, van Heijningen THM, van Kalken CK, Slovak ML, de Vries EGE, van der Valk P, Meijer CJLM, Pinedo HM. Overexpression of a M_r 110,000 vesicular protein in non-P-glycoprotein-mediated multidrug resistance. Cancer Res 1993, 53, 1475–1479
13. Scheffer GL, Wijngaard PLJ, Flens MJ, Izquierdo MA, Slovak ML, Pinedo HM, Meijer CJLM, Clevers HC, Scheper RJ. The drug resistance-related protein LRP is the human major vault protein. Nat Med 1995, 1, 578–582
14. Kedersha NL, Miquel M-C, Bittner D, Rome LH. Vaults. II. Ribonucleoprotein structures are highly conserved among higher and lower eukaryotes. J Cell Biol 1990, 110, 895–901
15. Rome L, Kedersha N, Chugani D: Unlocking vaults: organelles in search of a function. Trends Cell Biol 1991, 1, 47–50
16. Izquierdo MA, Shoemaker RH, Flens MJ, Scheffer GL, Wu L, Prather TR, Scheper RJ. Overlapping phenotypes of multidrug resistance among panels of human cancer-cell lines. Int J Cancer 1996, 65, 230–237
17. Izquierdo MA, Scheffer GL, Flens MJ, Giaccone G, Broxterman HJ, Meijer CJLM, van der Valk P, Scheper RJ. Broad distribution of the multidrug resistance-related vault lung resistance protein in normal human tissues and tumors. Am J Pathol 1996, 148, 877–887
18. Filipits M, Pohl G, Stranzl T, Suchomel RW, Scheper RJ, Jäger U, Geissler K, Lechner K, Pirker R. Expression of the lung resistance protein predicts poor outcome in de novo acute myeloid leukemia. Blood 1998, 91, 1508–1513
19. Kaplan EL, Meier P. Nonparametric estimation from incomplete observations. J Am Stat Assoc 1958, 53, 457–481
20. List AF, Spier CS, Grogan TM, Johnson C, Roe DJ, Greer JP, Wolff SN, Broxterman HJ, Scheffer GL, Scheper RJ, Dalton WS. Overexpression of the major vault transporter protein lung-resistance protein predicts treatment outcome in acute myeloid leukemia. Blood 1996, 87, 2464–2469
21. Ghaddar HM, Plunkett W, Kantarjian HM, Pierce S, Freireich EJ, Keating MJ, Estey EH. Long-term results following treatment of newly-diagnosed acute myelogenous leukemia with continuous-infusion high-dose cytosine arabinoside. Leukemia 1994, 8, 1269–1274
22. Lum BL, Fisher GA, Brophy NA, Yahanda AM, Adler KM, Kaubisch S, Halsey J, Sikic BI. Clinical trials of modulation of multidrug resistance. Cancer 1993, 72, 3502–3514
23. Pirker R, Keilhauer G, Raschack M, Lechner C, Ludwig H. Reversal of multi-drug resistance in human KB cell lines by structural analogs of verapamil. Int J Cancer 1990, 45, 916–919

# MRP EXPRESSION IN ACUTE MYELOID LEUKEMIA

An Update

Martin Filipits, Thomas Stranzl, Gudrun Pohl, Ralf W. Suchomel, Sabine Zöchbauer, Raoul Brunner, Klaus Lechner, and Robert Pirker

Divisions of Oncology and Hematology
Department of Internal Medicine I
University of Vienna Medical School
Währinger Gürtel 18, A-1090 Vienna, Austria

Keywords: acute myeloid leukemia, drug resistance, MRP, multidrug resistance, prognosis.

1. ABSTRACT

To determine the clinical significance of the multidrug resistance protein (MRP) in patients with de novo AML, we have studied MRP expression of leukemic cells at diagnosis and its association with clinical outcome in 127 patients. MRP expression was determined by immunocytochemistry by means of monoclonal antibodies QCRL-1/QCRL-3. MRP expression was low, intermediate and high in 30%, 46% and 24% of the patients, respectively. MRP expression was independent of age and sex of the patients, white blood cell count, FAB subtype, serum lactate dehydrogenase levels and karyotype aberrations. MRP expression had no impact on response to induction chemotherapy. The complete remission rates were 75%, 70% and 64% for patients with low, intermediate and high expression, respectively. Patients with intermediate or high MRP expression showed a trend toward shorter overall survival (p=0.09) as compared to patients with low MRP expression. MRP does not predict for response to induction chemotherapy but intermediate or high MRP expression might be associated with shorter overall survival of the patients.

2. INTRODUCTION

Drug resistance limits the efficacy of anticancer drugs in acute myeloid leukemia (AML). Multidrug resistance (MDR) is believed to be a major cause of resistance in this

Drug Resistance in Leukemia and Lymphoma III, edited by Kaspers *et al.*
Kluwer Academic / Plenum Publishers, New York, 1999.

disease. MDR1 gene expression has previously been shown to be an important prognostic factor in AML.[1-4] Patients expressing MDR1 RNA or P-glycoprotein in their leukemic cells at the time of diagnosis had lower complete remission rates and shorter duration of survival as compared to patients without MDR1 gene expression.[1-4]

Recently, other mechanisms resulting in the MDR phenotype have also been characterized.[5] The multidrug resistance protein (MRP) has been shown to mediate non-P-glycoprotein-mediated MDR of cell lines.[6,7] Drugs affected by MRP include anthracyclines and etoposide but not cytarabine.[8] In order to determine the clinical significance of MRP in AML, we studied MRP expression at diagnosis and its association with clinical outcome. The initial analysis of this study on 80 patients indicated no impact of MRP expression on clinical outcome.[9] Here we report an update of this study on a larger patient population and after longer follow-up.

3. PATIENTS AND METHODS

3.1. Patients

Between January 1990 and November 1997, 127 patients (67 females, 60 males) with de novo AML were admitted to this study (Table 1). The clinical data of the patients are summarized in Table 2. One-hundred-nineteen patients were treated with standard induction chemotherapy protocols, whereas 8 patients did not receive chemotherapy. Thirty-two patients received a DA protocol (daunorubicin 45 mg/m^2 daily on days 1–3, cytarabine 200 mg/m^2 daily by continuous infusion on days 1–7) and 71 patients received the DAE protocol (DA protocol plus etoposide 100 mg/m^2 daily on days 1–5). Five patients were treated with idarubicin plus cytarabine and three patients with intermediate-dose cytarabine. Eight patients with FAB subtype M3 received all-trans retinoic acid (ATRA) prior to chemotherapy. Response to induction chemotherapy was assessed according to standard criteria. Seventy-eight out of 83 patients in complete remission received consolidation therapy which consisted of either DA (n=25), DAE (n=28), intermediate-dose cytarabine (n=11), high-dose cytarabine (n=9), C-HAM (n=1), DAE followed by intermediate-dose cytarabine (n=3) or DAE followed by high-dose cytarabine (n=1). Twenty-two patients subsequently underwent bone marrow transplantation.

3.2. Leukemic Cells and Cell Lines

Leukemic cells were isolated from either peripheral blood or bone marrow aspirates by Ficoll-Paque (Pharmacia) gradient centrifugation. Smears were prepared and stored at -20°C until use.

Table 1. MRP expression in patients with AML

MRP expression	No. (%) of patients	
low	38	(30%)
intermediate	58	(46%)
high	31	(24%)

MRP expression of leukemic cells at diagnosis was determined by immunocytochemistry with QCRL-1/QCRL-3 as described in 'Patients and Methods' in 127 patients.

Table 2. MRP expression and clinical data of the patients

	All patients		Low MRP		Intermediate+high MRP		P
No. of patients	127		38	(30)	89	(70)	
Age (years)							
Median	61		63		60		NS*†
Range	15–88		15–88		17–83		
Sex							
Males	67		20	(30)	47	(70)	NS‡
Females	60		18	(30)	42	(70)	
White blood cell count							
Median	17000		8330		20760		NS†
Range	400–280700		780–280700		400–250000		
FAB subtype							NS§
M0	6		4	(67)	2	(33)	
M1	24		9	(38)	15	(62)	
M2	32		11	(34)	21	(66)	
M3	12		4	(33)	8	(67)	
M4	21		3	(14)	18	(86)	
M4Eo	7		0	(0)	7	(100)	
M5	15		3	(20)	12	(80)	
M6	6		3	(50)	3	(50)	
M7	1		0	(0)	1	(100)	
Not defined	3		1	(33)	2	(67)	
Lactate dehydrogenase (U/l)							
Median	435		361		463		NS†
Range	104–3800		104–2740		146–3800		
Karyotype							NS§
Good prognosis	24		5	(21)	19	(79)	
Intermediate prognosis	46		16	(35)	30	(65)	
Poor prognosis	46		14	(30)	32	(70)	
Not determined	11		3	(27)	8	(73)	
Induction therapy							
DA	32		3	(9)	29	(91)	0.06§
DAE	71		27	(38)	44	(62)	
IA	5		1	(20)	4	(80)	
ATRA + DA or DAE	8		4	(50)	4	(50)	
Intermediate-dose cytarabine + DAE	3		1	(33)	2	(67)	
None	8		2	(25)	6	(75)	
Bone marrow transplantation	22		5	(23)	17	(77)	NS‡

* NS = not significant
† Kruskal-Wallis test
‡ Chi-square test
§ Exact chi-square test
¶ Protocols and karyotype classification are described in 'Patients and Methods'

Cytospins of C1 and T5 cells were kindly provided by Drs. S.P.C Cole and R.G. Deeley (Queen's University, Kingston, Ontario, Canada).

3.3. Immunocytochemistry

Immunocytochemistry was performed as described.[10] Briefly, cells were fixed in cold acetone and incubated in 3% H_2O_2 in order to block endogenous peroxidase activity. Then cells were incubated for 2 h with a mixture (dilution 1:1000) of monoclonal antibodies QCRL-1 and QCRL-3.[11] Both antibodies were kindly provided by Drs. S.P.C Cole and R.G. Deeley (Queen's University, Kingston, Ontario, Canada). Antibody binding was detected by the avidin-biotin-peroxidase method as described.[10] The degree of expression was divided according to the percentage of staining leukemic cells into low (≤5%), intermediate (6–20%) and high (>20%) expression.

To ensure specificity of staining, several controls were performed. Firstly, C1 and T5 cells were used as negative and positive controls for MRP expression, respectively.[8] Secondly, negative controls for each sample were performed as described above but without monoclonal antibodies QCRL-1/QCRL-3. Thirdly, staining with irrelevant isotype-matched antibodies was performed as negative control in some cases.

3.4. Survival Analysis

Survival durations were estimated according to Kaplan-Meier.[12] Overall survival was measured from the time of diagnosis until the time of either death or last control. Disease-free survival was measured from the time of complete remission until the time of relapse or death. Patients who underwent bone marrow transplantation were censored at the time of transplantation.

3.5. Statistical Analysis

Frequencies were tested by chi-squared analysis. In addition, Kruskal-Wallis tests were performed. Comparisons of survival curves were done with the log-rank test.

4. RESULTS

MRP expression of leukemic cells obtained from either peripheral blood (n=78), bone marrow (n=82) or both sources (n=33) was determined by immunocytochemistry by means of monclonal antibodies QCRL-1/QCRL-3. The percentage of staining leukemic cells ranged from 0% to 78%. The results obtained from peripheral blood cells were similar to those from bone marrow cells. Low, intermediate and high MRP expression was observed in 38 (30%), 58 (46%) and 31 (24%) patients, respectively (Table 1).

Age and sex of the patients, white blood cell count, FAB subtype, serum lactate dehydrogenase levels and karyotype aberrations were not significantly different between patients with low MRP expression and those with intermediate or high MRP expression (Table 2).

Next, the relationship between MRP expression of the leukemic cells and response to induction therapy was determined. For all patients receiving chemotherapy (n=119), the complete remission rate was 70%. Early death (within four weeks after the begin of treatment) and resistant disease (after at least two treatment cycles) occurred in 14% and 12% of the patients, respectively. Five (4%) patients were not evaluable for response because

Table 3. MRP expression in relation to outcome of induction chemotherapy

	No. of patients	Complete remission		Resistant disease		Early death		Not evaluable	
No. of patients MRP positive patients	119	83	(70%)	14	(12%)	17	(14%)	5	(4%)
Low	36	27	(75%)	3	(8%)	4	(11%)	2	(6%)
Intermediate	55	38	(70%)	6	(10%)	10	(18%)	1	(2%)
High	28	18	(64%)	5	(18%)	3	(11%)	2	(7%)

Patients received induction chemotherapy as described in 'Patients and Methods'.
Chi-squared analysis with regard to complete remission revealed the following P-values:

	P-value
Low versus intermediate+high	0.4
Low+intermediate versus high	0.5
Low versus high	0.4
Low versus Intermediate	0.5
Intermediate versus high	0.7

they did receive only one cycle of chemotherapy which did not result in complete remission. The complete remission rates were 75%, 70% and 64% for patients with low, intermediate and high MRP expression, respectively (Table 3). The complete remission rate for patients with low MRP expression was 75% and for those with intermediate or high MRP expression 67% (p=0.4) (Table 3). The percentages of early death and resistant disease were also independent of MRP expression (Table 3).

Overall survival and disease-free survival were analysed in 119 and 83 patients, respectively. Relapses and deaths occurred in 50 and 85 patients, respectively. At a median follow up of 16 months, median overall survival was 13 months for the total study population. Median overall survival was 24, 9 and 12 months for patients with low, intermediate and high MRP expression, respectively (data not shown). Overall survival of patients with intermediate or high MRP expression was shorter than the survival of patients with low MRP expression (p=0.09) (Figure 1). Disease-free survival was independent of MRP expression (Figure 2).

5. DISCUSSION

In the present study, MRP expression of leukemic cells was low in 30%, intermediate in 46% and high in 24% of the patients. The level of MRP expression had no impact on response to induction chemotherapy but patients with intermediate or high expression showed a trend toward shorter overall survival as compared to patients with low expression.

Recently, a few studies on MRP expression in AML have been published.[13–21] The percentages of MRP RNA overexpression reported in these studies are similar to our percentage of high MRP expression. Zhou et al.[15] reported MRP RNA overexpression as compared to normal bone marrow in 9/51 (18%) patients with newly diagnosed AML. Burger et al.[17] found significantly elevated MRP RNA levels in 1/9 (11%) untreated patients and Ross et al.[16] in 6/24 (25%) patients. Nooter et al.[19] reported high MRP expression in 2/29

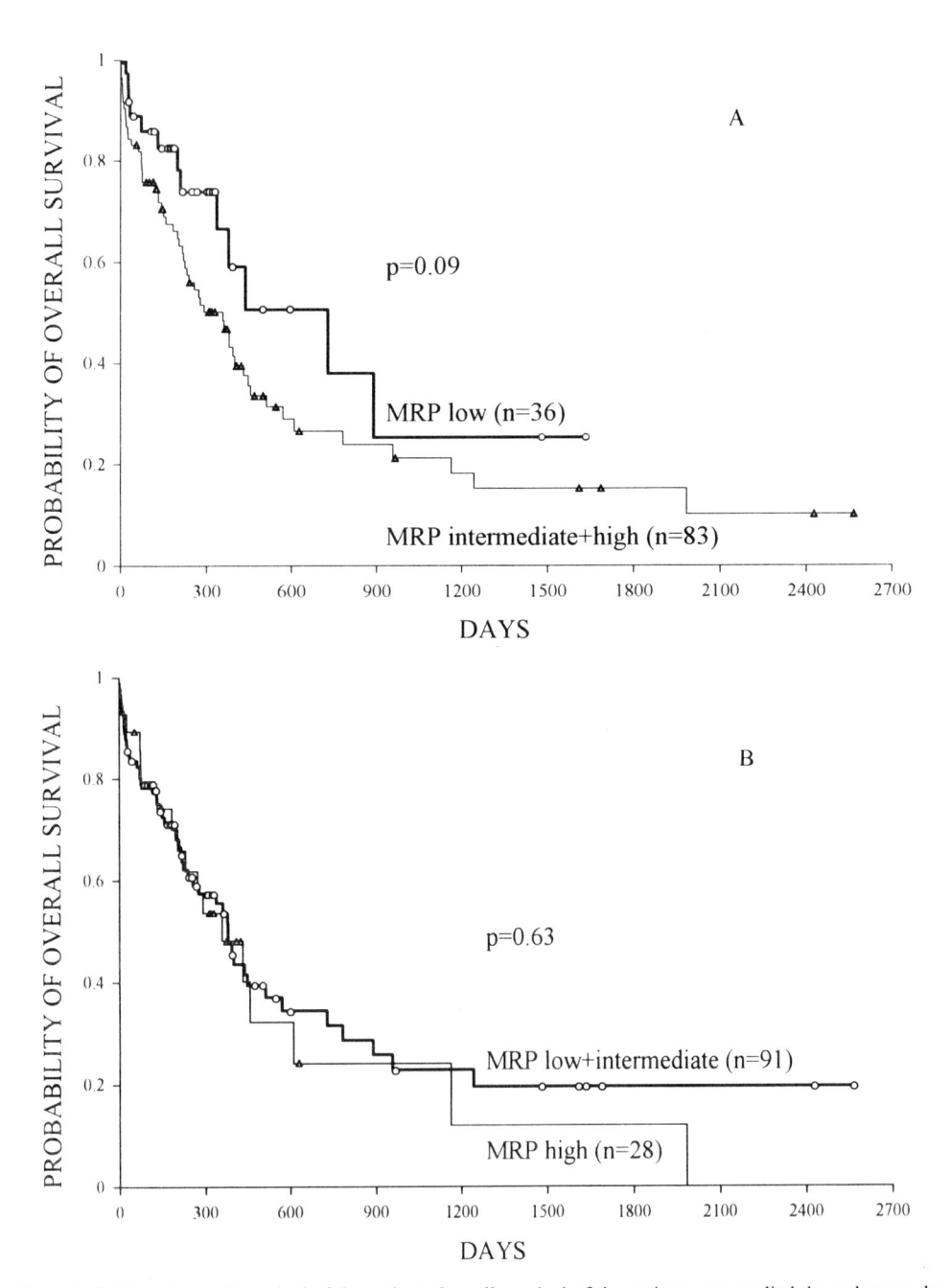

Figure 1. MRP and overall survival of the patients. Overall survival of the patients was studied dependent on the degree of MRP expression. Overall survival was calculated according to Kaplan-Meier [12] and curves were compared by the log-rank test.

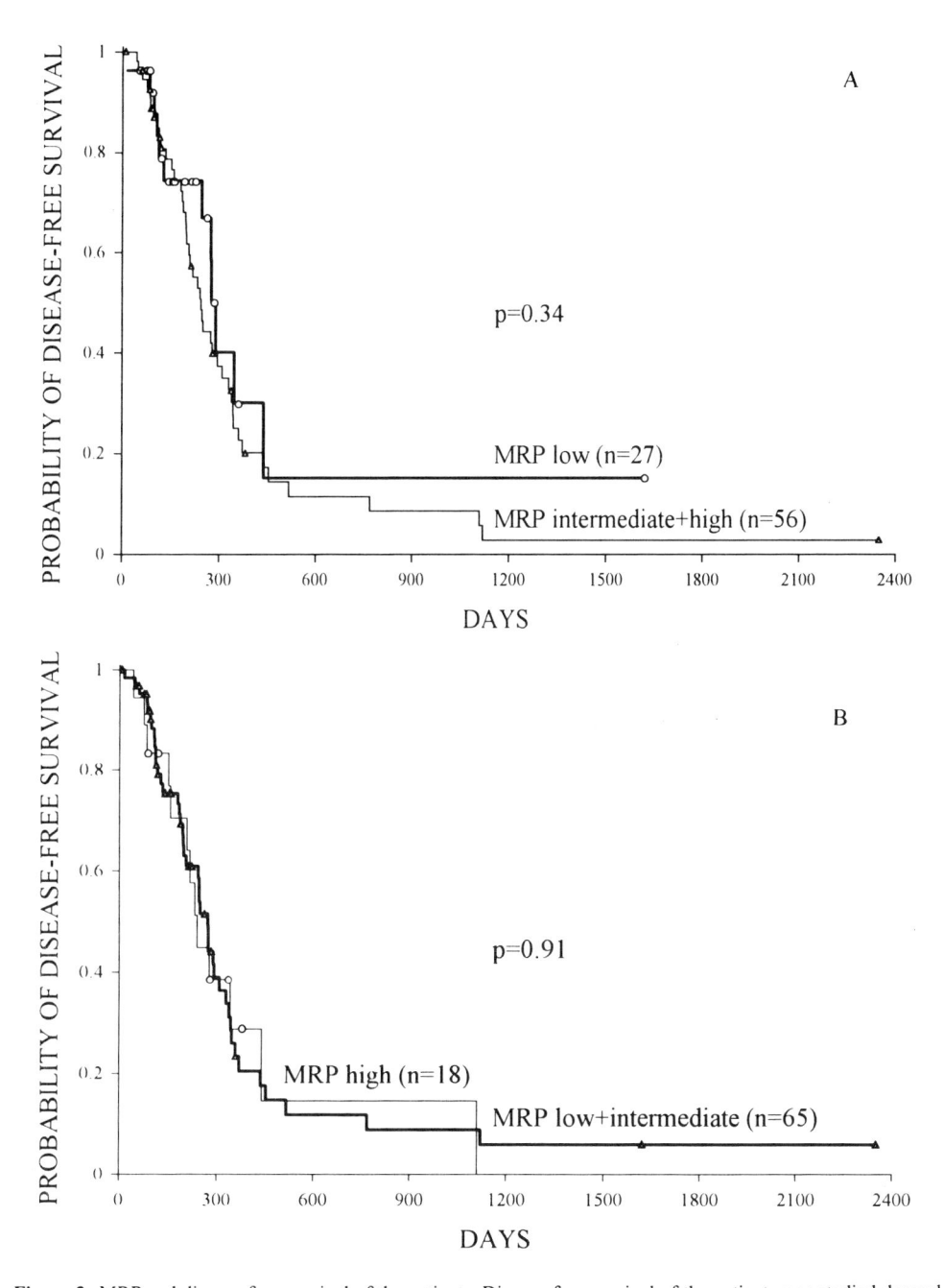

Figure 2. MRP and disease-free survival of the patients. Disease-free survival of the patients was studied dependent on the degree of MRP expression. Disease-free survival was calculated according to Kaplan-Meier [12] and curves were compared by the log-rank test.

(7%) untreated patients by means of a RNase protection assay and in 3/10 (30%) by means of immuno-cytochemistry with the monoclonal antibody MRPr1.

MRP RNA overexpression was significantly higher in secondary AML as compared to de novo AML[13] and tended to be higher in pretreated AML than in untreated AML in one[13] but not in another study.[19] In relapsed AML, MRP expression was higher than at the time of diagnosis in three studies,[14-16] with a statistical significant difference in one of these studies.[19]

In our study, MRP expression was not related to response to induction chemotherapy. Consistent with our data, no correlation between MRP RNA expression and response to chemotherapy was found in two other studies.[14,16] In contrast, some impact of MRP on clinical outcome was reported in three studies.[13,15,18] In two of these studies,[13,18] MRP RNA overexpression was more frequent in drug-refractory than in drug-sensitive patients but these differences did not reach the level of statistical significance. In the third study,[15] an impact of MRP on outcome was observed for P-gp negative patients.

Consistent with the lack of a relationship between MRP expression and response to induction chemotherapy, no impact of MRP expression on survival was observed in the intitial analysis of our study except that most patients surviving more than two years did not express high MRP levels.[9] In the present follow-up of our study, however, the group of patients with either intermediate or high expression showed a trend toward shorter survival. Thus the association between MRP and survival will have to be studied on a larger patient population in the future. Few studies on the relationship between MRP expression and survival have been reported by others.[14,21] In the study by Schneider et al., the duration of remission was independent of MRP RNA expression.[14] Deletion of the MRP gene was previously found in 5 out of 13 patients with inv(16) and was associated with longer overall survival and disease-free survival.[21] However, we did not observe a relationship between MRP expression and inv(16) in the present study.

Recently, a few studies evaluating the clinical significance of MRP gene expression in solid tumors have been published.[10,22-26] MRP overexpression of the tumors was associated with shorter survival in patients with either neuroblastoma[22] or breast cancer[23] and did predict for worse outcome of platin-based combination chemotherapy containing either vindesine or etoposide in patients with non-small-cell lung cancer.[24] In contrast, no associations between MRP expression and response to chemotherapy or survival were found in patients with ovarian carcinoma[25] or colorectal carcinoma.[26]

Other mechanisms of drug resistance are also active in AML.[27,28] In particular, the lung resistance protein (LRP) has recently been shown to be an important predictor of treatment outcome in AML.[29,30] Thus these mechanisms will have to be further evaluated with regard to their quantitative impact on clinical outcome in patients with AML.

In conclusion, MRP does not predict response to induction chemotherapy but intermediate or high MRP levels might be associated with shorter survival in AML.

ACKNOWLEDGMENTS

This study was supported by the 'Fonds zur Förderung der wissenschaftlichen Forschung' (project number P12264-MED).

REFERENCES

1. Pirker R, Wallner J, Geissler K, Linkesch W, Haas OA, Bettelheim P, Hopfner M, Scherrer R, Valent P, Havelec L, Ludwig H and Lechner K. MDR1 gene expression and treatment outcome in acute myeloid leukemia. J Natl Cancer Inst 1991, 83, 708–712

2. Marie J-P, Zittoun R and Sikic BI. Multidrug resistance (mdr1) gene expression in adult acute leukemias: correlations with treatment outcome and in vitro drug sensitivity. Blood 1991, 78, 586–592
3. Campos L, Guyotat D, Archimbaud E, Calmard-Oriol P, Tsuruo T, Troncy J, Treille D and Fiere D. Clinical significance of multidrug resistance P-glycoprotein expression on acute nonlymphoblastic leukemia cells at diagnosis. Blood 1992, 79, 473–476
4. Zöchbauer S, Gsur A, Brunner R, Kyrle PA, Lechner K and Pirker R. P-glycoprotein expression as unfavorable prognostic factor in acute myeloid leukemia. Leukemia 1994, 8, 974–977
5. Simon SM and Schindler M. Cell biological mechanisms of multidrug resistance in tumors. Proc Natl Acad Sci USA 1994, 91, 3497–3504
6. Cole SPC, Bhardwaj G, Gerlach JH, Mackie JE, Grant CE, Almquist KC, Stewart AJ, Kurz EU, Duncan AMV and Deeley RG. Overexpression of a transporter gene in a multidrug-resistant human lung cancer cell line. Science 1992, 258, 1650–1654
7. Grant CE, Valdimarsson G, Hipfner DR, Almquist KC, Cole SPC and Deeley RG. Overexpression of multidrug resistance-associated protein (MRP) increases resistance to natural product drugs. Cancer Res 1994, 54, 357–361
8. Cole SPC, Sparks KE, Fraser K, Loe DW, Grant CE, Wilson GM and Deeley RG. Pharmacological characterization of multidrug resistant MRP-transfected human tumor cells. Cancer Res 1994, 54, 5902–5910
9. Filipits M, Suchomel RW, Zöchbauer S, Brunner R, Lechner K and Pirker R. Multidrug resistance-associated protein in acute myeloid leukemia: no impact on treatment outcome. Clin Cancer Res 1997, 3, 1419–1425
10. Filipits M, Suchomel RW, Dekan G, Haider K, Valdimarsson G, Depisch D and Pirker R. MRP and MDR1 gene expression in primary breast carcinomas. Clin Cancer Res 1996, 2, 1231–1237
11. Hipfner DR, Gauldie SD, Deeley RG and Cole SPC. Detection of the M_r 190,000 multidrug resistance protein, MRP, with monoclonal antibodies. Cancer Res 1994, 54, 5788–5792
12. Kaplan EL and Meier P. Nonparametric estimation from incomplete observations. J Am Stat Assoc 1958, 53, 457–481
13. Hart SM, Ganeshaguru K, Hoffbrand AV, Prentice HG and Metha AB. Expression of the multidrug resistance-associated protein (MRP) in acute leukaemia. Leukemia 1994, 8: 2163–2168
14. Schneider E, Cowan KH, Bader H, Toomey S, Schwartz GN, Karp JE, Burke PJ and Kaufmann SH. Increased expression of the multidrug resistance-associated protein gene in relapsed acute leukemia. Blood 1995, 85, 186–193
15. Zhou D-C, Zittoun R and Marie J-P. Expression of multidrug resistance-associated protein (MRP) and multidrug resistance (MDR1) genes in acute myeloid leukemia. Leukemia 1995, 9, 1661–1666
16. Ross DD, Doyle LA, Schiffer CA, Lee EJ, Grant CE, Cole SPC, Deeley RG, Yang W and Tong Y. Expression of multidrug resistance-associated protein (MRP) mRNA in blast cells from acute myeloid leukemia (AML) patients. Leukemia 1996, 10, 48–55
17. Burger H, Nooter K, Zaman GJR, Sonneveld P, van Wingerden KE, Oostrum RG and Stoter G. Expression of the multidrug resistance-associated protein (MRP) in acute and chronic leukemias. Leukemia 1994, 8, 990–997
18. Schuurhuis GJ, Broxterman HJ, Ossenkoppele GJ, Baak JPA, Eekman CA, Kuiper CM, Feller N, van Heijningen THM, Klumper E, Pieters R, Lankelma J and Pinedo HM. Functional multidrug resistance phenotype associated with combined overexpression of Pgp/MDR1 and MRP together with 1-ß-D-arabinofuranosylcytosine sensitivity may predict clinical response in acute myeloid leukemia. Clin Cancer Res 1995, 1, 81–93
19. Nooter K, Westerman AM, Flens MJ, Zaman GJR, Scheper RJ, van Wingerden KE, Burger H, Oostrum R, Boersma T, Sonneveld P, Gratama JW, Kok T, Eggermont AMM, Bosman FT and Stoter G. Expression of the multidrug resistance-associated protein (MRP) gene in human cancers. Clin Cancer Res 1995, 1, 1301–1310
20. Legrand O, Perrot J-Y, Tang RP, Simonin G, Gurbuxani S, Zittoun R and Marie J-P. Expression of the multidrug resistance-associated protein (MRP) mRNA and protein in normal peripheral blood and bone marrow haemopoietic cells. Br J Haematol 1996, 94, 23–33
21. Kuss BJ, Deeley RG, Cole SPC, Willman CL, Kopecky KJ, Wolman SR, Eyre HJ, Lane SA, Nancarrow JK, Whitmore SA and Callen DF. Deletion of gene for multidrug resistance in acute myeloid leukaemia with inversion in chromosome 16: prognostic implications. Lancet 1994, 343, 1531–1534
22. Norris MD, Bordow SB, Marshall GM, Haber PS, Cohn SL and Haber M. Expression of the gene for multidrug-resistance-associated protein and outcome in patients with neuroblastoma. N Engl J Med 1996, 334, 231–238

23. Filipits M, Malayeri R, Suchomel RW, Pohl G, Stranzl T, Dekan G, Kaider A, Stiglbauer W, Depisch D and Pirker R. Multidrug resistance protein (MRP) is an independent prognostic factor in breast cancer. Submitted
24. Ota E, Abe Y, Oshika Y, Ozeki Y, Iwasaki M, Inoue H, Yamazaki H, Ueyama Y, Takagi K, Ogata T, Tamaoki N and Nakamura M. Expression of the multidrug resistance-associated protein (MRP) gene in non-small-cell lung cancer. Br J Cancer 1995, 72, 550–554
25. Izquierdo MA, van de Zee AGJ, Vermorken JB, van der Valk P, Belien JAM, Giaccone G, Scheffer GL, Flens MJ, Pinedo HM, Kenemans P, Meijer CJLM, de Vries EGE and Scheper RJ. Drug resistance-associated marker Lrp for prediction of response to chemotherapy and prognoses in advanced ovarian carcinoma. J Natl Cancer Inst 1995, 87, 1230–1237
26. Filipits M, Suchomel RW, Dekan G, Stiglbauer W, Haider K, Depisch D and Pirker R. Expression of the multidrug resistance-associated protein (MRP) gene in colorectal carcinomas. Br J Cancer 1997, 75, 208–212
27. Filipits M, Suchomel RW, Zöchbauer S, Malayeri R and Pirker R. Clinical relevance of drug resistance genes in malignant diseases. Leukemia 1996, 10, Suppl. 3, 10–17
28. Malayeri R, Filipits M, Suchomel RW, Zöchbauer S, Lechner K and Pirker R. Multidrug resistance in leukemias and its reversal. Leuk Lymphoma 1997, 23, 451–458
29. List AF, Spier CS, Grogan TM, Johnson C, Roe DJ, Greer JP, Wolff SN, Broxterman HJ, Scheffer GL, Scheper RJ and Dalton WS. Overexpression of the major vault transporter protein lung-resistance protein predicts treatment outcome in acute myeloid leukemia. Blood 1996, 87, 2464–2469
30. Filipits M, Pohl G, Stranzl T, Suchomel RW, Scheper RJ, Jäger U, Geissler K, Lechner, K and Pirker R. Expression of the lung resistance protein predicts poor outcome in de novo acute myeloid leukemia. Blood 1998, 91, 1508–1513

EVIDENCE FOR FUNCTIONAL DISCRIMINATION BETWEEN LEUKEMIC CELLS OVEREXPRESSING MULTIDRUG-RESISTANCE ASSOCIATED PROTEIN AND P-GLYCOPROTEIN

Zineb Benderra,[1] Hamid Morjani,[1] Aurélie Trussardi,[2] and Michel Manfait[1]

[1]Laboratoire de Spectroscopie Biomoléculaire
IFR 53, EA2063, UFR de Pharmacie
51 rue Cognacq Jay
51096 Reims cedex, France
[2]Institut Jean Godinot
Laboratoire de Biochimie
BP 171, 1 rue du Grl Koenig
51100 Reims, France

Keywords: Multidrug-resistance associated protein, P-glycoprotein, vacuolar H^+-ATPase, glutathione, anthracyclines, microspectrofluorometry.

1. ABSTRACT

Multidrug-resistance (MDR), caused by overexpression of either P-glycoprotein (Pgp) or the multidrug-resistance associated protein (MRP), is characterised by a decreased cellular drug accumulation. One form of MDR is the sequestration of the drug inside cytoplasmic vesicles followed by an a exocytotic and/or efflux process. In some studies, increased intracellular glutathione (GSH) has been associated with MDR. In this study, we examined the effects of 7-chloro-4-nitrobenz-2-oxa-1,3-diazole or NBD (a H^+-ATPase pump inhibitor) and buthionine sulphoximine or BSO (an inhibitor of GSH biosynthesis) on the subcellular distribution of daunorubicin or DNR in two leukemic homoharringtonine-resistant K562 cell lines, overexpressing MRP (K-H30) and Pgp (K-H300). DNR nuclear accumulation was carried out using microspectrofluorometry. Our results show that DNR nuclear accumulation and sensitivity of K-H30 cells were increased

Drug Resistance in Leukemia and Lymphoma III, edited by Kaspers *et al.*
Kluwer Academic / Plenum Publishers, New York, 1999.

by NBD and BSO whereas in K-H300 cells, NBD and BSO were unable to increase the DNR nuclear accumulation and sensitivity of these cells. This study demonstrates clearly that even if vesicular sequestration can happen in cells overexpressing MRP and Pgp proteins, only the MRP protein is able to extrude the drug through intracellular vesicles and efflux. In addition, GSH plays an important part in the pathway of drug transport in cells overexpressing MRP. Data entrain also the notion of functional discrimination between the MDR and MRP phenotype.

2. INTRODUCTION

A major obstacle impeding the success of chemotherapy is multidrug-resistance (MDR). Very often, the MDR phenotype is mediated by the P-glycoprotein (Pgp), the 170 KDa product of the mdr1 gene, which acts as an ATP-dependent drug efflux pump (1,2). Another MDR mechanism involves overexpression of the MRP protein (3), which has been identifed as a 190 KDa glycoprotein (4). Cell lines, which overexpress MRP usually display, reduced accumulation and increased efflux of drugs, which is ATP-dependent (3). The mechanism of action of MRP is less well defined than that of Pgp (5). Viable sensitive and resistant cells overexpressing Pgp or MRP, appear to sequester conventional anthracyclines differently (3,4,6). Sensitive cells display nuclear drug accumulation, whereas resistant cells show drug accumulation in cytoplasmic perinuclear vesicles. This vesicular sequestration in resistant cells is followed by an exocytotic or/and efflux process, which transports the drug to the exterior of the cell. Many studies have previously suggested that only the MRP protein is able to extrude the drug through intracellular vesicles (7). Glutathione (GSH) is widely distributed in animals, plants and microorganisms (8). The GSH and glutathione S-transferase (GST_s) play a primary role in cellular detoxification (9–11). Moreover, many studies indicate that GSH is a critical determinant in tumor cell resistance (12–14) by interacting with a wide range of drugs which become conjugated to glutathione S-conjugates (15). In order to understand the mechanisms of transport of DNR by MRP and Pgp proteins, we have examined the effects of 7-chloro-4-nitrobenz-2-oxa-1, 3 diazole (a H^+-ATPase pump inhibitor) and buthionine sulphoximine (an inhibitor of GSH biosynthesis) on cytotoxicity and nuclear accumulation of DNR using scanning confocal microspectofluorometry. This work was carried out on two sublines: K562 cells overexpressing MRP (K-H30) and Pgp (K-H300) (16).

3. MATERIALS AND METHODS

3.1. Cell Lines and Culture Conditions

The wild-type K562 (K562/WT) human myeloid cells, and the multidrug-resistant subclones K-H30, K-H100 and K-H300 were kindly supplied by Dr. J.P. Marie and Dr Anne-Marie Faussat (University of Paris, France). K-H30, K-H100 and K-H300 cells were established by the stepwise selection with increasing concentrations of homoharringtonine (HHT). K-H30, K-H100 and K-H300 cells were maintained by exposure to 30, 100 and 300 ng/ml of HHT respectively, for a period of 3 to 4 days every 3 weeks (16). Cells were grown in a 5% CO_2 atmosphere at 37°C, and RPMI-1640 medium (Gibco, Paris, France) supplemented with 10% foetal calf serum (Gibco) and 200 mM L-Glutamin (Sigma, St Quentin Fallavier, France).

3.2. Drugs and Chemicals

Daunorubicin (DNR), buthionine sulphoximine (BSO), homoharringtonine (HHT), 7 chloro-4-nitrobenz-2-oxa-1, 3 diazole (NBD) and 3-[4,5-dimethylthiazol-2-yl]-2,5-diphenyltetrazolium bromide (MTT) were obtained from Sigma (St Quentin Fallavier, France).

3.3. MTT Cytotoxicity Assay

Cytotoxicity experiments were performed using the MTT assay. Cells (100.000/ml) were exposed to drug (0.01–50 µM) at 37°C, with or without modulator at non toxic concentrations for 2 hours. Cells were washed and seeded (50.000/ml) in 96-well microplates for 72 hours. A solution of MTT (20 µl, 2.5 mg/ml) was added to each well for 3 hours. Medium was then discarded and 200 µl of DMSO were added to each well. Optical densities were measured at 540 nm using a "series 750 microplates reader" (Cambridge Technology, Watertown, MA). The 50% inhibitory concentration (IC_{50}) was determined as the drug concentration which resulted in a 50% reduction in cell viability. Resistance index (RI) was calculated by dividing the IC_{50} obtained for the resistant subline by the IC_{50} obtained for the K562 parental cell line.

3.4. RT-PCR analysis

Total cellular RNA was prepared using the guanidine isothiocyanate/acid/phenol method (17). mdr1, mrp and β2m transcripts were analysed by semi-quantitative RT-PCR using the following gene-specific oligo-nucleotide primers: MDR1 forward primer, 5'-CCCATCATTGCAATAGCAGG-3'; MDR1 reverse primer, 5'-GTTCAAACTTCTGCTCCTGA-3'; MRP forward primer, 5'-TCTCTCCCGA CATGACCGAGG-3'; MRP reverse primer, 5'-CCAGGAATATGCCCCGACTTC-3'; β2m forward primer, 5'-ACCCCCACTGAAAAAGATGA-3'; β2m reverse primer, 5'-ATCTTCAAACCTCCATGATG-3'. The β2m gene was used as an internal control. In brief, RT was performed using 1 µg of total RNA. Total cytoplasmic RNA was reverse transcribed using Moloney Murine Leukemia Virus reverse transcriptase (M-MLV reverse transcriptase, Gibco-BRL) according to the manufacturer's instructions. Aliquots representing 1/50 of cDNA template were diluted to 100 µl in Taq polymerase buffer containing: 1.5 mM $MgCL_2$, 0.25 mM dNTP, 0.6 and 0.3 µmole of primers MRP and β2m respectively, 1.5 U of DNA polymerase (Goldstar, EUROGENTEC). MRP PCR conditions were 94°C for 3 min followed by 32 cycles of 94°C for 45 sec, 61°C for 90 sec and 72°C for 90 sec then 1 cycle of 72°C for 10 min. For the MDR PCR the same concentration of cDNA were diluted to 100 µl in Taq polymerase buffer containing: 1.7 mM $MgCL_2$, 0.25 mM dNTP, 0.5 and 1 µmole of primers MDR and β2m respectively, 2.5 U of DNA polymerase (Goldstar, Eurogentec). MDR PCR conditions were 94°C for 30 sec followed by 35 cycles of 94°C for 50 sec, 57°C for 50 sec, 72°C for 20 sec then 1 cycle of 72°C for 10 min. Target (MRP, MDR) and control (β2m) gene sequence were coamplified in the same reaction. Following PCR, aliquots (10 µl) were subjected to electrophoresis on 2 % agarose gels and bands were visualised by UV transillumination using ethidium bromide staining prior to photography. Densitometry was performed using IMAGER of APPLIGEN ON-COR and the ratio between the target and control PCR products, for each cDNA sample, was determined by dividing the densitometric volume of the target electrophoretic band by that of the control band.

3.5. Confocal Laser Scanning Microspectrofluorometry

3.5.1. The Microspectrofluorometer. Fluorescence emission spectra from a microvolume of living cells were recorded using a confocal laser microspectrofluorometer (Dilor, Lille, France). An optical microscope Olympus BX40 equipped with 100X phase contrast water-immersion objective (Olympus UVFL 100PL, Japan) allowed the observation of the sample, the focussing of a 4 µW laser beam emitting at 457.9 nm (2065A model, Spectra Physics, Les Ulis, France) and the collection of the fluorescence emission in the 500–700 nm range through the same optics. The emission from a point is defected onto the entrance slit of the spectrograph where the emission signal was projected onto a CCD detector (Wright, Stonehouse, UK).

3.5.2. Nuclear drug Concentration Determination. The fluorescence emission spectrum from nuclei of K562 treated cells F (λ), can be expressed as a sum of the spectral contributions of free DNR, DNA-bound DNR and signal of nuclear autofluorescence (18).

$$F(\lambda) = C_f \cdot F_f(\lambda) + C_b \cdot F_b(\lambda) + C_n \cdot F_n(\lambda)$$

Where F_f and F_b are the fluorescence spectra of free and bound drug reffered to a unitary concentration. Taking this concentration into account, C_f and C_b represent intranuclear concentration of free and bound drug respectively, C_n is the contribution of autofluorescence responsible for the intrinsic nuclear spectrum F_n. In aqueous solution, each of these contributions has a characteristic spectral shape. The fluorescence yield in the free form was 40 times higher than that of the bound-DNA form. These spectral contributions lead to the concentrations of free and DNA-bound DNR. The sum of the values obtained gives the total nuclear concentration of DNR (18–20).

4. RESULTS

4.1. RT-PCR Analysis

In order to study involvement of Pgp and/or MRP in resistance of K562 cells, expression of mdr1 and mrp gene was studied in these cells using RT-PCR technique (Figure 1). When compared with parental K562 cells, K-H30 and K-H100 cells showed an increase in mrp gene, whereas in K-H300 cells mrp gene expression decreased when compared to K-H30 cells. As shown in Figure 1, we were unable to detect mdr1 gene in either K562/WT and K-H30 cells. The K-H100 and K-H300 cells expressed progressively higher amounts of mdr1 gene.

4.2. Cytotoxic Effect of DNR in K-H30 and K-H300 Cells

As shown in Table 1, the K-H30 cells were 4 fold resistant to DNR respectively when compared to wild-type K562/WT cells. However, The K-H300 cells were 45 fold resistant to DNR, when compared to wild-type K562/WT cells.

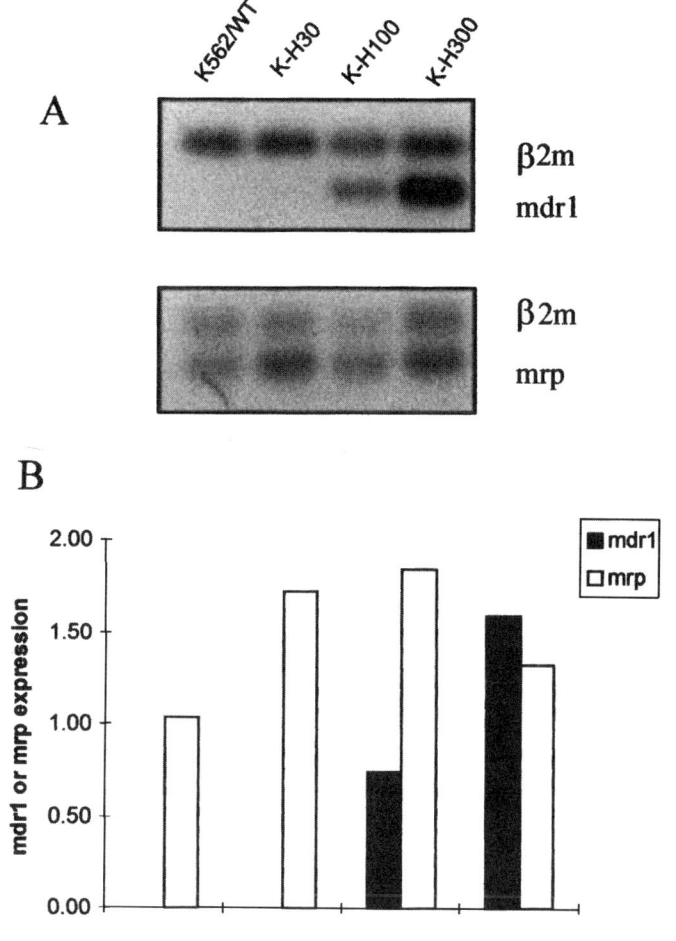

Figure 1. (A) quantitative PCR assay for mdr1 and mrp in sensitive parental cells (K562/WT) and multidrug-resistant subcolones K-H30, K-H100 and K-H300. (B) quantification of PCR (arbitrary unit). The ratio between the mdr1 or mrp and β2m mRNA gene is expressed as described in material and methods.

4.3. Effects of NBD on DNR Cytotoxicity and Nuclear Accumulation in K562 Cells

Incubation of K-H30 cells with NBD at non toxic concentrations leads to an increase of the DNR sensitivity of these cells. NBD had no effect on the cytotoxicity of DNR in K-H300 cells (Table 2).

The effects of NBD on DNR nuclear accumulation in HHT-resistant K562 sub-lines were investigated and results are shown in Figure 2 (top). In the absence of modulator, the nuclear accumulation of DNR in K562/WT, K-H30 and K-H300 cells was 193, 94 and 36 µM respectively. Co-incubation of the cells with 1 µM DNR and NBD at concentrations of 0.5 and 1 µM, restored the level of DNR nuclear accumulation in K-H30 cells to that in the K562/WT cells. NBD concentrations of 0.5 and 1 µM did not cause any increase of the nuclear accumulation of DNR in K-H300 cells.

Table 1. Cytotoxicity of DNR in K562/WT, K-H30 and K-H300 cells

Cell Line	IC50(µM)	Resistance index
K562/WT	0.1	—
K-H30	0.4	4
K-H300	4.5	45

IC50 (µM) is Drug concentration which induce 50% of growth inhibitory. RI (resistance index) is the ratio of IC50 (resistant cells) and IC50 (sensitive cells).

As shown in Figure 3 (top), NBD has no effect on nuclear accumulation of DNR in K562/WT and K-H300 cells. Treatment of K-H30 cells with NBD at a increasing concentrations of (0.2–1 µM) a progressive enhancement of DNR nuclear accumulation. NBD at 0.7 µM or greater concentrations, increased DNR nuclear accumulation to a level equal to that of K562/WT cells.

4.4. Effects of BSO on DNR Cytotoxicity and Nuclear Accumulation in K562 Cells

As shown in Table 3, BSO at 10 and 50 µM, decreased the resistance index value for DNR in K-H30 cells to 3.2 and 2.7 respectively. Moreover, 100 µM BSO decreased the level of DNR cytotoxicity in K-H30 cells to that in the K562/WT. Treatment of K-H300 cells with BSO had non effect on the cytotoxicity of DNR in these cells.

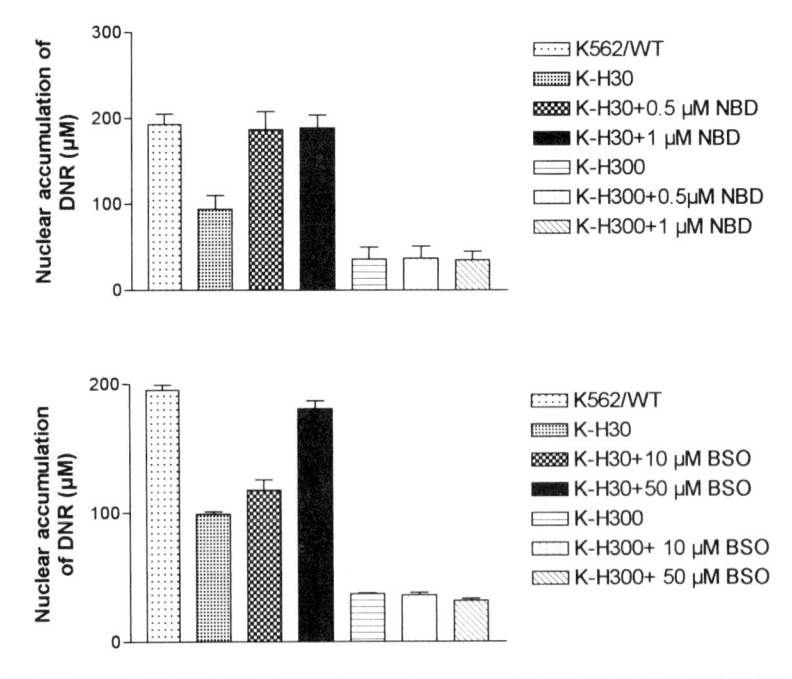

Figure 2. Effect of NBD (top) and BSO (bottom) on nuclear accumulation of DNR in K-H30 and K-H300 cells. Exponentially growing cells were incubated for 2 hours at 37°C with 1µM DNR in the presence or absence of NBD, washed in cold PBS before microspectrofluorometric analysis. Data are the mean ± standard deviation of three independent experiments.

Table 2. Residual resistance index values in K-H30 and K-H300 when treated with DNR IC50 and various concentrations of NBD

NBD (µM)	K-H30	K-H300
0.2	1.9	46.9
0.4	1.1	45.8
0.6	0.9	46.4

As shown in Figure 2 (bottom), treatment of K-H30 cells with 1 µM DNR and 10 µM BSO had a weak effect on DNR nuclear accumulation (117 µM). Treatment of these cells with 1 µM DNR and 50 µM BSO, caused a significant increase in nuclear accumulation of DNR (181 µM). BSO concentrations of 10 and 50 µM did not cause any increase of DNR nuclear accumulation in K-H300 cells. As shown in Figure 3 (bottom), NBD has no effect on nuclear accumulation of DNR in K562/WT and K-H300 cells. At various concentrations (3–50 µM), BSO caused a dose dependent increase of DNR nuclear accumulation in K-H30 cells. 100 µM BSO restored the level of DNR nuclear accumulation in K-H30 cells to that in the K562/WT cells.

5. DISCUSSION

HHT is an alkaloid isolated from the evergreen tree *Cephalotaxus harringtonia* native to the southern provinces of china (21). The results obtained on the multidrug resistant sublines of human myeloid leukemia K562 cells, established by exposure to different concen-

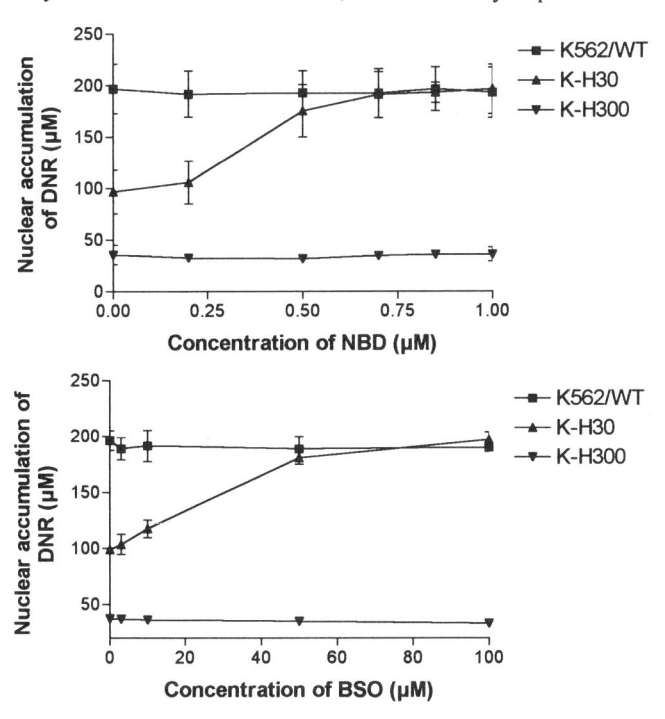

Figure 3. Effect of NBD (top) and BSO (bottom) at various concentrations on nuclear accumulation of DNR in K562/WT, K-H30 and K-H300 cells. Experimental conditions as in Figure 2.

Table 3. Residual resistance index values in
K-H30 and K-H300 when treated with DNR IC50 and
various concentrations of BSO

BSO (µM)	K-H30	K-H300
10	3.2	46.1
50	2.7	46.8
100	1.1	46.5

trations of HHT, suggest that multiple mechanisms of resistance are involved in the progressive HHT resistance (16). In the low-level resistant K-H30 cells, only overexpression of mrp gene was observed by northern-blot and RT-PCR analysis. In the intermediate-level resistant K-H100 and K-H200 cells both mrp and mdr genes were overexpressed, while in the high-level resistant K-H300 and K-H400 cells, mdr gene overexpression predominated. In a previous study, the redistribution of anthracyclines in viable resistant cells, is one of the major mechanisms of multidrug resistance (22). Sensitive cells display high nuclear drug uptake whereas in the resistant cells, anthracyclines are redistributed from the nucleus into cytoplasmic vesicles. This accumulation of anthracyclines into cytoplasmic vesicles is followed by an exocytotic and/or efflux process transporting the drug to the exterior of the cell. Marquardt and Center suggested a mechanism for drug extrusion from non-Pgp HL60/ADR cell line which involves intracellular vesicular transport (23). Many studies have indicated that the higher accumulation of anthracyclines in cytoplasmic vesicles of resistant cells may be driven by a more important pH gradient through the membrane of these organelles (24, 25). This pH gradient could be established by a vacuolar H^+-ATPase that was proposed to take an important part in the pathway of drug efflux from resistant cells (23). Results obtained in this study indicate that NBD was able to increase nuclear accumulation of DNR in cells overexpressing MRP (K-H30) and has no effect in cells overexpressing Pgp (K-H300). Moreover, NBD caused significant sensitisation of K-H30 cells to DNR whereas, the cytotoxicity of DNR in K-H300 cells remained unchanged.

In addition to H^+-ATPase pump, Cellular GSH play a primary role in cellular detoxification of electrophilic compounds (11). Moreover, in previous studies, elevated levels of GSH, together with increased activities of GST_s, may protect cells from cytotoxic drugs (12). The GST_s catalyse the conjugation reaction between reduced GSH and many xenobiotics (26). Elimination of the GS-X requires a specific ATP-dependent GS-X export pump termed GS-X pump (27). These data are consistent with MRP being a GSH conjugate transporter. In many studies, treatment of cells with BSO, an inhibitor of γ-glutamylcysteine synthetase, results in the depletion of GSH and increased sensitivity of cells to several drugs (28,29). Although pharmacological depletion of GSH results in sensitisation of some cells to cytotoxic drugs, it is unclear whether this is a direct consequence of GSH depletion or whether the two effects occur independently. In our study, in order to understand if the GSH plays an important role in Pgp and MRP mediated MDR, we have examined the effect of BSO on DNR distribution. Results obtained indicate that BSO was able to increase nuclear accumulation of DNR in cells overexpressing MRP (K-H30) and has no effect in cells overexpressing Pgp (K-H300). Moreover, as NBD, BSO caused significant sensitisation of K-H30 to DNR whereas, the cytotoxicity of DNR in K-H300 cells remained unchanged.

In conclusion, this study demonstrates clearly that even if vesicular sequestration can happen in cells overexpressing MRP and Pgp proteins, only the MRP protein is able to extrude the drug through intracellular vesicles and efflux. Finally, GSH plays an important part in the pathway of drug transport in cells overexpressing MRP. Data entrain also the notion of functional discrimination between the MDR and MRP phenotype.

ACKNOWLEDGMENTS

The authors are grateful to Dr JP Marie and Dr A-M Faussat for the kind gift of the K562 cell lines.

REFERENCES

1. Endicott JA, Ling V, The biochemistry of P-glycoprotein-mediated multidrug resistance, Annu Rev Biochem, 1989, 58, 137–171.
2. Gottesman MM, Pastan I, Biochemistry of multidrug resistance mediated by the multidrug transporter, Annu Rev Biochem, 1993, 62, 385–427.
3. Zaman GJR, Flens MJ, Van Leusden MR, De Haas M, Mulder HS, Lankelma J, Pinedo HM, Scheper RJ, Baas F, Broxterman HJ, Borst P, The human multidrug resistance-associated protein MRP is a plasma membrane drug efflux pump, Proc Nat Acad Sci (Wash), 1994, 91, 8822–8826.
4. Leier I, Jedlitschky G, Buchholz U, Cole SPC, Deeley RG, Keppler D, The MRP gene encodes an ATP-dependent pump for leukotriene C4 and structurally related conjugates, J Biol Chem, 1994, 269, 27807–27810.
5. Zaman GJ, Lankelma J, Van Tellingen O, Role of glutathione in the export of compounds from cells by the multidrug resistance-associated protein, Proc Nat Acad Sci (Wash), 1995, 92, 7690–7694.
6. Cole SPC, Sparks KE, Fraser K, Loe DW, Grant CE, Wilson GM, Deely RG, Pharmacological characterization of multidrug resistant MRP-transfected human tumor cells, Cancer Res, 1994, 54, 5902–5910.
7. Almquist KC, Low DW, Hipfner DR, Characterization of the M_r 190,000 multidrug resistance protein (MRP) in drug-selected and transfected human tumor cells, Cancer Res 1995, 55, 102–110.
8. Meister A, Anderson ME, Glutathione, Annu Rev Biochem, 1983, 52, 711–760.
9. Ishikawa T, Ali-Osman F, Glutathione-associated cis-diamminedichloroplatinum (II) metabolism and ATP-dependent efflux from leukemia cells, J Biol Chem, 1993, 268, 20116–20125.
10. Ishikawa T, Wright C, Ishizuka H, GS-X pump is functionally overexpressed in cis-diamminedichloroplatinum (II)-resistant human leukemia HL60 cells and down-regulated by cell differentiation, J Biol Chem, 1994, 269, 29085–29093.
11. Ishikawa T, Bao J, Yamane Y, Akimaru K, Frindrich K, Wright C, Kuo MT, Coordinated induction of MRP/GS-X pump and γ-glutamylcysteine synthetase by heavy metals in human leukemia cells. J Biol Chem, 1996, 271, 14981–14988.
12. Tew KD, Glutathione-associated enzymes in anticancer drug resistance, Cancer Res, 1994, 54, 4313–4320.
13. Lutzky J, Astor MB, Taub RN, Baker MA, Bhalla K, Gervasoni JE, Rosado M, Stewart V, Krishana S, Hindenburg AA, Role of glutathione and dependent enzymes in anthracyclines-resistant HL60/AR cells, Cancer Res, 1989, 49, 4120–4125.
14. Morrow CS, Cowan KH, Glutathione S-transferases and drug resistance, Cancer Cells, 1990, 2, 15–22.
15. Commandeur JNM, Stijntjes GJ, Vermeulen NPE, Enzymes and transport systems involved in the formation and disposition of glutathione S-conjugates, Pharmacol Rev, 1995, 47, 271–330.
16. Zhou DC, Ramond S, Viguie F, Faussat AM, Zittoun R, Marie JP, Sequential emergence of MRP-and MDR1-gene over-expression as well as MDR1-gene translocation in homoharringtonine-selected K562 human leukemia cell lines, Int J Cancer, 1996, 65, 365–371.
17. Chomczynski P, Sacchi N, Single-Step-method of RNA isolation by acid guanidiniumthiocynatephenol-chloroform extration, Anal Biochem, 1987, 162, 156–159.
18. Gigli M, Doglia S, Millot JM, Valentini L, Manfait M, Quantitative study of doxorubicin in living cell nuclei by microspectrofluorometry, Biochem Biophys Acta, 1988, 950, 13–20.
19. Gigli M, Rasoanaivo TWD, Millot JM, Jeannesson P, Rizzo V, Jardillier JC, Arcamone F, Manfait M, Correlation between growth inhibition and intranuclear doxorubicin and 4'-iododoxorubicin quantitated in living K562 cells by microspectrofluorometry, Cancer Res 1989, 49, 560–564.

20. Millot JM, Rasoanaivo TWD, Morjani H, Manfait M, Role of the aclacinomycin A-doxorubicin associated inreversal of doxorubicin resistance in K562 tumour cells, Br J Cancer 1989, 69, 678–684.
21. Zhou DC, Zittoun R, Marie JP, Homoharringtonine: an effective new natural product in cancer chemotherapy, Bull Cancer, 1995, 82, 987–995.
22. Coly HM, Amos PR, Twentyman PR, Workman P, Examination by confocal fluorescence imaging microscopy of the subcellular localisation of anthracyclines in parent and multidrug resistant cell lines, Br J Cancer, 1993, 67, 1316–1323.
23. Marquardt D, Center MS, Drug transport mechanism in HL60 cells isolated for resistance to adriamycin: evidence for nuclear drug accumulation in resistant cells, Cancer Res, 1992, 52, 3157–3163.
24. Schindler M, Grabski S, Hoff E, Simon SM, Defective pH regulation of acidic compartments in human breast cancer cells (MCF-7) is normalized in adriamycin-resistant cells (MCF-7 adr), Biochemistry, 1996, 35, 2811–2817.
25. Thiebault F, Currier SJ, Whitaker J, Haugland RF, Gottesman M, Pastan I, Willingham MC, Activity of the multidrug transporter results in alkalinisation of the cytosol: measurements of cytosolic pH by microinjection of a pH-sensitive dye, J Histochem Cytochem, 1990, 38, 685–690
26. Mannervik B, Danielson UH, Glutathione S-transferases-stucture and catalytic activity, CRC Crit Rev Biochem, 1988, 23, 283–337.
27. Ishikawa T, The ATP-dependent glutathione S-conjugate export pump, Trends Biochem Sci, 1992, 17, 463–468.
28. Hamilton TC, Winber MA, Louie KG, Batist G, Behrens BC, Tsuruo T, Grotzinger KR, Mckoy WM, Young RC, Ozols RF, Augmentation of adriamycin, melphalan and cisplatin cytotoxicity in drug-resistant and sensitive human ovarian carcinoma cell lines by buthionine sulfoximine mediated glutathione depletion, Biochem Pharmacol, 1985, 34, 2583–2586.
29. Mans DRA, Schuurhuis GJ, Treskes M, Lafleur MVM, Retel J, Pinedo HM, Lankelma J, Modulation by D, L-buthionine-S-R-sulphoximine of etoposide cytotoxicity on human non-small cell lung, ovarian and breast carcinoma cell lines, Eur J Cancer, 1992, 28A, 1447–1452.

18

BOTH Pgp AND MRP1 ACTIVITIES USING CALCEIN-AM CONTRIBUTE TO DRUG RESISTANCE IN AML

Ollivier Legrand,[*] Ghislaine Simonin, Jean-Yves Perrot, Robert Zittoun, and Jean-Pierre Marie

EA1529, Université Paris VI
Formation de Recherche Claude Bernard and Service d'hématologie
Hôpital Hôtel Dieu, Paris, France

Keywords: AML, MRP1, MDR1, LRP, calcein-AM, functional test.

1. SUMMARY

Thirteen cell lines with different levels of Pgp and MRP1 expression were used to assess the ability of calcein-AM uptake and calcein efflux to measure Pgp and MRP1 functions, respectively. There was a good correlation between MRP1 expression and the modulatory effect of probenecid (a specific modulator of MRP1) on the calcein efflux (r=0.91, p=0.0003) and between Pgp expression and the modulatory effect of CsA on calcein-AM uptake (r=0.96, p<0.0001). On light of the high correlations for both proteins, we tested calcein-AM uptake and efflux in fresh myeloid leukemic cells. In 53 AML patients, there was also a good correlation between MRP1 expression (measured by RT/PCR and by MRPm6 expression by flow cytometry) and the modulatory effect of probenecid on the calcein fluorescence (r=0.92, p<0.0001) and between Pgp expression as measured by UIC2 antibody binding on flow cytometry and the modulatory effect of CsA on calcein-AM uptake (r=0.83, p<0.0001). Pgp activity was higher in CD34+ leukemia than in CD34- leukemia (2.26±1.50 vs 1.46±1.21 respectively, p=0.003) and MRP1 activity was higher in CD34- leukemia than in CD34+ leukemia (1.77±0.40 vs 1.4±0.29 respectively,

---

[*] Correspondence to: Docteur Ollivier Legrand, Hôpital Hôtel-Dieu, 1 place du Parvis Notre Dame Service d'hématologie clinique, professeur Zittoun 75 181 Paris, Cedex 04, France Tel: (33) 1 42 34 82 66 Fax: (33) 1 42 34 82 54

Drug Resistance in Leukemia and Lymphoma III, edited by Kaspers *et al.*
Kluwer Academic / Plenum Publishers, New York, 1999.

p=0.004). Pgp expression and activity (p=0.004 and p=0.01, respectively), MRP1 activity (p=0.03) but not MRP1 expression were prognostic factors for achievement of CR. The effect of probenecid and CsA together were higher than the effect of either probenecid or CsA alone on calcein-AM uptake. These results suggest that functional testing (with calcein-AM±modulators) for the presence of both MRP1 and Pgp activities is of prognostic value and that MRP1 contributes to drug resistance in AML.

2. INTRODUCTION

Multidrug resistance (MDR) of some human cancers, particularly acute myeloid leukemia (AML), remains a major obstacle to successful chemotherapy. The best characterized resistance mechanism in AML is the one mediated by the MDR1 gene. MDR1 gene expression has been extensively studied in AML and has been shown to be associated with poorer outcome.[1] MDR1 gene expression has been also correlated with functional parameters (dye and drug uptake/efflux) measured by flow cytometry in AML. Several dyes (Rhodamine123, $DiOC_2$) and drugs (daunorubicin, doxorubicin) may be used to assess Pgp function. These functional tests correlate also with treatment outcome.[1] However, in several studies, discrepant cases were reported, with increased efflux and no significant MDR1 expression.[1] This suggests that alternative proteins, such as the more recently recognized multidrug resistance associated protein (MRP1)[2] or the lung resistance protein (LRP)[3] may contribute to the MDR phenotype. But the role and functionality of these two proteins are still discussed and unclear in AML.[4,5]

Cells exposed to calcein acetoxymethyl ester (calcein-AM) become fluorescent following the cleavage of calcein-AM by cellular esterases which produces a fluorescent derivate calcein. Pgp, the product of the multidrug transporter MDR1 gene, actively extrudes the calcein-AM, but not the fluorescent calcein.[6] On the other hand, fluorescent calcein and calcein-AM are extruded by the multidrug transporter MRP1.[7] Therefore, calcein-AM uptake (with specific modulator of Pgp) can be used to assess whether MDR1 is functional and calcein efflux can explore MRP1 activity. With this functional assay, the role and relative importance of Pgp and MRP1 can be clarified in AML.

In a recent study, Essodaigui et al.[8] have shown that calcein is much less efficiently transported by MRP1 than calcein-AM. Therefore, calcein-AM uptake (with specific modulators of Pgp and/or MRP) can be also used to assess whether MDR1 and/or MRP are functional.[6]

We have studied the relative importance of Pgp and MRP1 in AML using calcein-AM functional test. In addition, the correlation between this fluorescence-based flow cytometric functional assay and MDR proteins expression as well as the correlations between this functional assay and clinical or biological parameters were analysed.

3. MATERIALS AND METHODS

3.1. Cell Lines and Culture Conditions

The present study used 13 cell lines with different levels of MDR1, MRP1 and LRP (Table 1): A549 (given by S Chevillard, Institut Curie, Paris), a lung adenocarcinoma expressing spontaneously high level of MRP1; K562, a human erythroleukemia (gift from BI Sickic, Stanford, CA, USA) and K562/HHT30, K562/HHT100, K562/HHT200,

Table 1. MDR mRNA and MDR proteins expression (measured by RT/PCR and by flow cytometry, respectively), effect of probenecid on calcein efflux and effect of CsA on calcein-AM uptake for 13 cell lines

Cell lines	mRNA expression measured by RT/PCR† (Mean±SD)* MDR1	MRP1	Protein expression measured by flow cytometry†† (Mean±SD)* Pgp	MRP1	Effect of probenecid on calcein efflux††† (Mean±SD)*	Effect of CsA on calcein-AM uptake††† (Mean±SD)*
A549	0±0	1.11±0.39	1±0.03	2.88±0.24	1.51±0.08	1±0
K562	0±0.01	0.1±0.03	1±0.06	1.73±0.24	1.31±0.05	1±0.
HHT30	0.64±0.53	0.46±0.17	1.4±0.1	1.86±0.14	1.33±0.04	1±0
HHT100	0.93±0.68	0.08±0.07	6.8±1.5	1.65±0.11	1.23±0.08	4.9±1
HHT200	1.32±0.6	0.21±0.1	17.2±2.5	1.56±0.1	1.17±0.05	16.3±6.1
HHT300	2.65±1.06	0.33±0.39	71.3±7.2	1.84±0.18	1.25±0.11	39±7.5
HHT400	2.3±0.79	0.38±0.1	40.8±8.5	1.89±0.19	1.29±0.06	24.5±4.2
HL60	0±0.01	0.59±0.11	1.1±0.2	2.18±0.28	1.32±0.15	1±0.1
HL60 Pgp	8.74±2.16	0.38±0.03	125.3±18.9	1.49±0.22	1.2±0.05	46.7±9.9
HL60 MRP	0.4±0.51	2.14±0.24	2.5±0.6	5±2.4	1.85±0.13	10.9±8.1
CEM	0.5±0.24	0.21±0.05	2.2±0.5	1.58±0.4	1.28±0.04	1±0.2
CEM VLB	3.21±0.97	0.26±0.05	52.8±10.4	1.65±0.21	1.27±0.06	18.5±4.5
U937	0±0.02	0±0.03	1.2±0.4	1.07±0.13	1.17±0.02	1±0.1

* : The experiments were performed in triplicate, and at three different times.
† : The results were given as the ratio of : quantities of MDR mRNA product/ß2m mRNA product.
†† : Protein values were expressed as adjusted for control, i.e., as ratio of arithmetic mean fluorescence of UIC2/IgG2A control or MRPm6/IgG1 control.
††† : All the data are ratios of drug fluorescence with modulator divided by drug fluorescence without modulator after subtraction of the fluorescence of the control.

K562/HHT300, K562/HHT400, sublines of K562 developed in our laboratory which have been selected with 30, 100, 200, 300 and 400 ng/ml of homoharringtonine (HHT).[9] The other cell lines were HL60, a human promyelocytic leukemia, HL60/Pgp and HL60/MRP sublines of HL60, resistant to daunorubicin (gift by F Lacombe, Bordeaux, France and F Calvo, Hôpital Saint-Louis, France, respectively); the T lymphoblastic cell lines CEM and CEM/VLB (gift by F Calvo, Hôpital Saint-Louis, France) selected with 50 ng/ml of vinblastine.

3.2. Patients

Fifty three consecutive AML patients were analysed. Diagnosis was based on French-American-British (FAB) criteria.[10] For each patient, several clinical (age, sex, WHO performance status) and biological (WBC, cytogenetic, CD34) characteristics at diagnosis were analysed, as well as their response to treatment administered. Samples were considered positive for CD34 when more than 20% of the viable cells were stained with CD34 antibody (HPCA$_2$ clone, Becton Dickinson) in excess of the negative control. Patients were included in the EORTC Leukemia Cooperative Group protocols (AML10 or AML13 for younger or older patients respectively.

3.3. Fresh Leukemic Cells

Peripheral blood (31 patients) or bone marrow (22 patients) were collected after patients had given informed consent. All samples contained at least 70% of blasts before mononuclear cells isolation. Samples were analysed for proteins expression and function on the same day, within six hours. In the analysis of the fresh leukemic samples, the expression and function of MDR proteins were done with selected cells by CD34 antibody (two colors assays) or other markers (for examples CD33/CD7, CD33/CD2, CD33/CD19 or CD33/CD22 by three colors assays) if possible or with physical characteristics only if blast cells had no characteristic marker.

3.4. MRP1 and MDR1 mRNA Expression Measured by RT/PCR

The expression of MDR1 and MRP1 by RT/PCR was described elsewhere.[4,9,11] Variations between samples in the quantity of cDNA synthesis were normalized by the quantity of ß2 microglobulin (ß2m) in each sample. The results were calculated as the ratio : quantities of MDR mRNA product/ß2m mRNA product.

3.5. MRP1 and MDR1 Proteins Expression Measured by Flow Cytometry

Cells were permeabilized in 15% (v/v) lysing solution G (Becton Dickinson) in H2O and incubated for 15 minutes in PBS/BSA containing 1% (v/v) normal goat serum. Cells (5×10^5) were incubated for 1 hour at 4°C in 100 µl PSB/BSA 5% containing either the monoclonal antibody (MAbs) [UIC2 (1 µg/ml) (IgG2a) (Immunotech) or MRPm6 (2 µg/ml) (IgG1) (given by R.J. Scheper, Amsterdam, The Netherlands)] or the mouse isotype-matched control MAbs. Antibody binding was detected with R-phycoerythrin-labelled goat anti-mouse immunoglobulins (Immunotech, Marseille, France and Becton Dickinson, Grenoble, France) in accordance with the consensus recommendations of Beck et al.[12] Fluorescence was analysed on a FACSORT flow cytometer (Becton Dickinson, Grenoble, France). For each sample, 5000 events were collected. Protein values were expressed as adjusted for control, i.e., as ratio of arithmetic mean fluorescence of UIC2/IgG2A control or MRPm6/IgG1 control.[13] Correlations between MDR proteins expression and clinical, biological and clinical outcome were performed using MDR proteins expression, as a continuous variable in accordance with the different consensus.[12–14]

3.6. Functional Tests in Cell Lines and Fresh Leukemic Cells Using Rhodamine 123, Daunorubicin and Calcein-AM

3.6.1. Rhodamine 123. Cells (5×10^5) were stained with 200 ng/ml of Rh 123 for 20 minutes at 37°C in RPMI medium. The cells were washed twice in PBS and resuspended in Rh 123 free medium and allowed to efflux for 60 minutes at 37°C, either with or without modulators of MDR1 (cyclosporin A [CsA] 2µM) or MRP1 (probenecid 2 mM).[13,15,16] At the indicated times, 1×10^4 cells were taken for flow cytometry analysis. Samples were analysed on a FACSORT flow cytometer (Becton Dickinson). Cells from each subline which had not been exposed to Rh 123 were used as controls.

3.6.2. Daunorubicin. The same technique was used for anthracyclin and Rh 123. Briefly, cells were stained with 10^{-6}M of DNR for 30 minutes at 37°C, then resuspended in anthacyclin free medium for 1 hour at 37°C, either with or without modulators.

3.6.3. Calcein-AM. Cells were incubated with 0.1 µM of calcein-AM for 15 minutes at 37°C in RPMI medium with or without modulators. Cells were washed twice in cold PBS and samples were analysed on FACSORT flow cytometer (uptake of calcein-AM with CsA for MDR1 analysis). Cells were resuspended in calcein-AM free medium and allowed to efflux for 90 minutes at 37°C either with or without modulators (for MRP1 analysis). All samples were analysed without fixation. When we measured non fluorescent calcein-AM uptake with CsA (Pgp function), we assessed the amount of fluorescent calcein that had been converted from non fluorescent calcein-AM. Clearly, when the Pgp pump was active, then less calcein-AM was retained and less converted to fluorescent calcein. Similary, once converted we measured the amount extruded during the efflux assay (MRP1 function). We have also analysed calcein-AM uptake (± modulators of MRP1 and/or Pgp) to assess the relative role of these two proteins.

All the data were calculated as the ratio of drug fluorescence with modulator divided by drug fluorescence without modulator after subtraction of the fluorescence of the control.

3.7. Statistical Analysis

Clinical and biological factors were investigated for their influence on remission rate by the chi2 or Fisher's exact tests for binary variables and by the Mann Whitney U test for continuous values. Correlations among levels of expression of continuous values were estimated using the Spearman rank coefficient.

4. RESULTS

4.1. Correlations for 13 Cell Lines between RT/PCR and Flow Cytometry, for MRP1 and MDR1 Expression

Results of MDR1 and MRP1 expression measured by RT/PCR and flow cytometry are shown in Table 1. Correlation between RT/PCR and flow cytometry was good (r=0.94, p=0.0005 for MRP1 and r=0.96, p<0.0001 for MDR1).

4.2. Correlations for 13 Cell Lines between MRP1 and MDR1 Expression and Functional Tests Using Rhodamine 123, Daunorubicin, and Calcein AM

Relations between Pgp expression (UIC2) and the modulatory effects of CsA on the Rh 123 (r=0.82, p=0.002), daunorubicin (r=0.65, p=0.01) and calcein-AM (r=0.96, p<0.0001) uptake are reported in Figure 1 and Table 1. The relation between MRP1 expression (MRPm6) and the modulatory effects of probenecid on calcein efflux is shown in Figure 2 (r=0.91, p=0.0003) and Table 1. There was no correlation, neither between MRP1 expression and the effects of probenecid on Rh123 and DNR uptake or efflux nor between Pgp expression and the modulatory effect of probenecid on the three probes used. An example is shown in Figure 3.

4.3. Correlations for Fresh Leukemic Cells between MRP1 and MDR1 Expression and Functional Tests Using Rhodamine 123, Daunorubicin, and Calcein AM

Figure 4A illustrates the relation between MRP1 expression measured by flow cytometry and the modulatory effect of probenecid on calcein efflux (r=0.92, p<0.0001). Figure 4B illustrates the relation of Pgp expression, as measured with UIC2 antibody, with

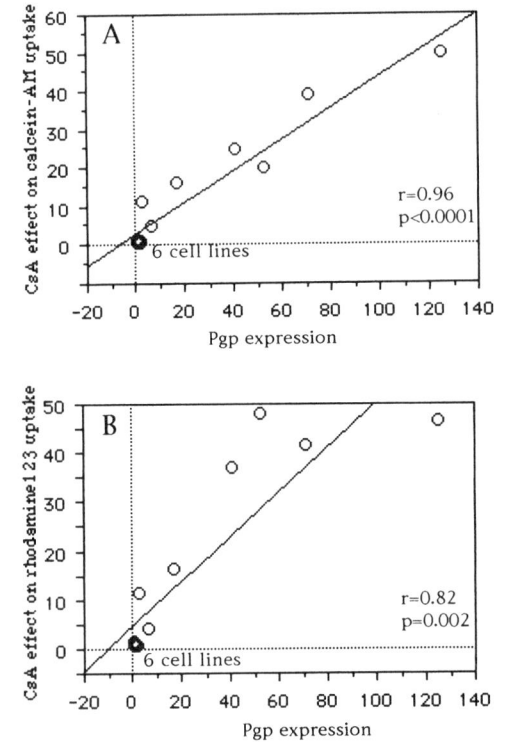

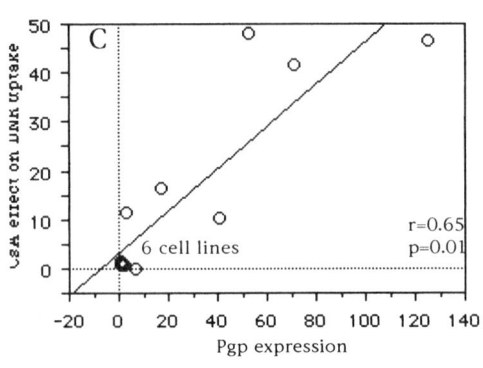

Figure 1. Correlations for 13 cell lines, between Pgp expression (measured by flow cytometry) and the modulatory effect of CsA on calcein-AM uptake (A), between Pgp expression and the modulatory effect of CsA on rhodamine123 uptake (B) and between Pgp expression and the modulatory effect of CsA on daunorubicin uptake (C).

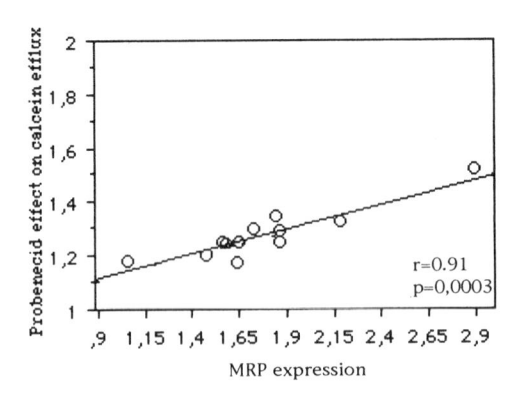

Figure 2. Correlation for 13 cell lines, between MRP1 protein expression (measured by flow cytometry) and the modulatory effect of probenecid on calcein efflux.

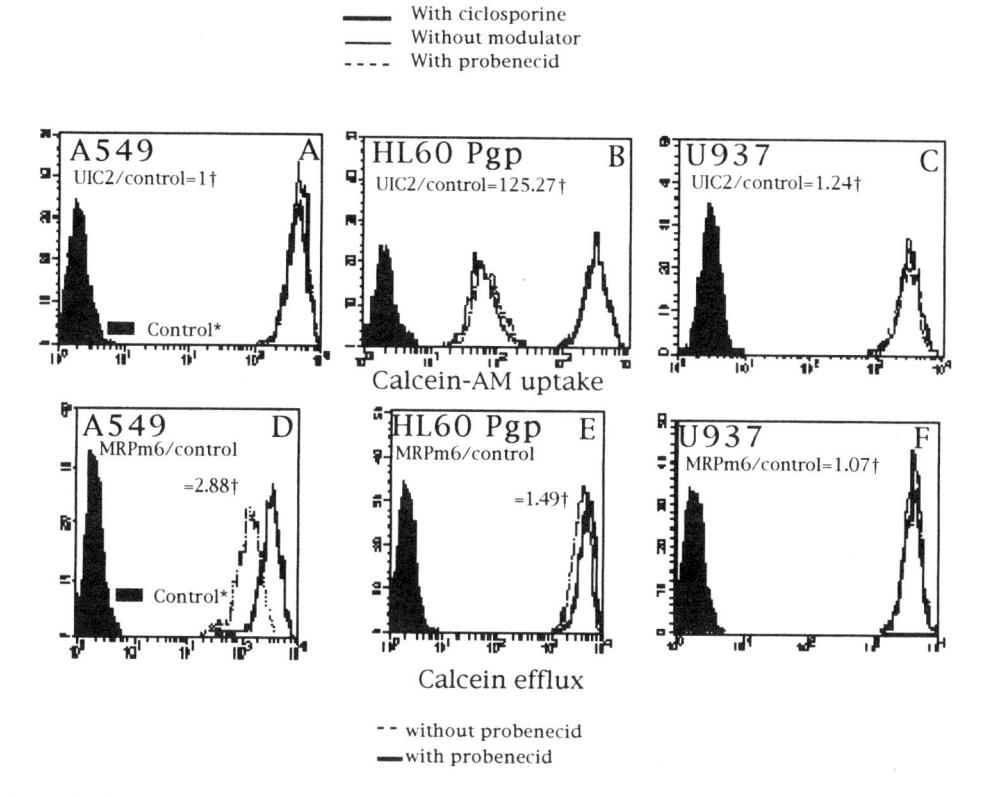

Figure 3. Flow cytometric histograms showing functional incorporation of calcein-AM, in A549 (A), in HL60 Pgp (B) and in U937 (C) cell lines, with CsA (bold line), with probenecid (dotted line) and without modulator (normal line). For A549 and U937 cell lines, the three histograms are superimposed. Flow cytometric histograms showing functional efflux of fluorescent calcein, in A549 (D), in HL60 Pgp (E) and in U937 (F) cell lines with probenecid (bold line) and without probenecid (dotted line). For U937 cell line, the two histograms are superimposed. Pgp and MRP1 expressions (measured by flow cytometry) of each cell line are noted on the figures. * Controls : autofluorescence of the cells that were not exposed to calcein-AM.

the modulatory effect of CsA on calcein-AM uptake (r=0.83, p<0.0001). See four examples Figure 5. For MDR1, we found a correlation between expression of Pgp (measured by flow cytometry) and the modulatory effect of CsA on Rh123 and DNR uptake (r=0.77, p=0.005 and r=0.65, p=0.01 respectively). There was no correlation between MRP1 expression (measured by flow cytometry) and the modulatory effect of probenecid on Rh123 or DNR uptake or efflux (data not shown).

4.4. MRP1 and MDR1 Expression in Fresh Leukemic Samples and Comparison with Clinical and Biological Parameters

There was no correlation between the expression of the two proteins studied. CD34+ leukemic cells expressed more Pgp and less MRP1 than CD34- leukemic cells (CD34+: 2.26 ± 0.79 vs CD34-: 1.46 ± 0.53, p = 0.03 for Pgp; CD34+: 1.4 ± 0.29 vs CD34-: 1.77 ± 0.40, p = 0.004 for MRP1). In the same way, the modulatory effect of CsA on calcein-AM uptake (which measures Pgp function) was more important in CD34+ leukemia than in

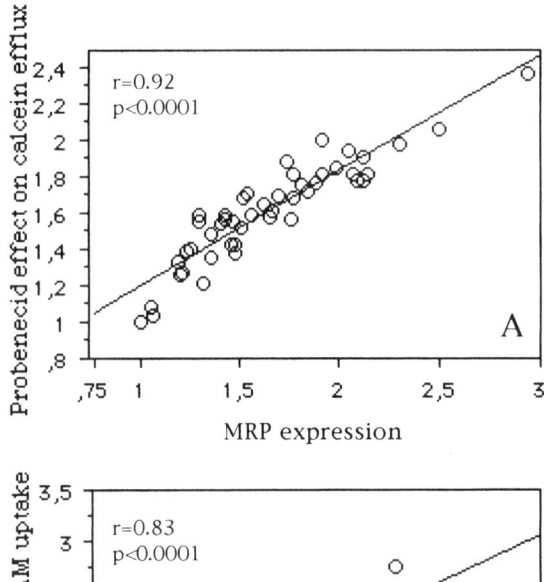

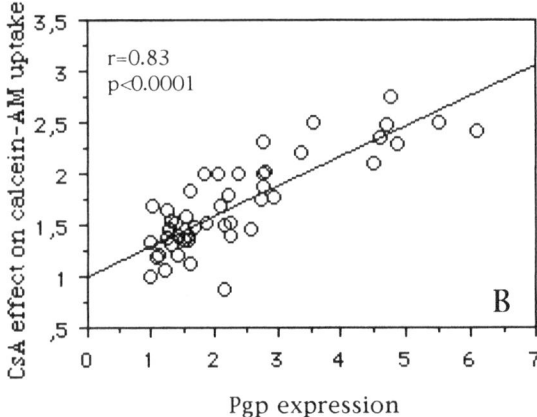

Figure 4. Correlation for fresh leukemic cells, between MRP1 expression (measured by flow cytometry) and the effect of probenecid on calcein efflux (A). Correlation for fresh leukemic cells, between Pgp expression (measured by flow cytometry) and the effect of CsA on calcein-AM uptake (B).

CD34- leukemia (2.01 ± 0.49 vs 1.69 ± 0.41, p = 0.02, respectively). On the other hand, the modulatory effect of probenecid on calcein efflux (which measures MRP1 function) was more important in CD34- leukemia than in CD34+ leukemia (1.70 ± 0.27 vs 1.26 ± 0.22, p = 0.02, respectively). Patients older than 60 expressed more Pgp, but not more MRP1 than younger patients (2.21 ± 0.45 vs 1.47 ± 1.19 for Pgp).

4.5. Prognostic Factors for Response to Therapy

Thirty two (60%) out of 53 patients achieved a complete remission. The prognostic factors for achievement of CR are summarized in Table 2 and Figure 6. Age was the only predictive clinical parameter for achievement of CR (p = 0.05). Among laboratory parameters, CR rate was significantly associated with CD34 and Pgp expression, with cytogenetic, with functional uptake of calcein-AM and with functional efflux of calcein. CR rate significantly decreased with increasing Pgp expression (p = 0.004), with increasing expression of CD34 (p = 0.01) and with unfavorable cytogenetics (p = 0.02). But CR rate was not associated with MRP1 (p = 0.07) expression. CR rate was also significantly worse in patients with an important modulatory effect of CsA on calcein-AM uptake (which measures Pgp function) and with an important modulatory effect of probenecid on calcein efflux (which analyses MRP1 function) (p = 0.01 and p = 0.03, respectively).

Figure 5. Four examples of fresh leukemic samples. First example, with high Pgp expression (a) and with high MRP1 expression (b) (measured by flow cytometry). There is an important modulatory effect of CsA on calcein-AM uptake (A) and an important effect of probenecid on calcein efflux (B). Second example, with no Pgp expression (c) and with a weak MRP1 expression (d). There is no modulatory effect of CsA on calcein-AM uptake (C) and a little modulatory effect of probenecid on calcein efflux (D). Third and fourth examples with high Pgp expression (e and g) and no MRP1 expression (f and h). In these two examples, there is an important modulatory effect of CsA on calcein-AM uptake (E and G) and no modulatory effect of probenecid on calcein efflux (F and H). * Controls : autofluorescence of the cells that were not exposed to calcein-AM. † We used the ratio : MDR MAbs (UIC2 or MRPm6) fluorescence divided by control MAbs (mouse isotype-matched control monoclonal antibodies, IgG2A for UIC2 and IgG1 for MRPm6) fluorescence. †† All the data were calculated as the ratio of drug fluorescence with modulator divided by drug fluorescence without modulator after subtraction of the fluorescence of the control.

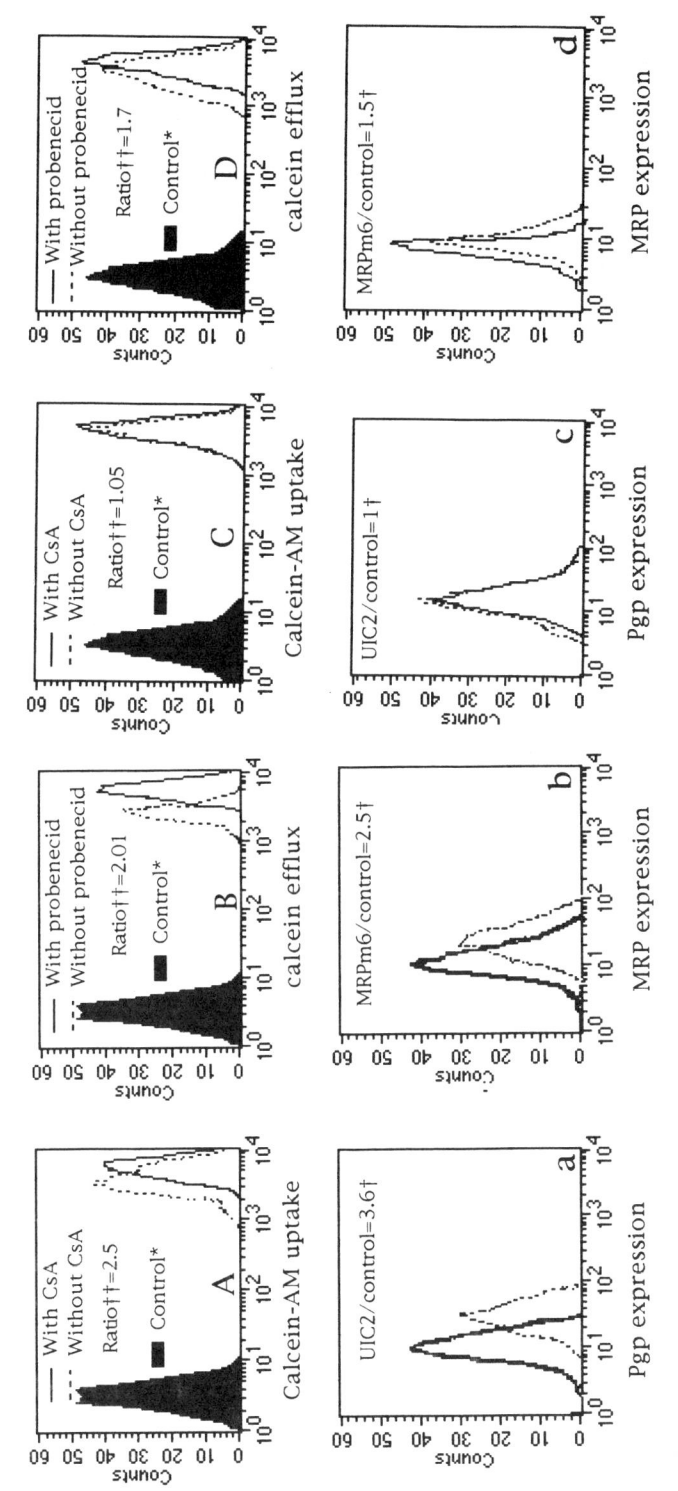

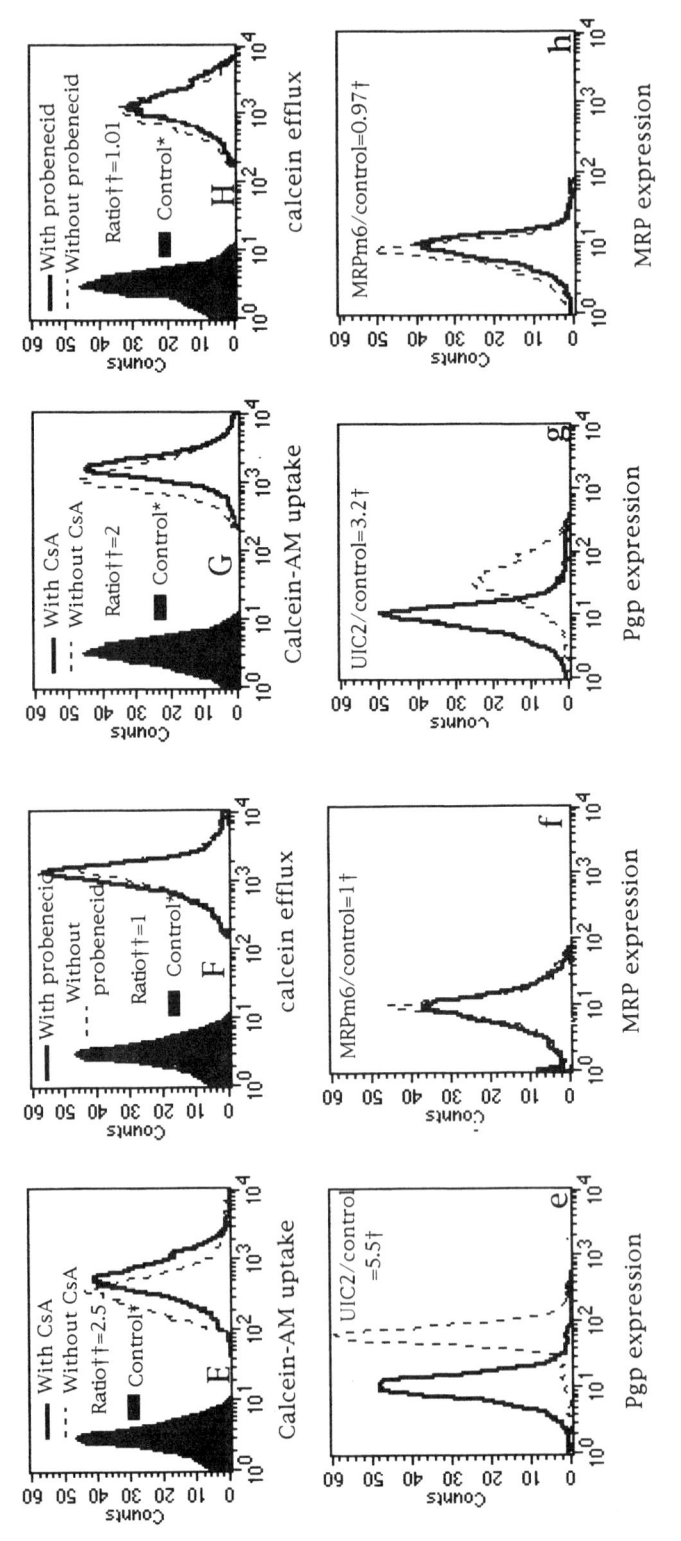

Figure 5. (*Continued*)

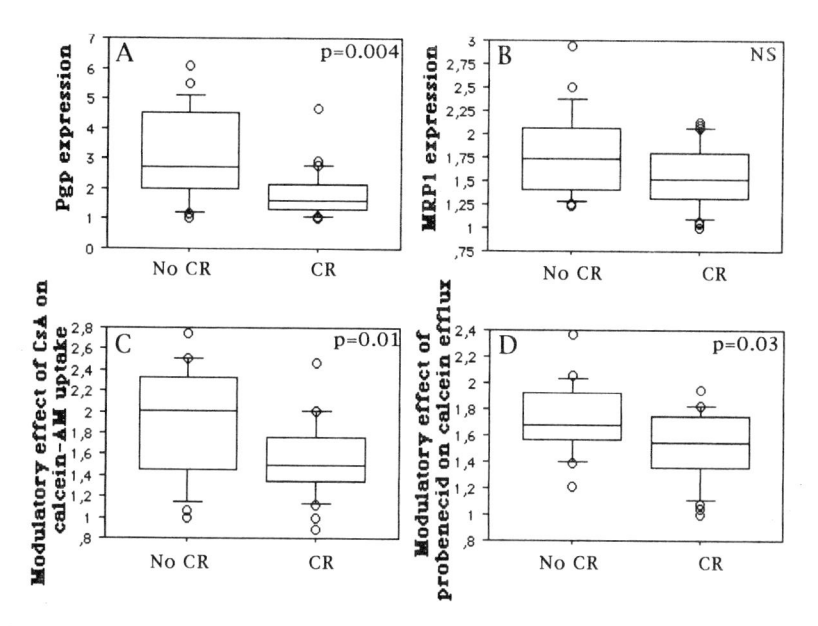

Figure 6. MDR prognostic factors with or without influence on the achievement of CR : Pgp expression (A) and MRP1 expression (B) (measured by flow cytometry), modulatory effect of CsA on calcein-AM uptake (C) and modulatory effect of probenecid on calcein efflux (D).

Table 2. Prognostic factors for achievement of CR for 53 AML patients

Parameters	Patients who achieved CR (32 patients)	Patients who did not achieve CR (21 patients)	P value
MDR parameters			
Pgp (measured by flow cytometry)	1.81±0.79	3.01±1.51	p=0.004
Modulatory effect of CsA on calcein-AM uptake	1.53±0.34	1.90±0.51	p=0.01
Modulatory effect of CsA on rhodamine 123 uptake*	1.51±0.95	2.21±1.12	p=0.02
Modulatory effect of CsA on daunorubicin uptake *	1.10±0.52	1.98±0.85	p=0.04
MRP1 (measured by flow cytometry)	1.55±0.33	1.78±0.45	NS
Modulatory effect of probenecid on calcein efflux	1.53±0.25	1.73±0.27	p=0.03
Other parameters			
Age (yo)	52±19	59±19	p=0.05
CD34+ patients (%)#	52%	85%	p=0.01
Unfavorable cytogenetic	2%	28%	p=0.02

#Samples were considered positive for CD34 when more than 20% of viable cells were stained with CD34 antibody in excess of the negative control.
*Only 49 patients were tested.

4.6. Respective Role of Both MRP1 and Pgp Activities Using Calcein-AM Uptake in Fresh Leukemic Samples

We analysed the functionality of both MRP1 and Pgp using calcein-AM uptake ± modulators of MRP1 (2mM of probenecid) or of Pgp (2µM of cyclosporinA) in 34 adult AML patients. We compared these results with the effect of CsA *and* probenecid on calcein-AM uptake. The effect of probenecid and CsA together were higher than the effect of

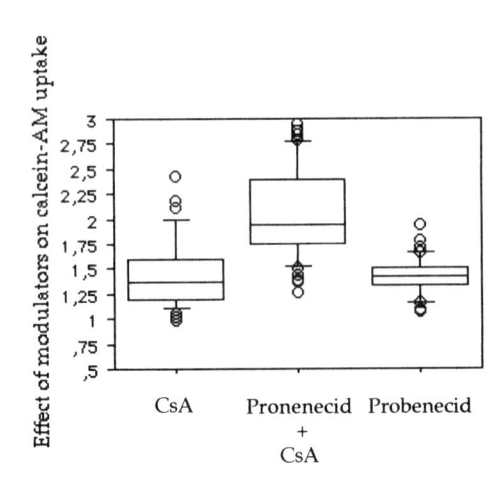

Figure 7. Effect and comparison of modulators on calcein-AM uptake. Between probenecid and probenecid + CsA (p<0.0001); between CsA and probenecid + CsA (p<0.0001); between CsA and probenecid (p=0.73).

either probenecid or CsA alone on calcein-AM uptake (Figure 7). In addition, the difference, between responders and patients with refractory disease, on calcein-AM uptake was higher when both probenecid and CsA were used together than when either probenecid or CsA was used alone (Table 3).

5. DISCUSSION

In different tumour cell lines with various levels of MDR proteins, we have confirmed that calcein-AM was a specific and sensitive probe for MRP1 and Pgp functions.[6,17-19] Probenecid, a specific and effective chemosensitizer of MRP1,[16] was used to modulate the calcein efflux and CsA was used to modulate the calcein-AM uptake. Although calcein-AM was actively extruded by MRP1 and Pgp, calcein-AM ± CsA (at 2μM) provided in cell lines a functional test as specific and sensitive as Rh123 ± CsA, the most specific and sensitive Pgp functional test.[12] All our results concerning calcein-AM uptake were calculated as the ratio of calcein-AM uptake with CsA (a specific modulator of Pgp, at 2μM) divided by calcein-AM uptake without CsA. For that reason, we analysed only Pgp function and no MRP1 function. These results encouraged us to test calcein-AM in fresh myeloid leukemic cells.

In myeloid leukemic cells, we showed that calcein-AM (± CsA, 2μM) provided also a sensitive and specific functional test which was strongly correlated with Pgp expression. This test was as specific and sensitive as functional tests using Rh123 and DNR in AML samples. Pgp expression and the modulatory effect of CsA on calcein-AM uptake were correlated with achievement of CR, the presence of CD34 and age. These findings, and particularly the fact that Pgp might limit the effectiveness of chemotherapy in CD34+ AML patients, were already noted.[20]

The functional test using calcein-AM (efflux of calcein and effect of probenecid, a specific modulator of MRP1, on calcein efflux) was strongly correlated with MRP1 expression in AML. Therefore, calcein-AM after cleavage by cellular esterase to fluorescent calcein was a specific and sensitive MRP1-probe. So, calcein-AM might be used to probe

Table 3. Achievement of complete remission and effect of modulators on calcein-AM uptake

Parameters	Patients who achieved CR (21 patients)	Patients who did not achieve CR (refractory patients) (13 patients)	P value[†]
Modulatory effect of CsA + probenecid on calcein-AM uptake	1.55±0.34	2.3±0.51	p=0.005
Modulatory effect of CsA on calcein-AM uptake	1.19±0.54	1.52±0.70	p=0.02
Modulatory effect of probenecid on calcein-AM uptake	1.25±0.12	1.45±0.21	p=0.04

[†]Using Mann Whitney U test.

specifically both MRP1 and Pgp activities. Singularly, expression of MRP1 measured by RT/PCR and flow cytometry was not a prognostic factor for achievement of CR, but probenecid effect on calcein efflux (which measures MRP1 function) was predictive for achievement of CR, in our data. Several studies support the hypothesis that MRP1 functions as a glutathione S-conjugate carrier.[21] Therefore, the MRP1 function is dependent on glutathione level. This may explain a dissociation between MRP1 expression which was not a prognostic factor and MRP1 function which was a prognostic factor for achievement of CR. Nevertheless, in our study there was a striking correlation between these two parameters (MRP1 expression and function). A few patients with high expression of MRP1 had a weak effect of probenecid on calcein efflux. Perhaps these results may explain this small difference between clinical outcome and MRP1 expression correlation (p = 0.07) and between clinical outcome and MRP1 function correlation (p = 0.03). This emphasizes also the facts that the functional test (with calcein-AM ± probenecid) is essential in the understanding of the MRP1 role, and that MRP1 contributes to MDR mechanism in AML. As for Pgp, it is important to look for dissociation between protein and function.[1] In addition to inhibition of calcein efflux, probenecid may be associated with an increased accumulation of daunorubicin and vincristine and with the correction of the altered distribution of daunorubicin.[16] The concentrations of probenecid (from 0.01 to 2 mM) that reverse MRP1 function are clinically achievable in vivo,[16] without major toxicity. These results suggest that probenecid is a good modulator for MRP1 activity and a potential candidate for clinical use to reverse MDR associated MRP1.

But, Pgp and MRP1 also actively extrude the calcein-AM.[6,8] Therefore, calcein-AM uptake (with specific modulators of Pgp and/or MRP) can assess both the functionality of Pgp and MRP1.The effect of probenecid and CsA together were higher than the effect of either probenecid or CsA alone on calcein-AM uptake. In addition, the difference, between responders and patients with refractory disease, on calcein-AM uptake was higher when both probenecid and CsA were used together than when either probenecid or CsA was used alone. Therefore, when in the same cell Pgp and MRP were blocked, there was an higher retention of calcein-AM than when we used either CsA (a modulator of Pgp only) or probenecid (a modulator of MRP only) alone.

MRP1 was overexpressed in CD34- AML when compared to CD34+ AML. These findings indicate that the MRP1 phenotype may limit the effectiveness of chemotherapy in CD34- AML and not in CD34+ AML. In accordance with this result, we and others have shown that the level of MRP1 expression in CD34+ normal hemopoietic cells and CD34+ leukemic cells are similar to those observed in sensitive cell lines,[11,22] but that MRP1 is overexpressed in more mature cells.[11,22]

In conclusion (i) Calcein-AM may be used in fresh leukemic cells to probe specifically both MRP1 and Pgp activities. (ii) With these functional assays the role of Pgp have been confirmed in AML. (iii) In the light of these results, Pgp function but also MRP function are implicated in resistance to chemotherapy in AML patients (iv) Therefore functional test (with calcein-AM±probenecid) is an essential tool for one to understand the MRP1 role in AML.

REFERENCES

1. Marie J-P, Zhou DC, Gurbuxani S, Legrand O, Zittoun R: MDR1/P-glycoprotein in haematological neoplasms. Eur J Cancer 32A: 1034, 1996.
2. Cole SPC, Bhardwaj G, Gerlach JH, Mackie JE, Grant CE, Almquist KC, Kurz EU, Duncan AM, Deeley RG: Overexpression of a transporter gene in a multidrug-resistant human lung cancer cell line. Science 258: 1650, 1992
3. Scheper RJ, Broxterman HJ, Scheffer GL, Kaaijk P, Dalton WS, van Heijningen TH, van Kalken CK, Slovak ML, de Vries EG, van der Valk P, Meijer CJLM, Pinedo HM: Overexpression of a Mr 110,000 vesicular protein in non-P-glycoprotein-mediated multidrug resistance. Cancer Res 54: 357, 1993.
4. Zhou DC, Zittoun R, Marie J-P: expression of multidrug resistance associated protein (MRP1) and multidrug resistance (MDR1) genes in acute myeloid leukemia. Leukemia 9: 1661, 1995.
5. List AF, Spier CS, Grogan TM, Jonhson C, Roe DJ, Greer JP, Wolff SN, Broxterman HJ, Scheffer GL, Scheper RJ, Dalton WS: Overexprression of the major vault transporter protein lung-resistance protein predicts treatment outcome in acute myeloid leukemia. Blood 87: 2464, 1996
6. Homolya L, Hollo Z, Germann UA, Pastan I, Gottesman MM, Sarkadi B: Fluorescent cellular indicators are extruded by the multidrug resistance protein. J Biol Chem 268: 21 493, 1993.
7. Feller N, Broxterman HJ, Wahrer DC, Pinedo HM: ATP-dependent efflux of calcein by the multidrug resistance protein (MRP1): no inhibition by intracellular glutathione depletion. FEBS Lett 368: 385, 1995.
8. Essodaigui M, Broxterman HJ, Garnier-Suillerot A: Kinetic analysis of calcein-acetoxymethylester efflux mediated by the multidrug resistance protein and P-glycoprotein. Biochemistry 37: 2243, 1998
9. Zhou DC, Ramond S, Viguié F, Faussat AM, Zittoun R, Marie J-P : Progressive resistance to homoharringtonine in human myeloleukemia K562 cells : relationship to sequential emergence of MRP and MDR1 gene overexpression and MDR1 gene translation. Int J Cancer 65: 365, 1996
10. Bennett JM, Catovsky D, Daniel MT, Flandrin G, Galton DAG, Gralnick NR, Sultan C: Proposed revised criteria for the classification of acute myeloid leukemia. Ann Intern Med 103: 620, 1985.
11. Legrand O, Perrot J-Y, Tang RP, Simonin G, Gurbuxani S, Zittoun R, Marie J-P: Expression of the multidrug resistance-associated protein (MRP) mRNA and protein in normal peripheral blood and bone marrow haemopoietic cells. Br J Haematol 94: 23, 1996.
12. Beck WT, Grogan TM, Willman CL, Cordon-Cardo C, Parham DM, Kuttesch JF, Andreeff M, Bates SE, Berard CW, Boyett JM, Brophy NA, Broxterman HJ, Chan HSL, Dalton WS, Dielt M, Fojo AT, Gascoyne RD, Head D, Houghton PJ, Kumar Svrivastava D, Lehnert M, Leith CP, Paietta E, Pavelic ZP, Rimsza L, Roninson IB, Sikic BI, Twentyman PR, Warnke R, Weinstein R: Methods to detect P-glycoprotein-associated multidrug resistance in patient tumors: consensus recommendations. Cancer Res 56: 3010, 1996.
13. Marie J-P, Huet S, Faussat A-M, Perrot J-Y, Chevillard S, Barbu V, Bayle C, Boutonnat J, Calvo F, Campos-Guyotat L, Colosetti P, Cazin J-L, De Cremoux P, Delvincourt C, Demur C, Drenou B, Fenneteau O, Feuillard J, Garnier-Suillerot A, Genne P, Gorisse M-C, Gosselin P, Jouault H, Lacave R, Le Calvez G, Léglise M-C, Léonce S, Manfait M, Maynadié M, Merle-Béral H, Merlin J-L, Mousseau M, Morjani H, Picard F, Pinguet F, Poncelet P, Racadot E, Raphael M, Richard B, Rossi J-F, Schlegel N, Vielh P, Zhou DC, Robert J. French Network of the Drug Resistance Intergroup, and Drug Resistance Network of 'Assistance Publique-Hôpitaux de Paris': Multicentric evaluation of the MDR phenotype in leukemia. Leukemia 11: 1086, 1997.
14. Marie J-P, Legrand O, Perrot J-Y, Chevillard S, Huet S, Robert J: Measuring multidrug resistance expression in human malignancies: elaboration of consensus recommendations. Semin hematol 34: 63, 1997.
15. Barrand MA, Bagrij T, Neo SY: Multidrug resistance-associated protein: a protein distinct from P-glycoprotein involved in cytotoxic drug expulsion. Gen Pharmacol 28: 639, 1997.
16. Gollapudi S, Kim CH, Tran BN, Sangha S, Gupta S: Probenecid reverses multidrug resistance in resistance-associated protein-overexpressing HL60/AR and H69/AR cells but not in P-glycoprotein-overexpressing HL60/Tax and P388/ADR cells. Cancer Chemother Pharmacol 40: 150, 1997.

17. Homolya L, Hollo M, Muller M, Mechetner EB, Sarkadi: A new method for a quantitative assessment of P-glycoprotein-related multidrug resistance in tumour cells. Br J Cancer 73: 849, 1996.
18. Hollo Z, Homolya L, Hegedus T, Sarkadi B: Transport properties of the multidrug resistance-associated protein (MRP) in human tumour cells. FEBS Lett 383: 99, 1996.
19. Hollo Z, Homolya L, Davis CW, Sarkadi B: Calcein accumulation as a fluorometric functional assay of the multidrug transporter. Biochim Biophys Acta 1191: 384, 1994.
20. Te Boekhorst PAW, de Leeuw K, Schoester M, Wittebol S, Nooter K, Hagemeijer A, Löwenberg B, Sonneveld P: Predominance of functional multidrug resistance (MDR-1) phenotype in CD34+ acute myeloid leukemia cells. Blood 82: 3157, 1993.
21. Müller M, Meijer C, Zaman GJR, Borst P, Scheper RJ, Mulder NH, de Vries EGE, Jansen PLM: Overexpression of the gene encoding the multidrug resistance-associated protein results in increased ATP-dependent glutathione S-conjugate transport. Proc Natl Acad Sci 91: 13033, 1994.
22. Schneider E, Cowan KH, Bader H, Toomey S, Schwartz GN, Karp JE, Burke PJ, Kaufmann SH: increased expression of the multidrug resistance associated protein gene in relapsed acute leukemia. Blood 85: 186, 1995.

ABSOLUTE LEVELS OF MDR-1, MRP, AND BCL-2 MRNA AND TUMOR REMISSION IN ACUTE LEUKEMIA

T. Köhler,[1] S. Leiblein,[2] S. Borchert,[1] J. Eller,[1] A.-K. Rost,[3] D. Laßner,[1] R. Krahl,[2] W. Helbig,[2] O. Wagner,[1] and H. Remke[1]

University of Leipzig Medical School
[1]Departments of Clinical Chemistry and Pathobiochemistry
Division of Molecular Biology
[2]Center of Internal Medicine
Division of Hematology
[3]IZKF Leipzig, Germany

Keywords: Acute leukemia, drug resistance, MRP, mdr-1, bcl-2, gene expression, quantitative PCR.

1. ABSTRACT

Mononuclear cells prepared from peripheral blood or bone marrow of 119 AML and 28 ALL patients prior and following therapy were analyzed for absolute transcript levels of the chemoresistance genes mdr-1 and MRP, and the proto-oncogene bcl-2, by validated contamination-protected quantitative RT-PCR. In newly diagnosed AML mainly tumors of the granulocytic lineage (FAB M1-M2) expressed increased mdr-1 mRNA amounts. The MRP gene was expressed in all investigated samples without relation to a particular FAB class. High initial expression of both genes did not confer a poor prognosis even at high number of CD34$^+$ cells. Data compared prior to and after therapy start (paired samples) revealed that AML patients who did not respond to therapy (NR) expressed increased levels of mdr-1 mRNA, as well as MRP and bcl-2 cDNA normalized to GAPDH reference transcripts, when compared to patients achieving complete remission (CR; p=0.003, 0.008 and 0.0005, respectively). In ALL-NR the mdr-1 and bcl-2 genes were entirely more active after induction chemotherapy. Arbitrary cut-off values were established in order to delimit pathological from non-pathological gene expression. 59% of studied AML and 33% of ALL-NR exceeded the arbitrary values (mdr-1: >2 amol/μg RNA, MRP: >10 zmol/amol

GAPDH, bcl-2: >5 zmol/amol GAPDH) for one and 11% of AML-NR for two parameters. Only 17% of the AML-CR and none of the ALL-CR group were above these limits. The results indicate that high individual activity of usually one, rarely two of the investigated genes might be associated with poor clinical outcome in treated acute leukemia.

2. INTRODUCTION

Despite of enormous advances in combination chemotherapy treatment it remains a sad reality that about 20–40 percent of adult patients suffering from acute myeloid leukaemia (AML) and up to 20 percent of acute lymphoblastic leukemia (ALL) patients do not achieve complete remission or relapse after initial remission. Therefore, the question remains, which molecular mechanisms may underly the clinical phenomenon of refractoriness or relapse. Particularly the "classical" multidrug resistance (MDR) has drawn specific attention. MDR is characterized by overexpression of some members of the ABC transporter protein superfamily, e.g. P-glycoprotein coded by the mdr-1 gene (1,2), the multidrug resistance-associated protein (MRP, 3–6), the lung-resistance-related protein (LRP) (1,7–9) and the anthracycline resistance-associated protein (10). However, there is also growing evidence that apoptotical or regrowth resistance, which is characterized by an imbalance between mechanisms inducing or inhibiting apoptosis mediated by members of the bcl-2 superfamily (1,11,12) may be associated with poor clinical response.

Unfortunately, no standardized methods are available to assess absolute expression rates of MDR related genes. Therefore, reports which provide reliable information about the functional overexpression of these genes are rare and applied mostly to the analysis of a relatively small number of patients (13,14). Therefore, gene expression studies in clinical samples are a controversial issue, and a complex of questions remains unanswered, e.g. which gene expression may be correlated to poor clinical outcome, and, which expression levels in leukemic blast cells constitute clinically relevant overexpression.

Samples of AML and ALL patients involved in a study coordinated by the East-German Hematology and Oncology Study Group (OSHO) were analyzed for absolute amounts of mdr-1, MRP and bcl-2 transcripts by validated quantitative RT-PCR. To reveal the clinical significance of data measured at presentation and following treatment, the results were compared between different patient groups and disease stages including morphological characterization by French-American-British (FAB) classification and detection of the CD34 differentiation antigen.

3. MATERIALS AND METHODS

3.1. Patient Characteristics and Treatment

Peripheral blood or bone marrow (BM) aspirates were collected from 119 AML and 28 ALL patients, classified according to the French-American-British (FAB) classification at the time of initial diagnosis (AD) or at relapse prior, and 85 AMLs and 24 ALLs following treatment (Tx). Patients were treated by standard chemotherapy protocols and were judged to have achieved CR when the BM showed regeneration with ≤5% blasts. Patients who died from toxic complications were considered not eligible for evaluation. All other patients were indicated nonresponsive. 75 AML and 24 ALL samples were available both AD and during Tx. $CD34^+$ cells were counted with a FACscan™ flow cytometer (Becton Dickinson, San Jose, CA, USA).

3.2. Clinical Sample Preparation and Cell Lines

Mononuclear cells from blood or BM samples were collected after separation on lymphocyte separation medium (density 1.077 g/mL; Boehringer Mannheim, FRG), and homogenized with 2 mL of RNAzol "B" (Tel-Test, Friendswood, TX, USA). As reference cell line the high-level multidrug resistant human T-lymphoblastoid cell line CCRF ADR5000, drug selected by adriamycin as described earlier (15), and the subline CCRF ADR10000 were used. RNA was extracted according to the manufacturers instructions, and dissolved in RNase-free H_2O. cDNA was synthesized from 1-µg RNA aliquots in a 20-µL standard reaction mixture (27). RNA and cDNA samples were stored at -80°C until use.

3.3. Quantitative RT-PCR and PCR Product Detection

Primers used for amplification of mdr-1, MRP, and glyceraldehyde-3-phosphate dehydrogenase (GAPDH) were described earlier (16,17). Bcl-2 primers were BCL2PR1 (5'-CTTTTGCTGTGGGGTTTTG-3') and BCL2PR2 (5'-CTTCTCCTTTTGGGGCTTTT-3'). Mdr-1 standard cRNA was synthesized and purified as described (17). Working solutions were prepared with RNase-free H_2O, supplemented with 100 ng/µL *Escherichia coli* carrier tRNA (Boehringer Mannheim). Bcl-2 competitor DNA fragments were synthesized *in vitro* by generating a single G→C base exchange at residue 3877 yielding an unique *Hha*I restriction site 26 bp upstream from the 3'-end of final PCR product.

Competitor DNA fragments developed for quantitation of MRP and GAPDH cDNA were prepared, calibrated and stored as described (16). cDNA aliquots prepared from clinical samples were at first screened for mdr-1 mRNA. 1–2 µg of positively evaluated RNA were amplified using a r*Tth* reverse transcriptase kit (Perkin-Elmer, Norwalk, CT, USA). Aliquots of mdr-1 cRNA (0.08–41.8 attomoles [10^{-18} moles, amol] per tube) were amplified separately to generate a calibration curve, PCR products were detected by PCR-ELISA (17). MRP, GAPDH and bcl-2 cDNAs were quantified separately by amplifying aliquots of reverse transcribed RNA in 50-µL, carryover protected standard competitive PCR reaction mixtures (16). Competitive MRP and bcl-2 cDNA amplifications were performed in triplicate by coamplifying 9.75, 2.93 and 0.98 zeptomoles (10^{-21} moles, zmol) of MRP, and 16.39, 3.38 and 1.31 zmol of bcl-2 competitor DNA fragment per tube with 35 cycles (MRP: 94°C for 30 s, 53°C for 30 s, 72°C for 1 min; bcl-2: 94°C for 30 s, 55°C for 30 s, 72°C for 1 min). GAPDH cDNA was measured in duplicate by co-amplification of 4.26 and 2.13 amol of a 355 bp heterologous competitor DNA subsequence of pMS1 plasmid (17) with 22 cycles (94°C for 30 s, 58°C for 30 s, 72°C for 45 s). MRP and GAPDH fragments were separated and quantified by high performance liquid chromatography (HPLC). 10-µL aliquots of bcl-2 PCR product were subjected to restriction digestion with 5 U of *Hha*I for 1 h at 37°C prior to electrophoresis through a 2.5% agarose gel. The stained bands were scanned using a GelPrint Video Documentation Workstation (MWG-Biotech, Ebersberg, FRG). The areas under the individual peaks obtained by HPLC or densitometry were used to determine the target/competitor ratios used for calculation of initial cDNA input (17).

3.4. Statistical Analyses

Differences between patients groups regarding quantitative mdr-1, MRP, and bcl-2 data and disease stages were performed by means of the nonparametric Mann-Whitney U-

4. RESULTS

4.1. Quality Assurance of Quantitative PCR Protocols

Four contamination-protected quantitative PCR protocols were developed. Mdr-1 mRNA amplified in duplicate was calculated from a reference curve prepared with separately amplified defined amounts of standard mdr-1 cRNA. In contrast, MRP, bcl-2, and GAPDH transcripts were quantified by competitive PCR using calibrated, double-stranded competitor DNA fragments. The overall dynamic range of each method was about 5×10^2 to 10^3 estimated by either titration of a constant cDNA amount with known competitor amounts, or by titration of known competitor amounts with cDNA dilution series. Since the measurement of cDNA amounts was found to be independent of added competitor concentration, analysis of MRP and bcl-2 transcripts in clinical samples was performed in triplicate, whereas GAPDH cDNA was measured in duplicate. Data corrected for absolute copies of reference GAPDH cDNA were sufficiently reproducible (MRP: mean ± 46%; bcl-2: mean ± 27%). The mdr-1 PCR-ELISA protocol yielded an variability ranging from 21 to 35%. Although absolute quantitation of gene expression reveals the relative activity of genes, not of proteins, a correlation between mdr-1 mRNA levels and drug efflux properties of the adriamycin resistant CCRF sublines was found: the higher the tolerated drug concentration in the medium (5 vs. 10 µg/ml for ADR5000 vs. ADR10000, respectively), the higher the number mdr-1 transcripts in the cell (166.64 ± 58.68 vs. 1296 ± 266 amol/µg RNA).

4.2. Mdr-1, MRP, and Bcl-2 Transcript Levels in Control, AML, and ALL Mononuclear Cells

Thirty-eight percent of AML and 32% of ALL samples were found to contain detectable mdr-1 mRNA amounts at the time of tumor presentation. AML M1+M2 leukemia with predominant granulocytic differentiation pathway were characterized by the highest mdr-1 mRNA amounts (Figure1). In ALL, the mdr-1 gene activity was lower compared to AML, and usually below 3.5 amol/µg RNA. Highest individual values were found in ALL-L2. In contrast, the MRP gene was expressed constitutively in all samples. No correlation between average MRP expression and FAB classification was found by statistical data analysis.

Paired samples, the first obtained at diagnosis and the second following induction treatment, were used to calculate Δmdr-1 and ΔMRP values. Differences were higher in AML-NR compared to AML-CR for both the mdr-1 mRNA (p=0.003), and MRP cDNA levels given relative to GAPDH reference gene transcripts (p=0.008) (Figure 2). Therefore, an average increase in mdr-1 and MRP gene activity was associated with therapy-resistance in AML. Samples from resistant ALL contained higher Δmdr-1 mRNA values compared to CR (p=0.008), whereas ΔMRP levels did not correlate with outcome of therapy (p=0.47).

To assess the risk of therapy failure already at the time of leukemia presentation, mdr-1 and MRP data were correlated to the percentage of CD34⁺ cells contained in the

Absolute Levels of Mdr-1, MRP, and Bcl-2 mRNA

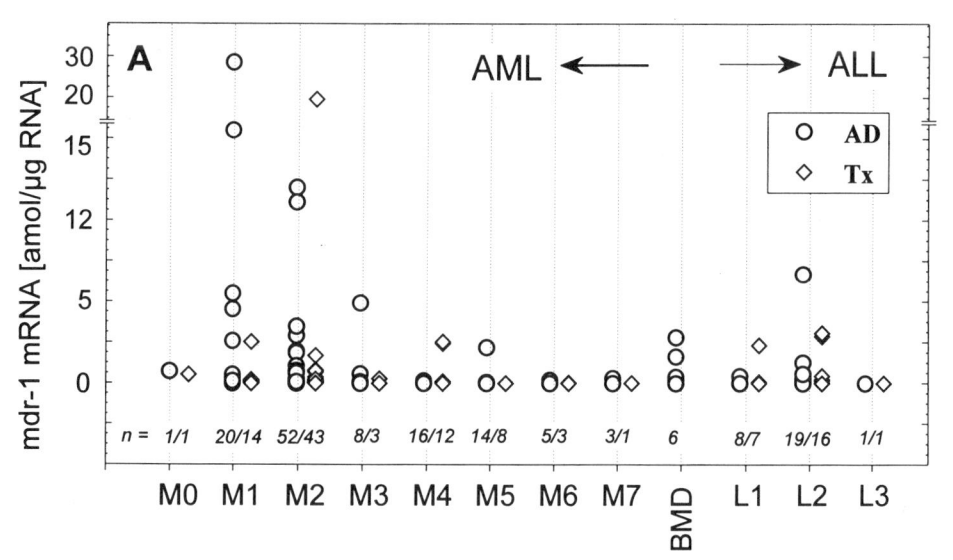

Figure 1. Mdr-1 gene expression in newly diagnosed and treated acute leukemia. Mdr-1 mRNA levels from AML and ALL samples collected prior (circles) and following induction chemotherapy (rhombs) measured by PCR-ELISA are plotted versus FAB classes (AML: M0-M7; ALL: L1-L3). Values >1 amol/µg RNA appeared more frequent in AML M1 (p=0.03) and M2 (p=0.17) compared to M4. BMD = bone marrow donors, n = number of analyzed samples AD/Tx.

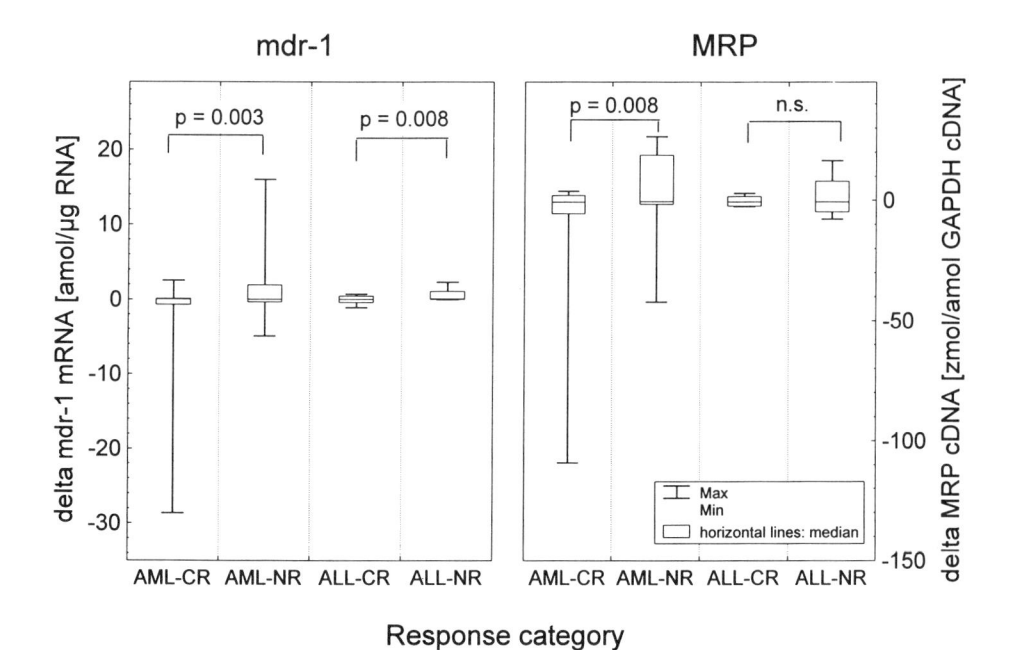

Figure 2. Correlation of mdr-1 and MRP expression with therapy response. From 75 AML (41 CR, 34 NR) and 28 ALL patients (17 CR, 11 NR) receiving at least one course of induction therapy data from paired samples were calculated (i.e. post-therapy minus prior-therapy values) and presented in box plots showing median and 90th percentile of each parameter relative to the response category. Statistical evaluation was performed by means of Mann-Whitney U-test.

sample AD. Neither high initial expression of the mdr-1 nor MRP gene did absolutely confer a poor prognosis of AML or ALL treatment even in the presence of an elevated number of CD34⁺ cells.

Mdr-1 mRNA plotted versus MRP and bcl-2 expression determined from the same sample showed that either the mdr-1 or MRP or bcl-2 gene were predominantly transcribed in AML and ALL (Figure 3). Therapy resistant AML and ALL samples showed significantly elevated overall mRNA levels of the "regrowth resistance" marker bcl-2 compared to those of patients achieving CR (AML: $p=0.0005$; ALL: $p=0.04$). Whereas either the bcl-2 or the MRP pathways appeared to be the preferred mechanisms in AML, an increased bcl-2 expression was associated with poor response in ALL.

Arbitrary cut-off values were established from the levels obtained from normal BM, and were 2 amol/µg RNA for mdr-1, 10 zmol/amol GAPDH cDNA for MRP, and 5 zmol/amol GAPDH cDNA for bcl-2. As demonstrated in Table 1, 59% of the AML-NR group, but only 17% of the AML-CRs expressed at least one of the three transcripts above the cut-offs. This difference was statistically significant in AML ($p=0.03$) but not in ALL.

5. DISCUSSION

Quantitative PCR assays have been applied for estimation of gene expression, because they allow the measurement of absolute numbers of investigated transcripts, provide reliable information about functional overexpression of a gene, and may serve for feasible comparison of results obtained by different studies (13,14). Samples of AML and ALL patients were analyzed for MDR related transcripts in order to find relationships between molecular parameters and clinical impact. In general, higher average activities of studied

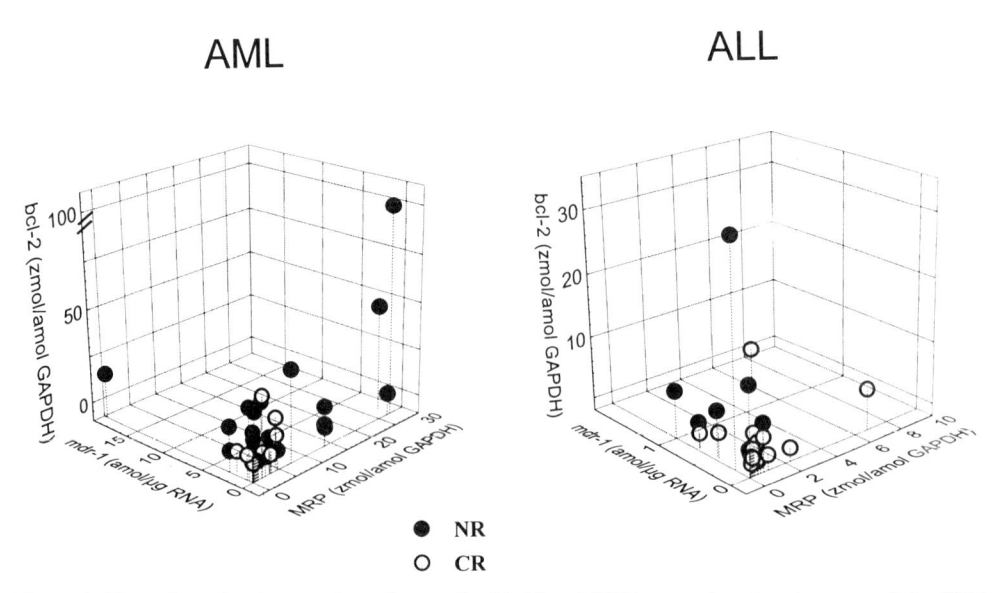

Figure 3. Three-dimensional comparison of normalized bcl-2 and MRP expression plotted versus mdr-1 mRNA content. Gene expression data of 24 AML and 18 ALL patients achieving CR (open circles), and 37 AML and 12 ALL samples from patients who never achieved remission (closed circles) are shown. Each point represents expression data measured in an unique sample.

Table 1. AML and ALL patients who overexpressed 1, 2, or all investigated transcripts (i.e. mdr-1, MRP, bcl-2) above the arbitrary cut-off values compared with therapy outcome

Investigated transcripts > cut-off (No.)	AML NR	AML CR	P value	ALL NR	ALL CR	P value
1	22/37 (59%)	4/24 (17%)	0.03*	4/12 (33%)	2/18 (11%)	n.s.*
2	4/37 (11%)	0/24	n.s.*	0/12	0/18	n.s.*
3	0	0		0	0	

11% of AML-NR group but none of ALL-NRs exceeded the arbitrary values for two parameters, whereas all three transcripts were never simultaneously increased. P-values obtained by Pearson's χ^2 test, n.s.: not significant.

genes were found in AML, which might contribute to the poorer prognosis of AML compared to ALL (18). Data generated by subtraction of values obtained prior from that after the initial cycles of treatment indicate the diagnostic value of both mdr-1 and MRP transcript amounts with regard to discrimination between efficient and poor remission in AML and partly in ALL. Nevertheless, the value of this observation appears to be limited, particularly for mdr-1, since all patients were treated with the antimetabolites ARA-C and the anthracycline IDA which are probably not or incompletely transported by P-glycoprotein (1). However, MRP is believed to be a potent ARA-C transporter (Dr. W.A. Evans, talk on the 3rd Symposium), which might explain the preference of that pathway particularly in resistant AML, which was observed earlier (4,5). Interestingly, and parallel to findings from the drug resistant cell lines, classical MDR in acute leukemia was characterized by one predominant drug efflux mechanism, due to either increased expression of the mdr-1 or MRP coded drug efflux pump. An inverse correlation between mdr-1, MRP, and/or LRP levels is consistant with findings of Stein et al. (9), Xu et al. (14) and Michieli et al. (8), who showed that the ability to accumulate a drug was impaired already by overexpression of one resistance gene, whereas the drug efflux was not further enhanced by a second mechanism. Arbitrary cut-off values for MDR gene expression defined to delimit pathological from non-pathological gene expression indicate again a high prevalence of a single defense mechanism. Out of the NR groups about two third of the AMLs and one fifth of ALLs overexpressed one, whereas only 11% of AML and none of the ALL group overexpressed two or more of the studied genes.

Besides classical MDR, regrowth resistance has gained interest as a novel approach for determination of chemosensitivity, since high expression of the bcl-2 proto-oncogene in AML cells has been associated with poor response to therapy (12,19–21). Our experiments confirm these observations. Interestingly, increased overall expression of the bcl-2 gene was particularly found in those samples containing neither detectable mdr-1 nor MRP mRNA. The preference of bcl-2 survival pathway in treated AML may be the result of G-CSF administration, which may also enhance the proliferation of tumor cells by decreasing the in vitro and in vivo cytotoxic effects of doxorubicin and etoposide (22) or ARA-C (23).

A multivariable model to evaluate treatment response in regard to MDR gene levels, disease type and survival duration is now in progress.

ACKNOWLEDGMENTS

The authors wish to thank Drs. Volker Gekeler, Byk-Gulden GmbH, Konstanz, and Heyke Diddens, Medical Laser Center Lübeck for the drug resistant T-lymphome cell lines, and Dr. S. Kasimir-Bauer, University Essen for the BMD samples. We also thank Dr. H. Garn, Institute of Immunology, Philipps-University of Marburg, FRG, for providing us with the GAPDH primer sequences, and Dr. D. Hasenclever, IMISE Leipzig, for statistical advise. We are greatful to G. Bönisch and C. Weishäupl for their skilled technical assistance. This work was supported by OSHO.

REFERENCES

1. McKenna SL, Padua RA. Multidrug resistance in leukaemia. Br J Haematol 19997; 96: 659–674.
2. Licht T, Pastan I, Gottesman MM, Herrmann F. The multidrug-resistance gene in gene therapy of cancer and hematopoietic disorders. Ann Hematol 1996; 72: 184–193.
3. Cole SPC, Bhardway G, Gerlach JH, Mackie JE, Grant CE, Almquist KC. Overexpression of a transporter gene in a multidrug-resistant human lung cancer cell line. Science 1992; 258: 1650–1653.
4. Hart SM, Ganeshaguru K, Hoffbrand AV, Prentice HG, Mehta AB. Expression of the multidrug resistance-associated protein (MRP) in acute leukemia. Leukemia 1994; 8: 2163–2168.
5. Schneider E, Cowan KH, Bader H, Toomey S, Schwartz GN, Karp JE, Burke PJ, Kaufmann SH. Increased expression of the multidrug resistance-associated protein gene in relapsed acute leukemia. Blood 1995; 85: 186–193.
6. Nooter K, Burger H, Stoter G: Multidrug resistance-associated protein (MRP) in haematological malignancies. Leuk Lymphoma 1996; 20: 381–387.
7. Scheffer GL, Wijngaard PL, Flens MJ, Izquierdo MA, Slovak ML, Pinedo HM, Meijer CJ, Clevers HC, Scheper RJ. The drug resistance-related protein LRP is the human major vault protein. Nat Med 1 1995; 578–582.
8. Michieli M, Damiani D, Ermacora A, Raspadori D, Michelutti A, Grimaz S, Fanin R, Russo D, Lauria F, Masolini P, Baccarani M. P-glycoprotein (PGP) and lung resistance-related protein (LRP) expression and function in leukaemic blast cells. Br J Haematol 1997; 96: 356–365.
9. Stein U, Walther W, Laurencot CM, Scheffer GL, Scheper RJ, Shoemaker RH. Tumor necrosis factor-alpha and expression of the multidrug resistance-associated genes LRP and MRP. J Natl Cancer Inst 1997; 89: 807–813.
10. Longhurst TJ, O'Neill GM, Harvie RM, Davey RA. The anthracycline resistance-associated (ara) gene, a novel gene associated with multidrug resistance in a human leukaemia cell line. Br J Cancer 1996; 74: 1331–1335.
11. Preisler HD, Raza A, Bonomi P, Taylor S, LaFolette S, Leslie W, Lincoln S. Regrowth resistance as a likely significant contributor to treatment failure in drug-sensitive neoplastic diseases. Cancer Invest 1997; 15: 358–368.
12. Kroemer G. The proto-oncogene Bcl-2 and its role in regulating apoptosis. Nature Med 1997; 3: 614–620.
13. Lyttelton MP, Hart S, Ganeshaguru K, Hoffbrand AV, Mehta AB. Quantitation of multidrug resistant MDR1 transcript in acute myeloid leukaemia by non-isotopic quantitative cDNA-polymerase chain reaction. Br J Haematol 1994; 86: 540–546.
14. Xu D, Knaust E, Pisa P, Palucka K, Lundeberg J, Arestrom I, Peterson C, Gruber A. Levels of mdr1 and mrp mRNA in leukaemic cell populations from patients with acute myelocytic leukaemia are heterogenous and inversely correlated to cellular daunorubicin accumulation. Br J Haematol 1996; 92: 847–854.
15. Gekeler V, Weger S, Probst H. MDR1/P-glycoprotein gene segments analyzed from various human leukemic cell lines exhibiting different multidrug resistance profiles. Biochem Biophys Res Commun 1990; 169: 796–802.
16. Köhler T, Rost A-K, Remke H. Calibration and storage of DNA competitors used for contamination-protected competitive PCR. BioTechniques 1997; 23: 722–726.
17. Köhler T, Laßner D, Rost A-K, Thamm B, Pustowoit B, Remke H. Quantitation of mRNA by polymerase chain reaction - Nonradioactive PCR methods. Springer -Verlag, Heidelberg, Germany, 1995.
18. Beck J, Niethammer D, Gekeler V. MDR1, MRP, topoisomerase II alpha/beta, and cyclin A gene expression in acute and chronic leukemias. Leukemia 1996; 10: 39–45.
19. Bradbury D, Zhu YM, Russell N. Regulation of Bcl-2 expression and apoptosis in acute myeloblastic leukaemia cells by granulocyte-macrophage colony-stimulating factor. Leukemia 1994; 8: 786–791.
20. Pallis M, Zhu YM, Russell NH. Bcl-x(L) is heterogenously expressed by acute myeloblastic leukaemia cells and is associated with autonomous growth in vitro and with P-glycoprotein expression. Leukemia 1997; 11: 945–949.

21. Campos L, Oriol P, Sabido O, Guyotat D. Simultaneous expression of P-glycoprotein and bcl-2 in acute myeloid leukemia blast cells. Leuk Lymphoma 1997; 27: 119–125.
22. Kondo S, Yin D, Takeuchi J, Morimura T, Oda Y, Kikuchi H. Bcl-2 gene enables rescue from in vitro myelosuppression (bone marrow cell death) induced by chemotherapy. Br J Cancer 1994; 70: 421–426.
23. Hu ZB, Minden MD, McCulloch EA: Post-transcriptional regulation of bcl-2 in acute myeloblastic leukemia: significance for response to chemotherapy. Leukemia 1996; 10: 410–416.

20

MULTIDRUG RESISTANCE PROTEIN MRP1, GLUTATHIONE, AND RELATED ENZYMES

Their Importance in Acute Myeloid Leukemia

Dorina M. van der Kolk,[1,3] Edo Vellenga,[1*] Michael Müller,[2] and Elisabeth G. E. de Vries[3]

[1]Division of Hematology
[2]Division of Gastroenterology and Hepatology
[3]Division of Medical Oncology
Department of Internal Medicine
University Hospital of Groningen, The Netherlands

1. ABSTRACT

Multidrug resistance (MDR), which is cross-resistance to structurally and functionally unrelated drugs such as anthracyclines, epipodophyllotoxins and vinca alkaloids, is a major cause of treatment failure in malignant disorders. Known mechanisms of MDR are overexpression of the ATP-dependent membrane proteins P-glycoprotein (P-gp) and multidrug resistance protein (MRP1), or an increased detoxification of compounds mediated by glutathione (GSH) or GSH related enzymes. MRP1 appeared to transport drugs conjugated to GSH and also unmodified cytostatic agents in presence of GSH. The relation between MRP1, GSH and enzymes involved in GSH metabolism or GSH dependent detoxification reactions recently has drawn a lot of attention. Coordinated induction of MRP1 and GSH related enzymes is reported in malignant cells after exposure to cytostatic agents.

Besides MRP1, a number of MRP1 homologs are identified, named MRP2, MRP3, MRP4, MRP5 and MRP6. The relation between MDR and expression of these MRP1 homologs is currently under research.

---

[*] Address for correspondence and reprint requests: E. Vellenga, M.D. Division of Hematology Department of Internal Medicine University Hospital P.O. Box 30.001 9700 RB Groningen The Netherlands Phone: +31–50–3612354 Fax: +31–50–3614862 E-mail: E.Vellenga@int.azg.nl

In human Acute Myeloid Leukemia (AML) the expression of MRP1 appears to be of potential importance. We demonstrated that AML blasts of patients express MRP1 protein and MRP1 and MRP2 mRNA. Furthermore a functional flow cytometric assay was developed to determine MRP functional activity. Since GSH and related enzymes have shown to play a critical role in MRP1 mediated transport of several anticancer drugs, both mechanisms should be studied in relation with each other. Further work on these interwoven mechanisms is needed to improve our understanding of MDR in leukemia.[*]

2. INTRODUCTION

Development of multidrug resistance (MDR) is a serious problem in the treatment of patients with cancer. MDR, which is cross-resistance to structurally and functionally unrelated drugs can occur as intrinsic in *de novo* tumors or as an acquired form in tumors which initially respond to chemotherapy but eventually show progression in spite of treatment. Drugs involved in MDR are the anthracyclines, vinca alkaloids, epipodophyllotoxins and taxenes.[1-3]

To escape from death, tumor cells can exert different strategies, thereby lowering the intracellular concentration of antitumor agents or making them unable to affect their target genes. The pathway of a cytostatic agent to reach its intracellular goal and subsequently to cause cell death can be underbroken at different levels. To date several of these mechanisms used by tumor cells, have been identified and it becomes more and more clear that some of these mechanisms are closely interwoven. A couple of MDR mechanisms that act at different points of the drug-pathway are: 1) *Multidrug resistance proteins*. Overexpression of ATP-dependent membrane proteins which transport drugs out of the cytoplasm into the extracellular medium or into intracellular vesicles, where they are unable to exert their task. The transport proteins thus far known to play a role in MDR are: P-glycoprotein (P-gp), a 170 kDa protein, encoded by the *MDR1* gene located on the long arm of chromosome 7.[5-7] Multidrug resistance protein (MRP1), which shares 15% amino acid identity with P-gp, is a 190 kDa protein, encoded by the *MRP1* gene, located on chromosome 16p13.[8-11] MRP2, also called cMOAT, is recently described to play a role in MDR, the *MRP2* gene is located on chromosome 10q24.[12]

The human major vault protein LRP is the most abundant component of the cellular organelles termed vaults, which are mainly present in the cytoplasm, but also in the nuclear membrane and nuclear pore complexes. LRP is a 110 kDa protein, the gene of which, like the *MRP1* gene, is located on chromosome 16p[13,14] and is probably involved in drug transport.[15] 2) *Detoxification*. Increased detoxification of compounds, mediated by glutathione (GSH) and enzymes involved in GSH metabolism or GSH dependent detoxification reactions, such as γ-glutamyl-cysteine-synthetase (γ-GCS) and glutathione S transferases (GST).[16-18] 3) *Drug targets*. Down-regulation of drug targets such as the nuclear enzyme DNA topoisomerase II, which plays an essential role in DNA replication and transcription.[19] 4) *Apoptosis*. Inhibition of drug-induced cell death, apoptosis, whereby the relative expressions of apoptosis accelerating and anti-apoptotic proteins of the CD95/FAS pathway, such as Bcl2, Bcl-X_L, Bcl-X_s, bad, bak, bax, FLICE and several additional caspases play a critical role.[20-23]

---

[*] Abbreviations used are: GSH: glutathione, γ-GCS: γ-glutamylcysteine synthetase, GSSG: reduced GSH, GR: GSH reductase, GST: GSH transferase.

This review will focus on the role of MRP1, GSH and related enzymes and their association, conjugation and transport by MRP1 in MDR, especially in Acute Myeloid Leukemia (AML).

3. MRP1

3.1. History

Although overexpression of P-gp has been associated with MDR in drug-selected cell lines and human tumors,[24-26] it does not in all cases explain the occurrence of MDR. The MDR cell line H69AR, derived from the drug sensitive parental cell line H69 by doxorubicin (DOX) selection, appeared to overexpress another protein of the ATP-binding cassette (ABC) transporter superfamily, namely the 190 kDa multidrug resistance protein MRP.[8,9] Furthermore transfection of an MRP expression vector in e.g. Hela cells has demonstrated that this protein is capable to confer resistance to drugs such as the epipodophyllotoxins and anthracyclines.[10,11,26] MRP1, as it is called nowadays because other MRP's have been identified, has been described to be overexpressed in other MDR cell lines, including the cell line GLC4/ADR[27] and the leukemia cell lines HL60/ADR,[28] U-937/A[29] and CEM/E.[30] When two groups demonstrated independently that MRP1 represents the GSH conjugate pump,[31-33] the relation between MRP1, GSH and enzymes involved in GSH metabolism or GSH dependent detoxification reactions, became an object of extensive investigation.

3.2. MRP1 Mediated Multidrug Resistance

The basic mechanism of action by which MRP1 confers resistance to multiple drugs is not well understood. The substrate specificity of the transporter appears to be quite broad since both cationic or neutral cytotoxic drugs as well as anionic compounds are transported by MRP1.[34] The biosynthetic release of endogenous leukotriene C4 (LTC4), synthetized in leukocytes through the conjugation of LTA4 with GSH,[35,36] is mediated by MRP1.[33] The finding of this and other physiological potential GSH conjugates to be transported as MRP1 substrates has led to the research of export of drug conjugates from cells by MRP1.

Double knockout of the *mrp1* gene in murine W9.5 embryonic stem cells, which totally abrogated mrp1 expression, resulted in increased drug sensitivity of etoposide (VP-16), teniposide, vincristine (VCR), DOX, daunorubicine (DNR) and sodium arsenite.[37] In another study increased sensitivity to the anticancer drug VP-16 in mice lacking the *mrp1* gene was reported.[38] The *mrp1* knock-out mice were viable and fertile but showed decreased inflammatory response, probably attributed to a decreased secretion of LTC4 from leukotriene-synthesizing cells.

3.3. MRP1 Homologs

Besides MRP1, a homolog of MRP1, the canalicular multispecific organic anion transporter (cMOAT) was cloned, also called MRP2, a new member of the ABC superfamily of transporters.[39] MRP2 expression was specifically enhanced in a cisplatin-resistant human head and neck cancer KB cell line. Although one group described MRP2 to be a splicing variant of MRP1,[40] the locus of the human *MRP2* gene was demonstrated on chromosome

10q24.[12] The amino acid sequence identity of human *MRP2* and *MRP1* is 49%. MRP2 is dominantly expressed in hepatocytes,[41] but MRP2 was also demonstrated at variable levels in AML blasts.[42] Recently, four new homologs of MRP1 were identified, named MRP3, MRP4, MRP5 and MRP6.[43] *MRP3*, located on chromosome17, is mainly expressed in the liver, like *MRP2*. MRP4 is expressed only at low levels in the lung, kidney, bladder and tonsil and is located on chromosome 13. MRP5, the gene of which is located on chromosome 3, is expressed in a number of tissues. *MRP6* is located next to *MRP1* on chromosome 16p13, and is almost 100% identical with the MRP-like half transporter called ARA.[44]

In cell lines selected for resistance several MRP-related genes can be upregulated. MRP2 appeared to be highly expressed in cell lines with ovarium, colon and epidermoid carcinoma origin. MRP3 and MRP5 are only overexpressed in a few cell lines, derived from epidermoid and ovarium carcinoma respectively. MRP4 was not overexpressed in any of the cell lines tested in that study. MRP2 levels correlated well with cisplatin but not with doxorubicin resistance in the resistant cell lines. No correlation was demonstrated between drug resistance and expression levels of MRP3, MRP4 and MRP5.

3.4. Membrane Topology of MRP1

MRP1 and P-gp, like several other bacterial and eukaryotic transporters belong to the ABC transporter proteins. Most of these proteins contain hydrophobic membrane spanning domains (MSD's) and cytoplasmic nucleotide binding domains (NBD's).[45] The mechanism by which P-gp and MRP1 transport drugs are apparently not the same, so it seems that protein-drug interactions are different between these transporters.[46,47]

The human MRP1, like the cystic fibrosis transmembrane conductance regulator (CFTR), contains a tandem repeat of six transmembrane helices, each followed by a NBD.[45,48] The C-terminal membrane-bound region is glycosylated and the N-terminal region of MRP1 contains an additional membrane-bound glycosylated area with four or five MSD's.[48]

Recently a study was published which suggested that the NH_2-terminal MSD of MRP1 contains an odd number of transmembrane helices, thus having an extracytosolic NH_2-terminus.[49] The functional significance of MRP1 N-glycosylation remains unclear since inhibition of N-linked glycosylation did not influence the transport function. Protein phosphorylation studies demonstrated that MRP1 is highly phosphorylated, primarily at serine residues.[50,51] In the presence of protein kinase C inhibitors MRP1 phosphorylation was inhibited in HL60/ADR cells, accompanied by a major increase in drug accumulation.[52] However it is not excluded that some protein kinase C inhibitors may be a substrate for MRP1 mediated transport, as has been described for P-gp.[53]

3.5. *MRP1* Gene Regulation

Little information is available regarding the regulation of *MRP1* gene transcription. The 5'-flanking DNA of the *MRP1* gene of HL60/ADR cells has been cloned.[54] Deletion mutant studies showed the promoter activity to be dependent on sequences between the nucleotides -91 to +103 in a GC-rich region of the *MRP1* genome. Sequence analysis indicated the presence of consensus domains for a number of regulatory elements, including AP-1, AP-2, SP1, ERE, GRE and CRE. The same group presented a study regarding the SP1 site which modulates the transcriptional activity of the *MRP1* gene.[55] Three SP1 consensus sites in the *MRP1* gene promoter were demonstrated to play a role in transcriptional activation of *MRP1* expression. But at present SP1 is not shown to be overexpressed in MRP1 overexpressing cells.

4. GSH AND RELATED ENZYMES

4.1. Synthesis and Recycling Pathways of GSH

GSH is a widely distributed non-protein thiol with a protective role in the cell.[56,57] It serves as a modulator of thiol-disulfide status of proteins, as a protector against oxidative stress and electrophilic compounds and as a transporter of endogenous and exogenous substances.[58]

The synthesis of GSH (Figure 1) in the cytosol takes place in two steps, catalyzed by the enzymes γ-glutamylcysteine synthetase (γ-GCS) and GSH synthetase (GS) respectively, whereby γ-GCS is the rate limiting enzyme. γ-GCS can be specifically inhibited by buthionine sulfoximine (BSO),[59] resulting in a reduction of GSH level up to 95%.[60] In response to oxidative stress GSH is dimerized and forms oxidized GSH (GSSG), which can be reduced again to monomeric GSH by GSH reductase (GR). The conjugation between GSH and a variety of endogenous and exogenous compounds can occur spontaneously but catalyzation by GSH transferases (GST) enhances these reactions. The MRP1 pump and also MRP2 are important mediators of GSH conjugate transport, but also GSSG and probably reduced GSH are substrates for these pumps.[12,31–33,64,69,70]

4.2. GSH in Drug Resistance

In recent years many studies presented GSH to be a critical determinant in cellular drug resistance to cytostatic drugs.[60–64] After the discovery of MRP1 to be identical to the GSH S-conjugate transporter[31–33] more and more attention is given to the role of GSH and

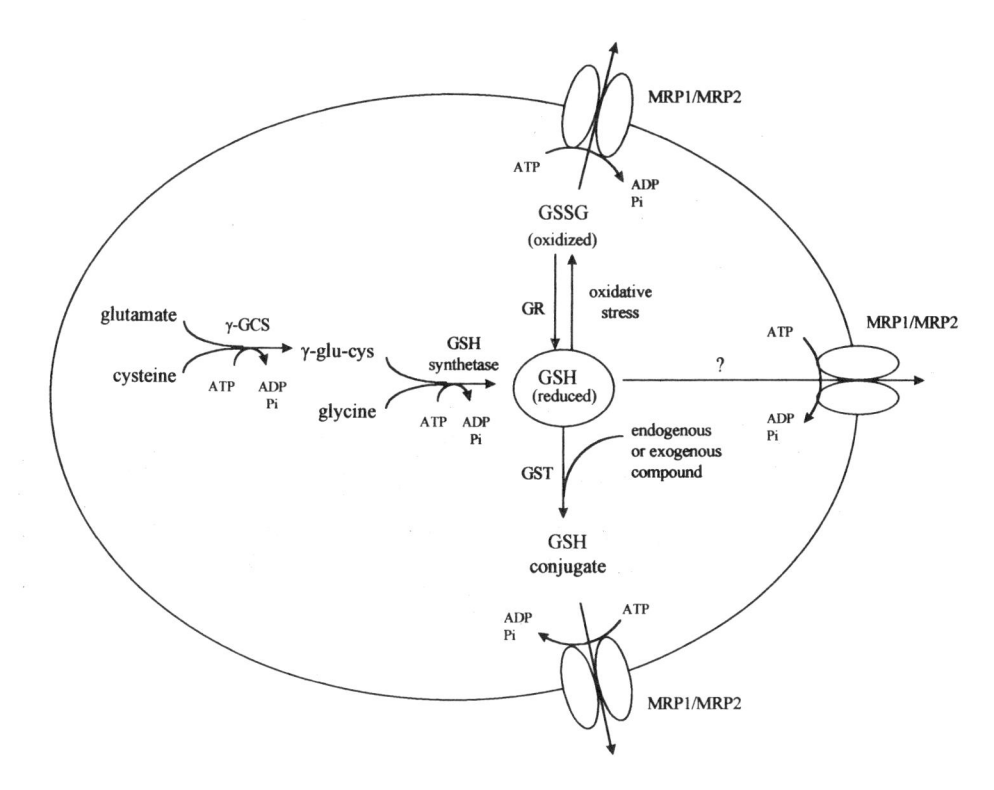

Figure 1. Schematic illustration of GSH metabolism.

enzymes involved in GSH metabolism or GSH dependent detoxification reactions, in drug transport by MRP1. Several reports have demonstrated that elevated levels of GSH and GST or GSH peroxidase may protect cells from anticancer agents such as the anthracyclines.[65] Resistance to DNR, VCR and Rh123 can be reversed in MRP1 overexpressing lung tumor cell lines by exposing these cells to BSO, the inhibitor of γ-GCS,[66] demonstrating that drug transport in MRP1 overexpressing cells can be regulated by GSH levels. Inhibition of GSH synthesis in the human myelogenous leukemia cell line HL60/AR also resulted in significant sensitization by DNR.[67] Disruption of the murine *mrp* gene led, besides increased sensitivity to VP-16, also to increased levels of GSH in *mrp*(-/-) mice.[68]

Although conjugation products of GSH and cytostatic drugs have not been demonstrated, there is evidence for a co-transport by MRP1 of natural product toxins such as VCR and VP-16, and GSH.[46,69] The mechanism by which this GSH-dependent transport takes place is unknown. It is possible that GSH may form reversible complexes and then can be co-transported with some cytostatic drugs.

5. RELATION BETWEEN MRP1 AND GSH

5.1 Coordinated Induction of MRP1 and GSH Related Enzymes

Since a correlation has been demonstrated between drug resistance and expression of GSH related enzymes, research has focussed on the mechanisms responsible for this. GST's can be induced by a number of chemicals.[70] Induction of gene expression can occur through elements in the promoter region of GST, like the xenobiotic response element (XRE) or the antioxidant response element (ARE), described in the promoter of the rat *GSTA2* gene.[71] Rat as well as human *GST*π and human γ-*GCS* genes are described to contain AP-1 sites in their promoter regions.[72-74] NF-κB binding sites have been identified in the 5'-upstream sequences of the γ-*GCS* gene[74] and also *GST* has been described to be under NF-κB control.[75]

Coordinated induction of MRP1 and γ-GCS has been reported by heavy metals in the cisplatin-resistant leukemia cell line HL-60/R-CP.[76] MRP mRNA levels could be induced within 30 h after incubation with cisplatin or heavy metals. Expression of γ-GCS was co-induced after 24 h cisplatin exposure, which resulted in an increase in intracellular GSH. This co-expression pattern was also shown in other tumor cell lines of different origin, including cervical carcinoma and small cell lung carcinoma cell lines, and in untreated tumor cells and normal mouse tissues.[77] It is also reported that the coordinated induction of MRP1 and γ-GCS can be transient. Treatment of human glioma cells with an alkylating antitumor agent resulted in elevated expression of MRP1 mRNA and γ-GCS mRNA, followed by a decrease in expression after the treatment.[78]

5.2. Functional Analyses and Modulation of MRP1

To study the drug efflux capacity of cells fluorescent probes are readily applicable. For P-gp the probes rhodamine 123[79] and calcein-AM[80] have been applied. MRP-mediated efflux can be studied using the fluorescent probe calcein[81] in combination with a specific inhibitor of MRP1. Calcein transport appeared to be ATP-dependent but GSH independent, since GSH depletion by exposing cells to BSO had no effect on the efflux of calcein. The use of calcein as a substrate for MRP1 gives the opportunity to study MRP1 function independently of the GSH status of the cell. To study the functional activity of MRP1 the fluorescent substrates should be used in combination with MRP1 modulators. A variety of MRP modulators are known, including the natural substrates for the transporter e.g. LTC4 or GSSG. But also other compounds can be applied such as the organic anion transport inhibitor probenecid[82] or the isoflavanoid tyrosine kinase inhibitor genistein.[82,83] However these compounds only inhibit MRP1 function at highly toxic concentrations. Additional inhibitors are the bisindolylmaleimide protein kinase C inhibitor GF109203X[84] and the ATP-ase inhibitor sodium orthovanadate.[31] A very effective MRP1 inhibitor appeared to be the LTD4 receptor antagonist MK-571.[85,86] Recently we developed a functional assay[42] to detect MRP activity using the substrate carboxyfluorescein diacetate (CFDA), which permeates the plasma membrane and upon cleavage of the ester bonds by intracellular esterases is transformed into the fluorescent anion carboxyfluorescein (CF).[87] MK-571 was used as inhibitor of MRP-mediated CF transport. Several tumor cell lines were studied, including the MRP1 overexpressing cell line GLC4/ADR and the *MRP1* transfected cell line S1(*MRP1*). The use of this assay appeared to be a very sensitive method to analyze GSH independent MRP function.

6. MDR IN AML

P-gp, MRP1 and also LRP expressions appear to be of potential importance in drug resistance in leukemia,[88–93] whereby MRP1 overexpression might precede the overexpression of P-gp in human myeloid leukemia cells.[29] But the relative contribution of each protein and the transport mechanisms by which they confer drug resistance are currently under investigation.

A number of studies have been published with regard to MRP1 mRNA and protein expression in AML cells and the results are diverse. Some studies suggest that MRP1 expression is a prognostic factor in AML[94] and show increased expression of MRP1 mRNA and protein in relapsed acute leukemia.[95,96] These data correlate nicely with in vitro experiments demonstrating an enhanced expression of MRP1 in time in response to e.g. cisplatin[77] or DNR[97] exposure. MRP1 mRNA and protein expression appeared to be inversely correlated with DNR accumulation in vitro.[97,98] An additional study showed that, although MRP1 protein was expressed at different levels in leukemic cells from de novo AML patients, the MRP1 protein expression did not predict for outcome of induction therapy or survival.[99] However limited data are available regarding the functional role of MRP1 in clinical drug resistance. Some AML subtypes are associated with an inversion in chromosome 16 (inv(16)), the chromosome on which the *MRP1* gene is located. AML patients with inv(16), most commonly patients with the French-American-British (FAB) classification M4Eo, have a relatively favorable prognosis. *MRP1* deletion is demonstrated in inv(16) AML and was associated with increased duration of disease-free survival, suggesting an important role for MRP1 in determining clinical outcome of AML patients.[100]

In our study[42] we demonstrated that AML blasts express MRP1 and MRP2 mRNA, and that MRP function, as determined by a flowcytometric assay using CF in combination with MK-571, correlated with MRP1 protein expression in these blast cells. AML patients with inv(16) showed relatively low MRP functionality, reflecting the decreased MRP1 pump function as result of the loss of the MRP1 gene on chromosome 16.

7. CONCLUSION

The overexpression of MRP1 is a mechanism by which cells can become multidrug resistant. To study the effects of MRP1 overexpression it is not only important to measure

MRP1 protein expression, but moreover it is necessary to analyze the functional drug efflux of MRP1. However, since GSH and related enzymes have shown to play a critical role in MRP1 mediated transport of several anticancer drugs, both mechanisms appear to be involved simultaneously and should be studied in relation with each other. Further work on these interwoven mechanisms is needed to improve our understanding of multidrug resistance in leukemia.

REFERENCES

1. Biedler JL, Riehm H. Cellular resistance to actinomycin D in Chinese hamster cells in vitro: cross-resistance, radioautographic, and cytogenetic studies. Cancer Res 1970, 30:1174–1184.
2. Dano K. Cross resistance between vinca alkaloids and anthracyclines in Ehrlich ascites tumour in vitro. Cancer Chemother Rep 1972, 56:701–708.
3. Ling B, Thompson LH. Reduced permeability in CHO cells as a mechanism of resistance to colchicine. J Cell Physiol 1974, 83:103–111.
4. Gros P, Neriah YB, Croop HM, Housman DE. Isolation and expression of a cDNA (mdr) that confers multidrug resistance. Nature 1986, 323:728–731.
5. Roninson IB, Chin JE, Choi KG, Gros P, Housman DE, Fojo A, Shen DW, Gottesman MM, Pastan I. Isolation of human mdr DNA sequences amplified in multidrug-resistant KB carcinoma cells Proc Natl Acad Sci USA 1986, 83:4538–4542.
6. Gerlach JH, Endicott JA, Juranka PF, Henderson G, Sarangi F, Deuchars KL, Ling V. Homology between P-glycoprotein and a bacterial haemolysin transport protein suggests a model for multidrug resistance. Nature 1986, 324:485–489.
7. Endicott JA, Ling V. The biochemistry of P-glycoprotein-mediated multidrug resistance. Ann Rev Biochem 1989, 58:13337–171.
8. Cole SPC, Bhardwaj G, Gerlach J, Mackie JE, Grant CE, Almquist KC, Stewart AJ, Kurz EU, Duncan AM, Deeley RG. Overexpression of a transporter gene in a multidrug-resistant human lung cancer cell line. Science 1992, 258:1650–1654.
9. Cole SPC, Deeley RG: Multidrug resistance-associated protein: sequence correction. Science 1993, 260:879.
10. Grant CE, Valdimarsson G, Hipfner DR, Almquist KC, Cole SPC, Deeley RG: Overexpression of multidrug resistance-associated protein (MRP) increases resistance to natural product drugs. Cancer Res 1994, 54:357–361.
11. Zaman GJR, Flens MJ, van Leusden MR, de Haas M, Mulder HS, Lankelma J, Pinedo HM, Scheper RJ, Baas F, Broxterman HJ et al. The human multidrug resistance-associated protein MRP is a plasma membrane drug-efflux pump. Proc Natl Acad Sci USA 1994, 91:8822–8826.
12. Taniguchi K, Wada M, Kohno K, Nakamura T, Kawabe T, Kawakami M, Kagotani K, Okumura K, Akiyama S, Kuwano M. A human canalicular multispecific organic anion transporter (cMOAT) gene is overexpressed in cisplatin-resistant human cancer cell lines with decreased drug accumulation. Cancer Res 1996, 56:4124–4129.
13. Scheper RJ, Broxterman HJ, Scheffer GL, Kaaijk P, Dalton WS, van Heijningen TH, van Kalken CK, Slovak ML, de Vries EGE, van der Valk et al. Overexpression of a M_r 110,000 vesicular protein in non-P-glycoprotein-mediated multidrug resistance. Cancer Res 1993, 53:1475–1479.
14. Scheffer GL, Wijngaard PLJ, Flens MJ, Izquierdo MA, Slovak ML, Pinedo HM, Meijer CJ, Clevers HC, Scheper RJ. The drug resistance-related protein LRP is the human major vault protein. Nature Med 1995, 1:578–582.
15. Izquierdo MA, Scheffer GL, Flens MJ, Schroeijers AB, van der Valk P, Scheper RJ. Major vault protein LRP-related multidrug resistance. Eur J Cancer 1996, 32A:979–984.
16. Peters WHM, Roelofs HMJ. Biochemical characterization of resistance to mitoxantrone and adriamycin in Caco-2 human colon adenocarcinoma cells: a possible role for glutathione S-transferases. Cancer Res 1992, 52:1886–1890.
17. Meijer C, Mulder NH, Timmer-Bosscha H, Sluiter WJ, Meersma GJ, de Vries EGE. Relationship of cellular glutathione to the cytotoxicity and resistance of seven platinum compounds. Cancer Res 1992, 52:6885–6889.
18. Tew KD. Glutathione-associated enzymes in anticancer drug resistance. Cancer Res 1994, 54:4313–4320.

19. Pommier Y, Kerrigan D, Schwartz RE, Swack JA, McCurdy A. Altered DNA topoisomerase II activity in Chinese hamster cells resistant to topoisomerase II inhibitors. Cancer Res 1986, 46:3075–3081.
20. Raff MC. Social controls on cell survival and cell death. Nature 1992, 356:397–400.
21. Fisher DE. Apoptosis in cancer therapy: crossing the threshold. Cell 1994, 78:539–542.
22. Hickman JA. Apoptosis and chemotherapy resistance. Eur J Cancer 1996, 32A:921–926.
23. Villa P, Kaufmann SH, Earnshaw WC. Caspases and caspase inhibitors. Trends Biochem Sci 1997, 22:388–393.
24. Nielsen D, Skovsgaard T. P-glycoprotein as multidrug transporter: a critical review of current multidrug resistant cell lines. Biochem Biophys Acta 1992, 1139:169–183.
25. Nooter K, Herweijer H. Multidrug resistance (mdr) genes in human cancer Br J Cancer 1991, 63:663–669.
26. Kruh GD, Chan A, Myers K, Gaughan K, Miki T, Aaronson SA. Expression complementary DNA library transfer establishes mrp as a multidrug resistance gene. Cancer Res 1994, 54:1649–1652.
27. Zijlstra JG, de Jong S, de Vries EGE, Mulder NH. Topoisomerases, new targets in cancer chemotherapy. Med Oncol & Tumor Pharmacother 1990, 7:11–18.
28. Krishnamachary N, Center MS. The MRP gene associated with a non-P-glycoprotein multidrug resistance encodes a 190-kDa membrane bound glycoprotein. Cancer Res 1993, 53:3658–3661.
29. Slapak CA, Mizunuma N, Kufe DW: Expression of the multidrug resistance associated protein and P-glycoprotein in doxorubicin-selected human myeloid leukemia cells. Blood 1994, 84:3113–3121.
30. Davey RA, Longhurst TJ, Davey MW, Belov L, Harvie RM, Hancox D, Wheeler H. Drug resistance mechanisms and MRP expression in response to epirubicin treatment in human leukaemia cell line. Leukemia Res 1995, 17:1–8.
31. Müller M, Meijer C, Zaman GJ, Borst P, Scheper RJ, Mulder NH, de Vries EGE, Jansen PLM. Overexpression of the gene encoding the multidrug resistance-associated protein results in increased ATP-dependent glutathione S-conjugate transport. Proc Natl Acad Sci USA 1994, 91:13033–13037.
32. Jedlitschky G, Leier I, Bucholz U, Center M, Keppler D. ATP-dependent transport of glutathione S-conjugates by the multidrug resistance-associated protein. Cancer Res 1994, 54:4833–4836.
33. Leier I, Jedlitschky G, Bucholz U, Cole SPC, Deeley RG, Keppler D. The MRP gene encodes an ATP-dependent export pump for leukotriene D4 and structurally related conjugates. J Biol Chem 1994, 269:27807–27810.
34. Hongxie S, Saptarski P, Breuninger LM, Ciaccio PJ, Laing NM, Helt M, Tew KD, Kruh GD. Cellular and in vitro transport of glutathione conjugates by MRP. Biochemistry 1996, 35:5719–5725.
35. Samuelsson B, Dahlén SE, Lindgren JA, Rouzer CA, Serhan. Leukotrienes and lipoxins: structures, synthesis and biological effects. Science 1987, 237:1171–1176.
36. Nicholson DW, Ali A, Klemba MW, Munday NA, Zamboni RJ, Ford-Hutchinson AW. Human leukotriene C4 synthase expression in dimethyl sulfoxide-differentiated U937 cells. J Biol Chem 1994, 267:17849–17857.
37. Lorico A, Rappa G, Flavell RA, Sartorelli AC. Double knockout of the MRP gene leads to increased drug sensitivity in vitro. Cancer Res 1996, 56:5351–5355.
38. Wijnholds J, Evers R, van Leusden MR, Mol CAAM, Zaman GJR, Mayer U, Beijnen JH, van der Valk M, Krimpenfort P, Borst P. Increased sensitivity to anticancer drugs and decreased inflammatory response in mice lacking the multidrug resistance-associated protein. Nature Med 1997, 11:1275–1279.
39. Müller M, Roelofsen H, Jansen PLM. Secretion of organic anions by hepatocytes: involvement of homologues of the multidrug resistance protein. Semin Liver Dis 1996, 16:211–220.
40. Mayer R, Kartenbeck J, Büchler M, Jedlitschky G, Leier I, Keppler D. Expression of the MRP gene-encoded conjugate export pump in liver and its selective absence from the canalicular membrane in transport-deficient mutant hepatocytes. J Cell Biol 1995, 131:137–150.
41. Keppler D, König J. Expression and localization of the conjugate export pump encode by the MRP2 (cMRP/cMOAT) gene in liver. FASEB J 1997, 11:509–516.
42. Van der Kolk DM, de Vries EGE, Koning JA, van den Berg E, Müller M, Vellenga E. Activity and expression of the multidrug resistance protein MRP1 and MRP2 in acute myeloid leukemia (AML) cells. Blood 1997, 90:801, Suppl.
43. Kool M, de Haas M, Scheffer GL, Scheper RJ, van Eijk MJT, Juijn JA, Baas F, Borst P. Analysis of expression of cMOAT (MRP2), MRP3, MRP4, and MRP5, homologs of the multidrug resistance-associated protein gene (MRP1) in human cancer cell lines. Cancer Res 1997, 57:3537–3547.
44. Longhurst TJ, O'Neill GM, Harvie RM, Davey RA. The anthracycline resistance-associated (ara) gene, a novel gene associated with multidrug resistance in a human leukaemia cell line. Br J Cancer 1996, 74:1331–1335.
45. Higgins CF. ABC transporters: From microorganisms to man. Annu Rev Cell Biol 1992, 8:67–113.

46. Loe DW, Almquist KC, Deeley RG, Cole SPC. Multidrug resistance protein (MRP)-mediated transport of leukotriene C4 and chemotherapeutic agents in membrane vesicles. Demonstration of glutathione-dependent vincristine transport. J Biol Chem 1996, 271:9675–9682.
47. Gottesmann MM, Pastan I. Biochemistry of multidrug resistance mediated by the multidrug transporter. Ann Rev Biochem 1993, 62:385–427.
48. Bakos E, Hegedüs T, Holló Z, Welker E, Tusnády GE, Zaman GJR, Flens MJ, Váradi A, Sarkadi B. Membrane topology and glycosylation of the human multidrug resistance-associated protein. J Biol Chem 1996, 271:12322–12326.
49. Hipfner DR, Almquist KC, Leslie EM, Gerlach JH, Grant CE, Deeley RG, Cole SPC. Membrane topology of the multidrug resistance protein (MRP). J Biol Chem 1997, 272:23623–23630.
50. Almquist KC, Loe DW, Hipfner DR, Mackie JE, Cole SPC, Deeley RG. Characterization of the M_r 190,000 multidrug resistance protein (MRP) in drug-selected and transfected human tumor cells. Cancer Res 1995, 55:102–110.
51. Loe DW, Almquist KC, Hipfner DR, Mackie JE, Cole SPC, Deeley RG. Characterization of the 190 kDa multidrug resistance protein (MRP) in drug-selected and transfected human tumor cells. Proc Am Assoc Cancer Res 1995, 36:322.
52. Ma L, Krishnamachary N, Center MS. Phosphorylation of the multidrug resistnace associated protein gene encoded protein P190. Biochemistry 1995, 34:3338–3343.
53. Epand RM, Stafford AR. Protein kinases and multidrug resistance. Cancer J 1993, 6:154–158.
54. Zhu Q, Center MS. Cloning and sequence analysis of the promoter region of the MRP gene of HL60 cells isolated for resistance to adriamycin. Cancer Res 1994., 54:4488–4492.
55. Zhu Q, Center MS. Evidence that SP1 modulates transcription activity of the multidrug resistance-associated protein gene. DNA Cell biol 1996, 15:105–111.
56. Fahey RC, Sundquist AR. Evolution of glutathione metabolism. Adv Enzymol Relat Areas Mol Biol 1991, 64:1–53.
57. Kosower NS, Kosower EM. The glutathione status in cells. Intern Rev Cytol 1978, 54:109–160
58. Ziegler DM. Role of reversible oxidation-reduction of enzyme thiols-disulfides in metabolic regulation. Annu Rev Biochem 1985, 54:305–329.
59. Griffith OW, Meister A. Potent and specific inhibition of glutathione synthesis by buthionine sulfoximine (S-n-butyl homocysteine sulfoximine) J Biol Chem 1979, 254:7558–7560.
60. Meister A. Glutathione deficiency produced by inhibition of its synthesis, and its reversal; applications in research and therapy. Pharmacol Ther 1991, 51:145–154.
61. Arrick BA, Nathan C. Glutathione metabolism as a determinant of therapeutic efficacy: A review. Cancer Res 1984, 44:4224–4232.
62. Ishikawa T, Ali-Osman F. Glutathione-associated cis-diamminedichloroplatinum(II) metabolism and ATP-dependent efflux from leukemia cells. J Biol Chem 1979, 254:7558–7560.
63. Ishikawa T. The ATP-dependent glutathione S-conjugate export pump. TIBS 1992, 17:463–468.
64. Zaman GJ, Lankelma J, van Tellingen O, Beijnen J, Dekker H, Paulusma C, Oude-Elferink RP, Baas F, Borst P. Role of glutathione in the export of compounds from cells by the multidrug-resistance-associated protein. Proc Natl Acad Sci USA 1995, 15:7690–7694.
65. Tew KD. Glutathione-associated enzymes in anticancer drug resistance. Cancer Res 1994, 54:4313–4320.
66. Versantvoort CHM, Broxterman HJ, Bagrij T, Scheper RJ, Twentyman PR. Regulation by glutathione of drug transport in multidrug-resistant human lung tumour cell lines overexpressing multidrug resistance-associated protein. Br J Cancer 1995, 72:82–89.
67. Lutzky J, Astor MB, Taub RN, Baker MA, Bhalla K, Gervasoni JE Jr, Rosado M, Stewart B, Krishna S, Hindenburg AA. Role of glutathione and dependent enzymes in anthracycline-resistant HL60/AR cells. Cancer Res 1989, 49:4120–4125.
68. Lorico A, Rappa G, Finch RA, YangD, Flavell RA, Sartorelli AC. Disruption of the murine MRP (multidrug resistance protein) gene leads to increased sensitivity to etoposide (VP-16) and increased levels of glutathione. Cancer Res 1997, 57:5238–5242.
69. Rappa G, Lorico A, Flavell RA, Sartorelli AC. Evidence that the multidrug resistance protein (MRP) functions as a co-transporter of glutathione and natural product toxins. Cancer Res 1997, 57:5232–5237.
70. Hayes JD, Pulford DJ. The glutathione S-transferase supergene family: regulation of GST and the contribution of the isozymes to cancer chemoprotection and drug resistance. Crit Rev Biochem Molec Biol 1995, 30:445–500.
71. Rushmore TH, King RG, Paulson KE, Pickett CB. Regulation of glutathione S-transferase Ya subunit gene expression: identification of a unique xenobiotic response element controlling inducible expression by planar aromatic compounds. Proc Natl Acad Sci USA 1990, 87:3826–3830.

72. Sakai M, Okuda A, Muramatsu M. Multiple regulatory elements and phorbol 12-O-tetradecanoate 13-acetate responsiveness of the rat placental glutathione transferase gene. Proc Natl Acad Sci USA 1988, 85:9456–9460.
73. Morrow CS, Cowan KH, Goldsmith ME. Structure of the human genomic glutathione S-transferase π gene. Gene 1989, 75:3–11.
74. Yao K-S, Godwin AK, Johnson SW, Ozols RF, O'Dwyer PJ, Hamilton TC. Evidence for altered regulation of γ-glutamylcysteine synthetase gene expression among cisplatin-sensitive and cisplatin-resistant human ovarian cancer cell lines. Cancer Res 1995, 55:4367–4374.
75. Moffat GJ, Bammler TK, McLaren AW, Driessen H, Finnstrom N, Wolf CR. Transcriptional regulation and structure/function analysis of the human and murine pi class GST genes. ISSX Workshop on glutathione S-transferases, London, Taylor and Francis, 1995.
76. Ishikawa T, Bao J-J, Yamane Y, Akimaru K, Frindrich K, Wright CD, Kuo MT. Coordinated induction of MRP/GS-X pump and γ-glutamylcysteine synthetase by heavy metals in human leukemia cells. J Biol Chem 1996, 271:14981–14988.
77. Kuo MT, Bao J-J, Furuichi M, Yamane Y, Gomi A, Savaraj N, Masuzawa T, Ishikawa T. Frequent coexpression of MRP/GS-S pump and γ-glutamylcysteine synthetase mRNA in drug-resistant cells, untreated tumor cells, and normal mouse tissues. Biochem Pharmacol 1998, 55:605–615.
78. Gomi A, Shinoda S, Masuzawa T, Ishikawa T, Kuo MT. Transient induction of the MRP/GS-X pump and γ-glutamylcysteine synthetase by 1-(4-amino-2-methyl-5-pyrimidinyl)methyl-3-(2-chloroethyl)-3-nitrosourea in human glioma cells. Cancer Res 1997, 57:5292–5299.
79. Lampidis TJ, Munck JN, Krishnan A, Tapiero H. Reversal of resistance to rhodamine in adriamycin-resistant Friend leukemia cells. Cancer Res 1985, 45:2626–2631.
80. Holló Z, Homolya L, Davis CM, Sarkadi B. Calcein accumulation as a fluorometric functional assay of the multidrug transporter. Biochym Biophys Acta 1994, 1191:384–388.
81. Feller N, Kuiper CM, Lankelma J, Ruhdal JK, Scheper RJ, Pinedo HM, Broxterman HJ. Functional detection of MDR1/P170 and MRP/P190-mediated multidrug resistance in tumour cells by flow cytometry. Br J Cancer 1995, 72:543–549.
82. Leier I, Jedlitschky G, Buchholz U, Keppler D. Characterization of the ATP-dependent leukotriene C4 export carrier in mastocytoma cells. Eur J Biochem 1994, 220:599–606.
83. Akiyama T, Ishida J, Nakagawa S, Ogawara H, Watanabe S, Itoh N, Shibuya M, Fukami Y. Genistein, a specific inhibitor of tyrosine-specific protein kinases. J Biol Chem 1987, 262:5992–5995.
84. Gekeler B, Boer R, Ise W, Sanders KH, Schachtele C, Beck J. The specific bisindolylmaleimide PKC-inhibitor GF109203X efficiently modulates MRP-associated multiple drug resistance. Biochem Biophys Res Commut 1995, 206:119–126
85. Jones TR, Zamboni R, Belley M, Champion E, Charette L, Ford-Hutchinson AW, Frenette R, Gauthier J-Y, Leger S, Masson P, McFarlane S, Piechuta H, Rokach J, Williams H, Young RN. Pharmacology of L-660,711 (MK-571): a novel potent and selective leukotriene D4 receptor antagonist. Can J Physiol Pharmacol 1989, 67:17–28.
86. Gekeler V, Ise W, Sanders KH, Ulrich WR, Beck J. The leukotriene LTD4 receptor antagonist MK-571 specifically modulates MRP associated multidrug resistance. Biochem Biophys Res Commun 1995, 208:345–352.
87. Breeuwer P, Drocourt JL, Bunschoten N, Zwietering MH, Rombouts RM, Abee T. Characterization of uptake and hydrolysis of fluorescein diacetate and carboxyfluorescein diacetate by intracellular esterases in Saccharomyces cerevisae, which result in accumulation of fluorescent product. Appl Environ Microbiol 1995, 61:1614–1619.
88. Schuurhuis GJ, Broxterman HJ, Ossenkoppele GJ, Baak JPA, Eekman CA, Kuiper CM, Feller N, van Heyningen THM, Klumper E, Pieters R, Lankelma J, Pinedo HM. Functional multidrug resistance phenotype associated with combined overexpression of Pgp/MDR1 and MRP together with cytosine-arabinoside sensitivity may predict clinical response in acute myeloid leukemia. Clin Cancer Res 1995, 1: 81–93.
89. Ross DD, Doyle LA, Schiffer CA, Lee EJ, Grant CE, Cole SPC, Deeley RG, Yang W, Tong Y. Expression of multidrug resistance-associated protein (MRP) mRNA in blast cells from acute myeloid leukemia (AML) patients. Leukemia 1996, 10: 48–55.
90. List AF. Role of multidrug resistance and its pharmacological modulation in acute myeloid leukemia. Leukemia 1996, 10: 937–942.
91. Legrand O, Perrot J-Y, Tang RP, Simonin G, Gurbuxani S, Zittoun R, Marie J-P. Expression of the multidrug resistance-associated protein (MRP) mRNA and protein in normal peripheral blood and bone marrow haematopoietic cells. Br J Haematol 1996, 94: 23–33.
92. Marks DC, Su GMI, Davey RA, Davey MW. Extended multidrug resistance in haematopoietic cells. Br J Haematol 1996, 95: 587–595.

93. Izquierdo MA, Scheffer GL, Flens MJ, Schroeijers AB, van der Valk P, Scheper RJ. Major vault protein LRP-related multidrug resistance. Eur J Cancer 1996, 32A:979–984.
94. Hart SM, Ganeshaguru K, Hoffbrand AV, Prentice HG, Mehta AB. Expression of the multidrug resistance-associated protein (MRP) in acute leukemia. Leukemia 1994, 12:2163–2168.
95. Schneider E, Cowan KH, Bader H, Toomey S, Schwartz GN, Karp JE, Burke PJ, Kaufmann SH. Increased expression of the multidrug resistance-associated protein gene in relapse acute leukemia. Blood 1995, 1:186–193.
96. Zhou D-C, Zittoun R, Marie J-P. Expression of multidrug resistance-associated protein (MRP) and multidrug resistance (MDR1) genes in acute myeloid leukemia. Leukemia 1995, 9:1661–1666.
97. Xu D, Knaust E, Pisa P, Palucha K, Lundeberg J, Areström I, Peterson C, Gruber A. Levels of mdr1 and mrp mRNA in leukaemic cell populations from patients with acute myelocytic leukaemia are heterogenous and inversely correlated to cellular daunorubicin accumulation. Br J Haematol 1996, 92:847–854.
98. Ross DD, Doyle LA, Schiffer CA, Lee EJ, Grant CE, Cole SPC, Deeley RG, Yang W, Tong Y. Expression of multidrug resistance-associated protein (MRP) mRNA in blast cells from acute myeloid leukemia (AML) patients. Leukemia 1996, 10:48–55.
99. Filipits M, Suchomel RW, Zöchbauer S, Brunner R, Klechner, Pirker R: Multidrug resistance-associated protein in acute myeloid leukemia: No impact on treatment outcome. Clin Canc Research 1997, 3:1419–1425.
100. Kuss BJ, Deeley RG, Cole SPC, Willman CL, Kopecky KJ, Wolman SR, Eyre HJ, Lane SA, Nancarrow JK, Whitmore SA, Callen DF. Deletion of gene for multidrug resistance in acute myeloid leukaemia with inversion in chromosome 16: prognostic implications. Lancet 1994, 343:1531–1534.

21

GLUTATHIONE AND THE REGULATION OF CELL DEATH

A. G. Hall

Paediatric Oncology
Cancer Research Unit
Newcastle University
Newcastle Upon Tyne, United Kingdom

Keywords: Glutathione, apoptosis, transferases, MRP, resistance, alkylating.

1. ABSTRACT

The association of elevated levels of glutathione and glutathione S-transferases with the development of resistance to alkylating agents was established more than 10 years ago. Although numerous similar reports have appeared since this time work in this area has tended to dwindle as interest has become focused on more fashionable areas of drug resistance research. However, over the past 3 or 4 years there has been a revival of interest in the study of glutathione and glutathione utilising enzymes driven by recent discoveries which have implicated redox balance as an important regulator of cell death and transmembrane drug transport. In this brief review I highlight some of the more rapid areas of advance.

2. PROTECTION AGAINST ELECTROPHILIC DRUGS

Glutathione (γ-glutamylcysteinylglycine, GSH) (Figure 1) is the most abundant non-protein thiol in the cell and, as such, is crucial in the generation of a reducing environment within the cytoplasm.[1] This ensures that protein sulfhydryl groups are maintained in a reduced state and that a variety of reactive oxygen species, generated as an inevitable by-product of aerobic respiration, are rapidly detoxified before they can cause serious damage to macromolecules such as membrane lipids and DNA. Early studies also indicated that GSH plays an important part in the protection of cells against electrophilic compounds through the formation of glutathione conjugates. Such reactions have been shown to occur both spontaneously and in reactions catalysed by a large multigene family of glutathione

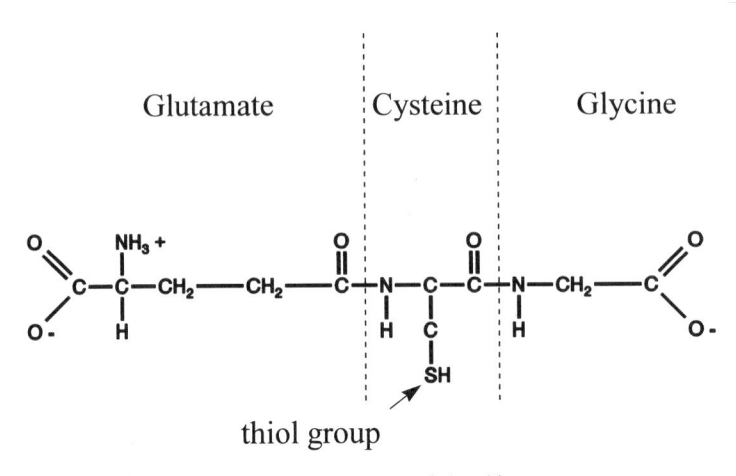

Figure 1. The structure of glutathione.

S-transferases (GSTs). GSTs have been found in a wide range of organisms and probably evolved to detoxify toxic foreign compounds (xenobiotics) at an early stage in phylogeny. As enzymes with very low substrate specificity they are well suited to the task of inactivating a wide range of toxins, all be it with low enzymic efficiency. This low catalytic rate is compensated by a high level of expression. For example in the liver, GST may account for up to 5% of total cytosolic protein.

The bifunctional alkylating agents, chlorambucil and melphalan, are known to be one group of toxic electrophiles which can form glutathione conjugates and act as substrates for the GSTs. Increased levels of GSH and GST have been associated with resistance to these drugs in a number of cell line and tumour biopsy studies. In addition both reduction in GSH as a result of inhibition of synthesis using buthionine sulfoximine (BSO) or inhibition of GST activity using compounds such as ethacrynic acid or indomethacin have been shown to potentiate their cytotoxic effects.[2] Direct evidence for the formation of drug conjugates in intact cells has not, however, been forthcoming and some doubt must remain as to the importance of this process *in vivo*.

3. GSTs AS BINDING PROTEINS

One of the first roles identified for the GSTs was as an intracellular binding protein. For this reason alpha class GST was originally dubbed "ligandin" in recognition of its ability to sequester potential intracellular toxins such as bilirubin. X-ray crystallography has indicated that the ligandin binding site probably lies in the cleft between the 2 monomeric units which form the native enzyme. Recently, however, it has been suggested that sequestration may also occur at the active site with certain compounds such as chlorambucil being released at a very low rate.[3] Unlike the case in most enzyme mediated reactions in this unusual situation the concentration of the enzyme becomes a factor in the determination of the end-point of the reaction rather than simply the rate at which it occurs (Figure 2). Drug sequestration may help to explain why drug-GSH conjugates have been difficult to identify in intact cells. It also implies that the amount of GST present, rather than the enzyme activity alone, may be important in the determination of the extent of drug resistance.

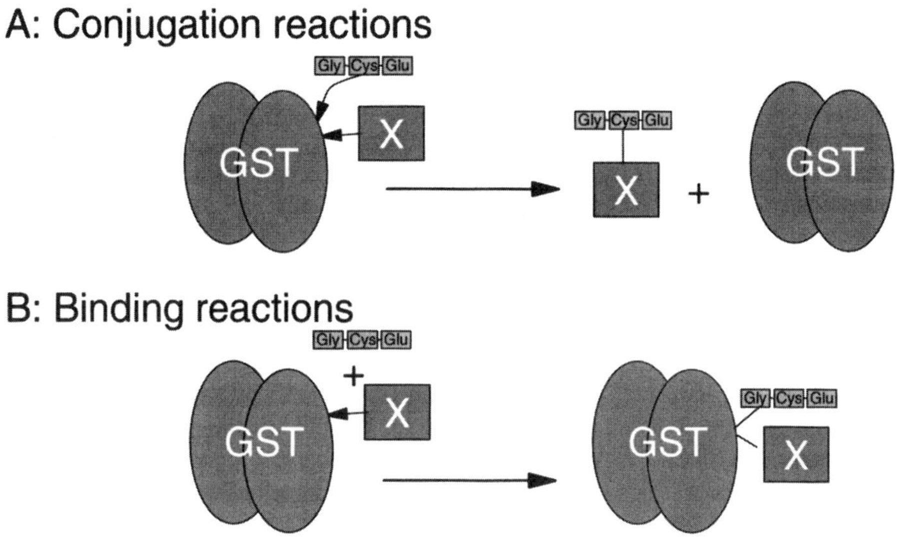

A: Conjugation reactions

B: Binding reactions

Figure 2. The action of GST as a binding protein. The upper diagram indicates the action of GST as a normal catalyst where X is an electrophilic compound. The lower diagram indicates GST acting as a binding protein, sequestering GSH conjugates. In this case X may be compounds such as bilirubin (binding between the monomeric units) or chlorambucil-GSH conjugates (binding at the active site). In the latter case the concentration of the enzyme influences the end point of the reaction.

4. GSH AND THE FUNCTION OF MRP

As mentioned above GSH research received a boost from the discovery that the multidrug-resistance associated protein, MRP, can act as a transporter of glutathione conjugates and that the MRP phenotype can be reversed by BSO. At present, however, many of the details which link MRP with GSH homeostasis are unclear. For example, although BSO will reverse resistance to vincristine and adriamycin there is no direct evidence that these drugs will form GSH conjugates. It seems more likely that GSH, through alteration in the intracellular redox state, regulates MRP function through the action of a molecular gating mechanism (Figure 3). This is, however, as yet unproven although the manipulation of intracellular GSH for the reversal of the MRP phenotype remains an attractive target for new drug development.

5. GSH AND THE CONTROL OF APOPTOSIS

Much recent excitement in the field of GSH research has centred around the observation that the generation of reactive oxygen species (ROS) appears to be involved in many forms of apoptosis and that mitochondria may be important mediators of this process. The involvement of ROS in the late, effector, stages of apoptosis, beyond the "point of no return", has been documented in many systems although the fact that this form of cell death can occur in anaerobic conditions and in cells with absent aerobic respiration implies that their formation is not a universal feature. The involvement of ROS in earlier, initiation phases of apoptosis is more controversial. There is, however, good evidence that, at least in some systems, the generation of free oxygen radicals is a central process in the triggering of cell death following for example FAS/APO-1 binding or exposure to tumour

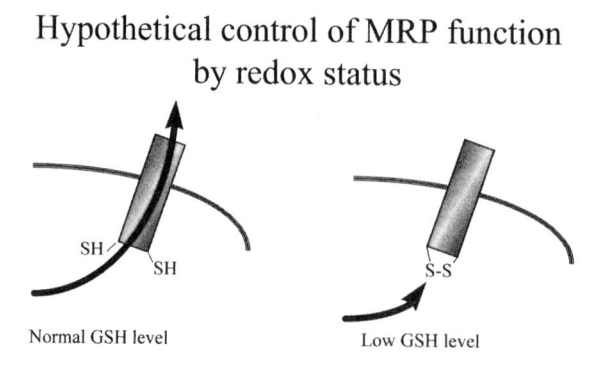

Hypothetical control of MRP function by redox status

Figure 3. The putative gating function of GSH in the regulation of MRP. With low GSH levels MRP function is reduced suggesting a possible "gating" function, possibly regulated by cysteine-rich sequences on the first cytoplasmic domain of the protein.

necrosis factor. This hypothesis is supported by a recent publication which suggests that p53 mediated apoptosis may involve the up-regulation of several genes involved in redox control, including microsomal GST and enzymes involved in GSH synthesis.[4]

The role of mitochondria in apoptosis has been the focus of much recent research interest and it has been suggested that this organelle may act as both a sensor and effector of apoptosis[5] An early event in the apoptotic cascade is the collapse of the mitochondrial transmembrane potential associated with the opening of pores within the mitochondrial membrane. This leads to the release of factors, including cytochrome c, which stimulate caspase activity and trigger the apoptotic pathway. It is possible that the opening of these pores will also lead to the release of mitochondrial GSH, an important regulator of ROS within this organelle. This would in turn be expected to lead to a rapid increase in cytoplasmic ROS and subsequent decrease in cytoplasmic GSH, as observed in many forms of apoptosis. It is possible that members of the bcl-2 family of proteins, important regulators of the apoptotic pathway, act to regulate the formation of mitochondrial pores and hence the initiation of the apoptotic cascade, although the role of these proteins in the control of mitochondrial GSH has not, as yet, been explored.

6. FUTURE DEVELOPMENTS

Much remains to be learnt of the way in which GSH regulates the intracellular redox potential during cell death. In the past too much emphasis has been placed on steady state levels of the tripeptide in the cytoplasm and insufficient attention has been given to the flux of GSH between mitochondrial, cytoplasmic and nuclear pools. In addition more remains to be learnt of the way in which GSH influences drug transport in cells with high levels of MRP expression. The revival of interest in this important pathway is now well established and the next few years promises to be very exciting for workers involved in this field.

ACKNOWLEDGMENTS

The support of the Leukaemia Research Fund is gratefully acknowledged.

NOTE ADDED TO TEXT

This is a modified version of an article which first appeared in the ECC newsletter in February 1998.

REFERENCES

1. Meister, A. Metabolism and function of glutathione. In "Glutathione: Chemical, biochemical and medical aspects" (D. Dolphin, R. Poulson, and O. Avramovic, Eds.), 1989, 367–474. Wiley, New York.
2. Hall, A., Robson, C. N., Hickson, I. D., Harris, A. L., Proctor, S. J., and Cattan, A. R. Possible role of inhibition of glutathione S-transferase in the partial reversal of chlorambucil resistance by indomethacin in a Chinese hamster ovary cell line. Cancer Res., 1989, 49, 6265–6268.
3. Meyer, D. J., Gilmore, K. S., Harris, J. M., Hartley, J. A., and Ketterer, B. Chlorambucil-monoglutathionyl conjugate is sequestered by human alpha class glutathione S-transferases. Br.J.Cancer, 1992, 66, 433–438.
4. Polyak, K, Xia, Y., Zweier, J.L., Kinzler, K.W. and Vogelstein, B. A model for p53-induced apoptosis. Nature, 1997, 389, 300–305.
5. Marchetti, P, Susin, S.A., Zamzami, N. and Kroemer, G. The mitochondrion as a sensor/effecter of oxidative stress during apoptosis. In "Oxidative stress in cancer AIDS and neurodegenerative diseases" (Montagnier, L, Olivier, R and Pasquier, C, Eds), 1998, 213–222. Marcel Dekker, New York.

EVIDENCE FOR THE INVOLVEMENT OF THE GLUTATHIONE PATHWAY IN DRUG RESISTANCE IN AML

J. M. Sargent,[1] C. Williamson,[1] A. G. Hall,[2] A. W. Elgie,[1] and C. G. Taylor[1]

[1]Haematology Research
Pembury Hospital
Kent TN2 4QJ, United Kingdom
[2]Paediatric Oncology
Medical School
Newcastle NE2 4HH, United Kingdom

Keywords: AML, drug resistance, glutathione, MRP, GSTµ, GSTα.

1. ABSTRACT

We have studied altered drug detoxification through the glutathione pathway as a possible mechanism of resistance in 38 patients with AML. GST α, µ and π expressions were determined using immunocytochemistry, the median percentages of positive cells being 73% (range 0–98), 55% (range 0–99) and 97% (range 80–100) respectively. MRP expression was measured using MRPm6 MoAb and flow cytometry. Results were expressed as the ratio of fluorescence associated with MRP over that of an isotype matched control (median, 1.32 ; range 0.95–2.15). Statistical analyses showed a significant increase in GSTα expression in blast cells showing *in vitro* resistance to doxorubicin, with a median value of 78% positive cells compared to 41% in the sensitive group (p<0.02). There was a significant reduction, however, in GSTµ expression from a median value of 60% in newly presenting patients to 40% in a group of patients who had received previous cytotoxic therapy (p<0.02). Interestingly, patients with high GSTµ expression appeared to co-express MRP (p<0.05). *In vitro* drug modulation studies, comparing the cytotoxic effect of doxorubicin ± ethacrynic acid at 6.5µM resulted in only one significant increase in sensitivity (2.6-fold), out of 22 comparisons. These results support the theory that altered detoxification through the glutathione pathway contributes towards drug resistance in AML.

Drug Resistance in Leukemia and Lymphoma III, edited by Kaspers *et al.*
Kluwer Academic / Plenum Publishers, New York, 1999.

Further studies using fresh blast cells are required to elucidate the importance of this mechanism for individual patients.

2. INTRODUCTION

Drug resistance remains a major problem in the management of acute myeloid leukaemia (AML). Identification of drug resistance before treatment is central to the understanding of the mechanisms involved. We have found the MTT assay to be a useful method to study drug resistance *in vitro* using fresh blast cells from patients.[1]

Several cellular mechanisms have been shown to confer drug resistance to leukaemic cells. Altered drug detoxification through the glutathione (GSH) pathway has been suggested as a major resistance mechanism in AML.[2] A family of multifunctional enzymes, the glutathione S-transferases (GSTs) promote the formation of drug-GSH conjugates which are then excreted from the cell by the ABC transporter, multidrug resistance associated protein (MRP).[3] Increased levels of GSH, GSTs and MRP have been found in resistant cell lines.[4]

Ethacrynic acid (ETH), which inhibits π class GST, has been shown to increase sensitivity to cytotoxic agents *in vitro* and has entered clinical trials as a potential resistance modulation agent.[5]

The aim of this study was to investigate the role of the GSH pathway in drug resistance using fresh blast cells from patients with AML.

3. METHODS

3.1. Patients

Samples derived from bone marrow or peripheral blood from 38 patients with AML were tested. Twelve patients had relapsed following previous chemotherapy. Blast cells were separated using density gradient centrifugation and a final cell suspension which contained >80% blasts was prepared in RPMI 1640.

3.2. Chemosensitivity Testing

Blast cells were exposed to 4 concentrations of cytotoxic drugs for 48h. Drugs tested included daunorubicin, doxorubicin, idarubicin, mitoxantrone, ara-C, 6-thioguanine and etoposide.

After drug exposure, cell survival was assessed using the MTT assay.[1] *In vitro* drug modulation studies were carried out on blast cells comparing the cytotoxic effect of doxorubicin (DOX) alone and in combination with ETH at a fixed dose of 6.5μM. The effect of the modifier was determined by comparing the area under the curve for DOX ± ETH using 2 tailed 't' test. The LC_{50} was calculated for each test and a sensitivity ratio of LC_{50} of DOX/ LC_{50} of DOX+ETH gave a measure of any modulation effect.

3.3. GST Expression

GST expression was determined using immunocytochemistry on cytospin preparations of the cells used for the MTT assay and three rabbit polyclonal antibodies raised against α, μ and π forms of the enzyme.[6] The standard APAAP technique was used and the percentage of positively staining cells was recorded.

3.4. MRP Expression

MRP expression was assessed using the MRPm6 MoAb and an indirect FITC labelling technique for flow cytometric analysis. An isotype matched control was run with every sample and results were expressed as the ratio of fluorescence associated with MRPm6 over that for the control. The doxorubicin resistant cell line HL60R was used as positive control.

3.5. Statistics

Non-parametrics methods were used when possible. Spearman's rank correlation coefficient was used to determine any relationships between parameters tested. The Mann Whitney U test was used to compare groups of patients.

4. RESULTS

4.1. GST Expression

There was marked variation in GSTα and μ expression between patients. Expression of GSTπ however, was similar throughout, all patients showing >80% cells staining positively (Figure 1). There was no correlation between the expression of any of the 3 isoforms in individual patients.

4.2. Correlation of GST Expression with *in Vitro* Chemosensitivity

There was a significant increase in GST α expression in blast cells showing *in vitro* resistance to DOX, where a median value of 78% positive cells compared to 41% in the sensitive group was observed ($p<0.02$).

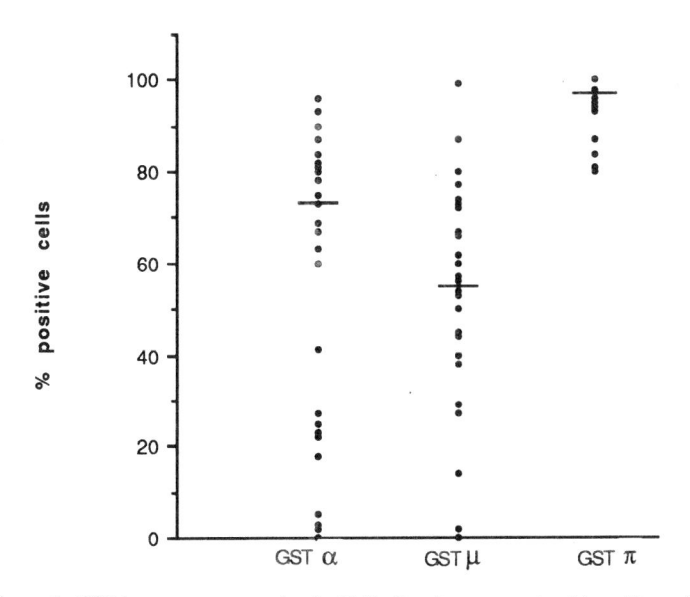

Figure 1. GST isoenzyme expression in AML. Results expressed as % positive cells.

4.3. Correlation of GST Expression with Clinical Parameters

There was a significant reduction in GSTμ expression, from a median value of 60% in newly presenting patients to 40% in the group of patients who had received previous cytotoxic therapy ($p<0.02$).

4.4. MRP Expression

The MRP status of 17 samples was assessed. The median ratio of fluorescence associated with test/control was 1.32 (range 0.95–2.15) There appeared to be a correlation between GSTμ expression and MRP expression ($p<0.05$).

4.5. *In Vitro* Modulation Studies

Only 1 of 22 comparisons demonstrated a significant increase (2.6-fold) in sensitivity to DOX on co-incubation with ETH.

5. DISCUSSION

Altered detoxification through the glutathione pathway has been postulated as a major mechanism of drug resistance in AML. The correlation we found between GST α expression and *in vitro* resistance to DOX suggests that this pathway is indeed involved and adds weight to previous reports of a correlation between resistance to doxorubicin and GST π.[7]

The finding of reduced GSTμ expression in patients who had received previous cytotoxic therapy is intriguing. GSTμ has recently been postulated as a possible modulator of cytochrome P450 transcription. Furthermore, high cytochrome P450 expression has been associated with poor prognosis in breast cancer.[8]

Our preliminary results demonstrated a correlation between two of the proteins involved in the glutathione pathway, namely GSTμ and MRP. This result suggests possible co-regulation of proteins involved in this pathway and would agree with previous studies where a relationship was established between low GSTμ expression and event free survival in ALL. This study demonstrated that 82% of patients with long term remissions were negative for GSTμ.[9]

Resistance modulation with ETH acid may only be effective in less than 5% of patients. Perhaps this is not surprising, since ETH is a π class GST inhibitor and there was no apparent correlation between GSTπ and sensitivity to DOX in this study.

Further investigations using fresh blast cells are required to elucidate the importance of this mechanism of resistance for individual patients.

ACKNOWLEDGMENTS

We are grateful for the support of the Kent Leukaemia and Cancer Equipment Fund, the EB Hutchinson Trust and the Leukaemia Research Fund, UK.

REFERENCES

1. Sargent JM, Taylor CG. Appraisal of the MTT assay as a rapid test of chemosensitivity in acute myeloid leukaemia. Br J Cancer, 1989, 60, 206–210.

2. McKenna SL, Padua RA. Multidrug resistance in leukaemia. Br J Haematol, 1997, 96, 659–674.
3. Barnouin K, Leier I, Jedlitschky G, Pourtier-Manzanedo A, Koing J, Lehmann W-D, Keppler D. Multidrug resistance protein-mediated transport of chlorambucil and melphalan congugated to glutathione. Br J Cancer, 1998, 77, 201–209.
4. Flens MJ, Izquierdo MA, Scheffer GL, Fritz JM, Meijer CJLM, Scheper RJ, Zaman GJR. Immunocytochemical detection of the multidrug resistance-associated protein MRP in human multidrug-resistant tumor cells by monoclonal antibodies. Cancer Res, 1994, 54, 4557–4563.
5. O'Dwyer PJ, LaCreta F, Nash S, Tinsley P, Schilder R, Clapper ML, Tew KD, Panting L, Litwin S, Comis RL, Ozols RF. Phase I study of thiotepa in combination with the glutathione transferase inhibitor ethacrynic acid. Cancer Res, 1991, 51, 6059–6065.
6. Ghazal-Aswad S, Hogarth L, Hall AG, George M, Sinha DP, Lind M, Calvert AH, Sunter JP, Newell DR. The relationship between tumour glutathione concentration, glutathione S-transferase isoenzyme expression and response to single agent carboplatin in epithelial ovarian cancer patients. Br J Cancer, 1996, 74, 468–473.
7. Samuels BL, Murray JL, Cohen MB, Safa AR, Sinha BK, Townsend AJ, Beckett MA, Weichselbaum RR. Increased glutathione peroxidase activity in a human sarcoma cell line with inherent doxorubicin resistance. Cancer Res, 1991, 51, 521–527.
8. Vaury C, Laine R, Noguiez P, de Coppet P, Jaulin C, Praz F, Pompon D, Amor-Gueret M. Human glutathione S-transferase M1 null genotype is associated with high inducibility of cytochrome P450 1A1 gene transcription. Cancer Res, 1995, 55, 5520–5523.
9. Hall AG, Autzen P, Cattan AR, Malcolm AJ, Cole M, Kernahan J, Reid MM. Expression of µ class glutathione S-transferase correlates with event free survival in childhood acute lymphoblastic leukemia. Cancer Res, 1994, 54, 5251–5254.

23

GLUTATHIONE IN CHILDHOOD ACUTE LEUKAEMIAS

P. Kearns,[1,2] R. Pieters,[1] M. M. A. Rottier,[1] A. J. P. Veerman,[1]
K. Schmiegalow,[3] A. D. J. Pearson,[2] and A. G. Hall[2]

[1]Department of Paediatric Haematology and Oncology
Free University Hospital
Amsterdam, The Netherlands
[2]Department of Paediatric Oncology
Medical School
University of Newcastle upon Tyne, United Kingdom
[3]Department of Haematology and Oncology
The Juliane Marie Centre
Copenhagen, Denmark

Keywords: Glutathione, childhood leukaemia, prognostic indicators, drug resistance.

1. ABSTRACT

In order to test the hypothesis that glutathione (GSH) is an important determinant of treatment response in childhood acute leukaemia, blast cell GSH levels were studied in a cohort of children with acute lymphoblastic (ALL) and acute myeloid (AML) leukaemia.

In both ALL and AML, several indicators of poor prognosis are well established but the underlying molecular mechanisms leading to resistant disease are still poorly understood. GSH is an intracellular thiol implicated in the development of cytotoxic drug resistance and appears to be involved in the control of cell proliferation and apoptosis.

In this study, total GSH was measured in cryopreserved blasts from 62 childhood ALL and 13 AML patients. In ALL, high GSH levels were associated with a relatively poor prognosis. A positive correlation was demonstrated between the GSH level and presenting white cell count (WCC). GSH levels were significantly higher in T lineage ALL compared with B lineage and in AML blasts compared with ALL.

These results are supportive of GSH as prognostic indicator in childhood leukaemia and may suggest one mechanism of treatment failure. They imply that it may be possible to improve chemosensitivity by the use of known modulators of GSH synthesis.

Drug Resistance in Leukemia and Lymphoma III, edited by Kaspers *et al.*
Kluwer Academic / Plenum Publishers, New York, 1999.

2. INTRODUCTION

Currently the 5 year survival in childhood ALL is 70–75% and in childhood AML around 50%. There are several well established indicators of prognosis including sex, age at initial presentation, presenting peripheral blood WCC and immunophenotype.[1] More recently *in vitro* drug sensitivity of leukaemic blasts has also been demonstrated as a useful indicator of prognosis.[2] These factors are valuable in development of risk adapted treatment protocols, however, there is still limited knowledge of the mechanisms by which these patient and disease characteristics lead to a poor response to therapy.

GSH is an intracellular thiol implicated in the development of cytotoxic drug resistance[3] and appears to be involved in the control of cell proliferation and apoptosis.[4,5] Many studies have demonstrated that elevated levels of GSH are associated with resistance to certain groups of cytotoxic agents, in particular the alkylating agents, anthracyclines and platinum drugs.[6] Much of this evidence arises from studies using cell lines.[3] In leukaemia, there have been few previous studies examining GSH in clinical samples and these have focused mainly on adult leukaemia[7,8] and included heterogeneous groups of chronic and acute leukaemias.[9] It has been found that GSH levels were higher in leukaemic cells compared with normal peripheral blood lymphocytes.[7,9] In addition, Maung et al.[8] demonstrated elevated GSH levels in patients who responded poorly to chemotherapy. In this study, we determined GSH levels in leukaemic blasts from children with acute leukaemia and examined the relationship with the established indicators of prognosis and with the risk of leukaemic relapse.

3. MATERIALS AND METHODS

Patient samples were from bone marrow or peripheral blood taken at initial diagnosis. Leukaemic blasts had been isolated on a Ficoll Isopaque gradient and cryopreserved in liquid nitrogen at -196°C. *In vitro* drug sensitivity for a panel of drugs currently used in the treatment of childhood acute leukaemia had been previously measured using the MTT assay as described by Pieters *et al.* 1991.[2] The panel of drugs tested were prednisolone, dexamethasone, daunorubicin, doxorubicin, 6-mercaptopurine, thioguanine, 400H-ifosfamide, cytarabine and vincristine. The cell pellets were thawed immediately prior to analysis for GSH, and kept at 4°C throughout sample preparation. Only cell pellets with greater than 90% blasts were analysed. Cell viability was tested by Trypan blue exclusion and only samples with greater than 85% viable cells were included in the analysis. The cells were lysed in 0.1% Triton-X (Sigma) and 10mM HCl. Total GSH was measured by the Tietze enzyme recycling method modified for application to leukaemic blast cell pellets as described by Kearns and Hall.[10] Protein determinations were performed by the Bradford method[11] using a commercially available kit.

Samples from 62 children with ALL were analysed The mean age was 77.4 months, (range 33–165 months). Fifty-one were B lineage leukaemia and 11 T lineage. Thirty-two patients were male and 30 female. Thirteen samples were from children with AML. The mean age was 106 months (range 12–194 months). This group comprised 10 male and 3 females.

4. RESULTS

The median GSH level in blasts from children with ALL was 6.54 nmol/mg protein (range 1.37–27.9 nmol/mg protein).The median GSH level was significantly higher in blasts from children with AML at 11.48 nmol/mg protein, range 5.5–16.4 nmol/mg pro-

Glutathione in Childhood Acute Leukaemias

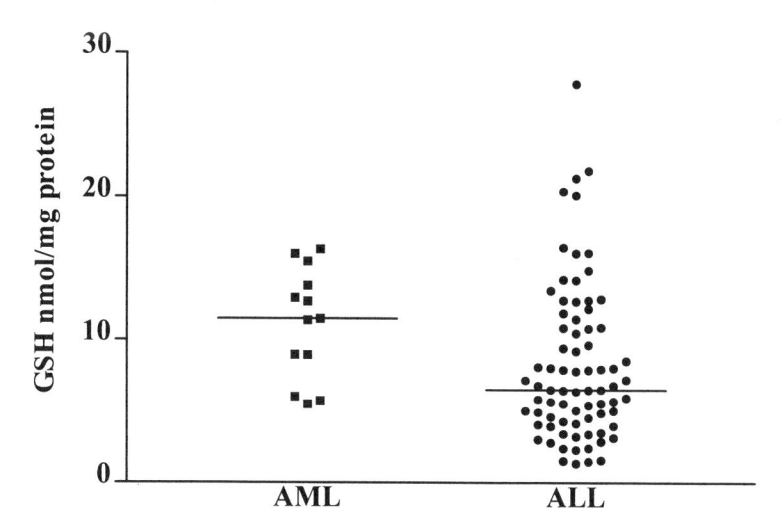

Figure 1. GSH levels in acute myeloid and acute lymphoblastic leukaemia. Median GSH level. Mann Whitney U test p=0.014.

tein, (Mann Whitney-U test p= 0.014) (Figure 1). In comparing the correlation between GSH levels and established indicators of prognosis, GSH levels were found to be 2.2 fold higher in T lineage ALL compared with B lineage cells. (Mann Whitney-U test p < 0.0001) (Figure 2).

There was also a significant correlation between presenting white cell count (WCC) and GSH level (Spearman Rank correlation coefficient, r =0.45, p=0.001) (Figure 3). No correlation was found between blast GSH level and gender or age at diagnosis (data not shown). GSH levels were weakly correlated with *in vitro* ifosfamide resistance in childhood ALL (Mann Whitney-U test p= 0.034), however in both ALL and AML, no correlation was demonstrated between GSH levels and *in vitro* sensitivity for the other cytotoxic drugs analysed.

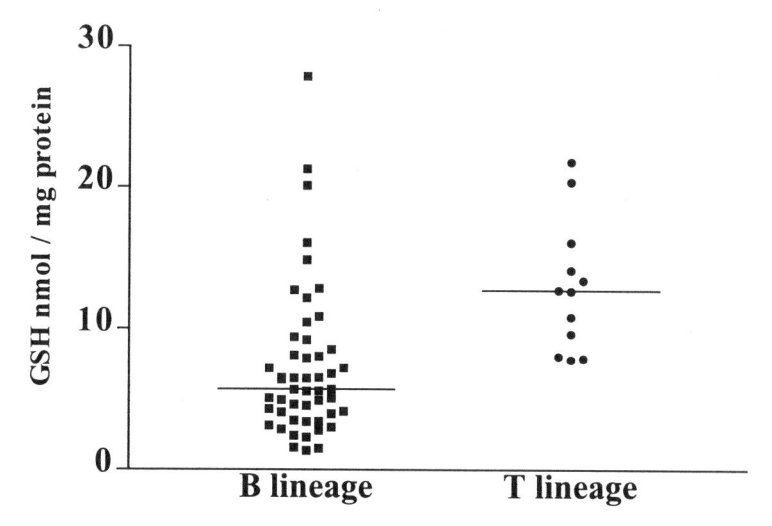

Figure 2. GSH levels and immunophenotype in childhood ALL. Median GSH level. Mann Whitney U test p < 0.0001.

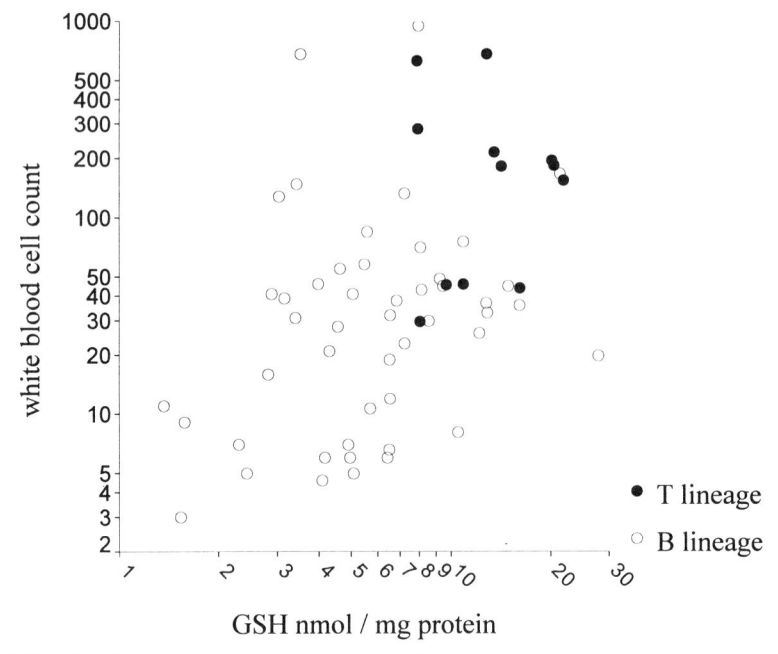

Figure 3. GSH levels and presenting white cell count in childhood ALL. Spearman rank correlation coefficient = 0.45, p = 0.001.

A high GSH level was defined as greater than the median value. In ALL, children with a high blast GSH concentration had a significantly greater risk of relapse (Log rank test p = 0.01) (Figure 4). All the T lineage samples fell into the high GSH group and the presenting WCC was significantly higher in those patients with high GSH (Mann Whitney U test p<0.0001). There was no significant difference in age at presentation between the two groups or in number of male and female patients. The AML group was too small and the follow up period too short for analysis of survival data at this stage.

5. DISCUSSION

Response to treatment in childhood AML is in general poor compared with ALL. In this study there were significantly higher GSH levels in AML blasts compared with ALL blasts. However, as the number of AML samples studied was small, it is not possible to make any conclusions on the clinical significance of this observation until further AML patients can be studied.

The correlation between blast GSH levels and established prognostic indicators was also examined. A high presenting WCC and T lineage immunophenotype are both markers of high risk of relapse in ALL[1]. In this study children with higher presenting WCC, also had greater GSH levels and this was independent of the positive correlation with T lineage immunophenotype. High GSH levels were also clearly associated with increased risk of relapse. This relationship was independent of age at presentation and sex but was not independent of presenting WCC. It is therefore proposed that blast GSH levels could provide an insight into the mechanism by which a high presenting peripheral WCC results in poor prognosis. There is increasing evidence to support the role of GSH in control of cell pro-

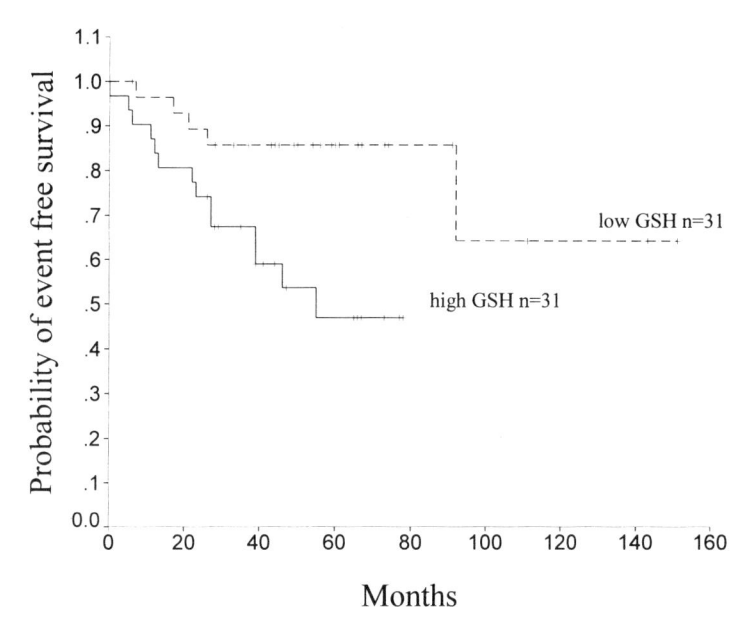

Figure 4. GSH levels and prognosis in childhood ALL. Kaplan Meier curve showing event free survival. The patients were divided into high and low GSH groups. High GSH level was defined as above the median value. Log rank tes p = 0.01.

liferation,[12,13] notably in the leukaemic cell line K562[14] and in peripheral blood lymphocytes.[15] Furthermore, pretreatment marrow proliferation rate has been proposed as an important prognostic parameter in childhood ALL.[16,17] Further investigation of the role of GSH in the control of cell cycle kinetics is warranted.

The correlation between blast GSH concentration and prognosis suggests that risk of relapse may be reduced by modulation of blast GSH levels. Buthionine S sulfoxamine (BSO) is known to decrease intracellular GSH via inhibition of γ-glutamylcysteine-synthetase, the rate limiting step in GSH synthesis. There are several studies demonstrating the use of BSO *in vivo*.[18–20] In phase 1 studies intracellular GSH levels were effectively reduced with tolerable side effects.[21] Phase 2 trials are currently underway studying the use of BSO in conjunction with alkylating agents in adult solid tumours. In view of the results of our study, the use of BSO to improve outcome in childhood leukaemia should be explored.

ACKNOWLEDGMENTS

This work was supported by the Leukaemia Research Fund, Great Ormond Street, London, UK.

REFERENCES

1. Cotes J. E., Kantarjian H. M. Acute lymphoblastic leukemia. A comprehensive review with emphasis on biology and therapy. Cancer, 1995, 76, 2393–2417.

2. Pieters R., Huismans D. R., Loonen A. H., Hahlen K., Van Der Does-Van Den Berg A., Van Wering E. R. and Veerman A. J. P. Relation of cellular drug resistance to long-term clinical outcome in childhood acute lymphoblastic leukaemia. Lancet, 1991, 338, 399–403.
3. O'Brien M. L. and Tew K. D. Glutathione and related enzymes in multidrug resistance. Eur. J. Cancer, 1996, 967–978.
4. Frischer H., Kennedy E. J., Chigurupati R. and Sivarajan M. Glutathione, cell proliferation, and 1,3-bis-(2-chloroethyl)-1-nitrosourea in K562 leukemia. Journal of Clinical Investigation, 1993, 92, 2761–2767.
5. Watson R. W. G., Rotstein O. D., Nathens A. B., Dackiw A. P. B. and Marshall J. C. Thiol-mediated redox regulation of neutrophil apoptosis. Surgery, 1996, 120, 150–158.
6. Ozols R. F., O'Dwyer P. J., Hamilton T. C. and Young R. C. The role of glutathione in drug resistance. Cancer Treat. Rev., 1990, 17, 45–50.
7. Ferraris A. M., Rolfo M., Mangerini R. and Gaetani G. F. Increased glutathione in chronic lymphocytic leukemia lymphocytes, Am. J. Hematol., 1994, 47, 237–238.
8. Maung Z. T., Reid M. M., Matheson E., Taylor P. R. A., Proctor S. J. and Hall A. G. Corticosteroid resistance is increased in lymphoblasts from adults compared with children: Preliminary results of in vitro drug sensitivity study in adults with acute lymphoblastic leukaemia. Br. J. Haematol., 1995, 91, 93–100.
9. Paydas S., Yuregir G. T., Sahin B., Seyrek E. and Burgut R. Intracellular glutathione content in leukemias. Oncology, 1995, 52, 112–115.
10. Kearns P. R. and Hall A. G. Microtitre plate technique for the measurement of glutathione in fresh and cryopreserved lymphoblasts using the enzyme recycling method. Methods in Molecular Medicine, 1999, (in press).
11. Bradford M. A rapid and sensitive method for the quantitation of microgram quantities of protein using the principle of protein-dye binding. Anal. Biochem., 976, 72, 248–254.
12. Terradez P., Asensi M., Lasso del la Vega M. C., Puertes I. R., Viña J. and Estrela J. M. Depletion of tumour glutathione *in vivo* by buthionine sulphoximine: Modulation by the rate of cellular proliferation and inhibition of cancer growth. Biochem. J., 1993, 292, 477–483.
13. Poot M., Teubert H., Rabinovitch P. S. and Kavanagh T. J. De novo synthesis of glutathione is required for both entry into and progression through the cell cycle. J. Cell. Physiol., 1995, 163, 555–560.
14. Frischer H., Kennedy E. J., Chigurupati R. and Sivarajan M. Glutathione, cell proliferation, and 1,3-bis-(2-chloroethyl)-1-nitrosourea in K562 leukemia. J. Clin. Invest., 1993, 92, 2761–2767.
15. Kavanagh T. J., Grossmann A., Jaecks E. P., Jinneman J. C., Eaton D. L., Martin G. M. and Rabinovitch P. S. Proliferative capacity of human peripheral blood lymphocytes sorted on the basis of glutathione content. J. Cell. Physiol., 1990, 145, 472–480.
16. Ngo E. O. and Nutter L. M. Status of glutathione and glutathione-metabolizing enzymes in menadione-resistant human cancer cells. Biochem. Pharmacol., 1994, 47, 421–424.
17. Scarffe J. H., Hann I. M., Evans D. I. K., Morris-Jones P., Palmer M. K., Lilleyman J. S. and Crowther D. Relationship between the pretreatment proliferative activity of marrow blast cells and prognosis of acute lymphoblastic leukaemia of childhood. Br. J. Cancer, 1980, 41, 764–771.
18. Siemann D. W. and Beyers K. L. In vivo therapeutic potential of combination thiol depletion and alkylating chemotherapy. British Journal of Cancer, 1993, 68, 1071–1079.
19. Medh R. D., Gupta V. and Awasthi Y. C. Reversal of melphalan resistance in vivo and in vitro by modulation of glutathione metabolism. Biochem Pharmacol., 1991, 42, 439–441.
20. Ozols R. F., Louie K. G., Plowman J., Behrens B. C., Fine R. L., Dykes D. and Hamilton T. C. Enhanced melphalan cytotoxicity in human ovarian cancer in vitro and in tumor-bearing nude mice by buthionine sulfoximine depletion of glutathione. Biochem Pharmacol., 1987, 36, 147–153.
21. O'Dwyer P. J., Hamilton T. C., Young R. C., LaCreta F. P., Carp N., Tew K. D., Padavic K., Comis R. L. and Ozols R. F. Depletion of glutathione in normal and malignant human cells in vivo by buthionine sulfoximine: clinical and biochemical results. J. Natl. Cancer Inst., 1992, 84, 264–267.

24

APOPTOSIS

Molecules and Mechanisms

Marina Konopleva,[1] Shourong Zhao,[1] Zhong Xie,[1] Harry Segall,[1] Anas Younes,[3] David F. Claxton,[1] Zeev Estrov,[2] Steven M. Kornblau,[1] and Michael Andreeff[1*]

[1]Department of Molecular Hematology and Therapy
[2]Department of Bioimmunotherapy
[3]Department of Lymphoma
Division of Medicine
M.D. Anderson Cancer Center
The University of Texas
Houston, Texas

Keywords: Apoptosis, programmed cell death (PCD), leukemia, lymphoma.

1. ABSTRACT

This review of the molecules and pathways involved in programmed cell death (apoptosis) discriminates triggers of apoptosis (e.g. chemotherapy, radiation, Fas ligation), modulators of apoptosis (e.g. Bcl-2 family members, Bcl-2 interacting proteins, Apafs, IAPs, and Fas/FasL modulators including FLICE and FLIPs), effectors (caspases 1–13) and cleavage substrates (e.g. PARP). Special consideration is given to the structure-function relationship of Bcl-2 family members and to their post-transcriptional modification. Brief references are made to the role of apoptotic pathway in leukemias and lymphomas and to strategies of modulating apoptotic pathways.

---

* Corresponding author: Michael Andreeff, M.D., Ph.D., Department of Molecular Hematology and Therapy, The University of Texas M.D. Anderson Cancer Center, 1515 Holcombe Boulevard, Box 81, Houston, Texas 77030 USA. Tel (713) 792-7260. Fax (713) 794-4747. E-mail: mandreef@notes.mdacc.tmc.edu.

Drug Resistance in Leukemia and Lymphoma III, edited by Kaspers *et al.*
Kluwer Academic / Plenum Publishers, New York, 1999.

2. INTRODUCTION

Apoptosis, or programmed cell death (PCD), is an active process in which an individual cell responding to internal and/or external cues commits suicide.[1,2] PCD is involved in many diverse homeostatic processes in multicellular organism, both during development and in the mature organism. Dysregulation of apoptosis can lead to pathological states involving cell accumulation, such as cancer, or cell loss, such as neurodegeneration.[3]

PCD is a genetically determined process. Cell death occurring during development of the nematode C. elegans involves the molecules CED-3 and CED-4, which are required for cell death to occur, and CED-9, which protects cells from death. In mammals, CED-3 homologs constitute a family of cystein proteases with aspartate specificity, formerly called the ICE (interleukin-1α-converting enzyme) family, and now designated caspases[4] that are the key effector proteins of apoptosis in mammalian cells.[5] The discovery that human Bcl-2 has functional and structural similarity to CED-9 demonstrated that programmed cell death in mammalian cells occurred by the same highly conserved mechanism as apoptosis in the nematode.[6,7]

The PCD cascade can be divided into several stages (Figure 1). Multiple signaling pathways lead from death triggering extracellular or intracellular agents to a central control and an execution stage. In this stage, the activation of CED3/caspases occurs, which leads to the characteristic "apoptotic" structural lesions accompanying cell death-cytoplasmic and chromatin condensation and DNA fragmentation. The caspases are zymogens: they exist as inactive polypeptides that can be activated by removal of the regulatory prodomain and assembled into the active heteromeric protease. Currently, the caspase family consists of 13 members, many of which have a proven role in inflammation or apoptosis. Caspases can be grouped into three subfamilies based on their specificities. Group I, or ICE subfamily of caspases (caspase 1, 4 and 5), prefer the tetrapeptide sequence WEHD and are believed to play a role mainly in inflammation, whereas members of group II (caspases 2,3 and 7) and group III (caspases 6, 8, 9, and 10) display a specificity for DexD and (I/L/V)ExD, respectively and are mainly involved in apoptosis.[8–10] The fact that caspases 8 and 10 each contain two N-terminal located death effector domains that enable them to associate with death receptors, places these two caspases most upstream in the apoptotic activation pathway.[11–13] In turn, caspase 3 appears to be the central executioner

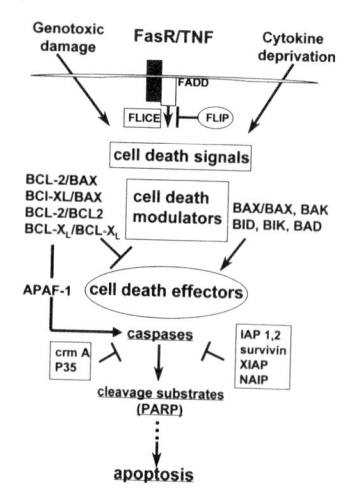

Figure 1. Schematic representation of the apoptotic cascade. Cell death signals include genotoxic damage, cytokine deprivation and Fas/FasL activation as triggers, Bcl-2 family members as modulators, caspases as effectors, and PAPR as cleavage substrates, leading to apoptosis. A more comprehensive list of molecules involved in initiation and control of apoptosis is shown in Table 1.

Apoptosis

Table 1. Triggers, modulators, effectors, and cleavage substrates involved in apoptotic pathways (also see Figure 1).

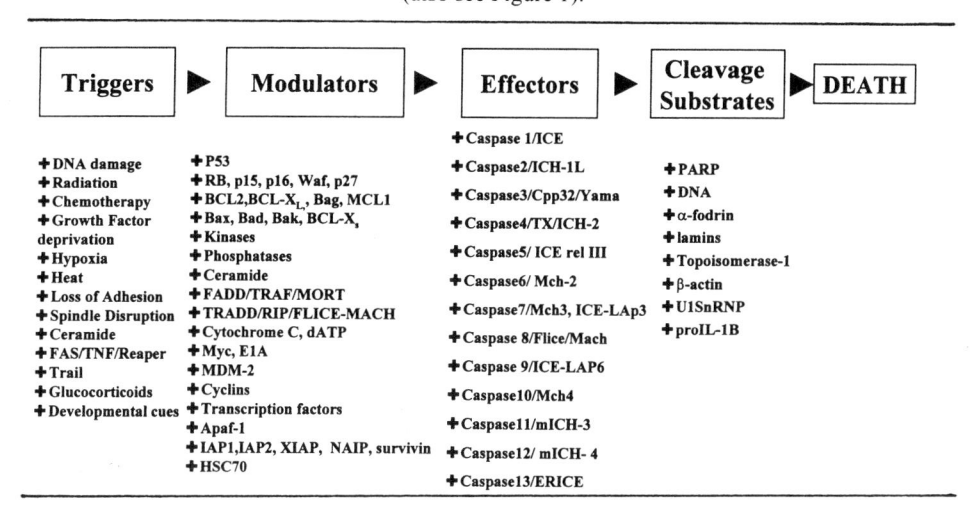

Triggers	Modulators	Effectors	Cleavage Substrates	→ DEATH
+DNA damage	+P53	+Caspase 1/ICE	+PARP	
+Radiation	+RB, p15, p16, Waf, p27	+Caspase2/ICH-1L	+DNA	
+Chemotherapy	+BCL2,BCL-X_L, Bag, MCL1	+Caspase3/Cpp32/Yama	+α-fodrin	
+Growth Factor deprivation	+Bax, Bad, Bak, BCL-X_s	+Caspase4/TX/ICH-2	+lamins	
+Hypoxia	+Kinases	+Caspase5/ ICE rel III	+Topoisomerase-1	
+Heat	+Phosphatases	+Caspase6/ Mch-2	+β-actin	
+Loss of Adhesion	+Ceramide	+Caspase7/Mch3, ICE-LAp3	+U1SnRNP	
+Spindle Disruption	+FADD/TRAF/MORT	+Caspase 8/Flice/Mach	+proIL-1B	
+Ceramide	+TRADD/RIP/FLICE-MACH	+Caspase 9/ICE-LAP6		
+FAS/TNF/Reaper	+Cytochrome C, dATP	+Caspase10/Mch4		
+Trail	+Myc, E1A	+Caspase11/mICH-3		
+Glucocorticoids	+MDM-2	+Caspase12/ mICH- 4		
+Developmental cues	+Cyclins	+Caspase13/ERICE		
	+Transcription factors			
	+Apaf-1			
	+IAP1,IAP2, XIAP, NAIP, survivin			
	+HSC70			

downstream in most studies,[14–17] and has also been shown to directly process pro-caspases-2, -6, -7, and -9.[18,19] For murine caspase 11 and 12, no human counterparts have been described so far. Recently, the isolation of human caspase 13 (ERICE) from the ICE subfamily was reported.[20] Activation of ERICE is mediated by caspase 8, suggesting the potential downstream role for active ERICE in caspase-8 mediated cell death. Caspases 2 and 3 were found to be prognostic factors in AML.[21]

3. TRIGGERS OF APOPTOSIS

3.1. Introduction

Many environmental, pharmocological or physiological stimuli can trigger apoptosis, a selection of which is shown in Table 1. In spite of their seemingly unrelated nature, they share downstream pathways that, although complex, are organized in unifying patterns that have very recently been elucidated. In a clinical context, these shared pathways provide rationale for the frequently observed resistance of tumors to multiple drugs and sometimes treatment modalities. Growth factors, which provide anti-apoptotic stimuli,[22] will trigger apoptosis when depleted from cytokine-dependent systems. Chemotherapeutic agents will exert their apoptogenic effects differentially in different cell types[23] depending on downstream signaling.

3.2. TNF/Receptor Family

Many death triggering signals are related to the TNF family that includes Fas ligand, TNF (tumor necrosis factor), lymphotoxin, CD30 ligand, CD40 ligand, CD27 ligand and TRAIL (TNF-related apoptosis-inducing ligand) (for review see Nagata, Cell[24]).

3.2.1. Fas and TNF Receptor Family. Fas (APO-1, CD95) is the receptor for FasL, and a member of the TNFR family (TNFR1, TNFR2, lymphotoxin-βR, NGFR (p75), CD40, CD27 and CD30, DR-3 (death-receptor 3) and others. The TNF induces apoptosis and activates the transcription factor NF-iB. Binding of FasL to Fas resulting in receptor trimerization[24,25] or cross-linking Fas with agonistic antibodies induces apoptosis. However, Fas/FasL interaction does not necessarily result in apoptosis[26,27] as downstream regulatory factors can suppress Fas/FasL death signaling. A novel cell-surface gene, toso, appears to be a negative regulator of Fas-mediated apoptosis in T cells, presumably through inhibition of caspase 8 processing[28]. Most other receptors in the TNF receptor family transduce stimulatory signals, although some of them (e.g. CD40,[29,30] CD30,[31] Apo3 ligand[32]) may also cause apoptosis.

A homologous 80 aminoacid domain in the cytoplasmic regions of Fas and TNFR1 has been designated the "death domain."[24] Adapter proteins (FADD/MORT1, and RAIDD) bind to these DD's via their own DD's.[33-36] A separate death effector domain (DED of FADD/MORT1) is required for propagation of the apoptotic signal. The DED of FADD/MORT1 binds to the prodomain of the caspase 8 FLICE/MACH, providing the connection of the Fas and TNFR1 death inducing signaling complex (DISC) and proteases.[37,38] Upon receptor trimerization with ligand, FADD/MORT1 recruits FLICE/MACH to the receptor, forming an active DISC which activates FLICE/MACH and thereby apoptosis. The recently described protein kinase RICK interacts with adapter molecule CLARP (caspase-like molecule known to bind FADD and FLICE) and promotes Fas-induced apoptosis.[39]

The CD95 system is an important regulator of T-cell cytotoxiciity. It has been suggested that tumor cells can evade immune attack by downregulating their CD95 receptors and by killing of activated lymphocytes through the expression of CD95L.[40] Such "immune privilege" has also been proposed for melanomas and colon cancers.[41,42]

In *lpr* (lymphoproliferation) and *gld* (generalized lymphoproliferative disease), which are loss of function mutations in the Fas and FasL genes, respectively, activated T cells, accumulate and cause autoimmune diseases. Conversely, overexpression of Fas can cause tissue destruction, e.g. hepatitis and in liver cirrhosis. FasL expressed on tumor cells can be cleaved and the soluble form of FasL can be found in sera from some but not all patients with malignancies[43] and may cause the multi-organ failure observed in cancer patients.

Fas can also be induced by many cytotoxic drugs[44,45] and it has been postulated that this is one of the mechanisms by which cytotoxic drugs kill cells.

Recently, a new family of six viral inhibitors (v-FLIPs for FLICE-inhibitory proteins) was described,[46] which interfere with apoptosis signaled through death receptors and which are present in several herpes viruses (including Kaposi's sarcoma-associated human herpesvirus-8), as well as in the tumorigenic human molluscipox virus.[47] v-FLIPs contain two death-effector domains which interact with the adaptor protein FADD, and this inhibits the recruitment and activation of the protease FLICE by the CD95 death receptor.[24,33,34] Cells expressing v-FLIPs are protected against apoptosis induced by CD95 or by the related death receptors TRAMP[48-50] and TRAIL-R. Protection of virus-infected cells against death-receptor-induced apoptosis may contribute to the oncogenicity of several FLIP-encoding viruses. The human cellular homolog, designated FLIP,[51] is predominantly expressed in muscle and lymphoid tissues. The short form, FLIPs, contains two death effector domains and is structurally related to the viral FLIP inhibiyors of apoptosis, whereas the long form, $FLIP_L$, contains in addition a caspase-like domain in which the active-centre cystein residue is substituted by a tyrosine residue.[51] FLIPs and $FLIP_L$ interact with the adaptor protein FADD and the protease FLICE, and potently inhibit apoptosis induced by all known human death receptors. FLIPL is expressed during the early stage of T-cell activation, but disappears when T cells become susceptible to Fas ligand-mediated apoptosis. High levels of FLIPL protein are also detectable in melanoma cell lines and in primary malignant melanomas but not in normal melanocytes, indicating that FLIP upregulation probably occurs during tumorigenesis.

3.2.2. TRAIL and Its Receptors. With the discovery of novel "death receptors" such as CAR1 and DR3 came the identification of a novel ligand that did not bind to any known receptor. This was called TRAIL ("TNF-related apoptosis inducing ligand" or APO2-L) (for review see[52]).

More recently, several receptors for TRAIL were identified, termed DR4, DR5, DcR1 and DcR2. Interestingly, DR4 did not bind to FADD or TRADD suggesting an alternative signaling machinery, differed from Fas. Indeed, DR4 and DR5 were found to activate caspases through FLICE2 (FADD-like interleukin-1β-converting enzyme2). Subsequently, non-signaling decoy receptors (DcR1, DcR2) were identified in normal human tissues, but not in most cancer cell lines examined. Their recognition of TRAIL may prevent TRAIL from binding to functional TRAIL receptors, therefore blocking and not transducing the cell death signal. The role of TRAIL in hematological malignancies has been recently examined and TRAIL was found to induce apoptosis in 27% of leukenias and lymphomas tested.[53] At this point in time, the definitive role(s) of TRAIL in apoptosis remains to be determined.

4. REGULATORS OF APOPTOSIS

4.1. Bcl-2 Family

The central control stage of the apoptotic machinery includes Bcl-2 family members (Bcl-2s) and associated proteins. The Bcl-2 family of proteins consists of both inhibitors and promoters of PCD, including the antiapoptotic proteins Bcl-X_L, Mcl-1, A1, Bcl-w and the proapoptotic proteins Bax, Bcl-X_S, Bad, Bik and Bid. Many of these proteins interact with each other through a complex network of homo- and heterodimers.[54,55] Bcl-2 can form heterodimers with the Bax, Bcl-X_L, Bcl-X_S, Mcl-1, and Bad proteins.[54–57] It is thought that the ratio of anti-apoptotic versus proapoptotic dimers is important in determining resistance of a cell to apoptosis. A recent paper emphasizes the crucial role of free, unbound Bcl-2 in the control of apoptosis.[58]

Antiapoptotic Bcl-X_L protein appears to have similar binding characteristics and has been shown to interact specifically with Bax, Bcl-X_S, Mcl-1, Bad, Bak, and itself, in addition to Bcl-2.[54,55] Bcl-X gene is highly related to Bcl-2.[59] Bcl-X transcripts are alternatively spliced into long (L) and short (S) forms. The protein product of the long form functionally resembles Bcl-2 as a potent inhibitor of cell death. In contrast to the Bcl-2 knockout mice, the Bcl-X knockout mice have an embryonic lethal phenotype with massive apoptosis in the brain, spinal cord and in the hematopoietic system.[60] The Bcl-X_S splice variant antagonizes cell death inhibition by the Bcl-X_L and Bcl-2 products.[59] Mcl-1 was identified based on increased expression in myeloblastic leukemia cells undergoing differentiation.[61] Mcl-1 can interact with Bax in hematopoietic FDC-P1 cells and can prolong cell viability under a variety of cytotoxic conditions.[62] Elevated expression of Mcl-1 was found at the time of leukemic relapse in AML and ALL.[63] Mcl-1 was also identified as

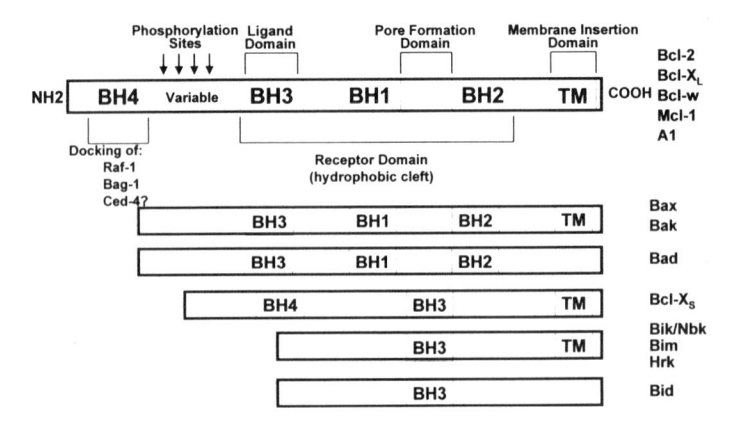

Figure 2. Molecular organization of Bcl-2 and members of this family. BH1–4=Bcl-2 homology regions 1–4. For details, see text.

a major prognostic factor in chronic lymphocytic leukemia (CLL).[64] Another Bcl-2 family member, A1, was isolated from mouse bone marrow induced to proliferate with GM-CSF, resembles an early response gene and is transcriptionally induced by GM-CSF.[65] Bcl-W was found to be expressed in a wide range of tissues and render cells refractory to certain apoptotic stimuli.[66]

Overexpression of proapoptotic proteins such as Bax and Bad counters the survival-promoting effect of Bcl-2 and Bcl-X_L. Bad can dimerize with Bcl-2 and Bcl-X_L; Bax also forms heterodimers with Bcl-2 and Bcl-X_L, although apparently with lower affinity than Bad. The Bax gene has been shown to encode alternatively splice variants;[67] a novel splice variant Bax-ω functions as a proapoptotic protein, but under conditions of constitutive overexpression, it can protect the cells from apoptotic cell death.[68] In acute lymphoblastic leukemias, a high incidence of Bax mutations was reported[69] which could explain the accumulation of immature blast cells.

4.2. Structure and Function of Bcl-2-Related Proteins

Recent structural analysis has clarified how Bcl-2-related proteins heterodimerize. Sequence comparison[66,70–72] had revealed four important Bcl-2 homology motifs: BH1, BH2 and BH3, present in both the anti- and pro-survival subfamilies, and BH4, present only in the former (Figure 3). Mutagenesis studies have shown that deletion of the *BH1* or *BH2* domain of Bcl-2 as well as certain amino acid substitution in these conserved domains abolish Bcl-2 function as a suppressor of cell death and also abrogate the ability of Bcl-2 to form heterodimers with Bax.[70,73] Similar mutations in the BH1 and BH2 domains of the antiapoptotic protein Bcl-X_L have the same effects on function and Bax binding.[55] These observations suggest that for Bcl-2 and Bcl-X_L to suppress apoptosis, they must be able to heterodimerize with Bax. A model for the regulation of cell survival by Bcl-2 family proteins has been suggested in which Bax homodimers comprise an active trigger for cell death. In the presence of an excess of Bcl-2 or Bcl-X_L, heterodimerization with Bax prevents the formation of toxic Bax homodimers, resulting in cell survival. The additional presence of Bad would than disrupt Bcl-2-Bax and Bcl-X_L-Bax heterodimers, liberating Bax once again to self-dimerize and promote death. However, in an equally plausible model, Bcl-2 and Bcl-X_L might be active repressors of cell death, and dominant heterodi-

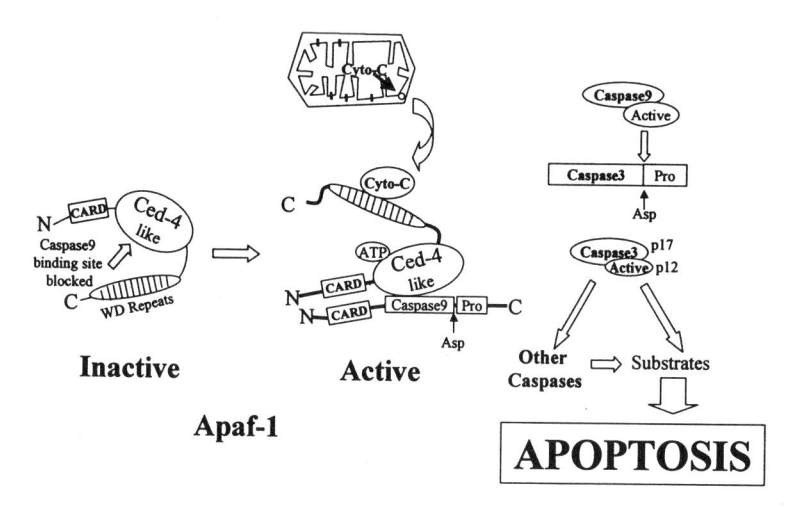

Figure 3. Cytochrome c activates cell death processes. Activation of caspase by cytochrome c is mediated by the CED-4 homolog Apaf-1.

merization with Bax or Bad may block the ability of the former molecules to prevent apoptosis. In favor of this model is the observation that specific mutations in Bcl-X_L that abrogate binding to Bax do not eliminate the ability of Bcl-X_L to prevent cell death.[74]

In contrast, the *BH3* domain was found to be important for functioning of proapoptotic members of Bcl-2 family. BH3 of Bax is required for both homodimerization and heterodimerization with Bcl-2.[72] Thus, the structural features of Bax that allow it to physically interact with other members of the Bcl-2 are strikingly different from Bcl-2, which does require BH1 and BH2 for heterodimerization with Bax, as well as for homodimerization with itself.[70,73]

The BH3 sequence is different in pro- and antiapoptotic proteins. Substituting BH3 of Bax for the corresponding domain of Bcl-2 converts the Bcl-2 protein from a death repressor to a death promoter.[75] Similarly, the region of Bak that contains the BH3 domain is sufficient for both heterodimerization with Bcl-X_L and for promoting apoptosis in mammalian cells.[71] Thus, Bak and presumably Bax, may encode a death effector domain in the vicinity of the BH3 region, or BH3 may merely serve as the binding site to interact with Bcl-2 and Bcl-X_L and neutralize their protective activity. In addition, the proapoptotic protein Bik contains a region with strong homology to the BH3 domain but lacks the BH1 and BH2 domains; however, it is able to bind Bcl-2 in a BH3-dependent manner.[76] A small novel protein, Bim, promotes apoptosis, with the BH3 domain being required for Bcl-2 binding and most of its toxicity.[77]

The three-dimentional structure of Bcl-X_L has recently been elucidated by X-ray cristallography and NMR spectroscopy.[78] The structure consists of two central hydrophobic α helices which are surrounded by amphiphatic helices. Three domains (BH1, 2 and 3) are in close spatial proximity and form an elongated hydrophobic cleft that may represent the binding site for other Bcl-2 family members. The second amphipathic helix of dimerized Bcl-2 family proteins inserts into this groove like a ligand binding to the receptor.[79,80] As the BH3 domain corresponds to this inserting α helix (ligand) but also forms part of the surface pocket (receptor), the implication is that Bcl-2 family members assume at least two conformations, with one dimerizing partner playing the role of the receptor and the

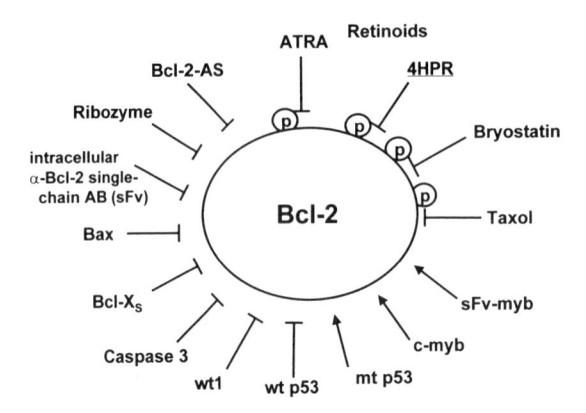

Figure 4. Activation and inhibition of Bcl-2: = activation, = inhibition, p = phosphorylation. For details, see text.

other that of the ligand. The propensity to adopt either a receptor or a ligand conformation may dictate whether a member of Bcl-2 family functions as an anti- vs a proapoptotic protein.[81,82]

All antiapoptotic members of the Bcl-2 protein family contain the *BH4* domain,[72] which is typically located near the N-terminus of these proteins and corresponds to the first amphipathic α helix in the crystal structure of the Bcl-X_L protein.[78] In contrast, the proapoptotic members of Bcl-2s lack BH4, with the exception of Bcl-X_S. Deletion mutants of Bcl-2 lacking the BH4 domain exhibit either loss of function or dominant-inhibitory activity, paradoxically promoting apoptosis,[73,75,83] thus indicating the functional significance of the BH4 domain. BH4 is not, however, required for binding to either Bax or wild-type Bcl-2 protein,[73] suggesting that it plays a role in some other aspects of Bcl-2 function. It is separated from the rest of the protein by a large unstructured loop and therefore may be able to swing away from the body of the protein for the purpose of interacting with several other proteins including Bag-1, the protein kinase Raf-1, the phosphatase calcineurin, p53-binding protein, and Nip1–3. In most cases, the functional significance of these interactions has not been explored. Recently, however, it has been reported that trough an interaction of the BH4 domain of Bcl-2 with the catalytic domain of Raf, Bcl-2 can target Raf-1 to the outer mitochondrial membrane, bringing it into proximity with a specific set of substrates.[84] The proapoptotic protein Bad represents at least one such substrate.[85,86] Activated Raf-1 efficiently phosphorylates Bad in vitro resulting in the persistent association of Bad with 14–3–3 in the cytosol.[87] Bad would be then be unavailable for interactions with Bcl-2 and Bcl-X_L, allowing the latter proteins to execute their anti-apoptotic function.[86,88] Antiapoptotic Bag-1 also binds Bcl-2 in a BH4-dependent manner. Presumably, anchored by the BH4 region of Bcl-2, Bag-1 can cause activation of the Raf-1 kinase, resulting in phosphorylation of Bad and therefore enhance protection from apoptosis (Figure 4).[86,89]

By virtue of its BH4 domain, Bcl-2 causes a redistribution of the Ca2+-dependent phosphatase calcineurin from the cytosol to intracellular membranes, preventing the interaction with phosphorylated nuclear factor of activated T-cells (NF-AT) or other substrates of calcineurin in the cytosol. Overexpression of calcineurin induces apoptosis in a Bcl-2-supressible manner,[90] presumably by dephosphorylation of Bad.

The Bcl-2/calcineurin interaction may also be relevant to the inhibition by Bcl-2 of cell *proliferation* as NF-AT-inducible genes are important for proliferation in some types of cells.[91,92] There is emerging evidence that Bcl-2 and its close relatives exert at least two distinct functions: they not only inhibit apoptosis but also restrain cell cycle entry.[93–98]

These two functions can be genetically separated as mutation of a conserved tyrosine residue (Y28) at the C-terminal end of the BH4 region does not effect the antiapoptotic activity of Bcl-2 but markedly reduces its ability to restrain re-entry of quiescent cells into the cell cycle.[99] The inhibitory effect of Bcl-2 on entry into the cell cycle may contribute to the indolent nature of lymphomas associated with Bcl-2 overexpression[100] and the better prognosis of patients whose breast cancer tissue shows abnormally high levels of Bcl-2 expression.[101] Likewise, patients with "poor prognosis" AML defined by certain cytogenetic abnormalities had significantly extended survival when high levels of Bcl-2 were determined at diagnosis (Andreeff et al., 1998 in press). Delayed cell cycle entry could result in longer times to relapse. However, the opposite was true for AML with "good prognosis" cytogenetics. Since most chemotherapeutic drugs target dividing cells, malignant cells expressing Bcl-2 are "doubly" protected: they are refractory to apoptosis and more likely to be quiescent.[102] An association between Bcl-X and prognosis in AML was recently suggested: a high ratio of Bcl-X_L to Bcl-X_S was associated with poor prognosis cytogenetics which identifies patients resistant to chemotherapy.[103]

4.3. Posttranscriptional Modifications: Phosphorylation of Bad and Bcl-2

Growth-factor regulated protein kinase phosphorylation of Bad was proposed as a possible mechanism for growth factor induced cell survival. The function of Bad is modulated by phosphorylation at two sites, serine 112 and serine 136.[84,86,88] However, Raf-1 and another kinase, PKC, phosphorylate Bad in vitro at serine residues other than Ser112 and Ser136, which suggests that Bad is not a physiological target of Raf-1 in vivo.[86] Recent findings demonstrate that activation of growth factor receptors can suppress apoptosis induced by Bad through a pathway involving a sequential induction of phosphoinositide-3'-OH kinase (PI3'K) activity, Akt activity, and finally Bad phosphorylation.[104,105] The PI3'K-Akt-Bad pathway may represent a general mechanism by which growth factors promote cell survival. In primary acute myelogenous leukemias, Bad was phosphorylated in 41/42 samples, perhaps reflecting the constitutive activation of survival pathways (Andreeff et al., 1998 in press).

The finding that the expression levels of Bcl-2s do not always predict the ability to resist death-promoting stimuli suggests the existence of Bcl-2-independent mechanisms regulating apoptosis. Several experiments have indicated that post-translational modification of Bcl-2s may play an important role in regulating their ability to promote cell survival. Bad phosphorylation in response to extracellular survival signals links the signaling transduction pathways and the function of Bcl-2 family proteins. The ability of the chemotherapeutic agent taxol to induce phosphorylation of Bcl-2 has been implicated as a mechanism by which it can promote death in face of high expression of Bcl-2.[106,107] Other drugs affecting the integrity of microtubules can also induce Bcl-2 phosphorylation; this novel function of Bcl-2 as a guardian of microtubule integrity allows elimination of the cells failing to complete mitosis.[108]

Deletion of a putative negative regulatory loop that contains the major serine/threonine phosphorylation sites in Bcl-2 enables Bcl-2 to promote cell survival under conditions where it is normally inactive.[109] Interestingly, CED-9 does not have a sufficient number of amino acids to encode a regulatory loop region[6] and may not need a specialized domain to post-translationally control its function. However, higher organisms seem to have acquired a more intricate system for regulating Bcl-2 function. As there are five serines and three threonines in the loop domain of Bcl-2, it is possible that there are multiple phosphorylation sites present in the loop. There can be also variations in the degree of phosphorylation. This fact could explain that serine phosphorylation of Bcl-2 has been reported to correlate with an increase in anti-apoptotic activity by two groups[110-112] and with a decrease by others.[106,109]

Additionally, Bcl-2 appears to be cleaved by proteases activated during apoptosis, which may explain the death of lymphocytes infected with HIV.[113] The loop domain of Bcl-2 and Bcl-X$_L$ is cleaved by caspases in vitro, in cells induced to undergo apoptotic cell death;[114,115] this cleavage releases a C-terminal product that lacks the BH4 domain and acts as a death effector therefore ensuring the inevitability of cell death. Thus, Bcl-2 may also be a downstream death substrate of caspases, suggesting the existence of a feedback loop between Bcl-2 and caspases.

4.4. Changes in Mitochondria during Apoptosis

One ground-breaking result in the past year that has changed the way we think about apoptosis includes the determination of the structure of the Bcl-2 family member Bcl-X$_L$ and its similarity to that of the pore forming domain of diphtheria toxin. The suggestion from these studies is that Bcl-2-related proteins may function as channels for ions, proteins, or both.[118] Now, direct evidence of ion-channel activity in vitro has been obtained from experiments in which the effects of recombinant Bcl-2 or Bcl-X$_L$ in synthetic lipid membranes were studied by using single-channel recordings from planar bilayers and by other approaches.[117,118] Although at present there is no direct evidence for in vivo channel formation, this phenomenon could explain cellular events associated with changes in mitochondria during apoptosis, particularly the mitochondrial 'megapore' opening which is associated with permeability transition and release of the apoptogenic protease activators cytochrome c and apoptosis-inducing factor (AIF) from mitochondria. Though varying among different cell types and particular members of the Bcl-2 family, in general, a large proportion of these protein molecules are associated with the outer mitochondrial membrane by virtue of their transmembrane domain.[119-121] Several observations suggest an important role for mitochondria in the control of apoptosis. For example, mitochondria isolated from cells induced to undergo apoptosis can stimulate apoptosis-like destruction of naive nuclei, whereas mitochondria purified from Bcl-2 overexpressing cells do not.[122] Interestingly, chemical inducers of mitochondrial megapore opening can induce normal mitochondria derived from healthy cells to liberate factors that result in the apoptosis-like destruction of nuclei.[122] Recently, this effect has been attributed to the release of cytochrome c and apoptosis-inducing factor (AIF) from mitochondria that can promote activation of proteases.[123,124] It has been hypothesized that the key function of Bcl-2-like proteins is to somehow retain cytochrome c in the mitochondria.[125,126] It remains to be determined whether the suppression of cytochrome c release by Bcl-2 reflects the ability of Bcl-2 either to block Bax channels or to transport cytochrome c back to the mitochondria.[125,126] However, Bcl-2 mutants lacking their C-terminal TM domain and therefore inefficiently associated with mitochondria retain partial antiapoptotic activity, suggesting that membrane targeting of Bcl-2 is not absolutely critical for its function.[67]

Although caspase activation usually occurs downstream of mitochondrial permeability transition, recent data indicate that caspases can also cause a dissipation of the mitochondrial inner transmembrane potential and therefore act upstream.[127,128] The membrane-permeabilizing effect of caspases is probably due to effects on specific protein substrates in the mitochondrial membranes; proteins of the Bcl-2 family may be the target of caspases. Thus, Bcl-2 is a caspase 3 substrate, and Bcl-X$_L$ is a caspase 1 substrate.[114,115]

These observations suggest that caspases and mitochondria can engage in a circular self-amplification loop that could accelerate or coordinate the apoptotic response.

4.5. Apoptosis Activating Factors (Apafs)

Of the Bcl-2/Bcl-X$_L$-binding proteins, CED-4 or its functional equivalent in mammalian cells is probably the most important. In C. elegans, this gene is believed to function downstream from CED-9 but upstream from CED-3.[129,130] Recent biochemical data support this concepts, as CED-3 and CED-4 can physically interact[131,132] most likely by virtue of their N-terminal domains, which both contain a motif designated a caspase recruitment domain (CARD)[133] (Figure 5). Furthermore, CED-9 as well as Bcl-X$_L$ can bind to C. elegans CED-4, which in turn binds to CED-3 or other caspases.[131,134–136] Indeed, CED-9, CED-4 and CED-3 can form a trimolecular complex.[131] Therefore, in C. elegans it appears that CED-4 is an adaptor protein that can receive an apoptotic signal, bind to pro-CED-3, and cause it to release its activated proteolytic domain. By binding to CED-4, CED-9 somehow prevents it from activating pro-CED-3.

Recently, X. Wang and coworkers have isolated a number of Apoptosis activating factors (Apaf 1–3).[137] Addition of dATP to these proteins results in cleavage and activation of the caspase-3 precursor. Earlier work had revealed Apaf-2 to be cytochrome c. Apaf-3 is a 45 kDa protein that has not yet been cloned. Apaf-1 was found to resemble CED-4. It has an amino-terminal CARD domain that may bind directly to caspase.[133] At the C-terminus of the protein is a large domain containing 12 WD-40 repeats. Such repeats usually mediate protein-protein interactions, and could in this case be involved in the physical interaction between Apaf-1 and Apaf-2/cytochrome c. Like CED-4, the peptide sequence of Apaf-1 contains regions that conform to the consensus for Walker A and B boxes, the nucleotide-binding p-loop motif. ATP may activate Apaf-1 by binding to this region.

The precise function of Bcl-2/CED-9-like proteins is still unknown. Presumably, Apaf-1 interacts with the caspase precursors via the CARD domain, in the presence of of dATP, allowing cleavage of the prodomain. Bcl-2-like proteins inhibit caspase activation by either binding directly to the adaptor protein (Apaf-1 or CED-4), or by preventing cytochrome c release, or both.[138] The death-promoting members of the Bcl-2 family (Bax, Bak) function by disrupting this biochemical interaction. The same mechanism is suggestive for the apoptosis induced by the "BH3 only" group of cell death activators, which in C. elegans includes Bik, Bid, Harakiri, Bad and a novel protein EGL-1.[139] Another possibility is that Bcl-2 may retain cytochrome c in the mitochondria indirectly. If cytochrome c is only one of a number of factors that can cause CED-4 to activate the caspases, induction of apoptosis by these alternate pathways might lead to a secondary loss of mitochondrial function, release of cytochrome c, and an amplification of the apoptotic cascade. In such a scenario, Bcl-2-like proteins would only act as CED-4 inhibitors, with their ability to prevent cytochrome c release being indirect, by inhibiting the initial, premitochondrial caspase activation.

In summary, CED-4 or human Apafs are likely to be critical for Bcl-2 function, enabling Bcl-2 to regulate the caspases. Proapoptotic members of the Bcl-2 family heterodimerize with Bcl-2 thereby displacing CED-4. Where CED-4/Apaf-1 binds to Bcl-2/Bcl-X$_L$ is unknown but the hydrophobic groove on the surface of the protein is a likely candidate thereby explaining the function of "BH3 only" proteins which can displace CED-4 from Bcl-X$_L$. Interactions with other proteins may be not as fundamental to the function Bcl-2s as CED-4 binding probably serves as supporting partner in different cellular contexts or circumstances-specific conditions. In addition, the regulation of mitochondrial permeability transition through Bcl-2s ion-channel activity might be important in some circumstances although the question remains whether it is a truly critical step in the apoptotic cascade or a secondary event.

4.6. Apoptosis Inhibitory Proteins (IAPs)

It now appears that another family of apoptotic suppressors has been identified through their homology with the baculovirus iap gene.[140–145] Several human cellular homologs have been isolated recently.[140,142,144] The human X-chromosome-linked IAP was shown to directly inhibit at least two members of the caspase family, caspase-3 and caspase-7, providing evidence for a mechanism of action for these mammalian cell-death supressors.[146] IAP genes display two distinct structural features. The first of these is a zinc binding domain known as a RING finger,[147] which has been also identified in a number of cellular proteins including the products of the protooncogenes c-cbl[148] and c-mpl,[149] as well as the recently described family of signal transducing molecules TRAF2[143,150] and CRAF1/CD40bp.[151–153] While RING domains have been found in several DNA binding proteins, they have not been shown to bind DNA, and probably act to mediate protein-protein interactions.[154] The second highly conserved feature of baculovirus IAP proteins is the presence of amino-terminal repeats of an 65 amino acid sequence termed a baculovirus IAP repeat (BIR). Both the BIR repeats and RING domains have been shown to be essential in preventing cell death in insect cells;[141] in XIAP, a single BIR2 domain was found to be sufficient for binding and inhibiting caspases-3 and −7.[155]

Loss of IAP-related genes may cause cell death in mammalian cells that express these genes. Consistent with this hypothesis, mutations in the NAIP gene are thought to contribute to spinal muscular atrophy.[142] This neurodegenerative syndrome results from the inappropriate death of motor neurons. In over two-thirds of the patients with the severe form of spinal muscular atrophy, there are deletions in the first two coding exons of NAIP. These deletions result in the loss of all of the first BIR and most of the second BIR domains. Thus it appears that the BIR domains are essential to the function of NAIP in maintaining motor neuron survival.

A new human gene survivin, encoding a structurally unique IAP apoptosis inhibitor, was recently described.[156] Survivin contains a single baculovirus IAP repeat and lacks a carboxy-terminal RING finger. Present during fetal development,[156,157] survivin is undetectable in terminally differentiated adult tissues. However, survivin is prominently expressed in transformed cell lines and in all the most common human cancers of lung, colon, pancreas, prostate, breast and in high-grade non-Hodgkin's lymphomas, suggesting survivin as a potential new target for apoptosis-based therapy.

5. MODULATION OF APOPTOSIS AS NOVEL STRATEGY IN CANCER TREATMENT

Although the precise contribution of apoptotic pathways to the pathophysiology and the resistance to drugs and radiation in many human tumors remains to be defined, major efforts are underway to modulate them. While anti-apoptotic strategies aim at reducing tissue damage in autoimmune diseases, stroke, myocardial infarction and hepatitis, to name a few, mostly by interfering with caspase activation, pro-apoptotic interventions have already been employed in cancer therapy. Because Bcl-2 has been extensively investigated it has become the target of many attempts to modulate it's expression and function. Figure

4 shows a variety of such approaches. Bcl-2 antisense oligonucleotides[158,159] are able to induce apoptosis in leukemia cell lines and primary samples, and enhance chemotherapy-induced apoptosis. This approach was already successfully implemented in a recent phase I study in lymphoma patients.[160] All-trans retinoid acid (ATRA) downregulates Bcl-2 and Bcl-X_L mRNA[161] and phosphorylates Bcl-2 with resulting loss of protective function[162] and enhances ARA-C when administrated after, but not before ARA-C.[161] Ribozyme directed against Bcl-2, intracellular anti-Bcl-2 single chain antibody (sFv),[163] Bax and Bcl-X_S inactivate Bcl-2's anti-apoptotic function. Bryostatin, Taxol and the retinoid-analog 4-HPR phosphorylate Bcl-2, but their precise modulation of apoptotic pathways remains to be determined. Figure 4 also denotes the negative regulations of Bcl-2 by wild type p53 and by the wt1 gene. Mutated p53, c-myb and sFv-myb have been reported to activate Bcl-2. Interestingly, caspase 3 cleaves Bcl-2 into fragments that exert pro-apoptotic activity.[114]

Some of these approaches will likely mature from in vitro tools to study the role of Bcl-2 in apoptosis to clinically useful drugs in cancer therapy. Other molecules in the apoptotic pathway will also be targeted and may allow a more rational development of cancer therapy by optimizing the known effects of established anti-cancer drugs through specific downregulation of anti-apoptotic and/or upregulation of pro-apoptotic pathways.

6. CONCLUSION

Following the discovery of apoptotic pathways in C. elegans, and the delineation of Fas/FasL signaling, several additional regulatory factors were identified in the mammalian cell-death pathway, with the emergence of FLIPs which inhibit the recruitment of FLICE by virtue of their similarity with death receptors, and with IAP family members that directly bind and inhibit caspases. The discovery of Apaf-1 as the mammalian CED-4 homolog has been a major step forward. However, our knowledge of the remarkably conserved key players in the apoptotic cascade continues to develop. The elucidation of the molecular mechanisms of apoptosis may therefore create the basis to manipulate the physiological cell death pathway and to interfere in diseases associated with hyper- or hypo-apoptosis.

ACKNOWLEDGMENT

The authors wish to thank Dr. J Reed for many excellent discussions and a successful, ongoing collaboration to dissect apoptotic pathways in leukemias. Supported in part by grants from the National Institutes of Health (PO1 CA55164, PO1 CA49639 and CA16672) and from the Stringer Professorship for Cancer Treatment and Research (M.A.).

REFERENCES

1. White E. Life, death, and the pursuit of apoptosis. Genes Dev 1996; 10(1):1–15
2. Yang E, Korsmeyer SJ. Molecular thanatopsis: a discourse on the BCL2 family and cell death. Blood 1996;88 (2):386–401
3. Thompson CB. Apoptosis in the pathogenesis and treatment of disease. Science 1995; 267 (5203): 1456–1462

4. Alnemri ES, Livingston DJ, Nicholson DW, Salvesen G, Thornberry NA, Wong WW, Yuan J. Human ICE/CED-3 protease nomenclature. Cell 1996;87(2):171
5. Yuan J, Shaham S, Ledoux S, Ellis HM, Horvitz HR. The C. elegans cell death gene ced-3 encodes a protein similar to mammalian interleukin-1 beta-converting enzyme. Cell 1993;75(4):641–652
6. Hengartner MO, Horvitz HR. Programmed cell death in Caenorhabditis elegans. [Review] [45 refs] Curr Opin Genet Dev 1994;4(4):581–586
7. Vaux DL, Weissman IL, Kim SK. Prevention of programmed cell death in Caenorhabditis elegans by human bcl-2. Science 1992;258(5090):1955–1957
8. Nicholson DW, Thornberry NA. Caspases: killer proteases. Trends Biochem Sci 1997; 22(8):299–306
9. Talanian RV, Quinlan C, Trautz S, Hackett MC, Mankovich JA, Banach D, Ghayur T, Brady KD, Wong WW. Substrate specificities of caspase family proteases. J Biol Chem 1997; 272(15):9677–9682
10. Thornberry NA, Rano TA, Peterson EP, Rasper DM, Timkey T, Garcia-Calvo M, Houtzager VM, Nordstrom PA, Roy S, Vaillancourt JP, Chapman KT, Nicholson DW. A combinatorial approach defines specificities of members of the caspase family and granzyme B. Functional relationships established for key mediators of apoptosis. J Biol Chem 1997; 272(29):17907–17911
11. Fernandes-Alnemri T, Armstrong RC, Krebs J, Srinivasula SM, Wang L, Bullrich F, Fritz LC, Trapani JA, Tomaselli KJ, Litwack G, Alnemri ES. In vitro activation of CPP32 and Mch3 by Mch4, a novel human apoptotic cysteine protease containing two FADD-like domains. Proc Natl Acad Sci U S A 1996; 93(15):7464–7469
12. Boldin MP, Goncharov TM, Goltsev YV, Wallach D. Involvement of MACH, a novel MORT1/FADD-interacting protease, in Fas/APO-1- and TNF receptor-induced cell death. Cell 1996; 85(6):803–815
13. Muzio M, Chinnaiyan AM, Kischkel FC, O'Rourke K, Shevchenko A, Ni J, Scaffidi C, Bretz JD, Zhang M, Gentz R, Mann M, Krammer PH, Peter ME, Dixit VM. FLICE, a novel FADD-homologous ICE/CED-3-like protease, is recruited to the CD95 (Fas/APO-1) death—inducing signaling complex. Cell 1996; 85(6):817–827
14. Faleiro L, Kobayashi R, Fearnhead H, Lazebnik Y. Multiple species of CPP32 and Mch2 are the major active caspases present in apoptotic cells. EMBO J 1997; 16(9):2271–2281
15. Martins LM, Kottke T, Mesner PW, Basi GS, Sinha S, Frigon N Jr, Tatar E, Tung JS, Bryant K, Takahashi A, Svingen PA, Madden BJ, McCormick DJ, Earnshaw WC, Kaufmann SH. Activation of multiple interleukin-1beta converting enzyme homologues in cytosol and nuclei of HL-60 cells during etoposide-induced apoptosis. J Biol Chem 1997; 272(11):7421–7430
16. MacFarlane M, Cain K, Sun XM, Alnemri ES, Cohen GM. Processing/activation of at least four interleukin-1beta converting enzyme-like proteases occurs during the execution phase of apoptosis in human monocytic tumor cells. J Cell Biol 1997; 37(2):469–479
17. Takahashi A, Hirata H, Yonehara S, Imai Y, Lee KK, Moyer RW, Turner PC, Mesner PW, Okazaki T, Sawai H, Kishi S, Yamamoto K, Okuma M, Sasada M. Affinity labeling displays the stepwise activation of ICE-related proteases by Fas, staurosporine, and CrmA-sensitive caspase-8. Oncogene 1997; 14(23):2741–2752
18. Srinivasula SM, Fernandes-Alnemri T, Zangrilli J, Robertson N, Armstrong RC, Wang L, Trapani JA, Tomaselli KJ, Litwack G, Alnemri ES. The Ced-3/interleukin 1beta converting enzyme-like homolog Mch6 and the lamin-cleaving enzyme Mch2alpha are substrates for the apoptotic mediator CPP32. J Biol Chem 1996; 271(43):27099–27106
19. Fernandes-Alnemri T, Takahashi A, Armstrong R, Krebs J, Fritz L, Tomaselli KJ, Wang L, Yu Z, Croce CM, Salveson G, et al. Mch3, a novel human apoptotic cysteine protease highly related to CPP32. Cancer Res 1995;55(24):6045–6052
20. Humke EW, Ni J, Dixit VM. ERICE, a novel FLICE-activatable caspase. Biol Chem 1998; 273(25):15702–15707
21. Estrov Z, Thall PF, Talpaz M, Estey EH, Kantarjian H, Andreeff M, Harris D, Van Q, Walterscheid M, Kornblau S. Caspase 2 and caspase 3 protein levels as predictors of survival in acute myelogenous leukemia. Blood 1998; 92(9):3090–3097
22. Lisovsky M, Estrov Z, Zhang X, Consoli U, Sanchez-Williams G, Snell V, Munker R, Goodacre A, Savchenko V, Andreeff M. Flt3 ligand stimulates proliferation and inhibits apoptosis of acute myeloid leukemia cells: regulation of Bcl-2 and Bax. Blood 1996;88(10):3987–3997
23. Consoli U, El-Tounsi I, Sandoval A, Snell V, Kleine HD, Brown W, Robinson JR, DiRaimondo F, Plunkett W, Andreeff M. Differential induction of apoptosis by fludarabine monophosphate in leukemic B and normal T cells in chronic lymphocytic leukemia. Blood 1998;91(5):1742–1748
24. Nagata S. Apoptosis by death factor. Cell 1997;88(3):355–365
25. Nagata S, Golstein P. The Fas death factor. Science 1995;267(5203):1449–1456
26. Munker R, Marini F, Jiang S, Savary C, Owen-Schaub L, Andreeff M. Expression of CD95(FAS) by gene transfer does not sensitize K562 to Fas-killing. Hematol Cell Ther 1997;39(2):75–78

27. Munker R, Andreeff M. Induction of death (CD95/FAS), activation and adhesion (CD54) molecules on blast cells of acute myelogenous leukemias by TNF-alpha and IFN-gamma. Cytokines Mol Ther 1996;2(3):147–159
28. Hitoshi Y, Lorens J, Kitada SI, Fisher J, LaBarge M, Ring HZ, Francke U, Reed JC, Kinoshita S, Nolan GP. Toso, a cell surface, specific regulator of Fas-induced apoptosis in T cells. Immunity 1998;8(4):461–471
29. Younes A, Snell V, Consoli U, Clodi K, Zhao S, Palmer JL, Thomas EK, Armitage RJ, Andreeff M. Elevated levels of biologically active soluble CD40 ligand in the serum of patients with chronic lymphocytic leukaemia. Br J Haematol 1998;100(1):135–141
30. Clodi K, Asgari Z, Macduff BM, Zhao S, Kliche K-O, Palmer JL, Cabanillas F, Andreeff M, Younes A. A potential autocrine loop involving CD40 ligand in B cell lymphoma. Submitted
31. Younes A, Consoli U, Snell V, Clodi K, Kliche KO, Palmer JL, Gruss HJ, Armitage R, Thomas EK, Cabanillas F, Andreeff M. CD30 ligand in lymphoma patients with CD30+ tumors. J Clin Oncol 1997;15(11):3355–3362
32. Marsters SA, Sheridan JP, Pitti RM, Brush J, Goddard A, Ashkenazi A. Identification of a ligand for the death-domain-containing receptor apo3. Curr Biol 1998; 8(9):525–528
33. Boldin MP, Varfolomeev EE, Pancer Z, Mett IL, Camonis JH, Wallach D. A novel protein that interacts with the death domain of Fas/APO1 contains a sequence motif related to the death domain. J Biol Chem 1995;270(14):7795–7798
34. Chinnaiyan AM, O'Rourke K, Tewari M, Dixit VM. FADD, a novel death domain-containing protein, interacts with the death domain of Fas and initiates apoptosis. Cell 1995;81(4):505–512
35. Chinnaiyan AM, Tepper CG, Seldin MF, O'Rourke K, Kischkel FC, Hellbardt S, Krammer PH, Peter ME, Dixit VM. FADD/MORT1 is a common mediator of CD95 (Fas/APO-1) and tumor necrosis factor receptor-induced apoptosis. J Biol Chem 1996; 271(9):4961–4965
36. Duan H, Dixit VM. RAIDD is a new 'death' adaptor molecule. Nature 1997 Jan 2;385(6611):86–89
37. Boldin MP, Goncharov TM, Goltsev YV, Wallach D. Involvement of MACH, a novel MORT1/FADD-interacting protease, in Fas/APO-1- and TNF receptor-induced cell death. Cell 1996;85(6):803–815
38. Muzio M, Chinnaiyan AM, Kischkel FC, O'Rourke K, Shevchenko A, Ni J, Scaffidi C, Bretz JD, Zhang M, Gentz R, Mann M, Krammer PH, Peter ME, Dixit VM. FLICE, a novel FADD-homologous ICE/CED-3-like protease, is recruited to the CD95 (Fas/APO-1) death—inducing signaling complex. Cell 1996;85(6):817–827
39. Inohara N, del Peso L, Koseki T, Chen S, Nunez G. RICK, a novel protein kinase containing a caspase recruitment domain, interacts with CLARP and regulates CD95-mediated apoptosis. J Biol Chem 1998;273(20):12296–12300
40. Strand S, Hofmann WJ, Hug H, Muller M, Otto G, Strand D, Mariani SM, Stremmel W, Krammer PH, Galle PR. Lymphocyte apoptosis induced by CD95 (APO-1/Fas) ligand-expressing tumor cells—a mechanism of immune evasion? Nat Med 1996; 2(12):1361–1366
41. Hahne M, Rimoldi D, Schroter M, Romero P, Schreier M, French LE, Schneider P, Bornand T, Fontana A, Lienard D, Cerottini J, Tschopp J. Melanoma cell expression of Fas(Apo-1/CD95) ligand: implications for tumor immune escape. Science 1996;274(5291):1363–1366
42. O'Connell J, O'Sullivan GC, Collins JK, Shanahan F. The Fas counterattack: Fas-mediated T cell killing by colon cancer cells expressing Fas ligand. J Exp Med 1996;184(3):1075–1082
43. Munker R, Midis G, Owen-Schaub L, Andreff M. Soluble FAS (CD95) is not elevated in the serum of patients with myeloid leukemias, myeloproliferative and myelodysplastic syndromes. Leukemia 1996;10(9):1531–1533
44. Friesen C, Herr I, Krammer PH, Debatin KM. Involvement of the CD95 (APO-1/FAS) receptor/ligand system in drug-induced apoptosis in leukemia cells. Nat Med 1996;2(5):574–577
45. Herr I, Wilhelm D, Bohler T, Angel P, Debatin KM. Activation of CD95 (APO-1/Fas) signaling by ceramide mediates cancer therapy-induced apoptosis. EMBO J 1997;16(20):6200–6208
46. Thome M, Schneider P, Hofmann K, Fickenscher H, Meinl E, Neipel F, Mattmann C, Burns K, Bodmer JL, Schroter M, Scaffidi C, Krammer PH, Peter ME, Tschopp J. Viral FLICE-inhibitory proteins (FLIPs) prevent apoptosis induced by death receptors. Nature 1997;386(6624):517–521
47. Senkevich TG, Bugert JJ, Sisler JR, Koonin EV, Darai G, Moss B. Genome sequence of a human tumorigenic poxvirus: prediction of specific host response-evasion genes. Science 1996;273(5276):813–816
48. Bodmer JL, Burns K, Schneider P, Hofmann K, Steiner V, Thome M, Bornand T, Hahne M, Schroter M, Becker K, Wilson A, French LE, Browning JL, MacDonald HR, Tschopp J. TRAMP, a novel apoptosis-mediating receptor with sequence homology to tumor necrosis factor receptor 1 and Fas(Apo-1/CD95). Immunity 1997;6(1):79–88

49. Kitson J, Raven T, Jiang YP, Goeddel DV, Giles KM, Pun KT, Grinham CJ, Brown R, Farrow SN. A death-domain-containing receptor that mediates apoptosis. Nature 1996;384(6607): 372–375
50. Chinnaiyan AM, O'Rourke K, Yu GL, Lyons RH, Garg M, Duan DR, Xing L, Gentz R, Ni J, Dixit VM. Signal transduction by DR3, a death domain-containing receptor related to TNFR-1 and CD95. Science 1996;274(5289):990–992
51. Irmler M, Thome M, Hahne M, Schneider P, Hofmann K, Steiner V, Bodmer JL, Schroter M, Burns K, Mattmann C, Rimoldi D, French LE, Tschopp J. Inhibition of death receptor signals by cellular FLIP. Nature 1997;388(6638):190–195
52. Golstein P. Cell death: TRAIL and its receptors. Current Biol 1997;7:R750-R753
53. Snell V, Clodi K, Zhao S, Goodwin R, Thomas EK, Morris SW, Kadin ME, Cabanillas F, Andreeff M, Younes A. Activity of TNF-related apoptosis-inducing ligand (TRAIL) in haematological malignancies. Br J Haematol 1997;99(3):618–624
54. Sato T, Irie S, Krajewski S, Reed JC. Cloning and sequencing of a cDNA encoding the rat Bcl-2 protein. Gene 1994;140(2):291–292
55. Sedlak TW, Oltvai ZN, Yang E, Wang K, Boise LH, Thompson CB, Korsmeyer SJ. Multiple Bcl-2 family members demonstrate selective dimerizations with Bax. Proc Natl Acad Sci USA 1995;92(17):7834–7838
56. Oltvai ZN, Milliman CL, Korsmeyer SJ. Bcl-2 heterodimerizes in vivo with a conserved homolog, Bax, that accelerates programmed cell death. Cell 1993;74(4):609–619
57. Yang E, Zha J, Jockel J, Boise LH, Thompson CB, Korsmeyer SJ. Bad, a heterodimeric partner for Bcl-XL and Bcl-2, displaces Bax and promotes cell death. Cell 1995;80(2):285–291
58. Otter I, Conus S, Ravn U, Rager M, Olivier R, Monney L, Fabbro D, Borner C. The binding properties and biological activities of bcl-2 and bax in cells exposed to apoptotic stimuli. J Biol Chem 1998;273(11):6110–6120
59. Boise LH, Gonzalez-Garcia M, Postema CE, Ding L, Lindsten T, Turka LA, Mao X, Nunez G, Thompson CB. bcl-x, a bcl-2-related gene that functions as a dominant regulator of apoptotic cell death. Cell 1993;74(4):597–608
60. Motoyama N, Wang F, Roth KA, Sawa H, Nakayama K, Nakayama K, Negishi I, Senju S, Zhang Q, Fujii S, et al. Massive cell death of immature hematopoietic cells and neurons in Bcl-x-deficient mice. Science 1995;267(5203)1506–1510
61. Kozopas KM, Yang T, Buchan HL, Zhou P, Craig RW. MCL1, a gene expressed in programmed myeloid cell differentiation, has sequence similarity to BCL2. Proc Natl Acad Sci USA 1993;90(8):3516–3520
62. Zhou P, Qian L, Kozopas KM, Craig RW. Mcl-1, a Bcl-2 family member, delays the death of hematopoietic cells under a variety of apoptosis-inducing conditions. Blood 1997;89(2):630–643
63. Kaufmann SH, Karp JE, Svingen PA, Krajewski S, Burke PJ, Gore SD, Reed JC. Elevated expression of the apoptotic regulator Mcl-1 at the time of leukemic relapse. Blood 1998;91(3):991–1000
64. Kitada S, Andersen J, Akar S, Zapata JM, Takayama S, Krajewski S, Wang HG, Zhang X, Bullrich F, Croce CM, Rai K, Hines J, Reed JC. Expression of apoptosis-regulating proteins in chronic lymphocytic leukemia: correlations with In vitro and In vivo chemoresponses. Blood 1998; 91(9):3379–3389
65. Lin EY, Orlofsky A, Berger MS, Prystowsky MB. Characterization of A1, a novel hemopoietic-specific early-response gene with sequence similarity to bcl-2. J Immunol 1993;151(4):1979–1988
66. Gibson L, Holmgreen SP, Huang DC, Bernard O, Copeland NG, Jenkins NA, Sutherland GR, Baker E, Adams JM, Cory S. bcl-w, a novel member of the bcl-2 family, promotes cell survival. Oncogene 1996;13(4):665–675
67. Oltvai ZN, Milliman CL, Korsmeyer SJ. Bcl-2 heterodimerizes in vivo with a conserved homolog, Bax, that accelerates programmed cell death. Cell 1993;74(4):609–619
68. Zhou M, Demo SD, McClure TN, Crea R, Bitler CM. A novel splice variant of the cell death-promoting protein BAX. J Biol Chem 1998;273(19):11930–11936
69. Meijerink JPP, Mensink EJBM, Wang K, Sedlak TW, Sloetjes AW, de Witte T, Waksman G, Korsmeyer SJ. Hematopoietic malignancies demonstrate loss-of-function mutations of bax. Blood 1998;91(8):2991–2997
70. Yin XM, Oltvai ZN, Korsmeyer SJ. BH1 and BH2 domains of Bcl-2 are required for inhibition of apoptosis and heterodimerization with Bax. Nature 1994;369(6478):321–323
71. Chittenden T, Flemington C, Houghton AB, Ebb RG, Gallo GJ, Elangovan B, Chinnadurai G, Lutz RJ. A conserved domain in Bak, distinct from BH1 and BH2, mediates cell death and protein binding functions. EMBO J 1995;14(22):5589–5596
72. Zha H, Aime-Sempe C, Sato T, Reed JC. Proapoptotic protein Bax heterodimerizes with Bcl-2 and homodimerizes with Bax via a novel domain (BH3) distinct from BH1 and BH2. J Biol Chem 1996;271(13): 7440–7444

73. Hanada M, Aime-Sempe C, Sato T, Reed JC. Structure-function analysis of Bcl-2 protein. Identification of conserved domains important for homodimerization with Bcl-2 and heterodimerization with Bax. J Biol Chem 1995;270(20):11962–11969
74. Cheng EH, Levine B, Boise LH, Thompson CB, Hardwick JM. Bax-independent inhibition of apoptosis by Bcl-XL. Nature 1996;379(6565):554–556
75. Hunter JJ, Bond BL, Parslow TG. Functional dissection of the human Bcl2 protein: sequence requirements for inhibition of apoptosis. Mol Cell Biol 1996;16(3):877–883
76. Boyd JM, Gallo GJ, Elangovan B, Houghton AB, Malstrom S, Avery BJ, Ebb RG, Subramanian T, Chittenden T, Lutz RJ, et al. Bik, a novel death-inducing protein shares a distinct sequence motif with Bcl-2 family proteins and interacts with viral and cellular survival-promoting proteins. Oncogene 1995;11(9):1921–1928
77. O'Connor L, Strasser A, O'Reilly LA, Hausmann G, Adams JM, Cory S, Huang OC. Bim: a novel member of the Bcl-2 family that promotes apoptosis. EMBO J 1998;17 (2):384–395
78. Muchmore SW, Sattler M, Liang H, Meadows RP, Harlan JE, Yoon HS, Nettesheim D, Chang BS, Thompson CB, Wong SL, Ng SL, Fesik SW. X-ray and NMR structure of human Bcl-xL, an inhibitor of programmed cell death. Nature 1996;381(6580):335–341
79. Sattler M, Liang H, Nettesheim D, Meadows RP, Harlan JE, Eberstadt M, Yoon HS, Shuker SB, Chang BS, Minn AJ, Thompson CB, Fesik SW. Structure of Bcl-xL-Bak peptide complex: recognition between regulators of apoptosis. Science 1997;275(5302): 983–986
80. Diaz JL, Oltersdorf T, Horne W, McConnell M, Wilson G, Weeks S, Garcia T, Fritz LC. A common binding site mediates heterodimerization and homodimerization of Bcl-2 family members. J Biol Chem 1997;272(17):11350–11355
81. Kiefer MC, Brauer MJ, Powers VC, Wu JJ, Umansky SR, Tomei LD, Barr PJ. Modulation of apoptosis by the widely distributed Bcl-2 homologue Bak. Nature 1995; 374(6524):736–739
82. Knudson CM, Tung KS, Tourtellotte WG, Brown GA, Korsmeyer SJ. Bax-deficient mice with lymphoid hyperplasia and male germ cell death. Science 1995;270(5233):96–99
83. Borner C, Martinou I, Mattmann C, Irmler M, Schaerer E, Martinou JC, Tschopp J. The protein bcl-2 alpha does not require membrane attachment, but two conserved domains to suppress apoptosis. J Cell Biol 1994;126(4):1059–1068
84. Wang HG, Rapp UR, Reed JC. Bcl-2 targets the protein kinase Raf-1 to mitochondria. Cell 1996;87(4):629–638
85. Yang E, Zha J, Jockel J, Boise LH, Thompson CB, Korsmeyer SJ. Bad, a heterodimeric partner for Bcl-XL and Bcl-2, displaces Bax and promotes cell death. Cell 1995; 80(2):285–291
86. Zha J, Harada H, Yang E, Jockel J, Korsmeyer SJ. Serine phosphorylation of death agonist BAD in response to survival factor results in binding to 14-3-3 not BCL-X. Cell 1996; 87(4):619–628
87. Muslin AJ, Tanner JW, Allen PM, Shaw AS. Interaction of 14-3-3 with signaling proteins is mediated by the recognition of phosphoserine. Cell 1996; 84(6):889–897
88. Gajewski TF, Thompson CB. Apoptosis meets signal transduction: elimination of a BAD influence. Cell 1996;87(4):589–592
89. Wang HG, Takayama S, Rapp UR, Reed JC. Bcl-2 interacting protein, BAG-1, binds to and activates the kinase Raf-1. Proc Natl Acad Sci USA 1996;93(14):7063–7068
90. Shibasaki F, McKeon F. Calcineurin functions in Ca(2+)-activated cell death in mammalian cells. J Cell Biol 1995;131(3):735–743
91. Linette GP, Li Y, Roth K, Korsmeyer SJ. Cross talk between cell death and cell cycle progression: BCL-2 regulates NFAT-mediated activation. Proc Natl Acad Sci USA 1996;93(18):9545–9552
92. Pietenpol JA, Papadopoulos N, Markowitz S, Willson JK, Kinzler KW, Vogelstein B. Paradoxical inhibition of solid tumor cell growth by bcl2. Cancer Res 1994;54(14): 3714–3717
93. Vaux DL, Cory S, Adams JM. Bcl-2 gene promotes haemopoietic cell survival and cooperates with c-myc to immortalize pre-B cells. Nature 1988;335(6189):440–442
94. Marvel J, Perkins GR, Lopez Rivas A, Collins MK. Growth factor starvation of bcl-2 overexpressing murine bone marrow cells induced refractoriness to IL-3 stimulation of proliferation. Oncogene 1994;9(4):1117–1122
95. Linette GP, Hess JL, Sentman CL, Korsmeyer SJ. Peripheral T-cell lymphoma in lckpr-bcl-2 transgenic mice. Blood 1995;86(4):1255–1260
96. Mazel S, Burtrum D, Petrie HT. Regulation of cell division cycle progression by bcl-2 expression: a potential mechanism for inhibition of programmed cell death. J Exp Med 1996;183(5):2219–2226
97. O'Reilly LA, Huang DC, Strasser A. The cell death inhibitor Bcl-2 and its homologues influence control of cell cycle entry. EMBO J 1996;15(24):6979–6990

98. Vairo G, Innes KM, Adams JM. Bcl-2 has a cell cycle inhibitory function separable from its enhancement of cell survival. Oncogene 1996;13(7):1511–1519
99. Huang DC, O'Reilly LA, Strasser A, Cory S. The anti-apoptosis function of Bcl-2 can be genetically separated from its inhibitory effect on cell cycle entry. EMBO J 1997;16(15):4628–4638
100. Cleary M, Rosenberg SA. The bcl-2 gene, follicular lymphoma, and Hodgkin's disease [editorial;comment]. J Natl Cancer Inst 1990;82(10):808–809
101. Lipponen P, Pietilainen T, Kosma VM, Aaltomaa S, Eskelinen M, Syrjanen K. Apoptosis suppressing protein bcl-2 is expressed in well-differentiated breast carcinomas with favourable prognosis. J Pathol 1995;177(1):49–55
102. Konopleva M, Zhao S, Jiang S, Snell V, Zhang X, Reed JC, Andreeff M. The antiapoptotic genes Bcl-X_L and Bcl-2 are overexpressed in quiescent leukemic progenitor cells. Blood (Suppl 1) 1997; 90:558a
103. Deng G, Lane C, Kornblau S, Goodacre A, Snell V, Andreeff M, Deisseroth AB. Ratio of bcl-xshort to bcl-xlong is different in good- and poor-prognosis subsets of acute myeloid leukemia. Mol Med 1998;4(3):158–164
104. del Peso L, Gonzalez-Garcia M, Page C, Herrera R, Nunez G. Interleukin-3-induced phosphorylation of BAD through the protein kinase Akt. Science 1997;278(5338):687–689
105. Datta SR, Dudek H, Tao X, Masters S, Fu H, Gotoh Y, Greenberg ME. Akt phosphorylation of BAD couples survival signals to the cell-intrinsic death machinery. Cell 1997;91(2):231–241
106. Haldar S, Jena N, Croce CM. Inactivation of Bcl-2 by phosphorylation. Proc Natl Acad Sci USA 1995;92(10):4507–4511
107. Srivastava RK, Srivastava AR, Korsmeyer SJ, Nesterova M, Cho-Chung YS, Longo DL. Involvement of microtubules in the regulation of bcl2 phosphorylation and apoptosis through cyclic AMP-dependent protein kinase. Mol Cell Biol 1998;18(6):3509–3517
108. Haldar S, Basu A, Croce CM. Bcl2 is the guardian of microtubule integrity. Cancer Res 1997;57(2):229–233
109. Chang BS, Minn AJ, Muchmore SW, Fesik SW, Thompson CB. Identification of a novel regulatory domain in Bcl-X(L) and Bcl-2. EMBO J 1997;16(5):968–977
110. May WS, Tyler PG, Ito T, Armstrong DK, Qatsha KA, Davidson NE. Interleukin-3 and bryostatin-1 mediate hyperphosphorylation of BCL2 alpha in association with suppression of apoptosis. J Biol Chem 1994;269(43):26865–26870
111. Chen CY, Faller DV. Direction of p21ras-generated signals towards cell growth or apoptosis is determined by protein kinase C and Bcl-2. Oncogene 1995;11(8):1487–1498
112. Cheng EH, Levine B, Boise LH, Thompson CB, Hardwick JM. Bax-independent inhibition of apoptosis by Bcl-XL. Nature 1996;379(6565):554–556
113. Strack PR, Frey MW, Rizzo CJ, Cordova B, George HJ, Meade R, Ho SP, Corman J, Tritch R, Korant BD. Apoptosis mediated by HIV protease is preceded by cleavage of Bcl-2. Proc Natl Acad Sci USA 1996;93(18):9571–9576
114. Cheng EH, Kirsch DG, Clem RJ, Ravi R, Kastan MB, Bedi A, Ueno K, Hardwick JM. Conversion of Bcl-2 to a Bax-like death effector by caspases. Science 1997;278 (5345):1966–1968
115. Clem RJ, Cheng EH, Karp CL, Kirsch DG, Ueno K, Takahashi A, Kastan MB, Griffin DE, Earnshaw WC, Veliuona MA, Hardwick JM. Modulation of cell death by Bcl-XL through caspase interaction. Proc Natl Acad Sci USA 1998;95(2):554–559
116. Reed JC. Double identity for proteins of the Bcl-2 family. Nature 1997;387(6635): 773–776
117. Minn AJ, Velez P, Schendel SL, Liang H, Muchmore SW, Fesik SW, Fill M, Thompson CB. Bcl-x(L) forms an ion channel in synthetic lipid membranes. Nature 1997;385(6614):353–357
118. Schendel SL, Xie Z, Montal MO, Matsuyama S, Montal M, Reed JC. Channel formation by antiapoptotic protein Bcl-2. Proc Natl Acad Sci USA 1997;94(10):5113–5118
119. Krajewski S, Tanaka S, Takayama S, Schibler MJ, Fenton W, Reed JC. Investigation of the subcellular distribution of the bcl-2 oncoprotein: residence in the nuclear envelope, endoplasmic reticulum, and outer mitochondrial membranes. Cancer Res 1993; 53(19): 4701–4714
120. Gonzalez-Garcia M, Perez-Ballestero R, Ding L, Duan L, Boise LH, Thompson CB, Nunez G. bcl-XL is the major bcl-x mRNA form expressed during murine development and its product localizes to mitochondria. Development 1994;120(10):3033–3042
121. Yang T, Kozopas KM, Craig RW. The intracellular distribution and pattern of expression of Mcl-1 overlap with, but are not identical to, those of Bcl-2. J Cell Biol 1995;128(6):1173–1184
122. Zamzami N, Susin SA, Marchetti P, Hirsch T, Gomez-Monterrey I, Castedo M, Kroemer G. Mitochondrial control of nuclear apoptosis [see comments]. J Exp Med 1996;183(4):1533–1544
123. Liu X, Kim CN, Yang J, Jemmerson R, Wang X. Induction of apoptotic program in cell-free extracts: requirement for dATP and cytochrome c. Cell 1996;86(1):147–157

124. Susin SA, Zamzami N, Castedo M, Hirsch T, Marchetti P, Macho A, Daugas E, Geuskens M, Kroemer G. Bcl-2 inhibits the mitochondrial release of an apoptogenic protease. J Exp Med 1996;184(4):1331–1341
125. Kluck RM, Bossy-Wetzel E, Green DR, Newmeyer DD. The release of cytochrome c from mitochondria: a primary site for Bcl-2 regulation of apoptosis. Science 1997;275 (5303):1132–1136
126. Yang J, Liu X, Bhalla K, Kim CN, Ibrado AM, Cai J, Peng TI, Jones DP, Wang X. Prevention of apoptosis by Bcl-2: release of cytochrome c from mitochondria blocked. Science 1997;275(5303):1129–1132
127. Marzo I, Brenner C, Zamzami N, Susin SA, Beutner G, Brdiczka D, Remy R, Xie ZH, Reed JC, Kroemer G. The permeability transition pore complex: a target for apoptosis regulation by caspases and bcl-2-related proteins. J Exp Med 1998;187(8): 1261–1271
128. Marzo I, Susin SA, Petit PX, Ravagnan L, Brenner C, Larochette N, Zamzami N, Kroemer G. Caspases disrupt mitochondrial membrane barrier function. FEBS Lett 1998; 427(2):198–202
129. Shaham S, Horvitz HR. Developing Caenorhabditis elegans neurons may contain both cell-death protective and killer activities. Genes Dev 1996;10(5):578–591
130. Shaham S, Horvitz HR. An alternatively spliced C. elegans ced-4 RNA encodes a novel cell death inhibitor. Cell 1996;86(2):201–208
131. Chinnaiyan AM, O'Rourke K, Lane BR, Dixit VM. Interaction of CED-4 with CED-3 and CED-9: a molecular framework for cell death. Science 1997;275(5303):1122–1126
132. Irmler M, Hofmann K, Vaux D, Tschopp J. Direct physical interaction between the Caenorhabditis elegans 'death proteins' CED-3 and CED-4. FEBS Letters 1997;406(1–2): 189–190
133. Hofmann K, Bucher P, Tschopp J. The CARD domain: a new apoptotic signalling motif. Trends Biochem Sci 1997;22(5):155–156
134. Spector MS, Desnoyers S, Hoeppner DJ, Hengartner MO. Interaction between the C. elegans cell-death regulators CED-9 and CED-4. Nature 1997;385(6617):653–656
135. Wu D, Wallen HD, Nunez G. Interaction and regulation of subcellular localization of CED-4 by CED-9. Science 1997;275(5303):1126–1129
136. Hu Y, Benedict MA, Wu D, Inohara N, Nunez G. Bcl-X_L interacts with Apaf-1 and inhibits Apaf-1-dependent caspase-9 activation. Proc Natl Acad Sci USA 1998;95:4386–4391
137. Zou H, Henzel WJ, Liu X, Lutschg A, Wang X. Apaf-1, a human protein homologous to C. elegans CED-4, participates in cytochrome c-dependent activation of caspase-3. Cell 1997;90(3):405–413
138. Vaux DL. CED-4—the third horseman of apoptosis. Cell 1997;90(3):389–390
139. Conradt B, Horvitz HR. The C. elegans protein EGL-1 is required for programmed cell death and interacts with the bcl-2-like protein CED-9. Cell 1998;93:519–529
140. Duckett CS, Nava VE, Gedrich RW, Clem RJ, Van Dongen JL, Gilfillan MC, Shiels H, Hardwick JM, Thompson CB. A conserved family of cellular genes related to the baculovirus iap gene and encoding apoptosis inhibitors. EMBO J 1996;15(11):2685–2694
141. Clem RJ, Miller LK. Control of programmed cell death by the baculovirus genes p35 and iap. Mol Cell Biol 1994;14(8):5212–5222
142. Roy N, Mahadevan MS, McLean M, Shutler G, Yaraghi Z, Farahani R, Baird S, Besner-Johnston A, Lefebvre C, Kang X, et al. The gene for neuronal apoptosis inhibitory protein is partially deleted in individuals with spinal muscular atrophy. Cell 1995;80(1):167–178
143. Rothe M, Pan MG, Henzel WJ, Ayres TM, Goeddel DV. The TNFR2-TRAF signaling complex contains two novel proteins related to baculoviral inhibitor of apoptosis proteins. Cell 1995;83(7):1243–1252
144. Uren AG, Pakusch M, Hawkins CJ, Puls KL, Vaux DL. Cloning and expression of apoptosis inhibitory protein homologs that function to inhibit apoptosis and/or bind tumor necrosis factor receptor-associated factors. Proc Natl Acad Sci USA 1996;93(10):4974–4978
145. Hay BA, Wassarman DA, Rubin GM. Drosophila homologs of baculovirus inhibitor of apoptosis proteins function to block cell death. Cell 1995;83(7):1253–1262
146. Deveraux QL, Takahashi R, Salvesen GS, Reed JC. X-linked IAP is a direct inhibitor of cell-death proteases. Nature 1997;388(6639):300–304
147. Lovering R, Hanson IM, Borden KL, Martin S, O'Reilly NJ, Evan GI, Rahman D, Pappin DJ, Trowsdale J, Freemont PS. Identification and preliminary characterization of a protein motif related to the zinc finger. Proc Natl Acad Sci USA 1993;90(6):2112–2116
148. Blake TJ, Shapiro M, Morse HC 3d, Langdon WY. The sequences of the human and mouse c-cbl proto-oncogenes show v-cbl was generated by a large truncation encompassing a proline-rich domain and a leucine zipper-like motif. Oncogene 1991; 6(4):653–657
149. de The H, Lavau C, Marchio A, Chomienne C, Degos L, Dejean A. The PML-RAR alpha fusion mRNA generated by the t(15;17) translocation in acute promyelocytic leukemia encodes a functionally altered RAR. Cell 1991;66(4):675–684

150. Song HY, Donner DB. Association of a RING finger protein with the cytoplasmic domain of the human type-2 tumour necrosis factor receptor. Biochem J 1995;309(Pt 3): 825–829
151. Hu HM, O'Rourke K, Boguski MS, Dixit VM. A novel RING finger protein interacts with the cytoplasmic domain of CD40. J Biol Chem 1994;269(48):30069–30072
152. Cheng G, Cleary AM, Ye ZS, Hong DI, Lederman S, Baltimore D. Involvement of CRAF1, a relative of TRAF, in CD40 signaling. Science 1995;267(5203):1494–1498
153. Sato T, Irie S, Reed JC. A novel member of the TRAF family of putative signal transducing proteins binds to the cytosolic domain of CD40. FEBS Letters 1995;358(2): 113–118
154. Borden KL, Boddy MN, Lally J, O'Reilly NJ, Martin S, Howe K, Solomon E, Freemont PS. The solution structure of the RING finger domain from the acute promyelocytic leukaemia proto-oncoprotein PML. EMBO J 1995;14(7):1532–1541
155. Takahashi R, Deveraux Q, Tamm I, Welsh K, Assa-Munt N, Salvesen GS, Reed JC. A single BIR domain of XIAP sufficient for inhibiting caspases. J Biol Chem 1998;273 (14):7787–7790
156. Ambrosini G, Adida C, Altieri DC. A novel anti-apoptosis gene, survivin, expressed in cancer and lymphoma. Nat Med 1997;3(8):917–921
157. Adida C, Crotty PL, McGrath J, Berrebi D, Diebold J, Altieri DC. Developmentally regulated expression of the novel cancer anti-apoptosis gene survivin in human and mouse differentiation. Am J Pathol 1998;152(1):43–49
158. Keith FJ, Bradbury DA, Yong-Ming Z, Russel NH. Inhibition of bcl-2 with antisense oligonucleotides induces apoptosis and increases the sensitivity of AML blasts to Ara-C. Leukemia 1995;9:131–138
159. Konopleva M, Tari A, López-Berestein A, Andreeff M. Inhibition of Bcl-2 with liposomal-delivered antisense oligonucleotides (AS-ODN) induces apoptosis and increases the sensitivity of primary acute myeloid leukemia (AML) cells and cell lines to cytosine arabinoside and doxorubicin. Blood 1997(Suppl 1);90:10, 494a
160. Webb A, Cunningham D, Cotter F, Clarke PA, Stefano PA, Ross P, Corbo M, Dziewanowska Z. Bcl-2 antisense therapy in patients with non-Hodgkin's lymphoma. The Lancet 1997;349:1137–1141
161. Andreeff M, Jiang S, Zhang X, Konopleva M, Estrov Z, Snell VE, Xie Z, Okcu MF, Sanchez-Williams G, Dong J, Estey EH, Champlin RE, Kornblau SM, Reed JC, Zhao S. Expression of bcl-2-related genes in normal and AML progenitors: changes induced by chemotherapy and retinoic acid. Leukemia 1999; in press
162. McCullogh EA. Phosphorylation of bcl-2 after exposure of human leukemic cells to retinoic acid. Blood (Suppl1)1997;90:494a
163. Piche A, Grim J, Rancourt C, Gomez-Navarro J, Reed JC, Curiel DT. Modulation of bcl-2 protein levels by an intracellular anti-bcl-2 single-chain antibody increases drug-induced cytotoxicity in the breast cancer cell line MCF-7. Cancer Res 1998;58:2134–2140

ACTIVATION OF APOPTOSIS PATHWAYS BY ANTICANCER DRUGS

Klaus-Michael Debatin

University Children's Hospital
Ulm, Germany

The first antitumor drug (aminopterin) was introduced into the treatment of childhood leukemia by Sidney Farber almost 50 years ago. In the past 20 years long term remission and cure has been achieved in 70-80% of patients with leukemia, using combination therapy with several anticancer drugs and high dose protocols. However, the widespread use of chemotherapy also has shown that certain tumors are chemosensitive while others are chemoresistant. Why is chemotherapy effective? Anticancer drugs have not been designed for a specific cellular or molecular target but have been identified in assays based on their capacity to inhibit proliferation and clonogenicity. Early concepts on how chemotherapy may kill tumor cells have focused on interference with either cellular metabolism or DNA synthesis. However the biochemical characterization of drug mediated inhibition of cellular proliferation has shown that most drugs hit various targets. Drugs efficiently used in cancer therapy include diverse chemical compounds such as antimetabolites (e.g. methotrexate, 5-fluorouracil), DNA damaging agents (e.g. cyclophosphamide, cisplatin, doxorubicine), mitotic inhibitors (e.g. vincristine), nucleotide analogs (6-mercaptopurine) or inhibitors of topoisomerases involved in DNA repair (e.g. etoposide). While cell death induced by anticancer agents has been considered to be a consequence of a block in proliferation or simply "toxicity", recent studies have shown that most anticancer agents induce apoptosis in target cells.

Recent data from different laboratories demonstrate that cell death induced in tumor cells by anticancer treatment involves key systems of the physiological apoptosis program.[1,2] Thus, chemosensitivity may reflect intact cellular pathways which are activated or participate in the death program, triggered by the exposure of the tumor cell to the drugs used for therapy. With the concept that some drugs may be cytotoxic through DNA-damage, p53, "the guardian of the genome", mutated in many tumors, has come into play suggesting that p53 may drive and activate the apoptosis machinery following treatment with e.g. DNA-damaging agents.[3-7] Thus p53 has been shown to be involved in various forms of apoptosis induced by cellular "stress"[3] and experimental systems using p53 knockout

Drug Resistance in Leukemia and Lymphoma III, edited by Kaspers *et al.*
Kluwer Academic / Plenum Publishers, New York, 1999.

mice have shown that a lack of p53 contributes to resistance of cells to DNA damaging agents and γ-irradiation. While p53 may represent a cellular masterswitch that regulates several distinct cellular responses, recent evidence suggests that key downstream elements of the apoptosis machinery are directly involved in apoptosis induced by anticancer drugs. Resistance towards chemotherapy in some cases has been found to be associated with increased levels of expression of anti-apoptotic molecules of the Bcl-2 family such as a Bcl-2 and Bcl-x$_L$.[8-13] While the levels of Bcl-2 expression e.g. in lymphoid tumors did not clearly correlate with clinical response to chemotherapy, reduced expression of Bax was found to be associated with poor outcome in breast cancer.[14-17] p53 has been found to transcribe expression of the proapoptotic bax gene following DNA-damage. Thus, some forms of chemotherapy-induced apoptosis mechanistically seem to involve upregulation of bax expression following p53 activation through DNA-damage, which leads to activation of the apoptosis program.[3,4,18]

Additions to this scenario now suggest an active role of the CD95 (APO-1/Fas) system in the process of drug-induced apoptosis. CD95, a member of the TNF/NGF superfamily, is constitutively expressed in many cells and can probably be induced in any tissue in the body by appropriate stimuli. Likewise, the CD95 ligand (CD95L) is also constitutively expressed in several cell types and may be induced e.g. in T cells after activation.[19-22] The CD95 system is one of the best characterized apoptosis pathways. Following crosslinking of the receptor by the multimeric ligand in the membrane bound or soluble form, a DISC (death inducing signalling complex) is formed that consists of the intracellular "death domains" of the receptor and the adapter molecule FADD. This complex recruites a chimeric adapter/caspase (caspase 8 or FLICE = FADD-like ICE) into the DISC, leading to activation of caspase 8 to cleave downstream caspases such as caspase 3 and substrates. While in some cells this pathway, using only a few signal molecules, directly leads to cell death (type I cells), in other cells (type II) mitochondrial function is critical for execution of the CD95 mediated death program.[23, 24]

The critical role of the CD95 system for growth control is best demonstrated in the immune system where genetically defined pathology that results from deficiencies in the receptor or the ligand is found.[19,25-28] During normal development of T- and B-cells, expression of CD95 is differentially regulated. While CD95 expression on hematopoietic stem cells is weak, the majority of thymocytes in mice and men express intermediate levels of CD95[29-33] although no definite role in negative selection of thymocytes has been demonstrated. Maturation of T-cells and export to the periphery as naive mature T-cells is associated with downregulation of the receptor which is re-expressed at high levels following activation.[34] B-cell precursors as well as circulating naive mature B-cells in the peripheral blood express only low levels of CD95.[29,33,35] Similar to T-cells, activation of mature B-cells in secondary lymphoid tissues *in vivo* is associated with increased levels of CD95. CD95 expression is found with advanced maturation of myeloid cells and high levels of CD95 can be induced on hematopoietic progenitors by activation e.g. through cytokines.

Corresponding to the apoptosis sensitive phenotype of CD95 positive activated T cells strong expression of CD95 and CD95 sensitivity is found in leukemic cells from patients with HTLV-I induced adult T-cell leukemia (ATL).[34,36-38] CD95 is also expressed in the majority of acute leukemias that represent precursor T-cell phenotypes such as in childhood T cell acute lymphoblastic leukemia/lymphoma.[39-41] However, most cells from patients with T-ALL are constitutively resistant towards CD95 induced apoptosis. A number of studies performed in hematologic malignancies, including precursor B-ALL, acute myeloid leukemia, chronic B-cell leukemia, chronic myelogenous leukemia, non-Hodgkin's lymphoma, Hodgkin's disease and plasma cell disorders, have found variable expression in these diseases.[42-51] While studies on constitutive expression of CD95 in clinical tumor samples may be misleading since exogenous stimuli may be able to upregulate receptor expression,[32] a favourable outcome for patients with CD95 positive AML undergoing chemotherapy as compared to CD95 negative AML has been found.[52]

Failure to upregulate CD95 expression or defects in the receptor, the ligand or signal molecules may result in apoptosis defects in tumor cells.[28] Blockade of CD95 mediated apoptosis *in vivo* may either be caused by the production of soluble receptor variants by alternative splicing that counteract the apoptosis inducing signal or alternatively may be due to mutations in the receptor. Increased levels of soluble CD95 have been found in tumor cell lines and in some patients with T- and B-cell leukemias but not in myeloid leukemias.[53-55] Mutations of the CD95 molecule in *lpr* mice and the CD95 ligand in *gld* mice constitute the first description of a pathology associated with an apoptosis gene defect.[19,28] However, neither *lpr* nor *gld* mice develop lymphoid or hematopoietic malignancy but rather suffer from a lymphoproliferative syndrome due to the inability to delete long term activated T-cells. The disease of *lpr* and *gld* mice is recapitulated in a group of patients with lymphoproliferation and autoimmunity in which mutations of the CD95 receptor, primarily located in the "death domain" of the molecule have been found.[25-28] Patients develop extensive lymphadenopathy and hepatosplenomegaly with autoimmune disease such as immune thrombocytopenia. In contrast, mutations of CD95 in pediatric T-ALL are rare.[56]

An important feature of apoptosis mediated by the CD95 system is the mechanism of autocrine suicide or paracrine death initially described for activated T cells.[57] Activation through T cell receptor triggering induces CD95L and upregulation of CD95 leading to interaction of the ligand with its receptor and subsequent initiation of the death program. In a similar way, doxorubicin and other anticancer drugs have been found to induce apoptosis which involves activation of the CD95/CD95L system in human leukemia T cell lines and other tumor cells.[58-62] Doxorubicin strongly stimulated CD95L messenger RNA and protein expression *in vitro* at concentrations relevant for therapy *in vivo*. CEM and Jurkat cells resistant to CD95-mediated apoptosis were also resistant to doxorubicin-induced apoptosis. Furthermore, doxorubicin-induced apoptosis was inhibited by blocking $F(ab)_2$ anti-APO-1 (anti-CD95) antibody fragments. Expression of CD95L mRNA and protein *in vitro* was also stimulated by other cytotoxic drugs such as methotrexate. Recent findings suggest that activation of other ligand/receptor driven amplifier systems initiated by death inducing ligands (DIL) such as TNF or TRAIL may also contribute to drug induced death [Herr, Jeremias and Debatin, submitted]. Cells treated with anticancer drugs may upregulate CD95 receptor expression in some cases.[59,60] In this respect upregulation of CD95 expression seems to be the crossroad where DNA damage, p53 accumulation and the apoptosis response meet. At least for some drugs DNA damage is considered to be an important contribution to the cytotoxic effect. The p53 protein may function by sensing damaged DNA and transcriptionally activating the expression of apoptosis promoting molecules such as CD95.[59] However upregulation of CD95L expression appears to be p53 independent. The molecular pathways triggered by anticancer drugs that lead to CD95L are not well understood. Recent evidence suggests that induction of CD95L expression by anticancer drugs may involve the cellular stress pathway.[64] Thus ceramide, which accumulates in response to different types of cellular stress such as chemo- and radiotherapy, induces expression of CD95L, cleavage of caspases and apoptosis. Phorbol ester treatment, known to antagonize ceramide generation and JNK/SAPK activity as well as γ-irradiation and CD95 mediated cytotoxicity downregulates doxorubicin-induced upregulation of CD95L, cleavage of CPP32 and cell death. Antisense CD95L inhibited ceramide- and cellular stress-induced apoptosis. Fibroblasts from type A Niemann-Pick patients (NPA), genetically deficient in ceramide synthesis fail to upregulate

CD95L expression and to undergo apoptosis after γ-irradiation or doxorubicin-treatment. However, JNK/SAPK activity was still inducible by doxorubicin in the NPA cells suggesting that activation of JNK/SAPKs alone is not sufficient for induction of the CD95 system and apoptosis. CD95L expression and apoptosis in NPA fibroblasts was restorable by exogenously added ceramide. In addition, NPA fibroblasts undergo apoptosis after triggering of CD95 with an agonistic antibody.

Activation of the caspase cascade is involved in most forms of apoptosis as a downstream effector system. Apoptosis induced in tumor cells by cytotoxic drugs such as cytarabine, doxorubicin, and methotrexate requires the activation of caspases, similar to the CD95 system.[65] Drug-induced activation of caspases was also found in *ex vivo*-derived T cell leukemia cells. Resistance to cell death could be mediated by a peptide caspase inhibitor (zVAD-fmk) or CrmA, a poxvirus-derived serpin. The peptide inhibitor was effective even when added several hours after drug treatment, indicating a direct involvement of caspases in the execution and not in the trigger phase of drug action. Drug-induced apoptosis was also strongly inhibited by antisense approaches targeting caspase-1 and -3, indicating that several members of this protease family were involved. CD95-resistant cell lines that failed to activate caspases upon CD95 triggering were cross-resistant to drug-mediated apoptosis. Thus, deficiencies in key apoptosis signalling systems like CD95L/CD95 may be involved in drug resistance. While caspase activation reflecting activation of apoptosis effector molecules has been found in most studies on drug induced apoptosis, a requirement for activation of the CD95 system could not always be demonstrated.[66,67] This may be explained by cell line differences, concentrations of the drugs used in the studies and/or redundancy in the system such as the participation of other death inducing ligand/receptor systems such as TRAIL or TNF or death receptor independent induction of cell death. Interestingly, activation of upstream (caspase 8) and downstream (caspase 3) effector caspases can be mediated by perturbance of mitochondria leading to permeability transition (PT) and release of apoptogenic molecules, such as cytochrome-c and AIF.[24] Perturbance of mitochondrial function is an essential part of the CD95 pathway in type II cells (see above). In addition, mitochondrial PT is also induced by several anticancer drugs and may be directly induced in a CD95 independent fashion, e. g. by betulinic acid, a newly discovered antitumor compound with exquisite specificity for neuroectodermal tumors.[68,] [Fulda, Susin, Kroemer and Debatin, submitted]

The demonstration of an involvement of apoptosis molecules in drug induced apoptosis sheds new light on the chemosensitivity of tumors. Thus, regardless of the primary target, activation of key effector pathways for apoptosis seems to be crucial for the anti-tumor effect of anticancer drugs (Figure 1). The initial trigger (phase I) may target diverse cellular functions such as metabolism, DNA or the mitotic apparatus. The cellular alteration is sensed by p53 and/or leads to activation of cellular stress programs (phase II) which in turn activate phase III events. These may include triggering of ligand/receptor (e.g. CD95) driven amplifier systems and/or mitochondrial alteration. Subsequent activation of the apoptosis program then leads to activation of downsteam caspases and subsequent cleavage of substrates. Alterations of the initial phase, the amplifier phase or the execution phase may lead to drug resistance. Thus, in addition to established mechanisms of drug resistance such as increased drug efflux by membrane pumps, failure to activate apoptosis programs due to mutations or functional alterations of key-molecules and pathways represents another mode of drug resistance in tumor cells.[65,69,70]

Induction of increased CD95 expression in tumor cells by cytotoxic drugs provides an additional aspect, since cytotoxic T-cells use the CD95 system as one of the key mechanisms to kill their target cells. Thus, tumor cells that express the CD95 receptor may be

Phase I →	Phase II →	Phase III →	Phase IV
Trigger	Sensor	Amplification	Execution
- DNA damage	- p53	- activation of DIL systems	- permeability transition
- metabolic inhibition	- stress pathway	(CD95, TRAIL, TNF)	- caspase activation
- microtubule disruption		- mitochondrial perturbance	- breakdown of cytoplasmic and nuclear substrates

Figure 1. Hypothetical sequence of apoptosis induction in response to chemotherapeutic agents.

turned into highly susceptible targets for killer cells (T cells, NK cells, LAK cells). Clinically relevant concentrations of diverse anticancer drugs such as cisplatin, doxorubicin, mitomycin, fluorouracil or camptothecin have been shown to induce CD95 expression in colon carcinoma cell lines and leukemic cell lines thereby strongly increasing the sensitivity for CD95 induced apoptosis by either an agonistic antibody, CD95L or activated killer cells.[71,72] This finding may explain why low dose chemotherapy is effective in certain tumors. For example, "maintenance" therapy is an indispensable element in the treatment of acute leukemias. The doses of methotrexate and 6-mercaptopurine used may be too low to mediate a direct cytotoxic effect but may be sufficient to sensitize the tumor cells for physiological apoptosis signals by upregulating expression of death regulators such as CD95. Likewise, 5-fluorouracil is successfully used in adjuvant therapy of colon carcinomas. This would suggest that chemotherapy not only has an immunosuppressive effect on the effector side but may also be immunomodulating at the side of the target cell.

In perspective the current studies on the interplay between cytotoxicity against tumors and apoptosis pathways will provide additional molecular understanding of sensitivity and resistance of tumor cells towards therapeutic intervention. The molecules and pathways critical for triggering of the cell death program may serve as targets for established and novel anticancer agents and treatment approaches.

REFERENCES

1. Dive C, Evans CA, Whetton AD. Induction of apoptosis – new targets for cancer chemotherapy. Cancer Biol (1992) 3: 417–427
2. Hannun YA. Apoptosis and the Dilemma of Cancer Chemotherapy. Blood (1997) 89, 6: 1845–1853
3. Levine AJ. p53, the cellular gatekeeper for growth and division. Cell (1997) 88: 323–331
4. Miyashita T, Krajewski S, Krajewska M, Wang HG, Lin HK, Liebermann DA, Hoffman B, Reed JC. Tumor suppressor p53 is a regulator of bcl-2 and bax gene expression *in vitro* and *in vivo*. Oncogene (1994) 9: 1799–1805
5. Lowe SW, Ruley HE, Jacks T, Housman DE. p53-dependent apoptosis modulates the cytotoxicity of anticancer agents. Cell (1993) 74: 957–967
6. Lowe SW, Bodis S, McClatchey A, Remington L, Ruley HE, Fisher DE, Housman DE, Jacks T. p53 Status and the Efficacy of Cancer Therapy *in Vivo*. Science (1994) 266: 807–810
7. Milner J. DNA damage, p53 and anticancer therapies. Nature Med (1995)1 (9): 879–880
8. Campana D, Coustan-Smith E, Manabe A, Buschle M, Raimondi SC, Behm FG, Ashmun R, Aricò M, Biondi A, Pui C-H. Prolonged Survival of B-Lineage Acute Lymphoblastic Leukemia Cells Is Accompanied by Overexpression of Bcl-2 Protein. Blood (1993) 81 (4): 1025–1031

9. Campos L, Rouault J-P, Sabido O, Oriol P, Roubi N, Vasselon C, Archimbaud E, Magaud J-P, Guyotat D. High Expression of Bcl-2 Protein in Acute Myeloid Leukemia Cells Is Associated With Poor Response to Chemotherapy. Blood (1993) 81 (11): 3091–3096
10. Miyashita T, Reed JC. Bcl-2 Oncoprotein blocks Chemotherapy-Induced Apoptosis in a Human Leukemia Cell Line. Blood (1993) 81 (1): 151–157
11. Dole MG, Jasty R, Cooper MJ, Thompson CB, Nuñez G, Castle VP. Bcl-x_L Is Expressed in Neuroblastoma Cells und Modulates Chemotherapy-induced Apoptosis. Cancer Res (1995) 55: 2576–2582
12. Minn AJ, Rudin CM, Boise LH, Thompson CB. Expression of Bcl-x_L can confer a multidrug resistance phenotype. Blood (1995) 86 (5): 1903–1910
13. Yang E, Korsmeyer SJ. Molecular thanatopsis: a discourse on the Bcl-2 family and cell death. Blood (1996) 88 (2): 386–401
14. Hermine O, Haioun C, Lepage E, d'Agay M-F, Briere J, Lavignac C, Fillet G, Salles G, Marolleau J-P, Diebold J, Reyes F, Gaulard P. Prognostic significance of Bcl-2 protein expression in aggressive non-Hodgkin's lymphoma. Blood (1996) 87: 265–272
15. Coustan-Smith E, Kitanaka A, Pui C-H, McNinch L, Evans WE, Raimondi SC, Behm FG, Aricò M, Campana D. Clinical relevance of BCL-2 overexpression in childhood acute lymphoblastic leukemia. Blood (1996) 87 (3): 1140–1146
16. Krajewski S, Blomqvist C, Franssila K, Krajewska M, Wasenius V-M, Niskanen E, Nordling S, Reed JC. Reduced expression of pro-apoptotic gene bax is associated with poor response rates to combination chemotherapy and shorter survival in women with metastatic breast adenocarcinoma. Cancer Res (1995) 55: 4471–4478
17. Bargou RC, Daniel PT, Mapara MY, Bommert K, Wagener C, Kallinich B, Royer HD, Dörken B. Expression of the bcl-2 gene family in normal and malignant breast tissue: low bax-α expression in tumor cells correlates with resistance towards apoptosis. Int J Cancer (1995) 60: 854–859
18. Miyashita T, Reed JC. Tumor Suppressor p53 Is a Direct Transcriptional Activator of the Human bax Gene. Cell (1995) 80: 293–299
19. Nagata S, Golstein P. The Fas death factor. Science (1995) 267: 1449–1456
20. Nagata S. Apoptosis by Death Factor. Cell (1997) 88: 355–365
21. Peter ME, Kischkel FC, Hellbardt S, Chinnaiyan AE, Krammer PH, Dixit VM. CD95 (APO-1/Fas)-associating signalling proteins. Cell Death Diff (1996) 3: 161–170
22. Krammer PH, Dhein J, Walczak H, Behrmann I, Mariani S, Matiba B, Fath M, Daniel PT, Knipping E, Westendorp MO, Stricker K, Bäumler C, Hellbardt S, Germer M, Peter ME, Debatin K-M. The role of APO-1 mediated apoptosis in the immune system. Immunol Rev (1994) 142: 175–191
23. Scaffidi C, Fulda S, Li F, Friesen C, Srinivasan A, Tomaselli KJ, Debatin K-M, Krammer PH, Peter ME. Two CD95 Signaling Pathways. EMBO J (1998) 17: 1675–1687
24. Kroemer G. The proto-oncogene bcl-2 and its role in regulating apoptosis. Nat Med (1997) 3, 6: 614–620
25. Rieux-Laucat F, Le Deist F, Hivroz C, Roberts IAG, Debatin K-M, Fischer A, De Villartay JP. Mutations in Fas Associated with Human Lymphoproliferative Syndrome and Autoimmunity. Science (1995) 268: 1347–1349
26. Fisher GH, Rosenberg FJ, Straus SE, Dale JK, Middelton LA, Lin AY, Strober W, Lenardo MJ, Puck JM. Dominant Interfering Fas Gene Mutations Impair Apoptosis in a Human Autoimmune Lymphoproliferative Syndrome. Cell (1995) 81: 935–946
27. Drappa J, Vaishnaw AK, Sullivan KE, Chu J-L, Elkon KB. Fas gene mutations in the Canale-Smith syndrome, an inherited lymphoproliferative disorder associated with autoimmunity. N Engl J Med (1996) 335: 1643–1649
28. Debatin K-M. Disturbances of the CD95 (APO-1/Fas) system in disorders of lymphohematopoietic cells. Cell Death Diff (1996) 3 (2): 185–189
29. Barcena A, Park SW, Banapour B, Muench MO, Mechetner E. Expression of Fas/CD95 and Bcl-2 by primitive hematopoietic progenitors freshly isolated from human fetal liver. Blood (1996) 88 (6): 2013–2025
30. Debatin K-M. APO-1 (CD95) and Bcl-2 Determinants of Cell Death in the Human Thymus. Res Immunol (1994) 56: 146–151
31. Debatin K-M, Süss D, Krammer PH. Differential expression of APO-1 on human thymocytes: implications for negative selection. Eur J Immunol (1994) 24: 753–758
32. Maciejewski J, Selleri C, Anderson S, Young NS. Fas Antigen Expression on CD34[+] Human Marrow Cells Is Induced by Interferon γ and Tumor Necrosis Factor α and Potentiates Cytokine-Mediated Hematopoietic Suppression *in vitro*. Blood (1995) 85 (11): 3183–3190
33. Stahnke K, Hecker S, Kohne E, Debatin K-M. CD95 (APO-1/Fas) mediated apoptosis in cytokine activated hematopoietic cells. Exp Hematol (1998) 26: 844–850

34. Klas C, Debatin K-M, Jonker RR, Krammer PH. Activation interferes with the APO-1 pathway in mature human T cells. Int Immunol (1993) 5: 625–630
35. DiGiuseppe JA, LeBeau P, Augenbraun J, Borowitz MJ. Multiparameter flow-cytometric analysis of Bcl-2 and Fas expression in normal and neoplastic hematopoiesis. Am J Clin Pathol (1996) 106 (3): 345–351
36. Debatin K-M, Goldman CK, Bamford R, Waldmann TA, Krammer PH. Monoclonal antibody-mediated apoptosis in adult T cell leukemia. Lancet (1990) 335: 497–500
37. Debatin K-M, Goldman CK, Waldmann TA, Krammer PH. APO-1 induced apoptosis of leukemia cells from patients with adult T cell leukemia. Blood (1993) 81: 2972–2977
38. Sugahara K, Yamada Y, Hiragata Y, Matsuo Y, Tsuruda K, Tomonaga M, Maeda T, Atogami S, Tsukasaki K, Kamihira S. Soluble and membrane isoforms of Fas/CD95 in fresh adult T cell leukemia (ATL) cells and ATL cell lines. Int J Cancer (1997) 72: 128–132
39. Kondo E, Yoshino T, Yamadori I, Matsuo Y, Kawasaki N, Minowada J, Akagi T. Expression of Bcl-2 protein and Fas antigen in non-Hodgkin's lymphoma. Am J Pathol (1994) 145: 330–337
40. Debatin K-M, Krammer PH. Resistance to APO-1 (CD95) induced apoptosis in T-ALL is determined by a Bcl-2 independent anti-apoptotic program. Leukemia (1995) 9: 815–820
41. Lücking-Famira KM, Daniel PT, Möller P, Krammer PH, Debatin K-M. APO-1 (CD95) Mediated Apoptosis in Human T-ALL Engrafted in SCID Mice. Leukemia (1994) 8: 1825–1833
42. Chauhan D, Kharbanda S, Ogata A, Urashima M, Teoh G, Robertson M, Kufe DW, Anderson KC. Interleukin-6 inhibits Fas-induced apoptosis and stress-activated protein kinase activation in multiple myeloma cells. Blood (1997) 89 (1): 227–234
43. Hata H, Matsuzaki H, Takeya M, Yoshida M, Sonoki T, Nagasaki A, Kuribayashi N, Kawano F, Takatsuki K. Expression of Fas/APO-1 (CD95) and apoptosis in tumor cells from patients with plasma cell disorders. Blood (1995) 86 (5): 1939–1945
44. Panayiotidis P, Ganeshaguru K, Foroni L, Hoffbrand AV. Expression and function of the Fas antigen in B chronic lymphocytic leukemia and hairy cell leukemia. Leukemia (1995) 9 (7): 1227–1232
45. Egle A, Villunger A, Marschitz I, Kos M, Hittmair A, Lukas P, Grünewald K, Greil R. Expression of Apo-1/Fas (CD95), Bcl-2, Bax and Bcl-x in myeloma cell lines: relationship between responsiveness to anti-Fas mab and p53 functional status. Br J Haematol (1997) 97: 418–428
46. Munker R, Lubbert M, Yonehara S, Tuchnitz A, Mertelsmann R, Wilmanns W. Expression of the Fas antigen on primary human leukemia cells. Ann Hematol (1995) 70 (1): 15–17
47. Selleri C, Sato T, Del Vecchio L, Luciano L, Barrett AJ, Rotoli B, Young NS, Maciejewski JP. Involvement of Fas-mediated apoptosis in the inhibitory effects of Interferon-α in chronic myelogenous leukemia. Blood (1997) 89 (3): 957–964
48. Dirks W, Schöne S, Uphoff C, Quentmeier H, Pradella S, Drexler HG. Expression and function of CD95 (Fas/APO-1) in leukaemia-lymphoma tumour lines. Br J Haematol (1997) 96: 584–593
49. Robertson MJ, Manley TJ, Pichert G, Cameron C, Cochran KJ, Levine H, Ritz J. Functional consequences of APO-1/Fas (CD95) antigen expression by normal and neoplastic hematopoietic cells. Leuk Lymphoma (1995) 17 (1-2): 51–61
50. Shima Y, Nishimoto N, Ogata A, Fujii Y, Yoshizaki K, Kishimoto T. Myeloma cells express Fas antigen/APO-1 (CD95) but only some are sensitive to anti-Fas antibody resulting in apoptosis. Blood (1995) 85 (3): 757–764
51. Wang D, Freeman GJ, Levine H, Ritz J, Robertson MJ. Role of the CD40 and CD95 (APO-1/Fas) antigens in the apoptosis of human B-cell malignancies. Br J Haematol (1997) 97: 409–417
52. Min YH, Lee S, Lee JW, Chong SY, Hahn JS, Ko YW. Expression of Fas antigen in acute myeloid leukaemia is associated with therapeutic response to chemotherapy. Br J Haematol (1996) 93: 928–930
53. Fellenberg J, Mau H, Scheuerpflug C, Ewerbeck V, Debatin K-M. Modulation of resistance to anti-APO-1 induced apoptosis in osteosarcoma cells by cytokines. Int J Cancer (1997) 72: 536–542
54. Knipping E, Debatin K-M, Stricker K, Heilig B, Eder A, Krammer PH. Identification of Soluble APO-1 in Supernatants of Human B- and T-Cell Lines and Increased Serum Levels in B- and T-Cell Leukemias. Blood (1995) 85: 1562–1569
55. Munker R, Midis G, Owen-Schaub L, Andreff M. Soluble Fas (CD95) is not elevated in the serum of patients with myeloid leukemias, myeloproliferative and myelodysplastic syndromes. Leukemia (1996) 10: 1531–1533
56. Beltinger CP, Kurz E, Böhler T, Schrappe M, Ludwig W-D, Debatin K-M. CD95(APO-1/Fas) mutations in childhood T-lineage acute lymphoblastic leukemia. Blood (1998) 91: 3943–3951
57. Dhein J, Walczak H, Bäumler C, Debatin K-M, Krammer PH. Autocrine T-cell suicide mediated by APO-1/Fas (CD95). Nature (1995) 373: 438–441
58. Friesen C, Herr I, Krammer PH, Debatin K-M. Involvement of the CD95 (APO-1/Fas) receptor/ligand system in drug induced apoptosis in leukemia cells. Nature Med (1996) 2 (5): 574–577

59. Müller M, Strand S, Hug H, Heinemann EM, Walczak H, Hofmann WJ, Stremmel W, Krammer PH, Galle P. Drug-induced apoptosis in hepatoma cells is mediated by the CD95 (APO-1/Fas) receptor/ligand system and involves activation of wild-type p53. J Clin Invest (1997) 99: 403–413
60. Fulda S, Sieverts H, Friesen C, Herr I, Debatin K-M. The CD95 (APO-1/Fas) system mediates drug induced apoptosis in neuroblastoma cells. Cancer Res (1997) 57: 3823–3829
61. Houghton JA, Harwood FG, Tillman DM (1997) Thymineless death in colon carcinoma cells is mediated via Fas signaling. Proc Natl Acad Sci USA 94: 8144–8149
62. Debatin K-M. Cytotoxic Drugs, Programmed Cell Death, and the Immune System: Defining New Roles in an Old Play. J Nat Cancer Inst (1997) 89: 750–751
63. Owen-Schaub LB, Zhang W, Cusack JC, Angelo LS, Santee SM, Fujiwara T, Roth JA, Deisseroth AB, Zhang W-W, Kruzel E, Radinsky R. Wild-type human p53 and a temperature-sensitive mutant induce Fas/APO-1 expression. Mol & Cell Biol (1995) 15, 6: 3032–3040
64. Herr I, Böhler T, Wilhelm D, Angel P, Debatin K-M. Activation of CD95 (APO-1/Fas) signaling by ceramide mediates cancer therapy-induced apoptosis. EMBO J (1997) 16 (20): 6200–6208
65. Los M, Herr I, Friesen C, Fulda S, Schulze-Osthoff K, Debatin K-M. Crossresistance of CD95- and drug-induced apoptosis as a consequence of deficient activation of caspases (ICE/Ced-3 proteases). Blood (1997) 90 (8): 3118–3129
66. Eischen CM, Kottke TJ, Martins LM, Basi GS, Tung JS, Earnshaw WC, Leibson PJ, Kaufmann SH. Comparison of apoptosis in wild-type and Fas-resistant cells: Chemotherapy-induced apoptosis is not dependent on Fas/Fas ligand interactions. Blood (1997) 90 (3): 935–943
67. Villunger A, Egle A, Kos M, Hartmann B, Geley S, Kofler R, Greil R. Drug-induced apoptosis is associated with enhanced Fas (APO-1/CD95) ligand expression but occurs independently of Fas (APO-1/CD95) signaling in human T-acute lymphatic leukemia cells. Cancer Res (1997) 57: 3331–3334
68. Fulda S, Friesen C, Los M, Scaffidi CA, Mier W, Benedict M, Nunez G, Krammer PH, Peter ME, Debatin K-M. Betulinic acid triggers CD95 (APO-1/Fas)- and p53-independent apoptosis via activation of caspases in neuroectodermal tumors. Cancer Res (1997) 57: 4956–4964
69. Friesen C, Fulda S, Debatin K-M. Deficient Activation of the CD95 (APO-1/Fas) System in drug-resistant cells. Leukemia (1997) 11: 1833–1841
70. Landowski TH, Gleason-Guzman MC, Dalton WS. Selection for drug resistance results in resistance to Fas-mediated apoptosis. Blood (1997) 89 (6): 1854–1861
71. Micheau O, Solary E, Hammann A, Martin F, Dimanche-Boitrel MT. Sensitization of cancer cells treated with cytotoxic drugs to Fas-mediated cytotoxicity. J Nat Cancer Inst (1997) 89: 783–789
72. Yoshihiro K, Zhou YW, Zhang XL, Chen TX, Tanaka S, Azuma E, Sakurai M. Fas/APO-1 (CD95)-mediated cytotoxicity is responsible for the apoptotic cell death of leukaemic cells induced by interleukin-2-activated T cells. Br J Haematol (1997) 96: 147–157

26

BCL-2 STIMULATES APOPTIN®-INDUCED APOPTOSIS

Astrid A. A. M. Danen-Van Oorschot,[1] Alex J. van der Eb,[1] and Mathieu H. M. Noteborn[1,2,*]

[1]Laboratory of Molecular Carcinogenesis
Department of Molecular Cell Biology
[2]Leadd BV, Wassenaarseweg 72
Leiden University Medical Center
2300 RA Leiden, The Netherlands

Keywords: anti-tumor therapy, Apoptin®, apoptosis, Bcl-2, BCR-ABL.

ABSTRACT

Apoptin, a protein encoded by an avian virus, induces apoptosis in various cultured human tumorigenic and/or transformed cell lines, e.g. in leukemia, lymphoma or EBV-transformed B cells. In such cells, Apoptin induces p53-independent apoptosis, and the proto-oncogene Bcl-2 accelerates this effect. The latter is surprising for, in general, Bcl-2 is known to inhibit e.g., p53-induced apoptosis. On the other hand, in normal non-transformed human cells, Apoptin is unable to induce apoptosis, even when Bcl-2 is over-expressed. In normal cells, Apoptin is found predominantly in the cytoplasm, whereas in tumor cells it is located in the nucleus. Cellular-localization studies showed that Apoptin is not located in mitochondria, indicating once more that Bcl-2 does not interfere with Apoptin in normal cells. In animal models Apoptin appears to be a safe and efficient anti-tumor agent. These data, in continuation with the observations that Apoptin is specifically stimulated by Bcl-2 in tumor cells, does not need p53, and is not inhibited by BCR-ABL in these cells, imply that Apoptin holds the promise of being the basis for anti-tumor therapy.

---

[*] Correspondence to: Dr Mathieu HM Noteborn, LEADD BV, P.O. Box 9503, 2300 RA Leiden, The Netherlands. Phone: 31 71 527 8736; Fax: 31 71 527 1736; e-mail: leadd@leadd.nl

1. INTRODUCTION

Apoptosis is a programmed physiological process for eliminating superfluous, altered or even malignant cells.[1] Apoptosis can be induced by many stimuli through different pathways, all of which seem to converge into one evolutionarily conserved process.[2] The over-all mechanism of apoptosis is still unclear, but several genes have already been identified as major elements of the process, such as the proto-oncogene Bcl-2. The latter belongs to an ever extending family of Bcl-2-like proteins, which either inhibit (e.g. Bcl-2) or accelerate (e.g. Bax) apoptosis.[3] Another crucial factor is the tumor suppressor p53, which induces or mediates the apoptosis signal. Non-functional p53 will result in tumor formation,[4] whereas over-expression of Bcl-2, (e.g., caused by chromosomal translocation) can result in development of tumors, such as leukemia, lymphoma or breast cancer.[3] Chronic myeloid leukemia is caused by a translocation involving the BCR and ABL genes. The ABL protein, a tyrosine-specific protein kinase constitutively activated by this translocation, inhibits apoptosis and causes tumor growth.[5]

Apoptosis plays an important role in tumor development, and can be exploited for therapeutic purposes. Many tumor cells have a disabling mutation in the decision-making machinery for apoptosis, but their execution system is still intact. This means that tumor cells will die if they are provided with an effective apoptotic signal. Both non-functional p53 and aberrant expression of Bcl-2 and BCR-ABL also hamper the treatment of cancer by chemotherapy or radiation.[6] More than 50% of the known tumor types, such as melanomas, lung cancer and a large number of lymphomas, lack functional p53 and (over-)express Bcl-2 or BCR-ABL. Patients with these types of cancer have a very low chance of responding to chemotherapy. In many research laboratories and clinics, new anti-tumor therapies are underway based on the induction of apoptosis and not inhibited by the lack of functional p53 and/or expression of anti-apoptotic genes.

In this report, the interaction of the apoptosis-inducing protein Apoptin with anti-apoptotic proteins Bcl-2 and BCR-ABL is described. In addition, the development of a first prototype anti-tumor therapy based on the expression of Apoptin will be discussed.

2. CELL DEATH INDUCED BY APOPTIN IS P53-INDEPENDENT AND IS NOT INHIBITED BY BCR-ABL

Expression of a single chicken anemia virus (CAV)-derived protein, Apoptin®, in transformed cells of chicken[7] and of human origin induces apoptosis.[8] Apoptin consists of 121 amino acids, and has no homologous viral or cellular counterparts. It has regions rich in proline and basic amino acids, and over-all contains a high percentage of serine and threonine residues.[9] Apoptin contains nuclear-localization and nuclear-export signals, which suggest that Apoptin can be located in the nucleus and/or cytoplasm (see below).

Zhuang et al. have shown that Apoptin does not need functional p53 to induce apoptosis. Transient expression of Apoptin in human tumor cells results in the induction of apoptosis by Apoptin to the same extent, independent of whether they contain wild-type p53, mutant p53 or no p53 at all. These results were corroborated by the finding that synthesis of the adenovirus Ad5 E1B-55K protein, an inhibitor of p53, does not decrease the apoptotic activity of Apoptin.[10]

Apoptin induces apoptosis in human K562 cells derived from acute myeloid leukemias, which produce a chimeric BCR-ABL protein.[11] From a therapeutic viewpoint, these properties of Apoptin are important. Many tumors express BCR-ABL and/or lack p53, and thus become resistant to chemotherapeutic agents.

3. BCL-2 ENHANCES APOPTIN-INDUCED APOPTOSIS IN TRANSFORMED CELLS

In our laboratory and many others, Bcl-2 has been shown to inhibit p53-mediated apoptosis.[12,13] On the other hand, Apoptin could still induce apoptosis in human malignant blood cells expressing high levels of endogenous Bcl-2. In lymphoblastoma-derived DoHH-2 cells, containing a high level of Bcl-2, Apoptin induced cell death even faster than in K562 cells, with a normal level of Bcl-2.[11]

We examined in more detail whether Bcl-2 enhances Apoptin activity. To that end, human Saos-2 cells were transiently transfected with plasmids encoding Apoptin and/or Bcl-2. Several days after transfection, Saos-2 cells transfected with both Apoptin and Bcl-2 underwent apoptosis to a significantly higher level than cells expressing Apoptin alone.[13,14] Apparently, Bcl-2 accelerates Apoptin-induced apoptosis in transformed mammalian cells, which is surprising since Bcl-2 is known to inhibit apoptosis, such as induced by the tumor-suppressor gene p53.[12]

Cells expressing Apoptin alone localize it in their nuclei.[15] In transfected cells expressing both Apoptin and Bcl-2, Apoptin is situated within the nucleus, whereas Bcl-2 is in the cytoplasm, just as when they are over-expressed separately. These results indicate that Apoptin does not change the cytoplasmic localization of Bcl-2 or vice versa, Bcl-2 does not change the nuclear localization of Apoptin.[13] Immunoprecipitation assays show that Bcl-2 does not co-precipitate with Apoptin, implying that no direct interaction between Apoptin and Bcl-2 exists (A. Den Hollander, unpublished data).

In summary, one can conclude that Bcl-2 plays an indirect role in the Apoptin-mediated reactions in tumor cells. It may be concluded that Apoptin should be especially effective in tumor cells over-expressing Bcl-2.

4. APOPTIN DOES NOT INDUCE APOPTOSIS IN NORMAL NON-TRANSFORMED HUMAN CELLS

Apoptin can induce apoptosis in cell lines derived from a great variety of human tumors, e.g. hepatomas, lymphomas, leukemias, melanomas, breast and lung tumors and colon carcinomas.[8] In contrary, Apoptin does not induce apoptosis in "normal" non-transformed human diploid cells, such as fibroblasts, keratinocytes, smooth muscle cells, T cells or endothelial cells. The possible cause for this phenomenon is that, in tumor cells, Apoptin is located in the nucleus, whereas in normal cells it is present in the cytoplasm. Long-term expression of Apoptin in normal human fibroblasts revealed that it has no toxic or transforming activity in these cells.[16]

It is not yet known whether transformed cells cannot recognize the nuclear export signal of Apoptin and "normal" cells can, or whether differential usage of the nuclear localization signals might be the explanation. An alternative cause might be differential modifications of Apoptin, such as phosphorylation, in tumorigenic/transformed cells versus normal cells. Transient transfection of normal human diploid cells with Apoptin and SV40 transforming large-T antigen resulted in apoptosis. Immuno-fluorescence analysis showed that, in these cells, Apoptin had moved from the cytoplasm into the nucleus. Apparently, mere expression of a transforming protein is sufficient to render normal cells susceptible to Apoptin, and the establishment of a stable transformed state is not required.[17]

In view of the data obtained with co-expression of SV40 large-T antigen and Apoptin, one might assume that over-expression of the proto-oncogene Bcl-2 in "normal" human cells will also force Apoptin to enter the nucleus resulting in the induction of apoptosis. We have reported that cells expressing Apoptin either alone or together with Bcl-2, did not undergo Apoptin-induced apoptosis.[16] Mitochondria are known to play a major role in Bcl-2-regulated apoptosis.[18] Staining of Apoptin-expressing cells with Mito-Tracker dye, which specifically stains mitochondria and a monoclonal antibody specific for Apoptin, however, shows that the majority of the Apoptin signal did not co-localize with the mitochondria.[14] These results prove again that Bcl-2 and Apoptin do not affect each other's activity in normal cells, whereas they do indirectly in transformed cells.

5. APOPTIN IS A PROMISING ANTI-TUMOR AGENT

Since Apoptin gene specifically induces apoptosis in (human) tumor cells, (in contrast to other agents) in spite of Bcl-2 over-expression, lack of functional p53 and/or expression of BCR-ABL, Apoptin may become an effective agent for anti-tumor therapy. At least, synthesis of Apoptin may decrease the effective dose of cytotoxic agents, resulting in a reduction of possible side-effects of chemo- and related anti-tumor therapies.

To allow efficient uptake of the Apoptin gene, one has to make viral vectors expressing the protein. In our laboratory, high titers of recombinant-Apoptin adenovirus have been produced by means of the PER.C6 helper cells.

A first series of in-vivo studies with rodents (A.M. Pietersen and M. Van der Eb, unpublished results) show that Apoptin is a candidate for safe and effective anti-tumor gene therapy. Toxicity studies with rats showed that recombinant adenovirus expressing Apoptin did not result in obvious abnormalities. Intra-tumoral infection of nude mice bearing subcutaneous human hepatomas with a single batch of recombinant Apoptin-adenovirus, resulted in reduction of tumor-growth and symptoms of regression. In contrast, control adenovirus did not reduce the tumor growth.

In conclusion, these features show that Apoptin holds the promise of being the basis for anti-cancer therapy.

ACKNOWLEDGMENTS

This research was partially made possible by research grants from The Netherlands Ministry of Economic Affairs, Aesculaap Beheer BV, Boxtel, the Dutch Cancer Foundation, Amsterdam, and Nuffic, The Hague, The Netherlands.

REFERENCES

1. Vaux DL, Strasser A. The molecular biology of apoptosis. Proc Natl Acad Sci USA 1996; 93: 2239–2244.
2. White E. Life, death and the pursuit of apoptosis. Genes Dev 1996; 10: 1–15.
3. Reed JC. Double identity for proteins of the Bcl-2 family. Nature 1997; 387: 773–776.
4. Levine AJ. p53, the cellular gatekeeper for growth and division. Cell 1997; 88: 323–331.
5. Hunter T. Oncoprotein networks. Cell 1997; 88: 333–346.

6. McDonnell TJ, Meyn RE, Robertson LE. Implications of apoptotic cell death regulation in cancer therapy. Sem Cancer Biol 1995; 6: 53–60
7. Noteborn MHM, Todd D, Verschueren CAJ, De Gauw HWFM, Curran WL, Veldkamp S, Douglas AJ, McNulty MS, Van der Eb AJ, Koch G. A single chicken anemia virus protein induces apoptosis. J Virol 1994; 68: 346–351.
8. Noteborn MHM, Danen-van Oorschot AAAM, Van der Eb AJ. The Apoptin® gene of chicken anemia virus in the induction of apoptosis in human tumorigenic cells and in gene therapy of cancer. In: Boulikas T, ed. Gene Therapy and Molecular Biology 1998; 1: 399–406.
9. Noteborn MHM, De Boer GF, Van Roozelaar D, Karreman C, Kranenburg O, Vos J, Jeurissen SHM, Zantema A, Hoeben RC, Koch G, Van Ormondt H, Van der Eb AJ. Characterization of cloned chicken anemia virus DNA that contains all elements for the infectious replication cycle. J Virol 1991; 65: 3131–3139.
10. Zhuang S-M, Shvarts A, Van Ormondt H, Jochemsen A-G, Van der Eb AJ, Noteborn MHM. Apoptin, a protein derived from chicken anemia virus, induces a p53-independent apoptosis in human osteosarcoma cells. Cancer Res 1995; 55: 486–489.
11. Zhuang S-M, Landegent JE, Verschueren CAJ, Falkenburg JHF, Van Ormondt H, Van der Eb AJ, Noteborn MHM. Apoptin, a protein encoded by chicken anemia virus, induces cell death in various human hematologic malignant cells in vitro. Leukemia 1995; 9 S1: 118–120.
12. Rao L, White E. Bcl-2 and the ICE family of apoptotic regulators: making a connection. Curr Opin Genet Dev 1997; 7: 52–58.
13. Danen-Van Oorschot AAAM, Den Hollander A, Takayama S, Reed J, Van der Eb AJ, Noteborn MHM. BAG-1 inhibits p53-induced but not Apoptin-induced apoptosis. Apoptosis 1997; 2: 395–402.
14. Danen-van Oorschot AAAM, Zhang Y, Erkeland S, Fischer DF, Van der Eb AJ, Noteborn MHM. The effect of Bcl-2 on Apoptin in normal cells versus transformed human cells. Leukemia 1999; In press.
15. Noteborn MHM, Van der Eb AJ, Koch G, Jeurissen SHM. VP3 of the chicken anemia virus (CAV) causes apoptosis. In: H.S. Ginsberg, F. Brown, R.M. Channock, R.A. Lerner, eds. Vaccines 93: Modern approaches to new vaccines including prevention of AIDS. Cold Spring Harbor, USA, CSHL Press 1993; 299–304.
16. Danen-van Oorschot AAAM, Fischer DF, Grimbergen JM, Klein B, Zhuang S-M, Falkenburg JHF, Backendorf C, Quax PHA, Van der Eb AJ, Noteborn MHM. Apoptin induces apoptosis in human transformed and malignant cells but not in normal cells. Proc Natl Acad Sci USA 1997; 94: 5843–5847.
17. Noteborn MHM, Zhang Y, Van der Eb, AJ. Apoptin specifically causes apoptosis in tumor cells and after UV-treatment in untransformed cells from cancer-prone individuals: A review. Mutation Research; 1998; 400: 447–455.
18. Kroemer G, Zamzani N, Susin SA. Mitochondrial control of apoptosis. Immunol Today 1997; 18: 44–51.

CD95 (FAS/APO-1) ANTIGEN IS A NEW PROGNOSTIC MARKER OF BLAST CELLS OF ACUTE LYMPHOBLASTIC LEUKAEMIA PATIENTS

A. Yu. Baryshnikov, E. R. Polosukhina, N. N. Tupitsin, N. V. Gavrikova,
L. Yu. Andreeva, T. N. Zabotina, S. A. Mayakova, V. I. Kurmashov,
A. B. Syrkin, Z. G. Kadagidze, D. Yu. Blochin, and Yu. V. Shishkin

Cancer Research Center
Russian Academy of Medical Sciences
Moscow, Russia

Keywords: CD95 (Fas/APO-1) antigen, apoptosis, acute lymphoblastic leukemia, IPO-4.

1. ABSTRACT

We analyzed CD95(Fas/APO-1) antigen expression on bone marrow blasts in 38 children with acute lymphoblastic leukemia (ALL) receiving a treatment in the Department of Leukaemias at the Cancer Research Center in 1987–1989 years (n = 22) and in 1994–1997 years (n = 16). CD95 antigen expression was studied by monoclonal antibodies (MoAbs) IPO-4 in indirect immunofluorescence analysis. CD95 antigen was expressed on 35.8±7.5% bone marrow blasts, most frequently (63.6%) in the clinically favourable Pre-B ALL. Only in this group CD95 antigen expression was correlated with CD10 antigen expression that has a positive influence to the time of complete remission in ALL patients. Our data showed that CD95 expression on blast cells is a favourable prognostic sign, associated with increased relapse-free and total survival. On the contrary, the absence of CD95 antigen on blasts is an unfavourable sign for disease evolution.

2. INTRODUCTION

Acute lymphoblastic leukemia (ALL) is one of the most widespread disorders of childhood. It comprises almost 75–80% of childhood acute leukemias. Modern combination chemotherapy produces complete remissions in a majority but not all patients. Therefore it is very important to discover features that have prognostic significance. It has been shown that expression of common ALL antigen (CALLA, CD10) has been associated with favourable outcome.[1] Expression of another antigen has diagnostic but not prognostic importance. In an attempt to identify additional factors of prognosis we studied the expression of CD95(Fas/APO-1) antigen on bone marrow blasts of ALL patients. CD95(fas/APO-1) antigen is a cell-surface protein. It belongs to the tumor necrosis factor and nerve growth factor receptor superfamily. CD95 crosslinking by the Fas ligand or an agonist anti-CD95 antibody can deliver a cell death signal. Some attempts to determine CD95 antigen expression and function in ALL were done. Kotani et al.[2] analyzed CD95 antigen expression and function on mononuclear cells in peripheral blood from 12 patients with T-ALL by flow cytometry. They found that cells from patients express CD95 more significantly than cells from healthy donors. In the majority of patients leukemic cells responded to Fas-mediated apoptosis. Lucking-Famira et al.[3] tried to use anti-CD95 MoAbs for T-ALL therapy. Human leukemic cells were transplanted in immunodeficient mice SCID line and anti-CD95 was injected. The treatment of mice in vivo by MoAbs induced apoptosis in most of leukemic cells, increasing the average life-expectancy of mice. Debatin K.M. et al.[4] found CD95 antigen expression on blastic cells in 21 of 30 children with T-ALL and 6 cell lines from T-ALL. No correlation between CD95 intensity expression and apoptosis sensitivity was found in T-cell cultures as well as in cells from patients. Debatin et al.[5] demonstrated that T-blasts from patients with T-leukaemia have very high levels of apoptosis. The aim of this work was the study of CD95 (Fas/APO-1) antigen on bone marrow blasts in children with ALL and the analysis of relapse-free survival and total survival time correlated with CD95 antigen expression.

3. MATERIALS AND METHODS

3.1. Patients

We examined 38 children with ALL receiving the treatment by programme 2 in the Department of Leukemia, Cancer Research Center in 1987–1989 (22 patients) (Table 1) and receiving the treatment by mBFM-90 in 1994–1997 (16 patients) (Table2).

3.2. Treatment

Twenty-two patients in 1987–1989 received treatment by programme 2 that consisted of induction therapy with PRED (prednisone) p.o. 40 mg/m2/day, VCR (vincristine) i.v. 1.5 mg/m2/week (max 2 mg) N4, DNR (daunorubicin) i.v. 30 mg/m2/week N4, L-ASP (L-asparaginase) i.m. 10000 ME/m2/day N8, CP (cyclophosphamide) i.v. 1000 mg/m2 N2, MTX (methotrexate) i.th. arabinoside) i.v. 100 mg/m2/day for 3–5 days, MTX (methotrexate) 500–1000 mg/m2 N3 weekly (i.v. 1/10 - 1 h, dosages age dependent 6–12 mg N5; consolidation regimen with ARA-C (cytosine arabinoside) i.v. 100 mg/m2/day for 3–5 days, MTX (methotrexate) 500–1000 mg/m2 N3 weekly (i.v. 1/10 - 1 h,9/10- 24 h) with Leucovorine 15 mg/m2 in 36 and 42 h., MTX (methotrexate) i.th. dosages age-dependent 6–12 mg N3; CNS (cranial) irradiation with 18–24 Gy; continuation therapy for 5 years with MTX p.o. 20 mg/m2/ weekly and reinduction protocols 1 time in 2–3 months with VCR (vincristine) i.v. 1.5 mg/m2/ week N2 and DNR (daunorubicin) i.v. 30 mg/m2/week N2, 1 times in 6 months with ARA-C (cytosine arabinoside) i.v. 100 mg/m2/day N5 and ARA-C (cytosine arabinoside) i.v. 100 mg/m2/day N5.

Table 1. Characteristics of 22 patients receiving the treatment by programme 2

Years of age	Sex	FAB- types	Risk group
0- 2: 2	F : 10	L1 - 4	Standard - 4
2- 6: 6	M : 12	L2 - 6	Medium - 13
6-10: 7		L1/L2- 6	High - 5
10-16: 7		L2/L1 - 5	
		L3 - 1	

Sixteen patients received modificate ALL-BFM-90 (MTX 1000 mg/m2) consisting of induction therapy—protocol 1, protocol M (high doses of the MTX 1000 mg/m2 N4, 6-MP p.o. 25 mg/m2/day 1–56 days); reinduction therapy—protocol 2, CNS (cranial) irradiation (18–24 Gy dosages) age dependent (<1 year - not, 1–2 years - 18, >2 - 24 Gy); and continuation therapy 104 weeks with 6-mercaptopurine p.o. 50 mg/m2/daily and MTX p.o. 20 mg/m2/ weekly.

3.3. Monoclonal Antibodies

We studied CD95 (Fas/APO-1) antigen expression using MoAbs IPO-4, which were produced and described by S.Sidorenko et al. (1987) as MoAbs against activation antigen. At the Fifth International Workshop and Conference on Human Leukocyte Differentiation Antigens in 1993 (Boston) they were characterised as MoAbs against CD95 antigen. We considered positive reaction if the percentage of CD95 positive cells was > 10%. To establish phenotypic subclassification of ALL we used MoAbs to CD5, CD7, CD10, CD3, CD19, HLA-DR, CD34 antigens. We also examined cytoplasmic and surface immunoglobulins.

3.4. Immunofluorescence Assay

Antigen expression was studied by indirect surface immunofluorescence assay on freshly isolated cells using flow cytometry (FACScan, Becton Dickinson). Bone marrow samples were isolated by sedimentation in 1% gelatin solution for 45 min. at 37°C and then the cells were resuspended in 0.5 ml of lysing solution (Becton Dickinson) for total lysis of erythrocytes, then washed three times in phosphate-buffered saline (PBS) and resuspended in PBS.

3.5. Indirect Immunofluorescence Technique

5×10^5 cells were incubated with 20 µl of MoAbs at room temperature for 30 min. After one washing with PBS they were stained with 20 µl FITC-conjugated sheep antiserum against mouse immunoglobulins for 30 min. at 4°C. After that the cells were washed

Table 2. Characteristics of 16 patients receiving the treatment by mBFM-90

Years of age	Sex	FAB-types	Risk group
0–2: 1	F : 7	L1–5	Standard-4
2–6: 12	M : 9	L2–6	Medium-8
6–10: 2		L1/L2–2	High-4
10–16: 1		L2/L1–2	
		L3–1	

twice and resuspended in PBS with 1% formalin and 0.1% sodium aside to be tested for reactivity by indirect immunofluorescence.

3.6. Measurement of Apoptosis

Apoptosis was assessed with the cytofluorometric analysis of hypodiploid DNA-labeled with propidium iodide (PI). 2×10^5 cells were washed in PBS and resuspended in 70% ethanol for 1 hour, after that they were centrifuged at 500 rpm for 7 min. Then the cells were resuspended in 1.0 ml of hypotonic fluorochrome solution (5 µg/ml PI, 0.1% sodium citrate, 0.1% Triton X100). After gentle mixing, cells were incubated at room temperature for 15 min. in the darkness. The PI fluorescence of stained DNA was measured with FACScan without further washings. FACS settings were designed to identify a distinct hypodiploid DNA region below the diploid G0/G1 DNA peak.

4. RESULTS

Table 3 presents the expression of antigens for phenotypic subclassification of ALL.

We studied the immunophenotype of all 38 patients using MoAbs and we found 6 immunological subtypes of ALL. Pro-B cell ALL was in 15.7% of children, Pre-Pre B - ALL in 57.8%, Pre-B - in 5.2%, B-ALL - in 2.6%, T-ALL - in 13.1% and "0" subtype - in 5.2%. We investigated CD95 antigen expression on bone marrow blast cells of ALL patients (Table 4).

CD95 was expressed on 35.8±7.5% bone marrow blasts of 38 children with total blastosis. Comparing the frequency of this antigen in different immunological subtypes we found that it is most frequently expressed in clinically most favourable Pre-Pre-B ALL subtype of ALL. In accordance with presence or absence of CD95 antigen on bone marrow blast surface we separated 38 children in 2 subgroups: CD95 positive and negative. CD95 positive comprised 1 child with Pro-B subtype of 6 diagnosed, 14 of 22 with Pre-Pre-B ALL, 1 patient with B-ALL, 2 of 5 patients with T-ALL, 1 of 2 with "0" subtype of ALL. The CD95 negative subgroup comprised 5 children with Pro-B ALL, 8 with Pre-Pre-B ALL, 3 with T-ALL and 1 with "0" ALL. Correlation analysis demonstrated that none of immunological, clinical and haematological features are correlated with CD95 antigen expression. However, we have found an interesting correlation in Pre-Pre-B ALL group between CD10 antigen expression and CD95 antigen one (r = 0.56, p<0.05). The incidence of relapses in CD95 positive group was 17.6%, and the remission was achieved in 82.3% of children. The median of relapse-free survival was not reached, because more than 50% of children in this group maintain remission. In 25% of patients the remission time was 23.7 months. On the contrary, in CD95 negative group the median of relapse-free survival was 19.5 months and we observed an increased incidence of relapses till 37.5%. In 25% of

Table 3. Immunophenotyping of ALL

Immuno-phenotype	CD19	CD10	CD3	CD5	CD7	CD34	HLA-DR	Ig
Pro-B	+	–	–	–	–	+/–	+	–
Pre-Pre-B	+	+	–	–	–	+/–	+	–
Pre-B	+	+	–	–	–	–	+	cyt
B	+	–	–	–	–	–	+	surf
T	–	+/–	+/–	+	+	+/–	+/–	–
0	–	–	–	–	–	+/–	+/–	–

Table 4. Immunological characteristics of ALL patients

Immuno-phenotype	Cases	Number of CD95 positive cases	Incidence (in % of positive cases)	Number of CD95 positive blasts(M±m)
Pro-B	6	1	16,6	21
Pre-Pre-B	22	14	63,6	
Pre-B	2	0	0	38,8±9,7
B	1	1	100	0
T	5	2	40	74,1
0	2	1	50	84,5±10,5
The whole	38	19	50	11

patients in this group the remission time was 7 months. It is important to note, that the differences in relapse-free survival between CD95 positive and CD95 negative are certain, valued by statistical tests: Gehan's Wilcoson-test p = 0.02; F-test p = 0.05; Cox's test p = 0.05. The differences in relapse-free survival were reflected in total survival of children with ALL (Figure 1).

In the CD95 positive group the median was not reached because 14 children (73.7%) are alive and 5 died (26.3%). In CD95 negative group the median is 25.5 months: 10 children died (52.6%), and 9 (47.3%) are alive. In 25% of patients in this group the total survival is 8.7 months. The analysis of results using Gehan's Wilcoson test and F-test showed that the differences between CD95 positive and CD95 negative groups are certain, with p = 0.05 and p = 0.027, respectively.

Total survival analysis is particularly interesting in the group of children (n = 22) that was observed in 1987–1997 years. 10-year survival analysis demonstrated that the survival median is 118.5 months and 75% of patients lived 123.5 months. In the CD95 negative group the total survival median is 24 months (Figure 2).

Relapse-free survival median in CD95 positive group is 115 months; in CD95 negative group it is 13.2 months. In 30% of children that received the treatment in 1994–1997

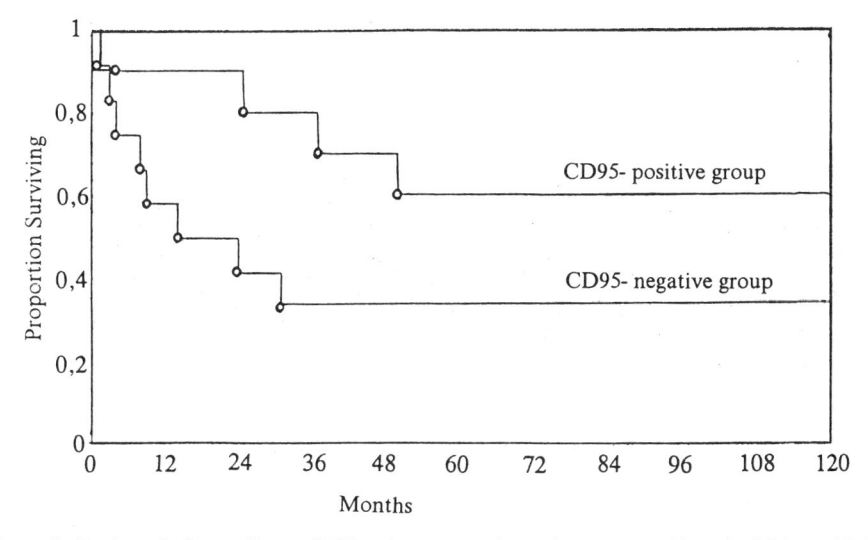

Figure 1. Total survival according to CD95 antigen expression on bone marrow blasts in children with ALL.

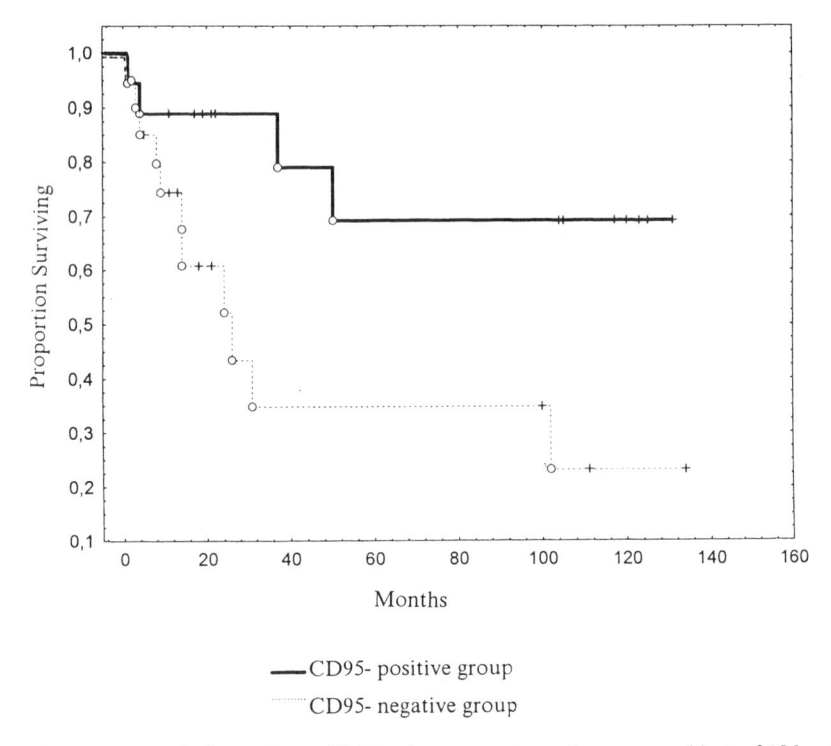

Figure 2. Ten-year survival according to CD95 antigen expression on bone marrow blasts of ALL patients.

years we valued the apoptotic cell rate during polychemotherapy according the program ALL-BFM-90. We measured the percentage of spontaneous apoptosis in bone marrow blasts before the treatment with BFM-90 and on the 15th day of control effectively polyhemotherapy. Spontaneous apoptosis was found in 8.6 ± 3.7% of blasts, and induced by polychemotherapy apoptosis of bone marrow cells on the 15th day was 79.2 ± 12.5% (Figure 3).

5. DISCUSSION

CD95 antigen, a surface cell receptor, belongs to the receptor TNF/NFG superfamily as nerve growth factor, tumor necrosis factor, antigens CD27, CD30 and CD40. CD95 antigen can transmit apoptotic signal by cross binding with CD95-ligand or anti-CD95 MoAbs. Recent studies showed that CD95 antigen may have an important role in controlling normal hemopoesis. Furthermore, CD95-mediated apoptosis may have a role in pathophysiology for some haematological diseases. In our work we have used original data to study CD95 antigen expression observed since 1987 in the Cancer Research Center by MoAbs IPO-4 which were included in CD95 differentiation cluster on the 5th International Workshop and Conference on Human Leukocyte Differentiation Antigens (1993, Boston). We studied Fas antigen expression on bone marrow blasts from children with ALL. Analysis of treated group since 1987 showed that according CD95 antigen expression there were two subgroups: CD95 positive and CD95 negative. It is important to notice that CD95 is often expressed in Pre-Pre-B ALL, the most prognostically favourable

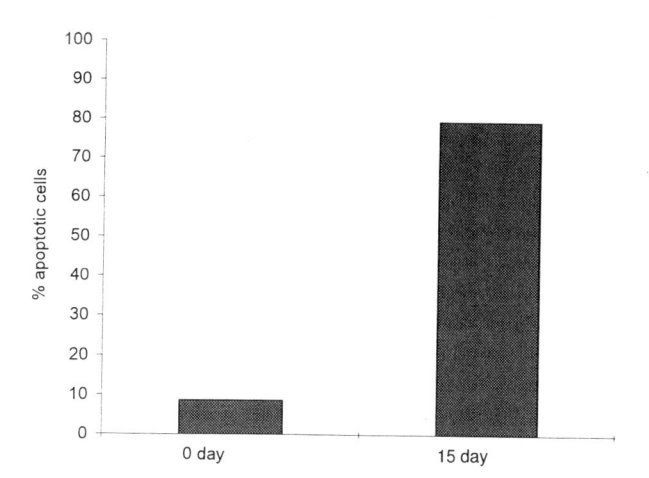

Figure 3. Induction apoptosis by polychemotherapy in bone marrow blasts of ALL patients.

type. In CD95 positive subgroup the 10-year total survival median was 118.5 months and in the CD95 negative subgroup, 24 months. So, CD95 antigen expression on blastic cells is a good prognostic sign, increasing the relapse-free and total survival. On the contrary, CD95 antigen absence on blast surface is an unfavourable sign in the evolution of disease. In the studied group of patients CD95 expression was not correlated with morphological types according FAB classification, risk of relapse, clinical indices, among which we analysed the dimensions of liver, spleen, lymph nodes, the presence or absence of anaemic, hemorragic and bone-joint syndromes in acute period, the absolute quantity of haemoglobin, leucocytes, platelets in peripheral blood. In the correlation analysis of immunological marker expression we showed that only in Pre-Pre-B ALL group CD10 antigen expression has a positive influence on complete remission time in patients with ALL and it is correlated with CD95 antigen expression. In CD95 expression analysis of bone marrow blasts from children that received a treatment in 1994–1997 years we can notice the highest expression in Pre-Pre-B ALL, and also a correlation with CD10 antigen expression on blasts and a good prognosis for relapse-free and total survival in CD95 positive subgroup. Statistical analysis of united subgroups shows certain differences between CD95 positive and CD95 negative subgroups for relapse-free and total survival. That was demonstrated with some independent methods of valuation. We can consider the presence of CD95 antigen as a favourable prognostic sign at the basis of cytostatic action mechanism found recently by C. Frisen et al.,[6] e.g., of doxorubicin and methotrexate that are used for induction and consolidation of remission in ALL. They showed that in leukaemic cells cytostatics can work through interaction CD95 receptor/CD95 ligand. Doxorubicin induces on cell surface the expression of CD95 ligand which is bound with CD95 receptor and so achieving the transmission of the death cell signal. This mechanism was found before in apoptosis of T-cells induced by MoAb against CD3/TCR complex of T-cell receptor antigen.[7,8] In T-cell of CEM line it was demonstrated that doxorubicin in therapeutic doses stimulates the mRNA CD95 ligand expression. Methotrexate also stimulates CD95 ligand expression in concentrations that are used in vivo for treatment. Probably, with this hypothesis it is possible to explain our results of apoptosis induction by chemotherapy on CD95 positive bone marrow blasts in children and a better prognosis for patients which blast cells express CD95 receptor. So, CD95 receptor/ligand system opens a new strategy for tumor chemotherapy.

Thanks to the work done since 1987 in the Cancer Research Center (to study CD95 antigen expression on bone marrow blasts in children with ALL) we can conclude that

CD95 antigen expression has a certain influence in increasing relapse-free and total survival. Also, that CD95 positive leukemic cell apoptosis can depend on capacities of cytostatics to induce cell death in leukemic cells through interaction of CD95 receptor and CD95 ligand.

ACKNOWLEDGMENTS

The authors would like to thank Prof. D. F. Gluzman, who courteously provided MoAbs IPO-4 for our investigations.

REFERENCES

1. Baryshnikov A.Yu., Kadagidze Z.G., Tupitsin N.N., Machonova L.A.. Immunological phenotype of leukemic cell. Moscow, 1989, 240.
2. Kotani-T; Aratake-Y; Kondo-S; Tamura-K; Ohtaki-S. Expression of functional Fas antigen on adult T-cell leukemia. Leuk-Res., 1994, 18(4), 305–310
3. Lucking-Famira KM; Daniel-PT; Moller-P; Krammer-PH; Debatin-KM APO-1 (CD95) mediated apoptosis in human T-ALL engrafted in SCID mice. Leukemia, 1994, 8(11), 1825–1833
4. Debatin K.-M., Goldman C.K., Waldman T.A., Krammer P.H. APO-1-induced apoptosis of leukemia cells from patients with adult T-cell leukemia, Blood, 1993, 81, 2972 - 2977
5. Debatin K.-M., Goldman C.K., Bamford R. et al. Monoclonal antibody mediated apoptosis in adult T cell leukemia, Lancet, 1990, 335, 447
6. Friesen-C; Herr-I; Krammer-PH; Debatin-KM .Involvement of the CD95 (APO-1/FAS) receptor/ligand system in drug-induced apoptosis in leukemia cells. Nat-Med.,1996, 2(5), 574–577
7. Brunner T., Mogil R.J., LaFase D.,Yoo N.J., Mahboubl A. Cell-autonomous Fas(CD95)/Fas-ligand interaction mediates activation-induced apoptosis in T-cell hybridomas, Nature,1995, 373, 441–444
8. Ju Shyr-Te, Panka D.J., Cui H., Ettinger R., Marshak-Rothstei. Fas(CD95)/FasL interactions required for programmed cell death after T-cell activation, Nature,1995, 373, 444–448

28

INHIBITION OF FAS/FAS-LIGAND DOES NOT BLOCK CHEMOTHERAPY-INDUCED APOPTOSIS IN DRUG SENSITIVE AND RESISTANT CELLS

Deborah S. Richardson,[*] Paul D. Allen, Stephen M. Kelsey, and Adrian C. Newland

Department of Haematology
St. Bartholomew's and Royal London School of Medicine, United Kingdom

1. ABSTRACT

It has been suggested that one means by which chemotherapeutic agents exert their effect on leukaemic cells, is via autocrine induction of fas-ligand which then binds to fas (CD95), activates the caspase pathway and results ultimately in apoptotic death. In order to test this hypothesis, we have treated leukaemic cell lines with various chemotherapeutic agents (idarubicin, etoposide, fludarabine and 2-CdA) with and without pre-treatment with fas (ZB4) and fas-ligand (NOK-1) blocking monoclonal antibodies. Cell cycle analysis and quantitation of apoptosis were performed by flow cytometry following propidium iodide staining. HL-60 cells were found to be sensitive to the induction of apoptosis with all drugs tested but were highly resistant to treatment with a fas-ligating antibody (CH11). Apoptosis was neither inhibited in parental CEM cells nor their mdr-expressing drug resistant counterpart, CEM/VLB100 by pre-treatment with either ZB4 or NOK1. In addition, CEM/VLB100 were slightly more sensitive to treatment with CH11 (100ng/ml) than parental CEM cells (% age apoptosis = 30.35 and 23.675, p=0.024) and at least as sensitive to recombinant fas-ligand (50 ng/ml) (% age apoptosis = 26.6 and 20.2, p=NS).

We conclude that it is unlikely that fas/fas-ligand interactions play a significant role in the induction of apoptosis by these chemotherapeutic agents in the leukaemic cell lines tested.

---

[*] Communicating author: Dr. Deborah Richardson. Address for communication: Department of Haematology, Royal London Hospital,Whitechapel Road, London E1 1BB UK, Telephone: 00 44 171 377 7000, Fax: 00 44 171 377 7016, E-mail: d.s.richardson@mds.qmw.ac.uk

Drug Resistance in Leukemia and Lymphoma III, edited by Kaspers *et al.*
Kluwer Academic / Plenum Publishers, New York, 1999.

2. INTRODUCTION

Despite differences in cellular targets, many chemotherapeutic agents used in the treatment of haematological malignancy have been shown to result in apoptosis or programmed cell death.[1-3] The critical pathways linking cellular damage to cell death are now being investigated and described, however, it remains unclear exactly how cytotoxic agents kill cells. The cellular receptor, fas (APO-1 or CD95), a member of the tumour necrosis factor (TNF) receptor family, has been shown to be involved in the induction and regulation of apoptosis in certain lymphoid cells, via binding of fas ligand,[4,5] resulting in activation of the caspase system and ultimately in the cleavage of death substrates including PARP.[6-8] Human adult T-cell leukaemia/lymphoma cells[9,10] and renal carcinoma cells have been shown to die in response to treatment with anti-fas antibody[11] and recently it has been suggested that doxorubicin-induced cytotoxicity might be mediated by fas/fas-ligand interactions in human leukaemia T-cells.[12] This study investigated the role of fas/fas-ligand interactions in the mechanism of action of various chemotherapeutic agents used in the treatment of leukaemia and lymphoma.

3. MATERIALS AND METHODS

3.1. Reagents

The following cytotoxic agents were used: idarubicin (Pharmacia, Milton Keynes, UK), etoposide (Bristol Myers Pharmaceuticals, Middlesex, UK), vinblastine (David Bull Laboratories, Warwick, UK), 2-chloro-2'-deoxyadenosine (CdA) (Sigma, Poole, Dorset, UK). Fludarabine desphosphate (F-ara-A) was kindly given by Prof. Varsha Gandhi of MD Anderson Cancer Center, Texas, and Schering AG, Berlin, Germany. Anti-Fas (CD95) clone CH-11 (fas-ligating) and ZB4 (fas-blocking) monoclonal antibodies were obtained from Immunotech, Marseille, France. NOK-1 mouse anti-human fas ligand monoclonal antibody (fas ligand neutralising antibody) was obtained from Pharmingen, San Diego, California, and recombinant human soluble fas ligand from Calbiochem, Cambridge, Massachusetts.

3.2. Cell Lines and Culture Conditions

The following cell lines were used in this study; HL-60, human myeloid leukaemia cells, obtained from the European Collection of Animal Cell Cultures (Salisbury, UK); CCRF-CEM, human T-lymphoblastic leukaemia cell line and its vinblastine-induced multidrug-resistant (MDR) counterpart, CEM/VLB100.[13,14] Cells were cultured in RPMI 1640 (Sigma), supplemented with 10% heat-inactivated fetal calf serum (Sigma), 2.0 mM L-glutamine (Sigma), 100U/ml penicillin and 100µg/ml streptomycin at 37°C in a 5% CO2 incubator. Cells were maintained at $2-7 \times 10^5$ cells/ml by subculture.

3.3. Incubation of Cells with CH11 or NOK1 and Cytotoxic Agents

Cells in exponential growth were seeded at 1×10^6/ml in 24 well plates (Costar) in 1ml volumes of supplemented medium. Cells were treated with either 0 or 1µg/ml ZB4 and control wells containing 100 ng/ml CH11 were also used. In separate experiments, cells were treated with 0 or 1µg/ml NOK1; control wells containing 50 ng/ml fas ligand were also used. Concentrations of CH11 and fas-ligand which induced apoptosis in CEM and CEM/VLB100 had been established in previous experiments. After 1 hour, various chemotherapeutic agents were added to the wells: idarubicin (0.1–1µg/ml), etoposide (2–20 µg/ml), or F-ara-A (20 µM) or CdA (10 µM). Plates included control wells without

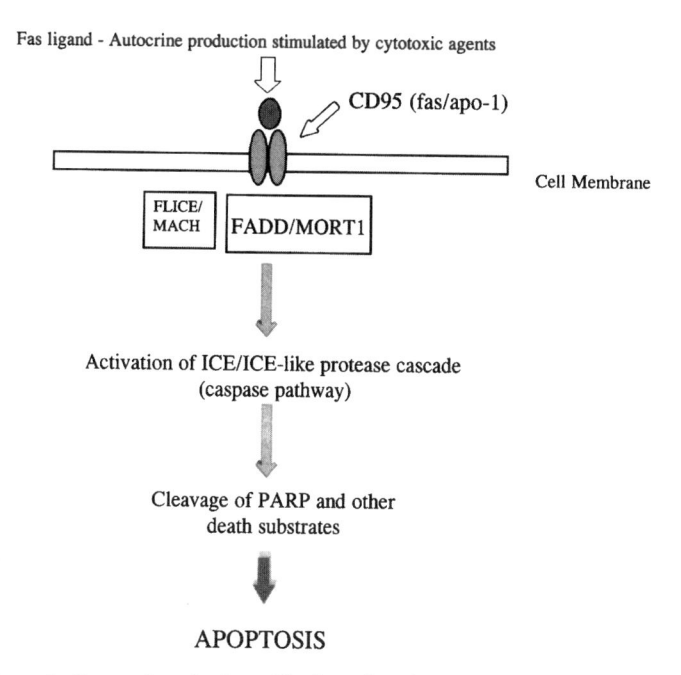

Figure 1. Proposed mechanism of fas dependent chemotherapy-induced apoptosis.

cytotoxic drug. After 24 hours 100 µl aliquots of cells were harvested and analysed for cell-cycle distribution and apoptosis.

3.4. Analysis of Apoptosis and Cell-Cycle Profile

Determination of apoptotic fraction and cell cycle analysis was performed by flow cytometry. Harvested cells were washed with Hanks' balanced salt solution (HBSS) and made permeable by re-suspension in ice-cold 70% ethanol and incubation at 4°C for 30 minutes. The cells were then washed and re-suspended in 1ml of HBSS containing 50 µg/ml propidium iodide and 200 µg/ml RNase type IIIA (Sigma). Cells were analysed 30 minutes after processing, using an EPICS Elite cytometer (Coulter Electronics, Luton, UK). Pulse processing using peak channel versus integral red channel signal was used to discriminate doublet and aggregated cells from single, diploid cells and to exclude debris. G0/G1, S and G2M fractions were identified from the resulting cell-cycle profiles and the percentage apoptotic cells in each sample was measured from the sub-G0/G1 fraction.[15]

3.5. Statistical Analysis

Results were analysed using the two-tailed, paired t-test.

4. RESULTS

4.1. Inhibition of Fas Does Not Prevent Chemotherapy-Induced Apoptosis in CEM or CEM/VLB100

Pre-treatment with ZB4 fas-blocking antibody inhibited CH11 induced apoptosis in both CEM and CEM/VLB100 cells, although ZB4 alone increased apoptosis above background in CEM/VLB100 cells. However, ZB4 did not inhibit chemotherapy-induced apoptosis in either cell line (Figures 2a and b).

4.2. Inhibition of Fas-Ligand Does Not Prevent Chemotherapy-Induced Apoptosis in CEM or CEM/VLB100

Pre-treatment with NOK1 fas ligand blocking antibody inhibited recombinant fas ligand induced apoptosis in both CEM and CEM/VLB100 cells. However, NOK1 did not inhibit chemotherapy-induced apoptosis in either cell line (Figures 3a and b).

4.3. HL-60 Cells Are Sensitive to Chemotherapy-Induced Apoptosis But Resistant to Fas-Ligation

In various experiments, HL-60 cells were shown to be highly sensitive to induction of apoptosis by various chemotherapeutic agents but were resistant to the induction of apoptosis by fas-ligation with CH11 (Tables 1 and 2).

4.4. Comparative Sensitivity of CEM and CEM/VLB100 to Treatment with Fas-Ligand or CH11

CEM/VLB100 were slightly more sensitive to treatment with CH11 (100 ng/ml) than parental CEM cells (percentage apoptosis = 30.35 and 23.68, respectively, p = 0.024) and at least as sensitive to recombinant fas-ligand (50ng/ml) (percentage apoptosis = 26.6 and 20.2, p = NS).

5. DISCUSSION

Various workers have suggested that fas/fas-ligand interactions might mediate cytotoxic-induced death in malignant cells, including human T-cell lymphoblastic leukaemia[12]

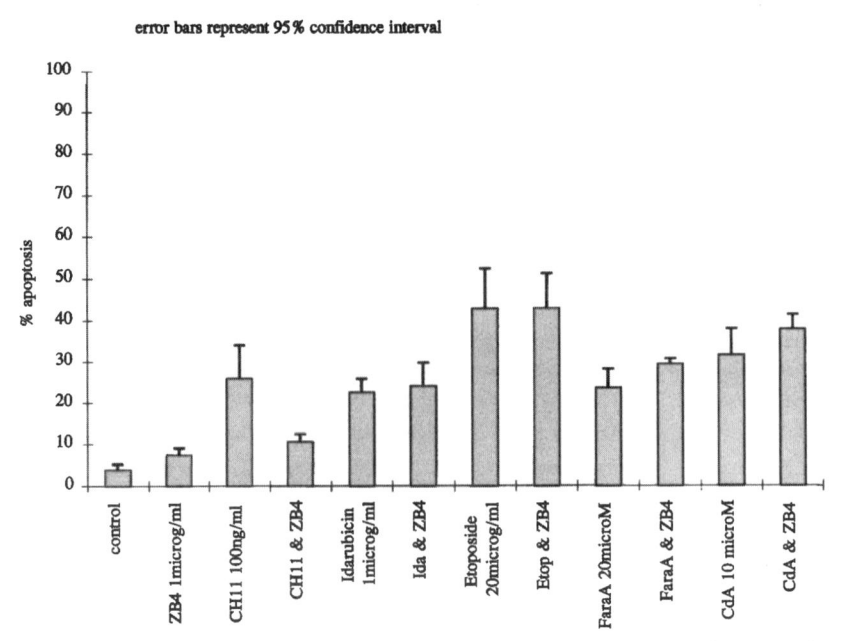

Figure 2a. Chemotherapy induced apoptosis and inhibition of fas with ZB4 in CEM at 24 hours. Results are from a minimum of 4 independent experiments.

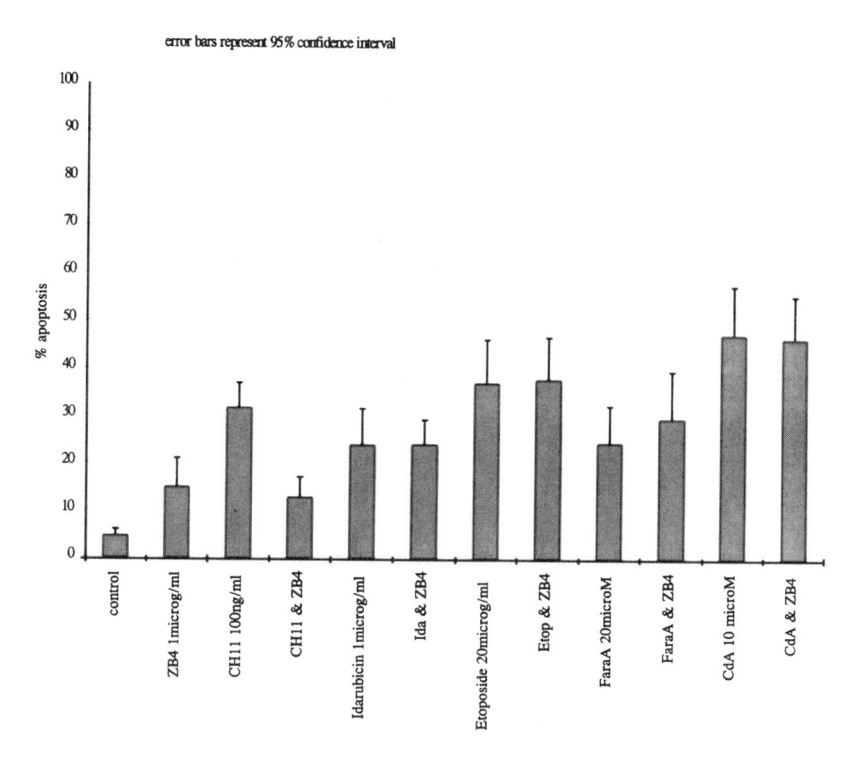

Figure 2b. Chemotherapy induced apoptosis and inhibition of fas with ZB4 in CEM/VLB100 at 24 hours. Results are from a minimum of 4 independent experiments.

and hepatoma cells,[16] suggesting that, at least in some tumours, the apoptotic pathway might be induced by a common mechanism, possibly involving release of fas-ligand in an autocrine and/or paracrine fashion and subsequent binding to and stimulation of the fas receptor. Fas-ligand messenger RNA[12] and protein[17] have been shown to increase in response to treatment with various anti-cancer drugs in human T-lymphoblastic leukaemia cells. All cytotoxic agents tested in this study (etoposide, idarubicin, fludarabine, CdA and vinblastine) induced apoptosis, as measured by flow cytometry, in the human mdr1 positive and negative T-lymphoblastic cell lines tested, however, it was not possible to block apoptosis by inhibition of either the fas receptor with the monoclonal antibody, ZB4 or by inhibition of fas-ligand with NOK1. These antibodies were able to block CH11 and recombinant fas-ligand induced apoptosis, respectively. These results concur with those of other groups who have also failed to inhibit chemotherapy-induced apoptosis by various strategies including overexpression of the cowpox virus protein, CrmA,[17] which specifically inhibits fas-mediated signalling,[18] or use of antibodies directed against fas[19,20] and fas-ligand.[17] Although the myeloid leukaemia cell line tested (HL-60) was sensitive to the

Table 1. Percentage apoptosis in HL-60 cells induced by incubation with various chemotherapeutic agents after 24 hours

Control	Idarubicin 0.1μg/ml	Etoposide 2 μg/ml	F-ara-A 20 μM	Vinblastine 1 μg/ml
5.58 ± 1.97	39.6 ± 14.28	54.8 ± 3.44	44.1 ± 5.62	25.58 ± 2.72

Means of 5 independent experiments are given ± 95% confidence interval.

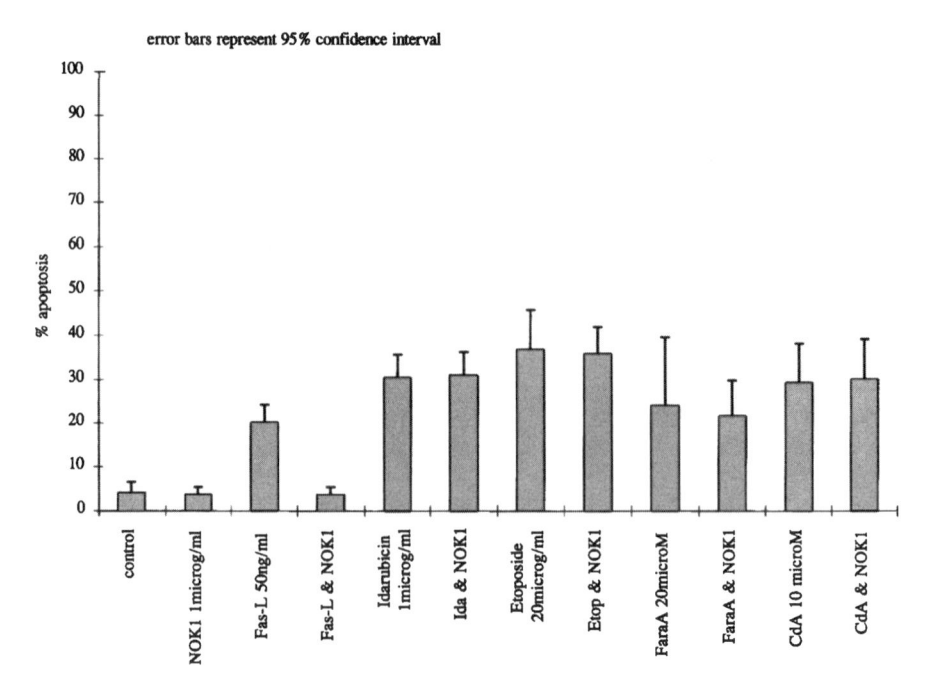

Figure 3a. Chemotherapy induced apoptosis and inhibition of fas-ligand with NOK-1 in CEM at 24 hours. Results are from 3 independent experiments.

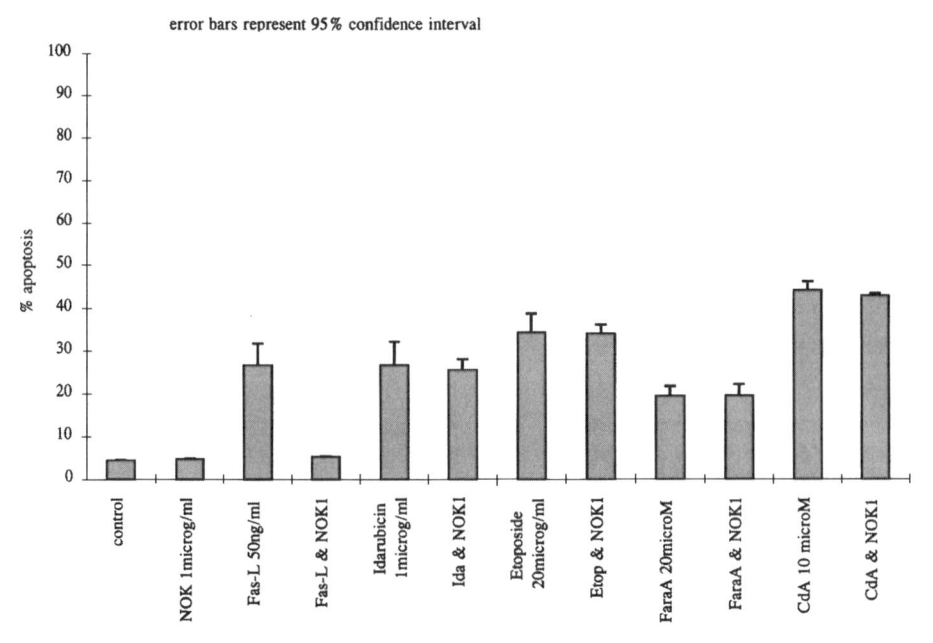

Figure 3b. Chemotherapy induced apoptosis and inhibition of fas-ligand with NOK-1 in CEM/VLB100 at 24 hours. Results are from 3 independent experiments.

Table 2. Percentage apoptosis in HL-60 cells induced by incubation with CH11 after 24 hours

Control	CH11 100ng/ml
8.8 ± 0.93	9.5 ± 0.4

Means of 3 independent experiments are given ± 95% confidence interval.

induction of apoptosis by chemotherapeutic agents, HL-60 cells were not sensitive to fas-ligation. CD95 has been shown to be expressed on a variety of cell lines however the majority of myeloid derived lines which express fas are resistant to anti-fas antibody-induced cell death,[21] suggesting that the fas receptor is non-functional or that the apoptotic pathway downstream of fas is defective in these cells. It has been suggested that CD95-mediated apoptosis in hepatoma cells is dependent on p53 activation[16] and it is known that HL-60 cells do not express p53;[22] failure of p53 expression might, therefore explain the lack of response to fas-ligation in HL-60 cells. There are conflicting reports on a correlation between sensitivity to fas-ligation and chemotherapy-induced apoptosis; Landowski and co-workers found that human myeloma (8226) and CEM cells selected for resistance to anthracenes, doxorubicin or mitoxantrone were also resistant to fas-mediated apoptosis[23] but Eischen and colleagues found that fas-resistant Jurkat cells underwent apoptosis that was indistinguishable from that of fas-sensitive parental cells after treatment with a wide range of chemotherapeutic agents.[20] In our experiments, the mdr1-expressing CEM/VLB100 cells were found to be at least as sensitive to fas-ligand and slightly more sensitive to fas-induced apoptosis as the parental CEM cells. At the relatively high doses of chemotherapy used, there was no significant difference in sensitivity to apoptosis in the two cell lines with the exception of CdA-treated CEM/VLB100 cells which were more sensitive than the parental CEM cells; CdA is not affected by the p-glycoprotein drug efflux pump.

It is becoming clear that there is unlikely to be one common means of activation of apoptosis by all chemotherapeutic agents in all malignant cells. It is also possible that differing mechanisms of activation will have varying importance at different drug dose levels. Despite this apparent complexity, increased understanding of the apoptotic "network" is likely to allow further therapeutic options in the treatment of malignancy.

ACKNOWLEDGMENTS

Deborah Richardson was a Leukaemia Research Fund Clinical Training Fellow, 1996–1997 and is grateful for their support. The following have generously given their support and advice; Sunira Patel, Tim Milne, Dr. Marion Macey and Dr. Denise Syndercombe-Court. I also wish to thank my medical colleagues and friends, for their patience, encouragement and forbearance, in particular, Drs. Steve Johnson, Juliet Mills, Vinod Parameswaran and Louise Hendry.

REFERENCES

1. Dive C, Wyllie AH. Apoptosis and cancer chemotherapy. In: Hickman JA, Tritton TR, eds. Cancer Chemotherapy. Oxford: Blackwell Scientific Publications; 1993:21–55.

2. Dive C, Hickman JA. Drug-target interactions: only the first step in the commitment to a programmed cell death? Br J Cancer. 1991, 64,192–196.
3. Kaufmann SH, Desnoyers S, Ottaviano Y, Davidson NE, Poirier GG. Specific proteolytic cleavage of poly(ADP-ribose) polymerase: an early marker of chemotherapy-induced apoptosis. Cancer Res. 1993, 53(17),3976–85.
4. Nagata S. Apoptosis by death factor. Cell. 1997, 88,355–365.
5. Krammer PH, Dhein J, Walczak H, Behrmann I, Mariani S, Matiba B, Fath M, Daniel PT, Knipping E, Westendorp MO, Stricker K, Bäumler C, Hellbardt S, Germer M, Peter ME, Debatin K-M. The role of APO-1-mediated apoptosis in the immune system. Immunol Rev. 1994, 142,175–191.
6. Schlegel J, Peters I, Orrenius S, Miller DK, Thornberry NA, Yamin TT, Nicholson DW. CPP32/apopain is a key interleukin 1 beta converting enzyme-like protease involved in Fas-mediated apoptosis. J Biol Chem. 1996, 271(4),1841–4.
7. Hasegawa J, Kamada S, Kamiike W, Shimizu S, Imazu T, Matsuda H, Tsujimoto Y. Involvement of CPP32/Yama(-like) proteases in Fas-mediated apoptosis. Cancer Res. 1996, 56(8),1713–8.
8. Casiano CA, Martin SJ, Green DR, Tan EM. Selective cleavage of nuclear autoantigens during CD95 (fas/APO-1)-mediated T cell apoptosis. J Exp Med. 1996, 184,765–770.
9. Debatin K-M, Goldmann CK, Bamford R, Waldmann TA, Krammer PH. Monoclonal antibody-mediated apoptosis in adult T-cell leukaemia. Lancet. 1990, 335,497–500.
10. Debatin K-M, Goldmann CK, Waldmann TA, Krammer PH. APO-1-induced apoptosis of leukemia cells from patients with adult T-cell leukaemia. Blood. 1993, 81,2972–2977.
11. Nonomura N, Miki T, Yokoyama M, Imazu T, Takada T, Takeuchi S, Kanno N, Nishimura K, Kojima Y, Okuyama A. Fas/APO-1-mediated apoptosis of human renal cell carcinoma. Biochem Biophys Res Commun. 1996, 229,945–951.
12. Friesen C, Herr I, Kramer PH, Debatin K-M. Involvement of the CD95 (APO-1/Fas) receptor/ligand system in drug-induced apoptosis in leukemia cells. Nature Med. 1996, 2,574–577.
13. Beck WT, Mueller TJ, Tanzer LR. Altered surface membrane glycoproteins in vinca alkaloid-resistant human leukemic lymphoblasts. Cancer Res. 1979, 39(6),2070–6.
14. Kartner N, Riordan JR, Ling V. Cell surface p-glycoprotein is associated with multidrug resistance in mammalian cell lines. Science. 1983, 221,1285–8.
15. Darzynkiewicz Z, Bruno S, Del Bino G, Gorczyca W, Hotz MA, Lassota P, Traganos F. Features of apoptotic cells measured by flow cytometry. Cytometry. 1992, 13,795–808.
16. Muller M, Strand S, Hug H, Heinemann EM, Walczak H, Hofmann WJ, Stremmel W, Krammer PH, Galle PR. Drug-induced apoptosis in hepatoma cells is mediated by the CD95 (APO-1/Fas) receptor/ligand system and involves activation of wild-type p53. J Clin Invest. 1997, 99(3),403–13.
17. Villunger A, Egle A, Kos M, Hartmann BL, Geley S, Kofler R, Greil R. Drug-induced apoptosis is associated with enhanced Fas (Apo-1/CD95) ligand expression but occurs independently of Fas (Apo-1/CD95) signaling in human T-acute lymphatic leukemia cells. Cancer Res. 1997, 57(16),3331–4.
18. Tewari M, Dixit M. Fas- and tumour necrosis factor-induced apoptosis is inhibited by the cowpox virus *crmA* gene product. J Biol Chem. 1995, 270,3255–3260.
19. Gamen S, Anel A, Lasierra P, Alava MA, Martinezlorenzo MJ, Pineiro A, Naval J. Doxorubicin-induced apoptosis in human T-cell leukemia is mediated by caspase-3 activation in a fas-independent way. FEBS Lett. 1997, 417(3),360–364.
20. Eischen CM, Kottke TJ, Martins LM, Basi GS, Tung JS, Earnshaw WC, Leibson PJ, Kaufmann SH. Comparison of apoptosis in wild-type and Fas-resistant cells: chemotherapy-induced apoptosis is not dependent on Fas/Fas ligand interactions. Blood. 1997, 90(3),935–43.
21. Dirks W, Schöne S, Uphoff C, Quentmeier H, Pradella S, Drexler HG. Expression and function of CD95 (fas/apo-1) in leukaemia-lymphoma tumour lines. Br J Haematol. 1997, 96,584–593.
22. Wolf D, Rotter V. Major deletions in the gene encoding the p53 tumor antigen cause lack of p53 expression in HL-60 cells. Proc Natl Acad Sci USA. 1985, 82,790–794.
23. Landowski TH, Gleason-Guzman MC, Dalton WS. Selection for drug resistance results in resistance to fas-mediated apoptosis. Blood. 1997, 89(6),1854–1861.

EFFECTS OF PARP INHIBITION ON DRUG AND FAS-INDUCED APOPTOSIS IN LEUKAEMIC CELLS

Deborah S, Richardson,[*] Paul D. Allen, Stephen M. Kelsey, and Adrian C. Newland

Department of Haematology
St. Bartholomew's and Royal London School of Medicine, United Kingdom

1. ABSTRACT

Poly (ADP-ribose) polymerase (PARP) is activated following binding to DNA strand breaks and is cleaved in cells undergoing apoptosis. Work predominantly in murine systems has suggested that inhibitors of PARP might potentiate the effects of chemotherapeutic agents and be used as adjuncts to cancer therapy. Therefore, we studied the role of PARP in drug-induced apoptosis in HL-60, myeloid leukaemia cells and found that pre-treatment with 3-aminobenzamide (3AB) or 6(5H)- phenanthridinone, inhibitors of PARP, resulted in resistance to, rather than potentiation of apoptotic death induced by DNA-damaging agents, idarubicin, etoposide and fludarabine, as determined by flow cytometry, following propidium iodide staining. 3AB treated CEM/VLB100, mdr-expressing human lymphoblastic leukaemia cells were also found to be more resistant to idarubicin compared to cells treated with idarubicin alone, however, apoptosis was not reduced in parental CCRF-CEM cells under the same conditions. Similar results were obtained using agents with primary modes of action which do not involve DNA damage, vinblastine and a fas-ligating antibody (CH11). The precise role of PARP has yet to be defined but might involve effects on cell cycle progression.

We conclude that PARP activation appears to be involved in apoptosis in certain leukaemic cell lines and that these effects are independent of lineage or p-glycoprotein. Constitutive failure to activate PARP might be responsible for conferring resistance to apoptosis.

---

[*] Communicating author: Dr. Deborah Richardson. Address for communication: Department of Haematology, Royal London Hospital, Whitechapel Road, London E1 1BB UK. Telephone: 00 44 171 377 7000, Fax: 00 44 171 377 7016 E-mail: d.s.richardson@mds.qmw.ac.uk

Drug Resistance in Leukemia and Lymphoma III, edited by Kaspers *et al.*
Kluwer Academic / Plenum Publishers, New York, 1999.

2. INTRODUCTION

ADP-ribosylation reactions were first described more than 30 years ago (reviewed[1]) but their role has yet to be fully understood. The metalloenzyme, PARP catalyses ADP-ribosylation of various proteins, including itself, by transfer of ADP-ribose from its substrate NAD⁺, to form ADP-ribose polymers which are subsequently degraded by poly(ADP-ribose) glycohydrolase.[2] The enzyme thus participates in post-translational self-modification (automodification) and heteromodification of other chromatin proteins.[3,4] PARP consists of three main functional elements,[5] a zinc finger DNA-binding domain,[6] an auto modification zone[7] and a carboxyl terminal catalytic domain[8] and is activated by DNA strand breaks.[4,9–11] Evidence points to a role for PARP in the cellular response to DNA damage.[12,13] It has been shown that PARP can bind melphalan-damaged DNA[14] and early reports suggested that PARP participates in repair of alkylation-induced damage to DNA by enhancement of DNA polymerase activity.[15] PARP may also activate DNA ligase activity.[16] Various chemical inhibitors of PARP have been described[17–20] and in L1210, murine leukaemia cells, treatment with 3AB prevented removal of single-strand breaks.[21] An alternative approach, using antisense RNA in HeLa cells showed that depletion of PARP resulted in a delay in DNA strand break rejoining, however the authors state that DNA repair capacity was re-established at a later time, indicating that the nuclear enzyme concentration may exceed the requirement for DNA repair.[22] More recent work has suggested that unmodified PARP molecules bind tightly to DNA strand breaks and then automodification of PARP allows the enzyme to be released and access for DNA repair enzymes to occur.[23] Inhibitors of PARP have been shown to potentiate the cytotoxicity of alkylating agents,[24–28] γ-irradiation,[24] bleomycin[29] and dexamethasone[30] in Chinese hamster ovary (CHO) and murine leukaemia and thymocyte cells. CHO mutants with decreased PARP activity have increased sensitivity to killing by alkylating agents.[31] Such reports have stimulated interest in modification of PARP activity as a means of potentiating chemotherapy and irradiation in the treatment of human malignancies;[32,33] with this in mind we investigated the effect of incubation with inhibitors of PARP on human leukaemia cells treated with various chemotherapeutic agents.

3. MATERIALS AND METHODS

3.1. Reagents

3AB and 6(5H)-phenanthridinone (6PA) were obtained from Sigma-Aldrich Company (Poole, Dorset, UK). 3AB was dissolved in sterile water and 6PA in dimethyl sulphoxide (DMSO) to achieve stock concentrations of 100mM and 10mM respectively. The final concentration of DMSO in culture did not exceed 0.5%. The following cytotoxic agents were used: idarubicin (Pharmacia, Milton Keynes, UK), etoposide (Bristol Myers Pharmaceuticals, Middlesex, UK.), vinblastine (David Bull Laboratories, Warwick, UK). Fludarabine desphosphate (F-ara-A) was kindly given by Prof. Varsha Gandhi of MD Anderson Cancer Center, Texas, USA and Schering AG, Berlin, Germany. Anti-Fas (CD95), clone CH-11 was obtained from Immunotech, Marseille, France.

3.2. Cell Lines and Culture Conditions

The following cell lines were used in this study; HL60, human myeloid leukaemia cells, obtained from the European Collection of Animal Cell Cultures (Salisbury, UK);

CCRF-CEM, human T-lymphoblastic leukaemia cell line and its vinblastine-induced multidrug-resistant (MDR) counterpart, CEM/VLB100.[34,35] Cells were cultured in RPMI 1640 (Sigma), supplemented with 10% heat-inactivated fetal calf serum (Sigma), 2.0mM L-glutamine (Sigma), 100U/ml penicillin and 100µg/ml streptomycin at 37°C in a 5% CO2 incubator. Cells were maintained at 2–7 × 10^5 cells/ml by subculture.

3.3. Incubation of Cells with 3AB or 6PA and Cytotoxic Agents

Cells in exponential growth were seeded at 1 × 10^6/ml in 24 well plates (Costar) in 1ml volumes of supplemented medium. Cells were incubated with either 3AB at concentrations of 0, 1 or 5mM or 6PA at concentrations of 0 or 50 µM. Control wells with DMSO 0.5% alone, were also used. After 1 hour, various chemotherapeutic agents were added to the wells: idarubicin (0.01–1µg/ml), etoposide (0.2–20 µg/ml), vinblastine (0.01–1 µg/ml) or F-ara-A (1,10 or 20 µM). Plates included control wells without cytotoxic drug. After 24–48 hours 100 µl aliquots of cells were harvested and analysed for cell-cycle distribution and apoptosis.

3.4. Incubation with CH-11

Cells were also incubated with 6PA (0 or 50 µM) prior to the addition of 100ng/ml CH-11 for 24 hours. Cells were then harvested and analysed as below.

3.5. Analysis of Apoptosis and Cell-Cycle Profile

Determination of apoptotic fraction and cell cycle analysis was performed by flow cytometry. Harvested cells were washed with Hanks' balanced salt solution (HBSS) and made permeable by re-suspension in ice-cold 70% ethanol and incubation at 4°C for 30 minutes. The cells were then washed and re-suspended in 1ml of HBSS containing 50 µg/ml propidium iodide and 200 µg/ml RNase type IIIA (Sigma). Cells were analysed 30 minutes after processing, using an EPICS Elite cytometer (Coulter Electronics, Luton, UK). Pulse processing using peak channel versus integral red channel signal was used to discriminate doublet and aggregated cells from single, diploid cells and to exclude debris. G0/G1, S and G2M fractions were identified from the resulting cell-cycle profiles and the percentage apoptotic cells in each sample was measured from the sub-G0/G1 fraction.[36]

3.6. Statistical Analysis

Results were analysed using the paired t-test.

4. RESULTS

4.1. 3AB Reduces Chemotherapy-Induced Apoptosis in HL60 and CEM/VLB100 Cells But Not Parental CEM

In HL60 cells, pre-treatment with 1 or 5mM 3AB reduced the percentage of cells undergoing apoptosis when subsequently treated with idarubicin or etoposide compared with those treated with cytotoxic agent alone. 3AB only produced a significant reduction in apoptosis in HL60 exposed to F-ara-A at the higher dose (5mM) (Figure 2). In cells treated with 3AB and idarubicin (Figure 3a and b) or etoposide, an increase in the S phase and G2M fractions was seen but in those treated with 3AB and F-ara-A, an increase in (G0)G1 cells occurred (Figure 4).

In contrast, no inhibition of apoptosis occurred in 3AB and idarubicin or etoposide-treated parental CEM cells and only a slight reduction of apoptosis in the F-ara-A treated CEM cells. The mdr-expressing CEM/VLB100 cells were more resistant to idarubicin and F-ara-A when pre-treated with 3AB but no effect was seen in etoposide treated cells (Table 1).

4.2. Pre-Treatment with 3AB Modifies the Induction of Apoptosis in Cells Incubated with the Microtubule-Disrupting Agent, Vinblastine

In HL60 cells treated with 3AB, at 24 hours apoptosis was reduced and this was associated with an increase in cells in the G2M phase of the cell cycle (Figure 5). In vinblastine-treated CEM cells at 48 hours, 3AB slightly reduced the percentage of cells undergoing apoptosis and again, a corresponding increase in G2M cells was seen. This effect was more marked in CEM/VLB100 cells (Figure 6).

4.3. Effects of Pre-Treatment with 6PA on Chemotherapy-Induced Apoptosis

HL60 cells pre-treated with 6PA were rendered more resistant to idarubicin, F-ara-A and vinblastine (Figure 7).

4.4. Effects of 6PA on CH-11 Induced Apoptosis

HL60 cells are resistant to the induction of apoptosis by CH-11. In CEM cells, 6PA has no effect on CH-11 induced apoptosis but in CEM/VLB100, apoptosis was reduced (Figure 8).

5. DISCUSSION

This study has shown that in HL-60 human myeloid leukaemia cells and CEM/VLB100 mdr-positive T-lymphoblastic leukaemia cells, treatment with a PARP in-

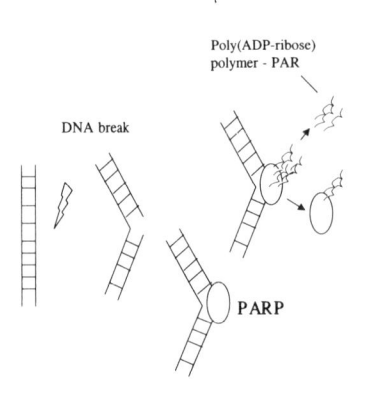

Figure 1. Poly(ADP-ribose) polymer (PAR) formation following DNA damage. Automodification of the PARP molecule occurs with subsequent release of PARP from the DNA strand break.

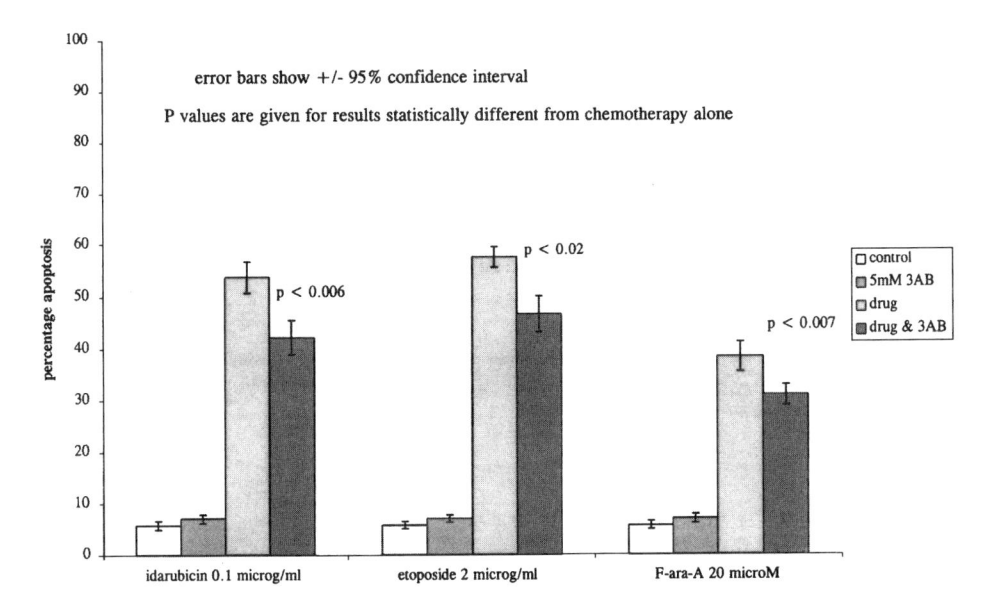

Figure 2. Effect of 3AB pre-treatment on chemotherapy-induced apoptosis in HL60. Results are from 4 independent experiments.

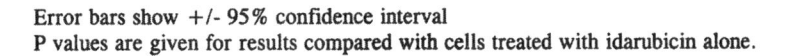

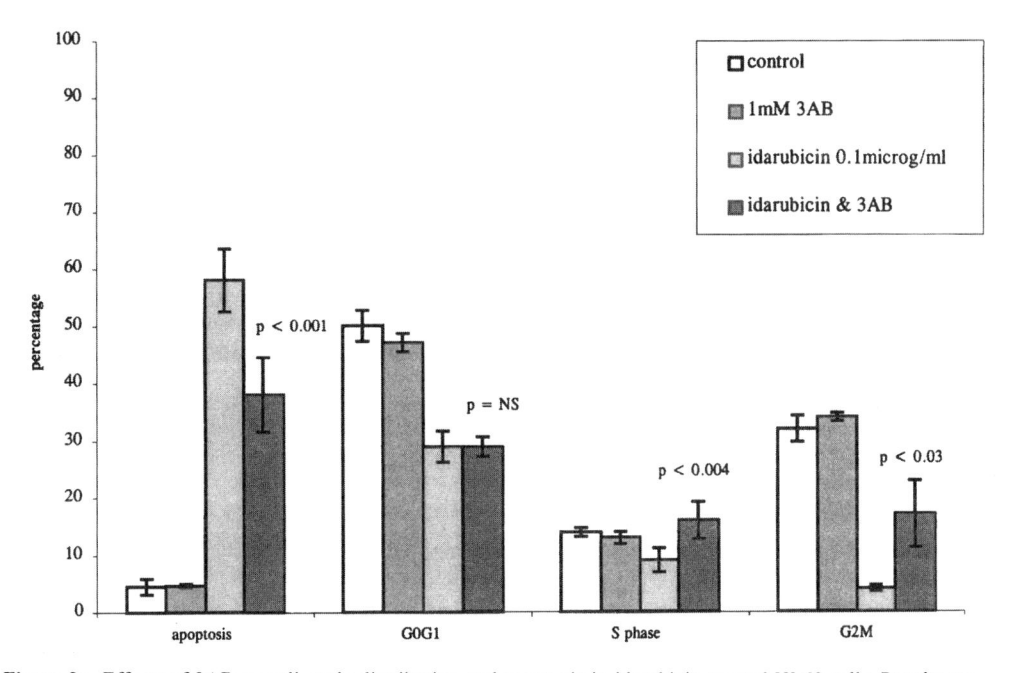

Figure 3a. Effects of 3AB on cell cycle distribution and apoptosis in idarubicin-treated HL60 cells. Results are from 4 independent experiments.

Figure 3b. Cell cycle profiles for idarubicin-treated HL60 cells.

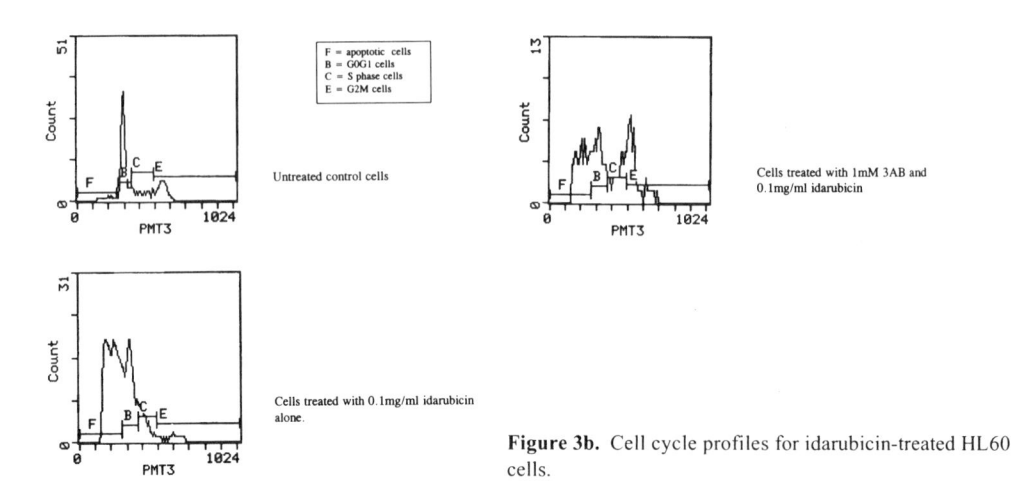

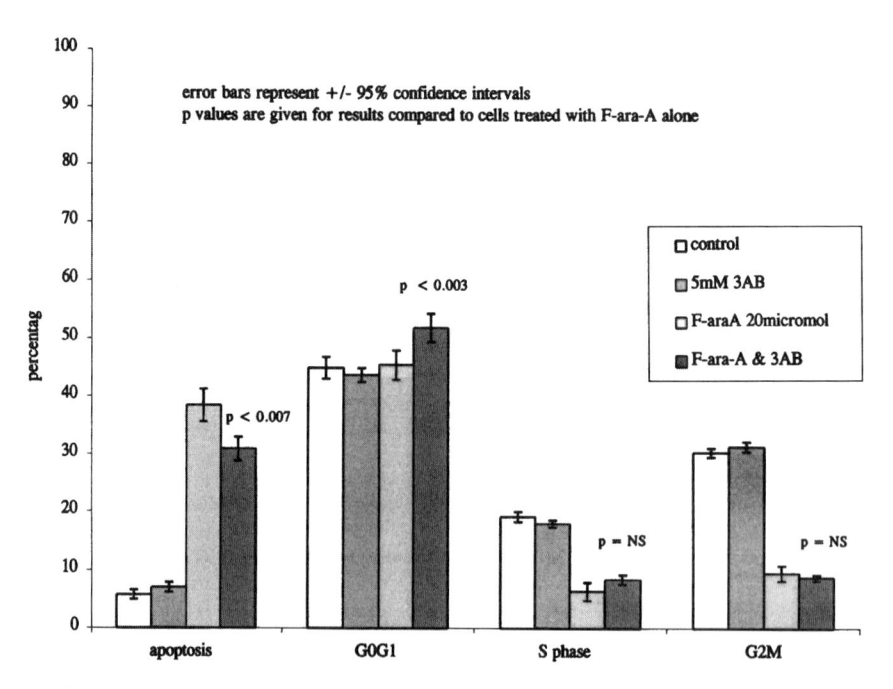

Figure 4. Effects of 3AB on cell cycle distribution and apoptosis in F-ara-A treated HL60 cells. Results are from 4 independent experiments. Results are from 4 independent experiments.

Table 1. Induction of apoptosis in CEM and CEM/VLB100 by various chemotherapeutic agents with and without pre-treatment with 3AB

	Control	1mM 3AB	5mM 3AB	Drug	Drug & 1mM 3AB	Drug & 5mM 3AB
CEM						
Idarubicin 1µg/ml	4.2 ± 1.1	3.6 ± 0.8	3.8 ± 0.8	27.1 ± 2.6	31.1 ± 4.4	28.0 ± 1.2
Etoposide 20µg/ml	4.2 ± 1.1	3.6 ± 0.8	3.8 ± 0.8	46.4 ± 7.0	47.7 ± 3.3	44.3 ± 3.1
F-ara-A 20µM	5.3 ± 1.9	4.6 ± 1.9	3.8 ± 0.8	32.6 ± 1.7	29.7 ± 1.9	24.1 ± 3.5
CEM/VLB100						
Idarubicin 1µg/ml	5.1 ± 0.9	4.4 ± 0.9	5.0 ± 1.6	39.1 ± 2.8	29.6 ± 1.7	22.3 ± 4.9
Etoposide 20µg/ml	5.1 ± 0.9	4.4 ± 0.9	5.0 ± 1.6	46.5 ± 4.9	45.1 ± 2.2	38.4 ± 4.3
F-ara-A 20µM	5.1 ± 0.9	4.4 ± 0.9	5.0 ± 1.6	40.7 ± 3.2	33.0 ± 4.6	27.3 ± 2.4

Results are the mean of 4 independent experiments +/- 95% confidence interval.

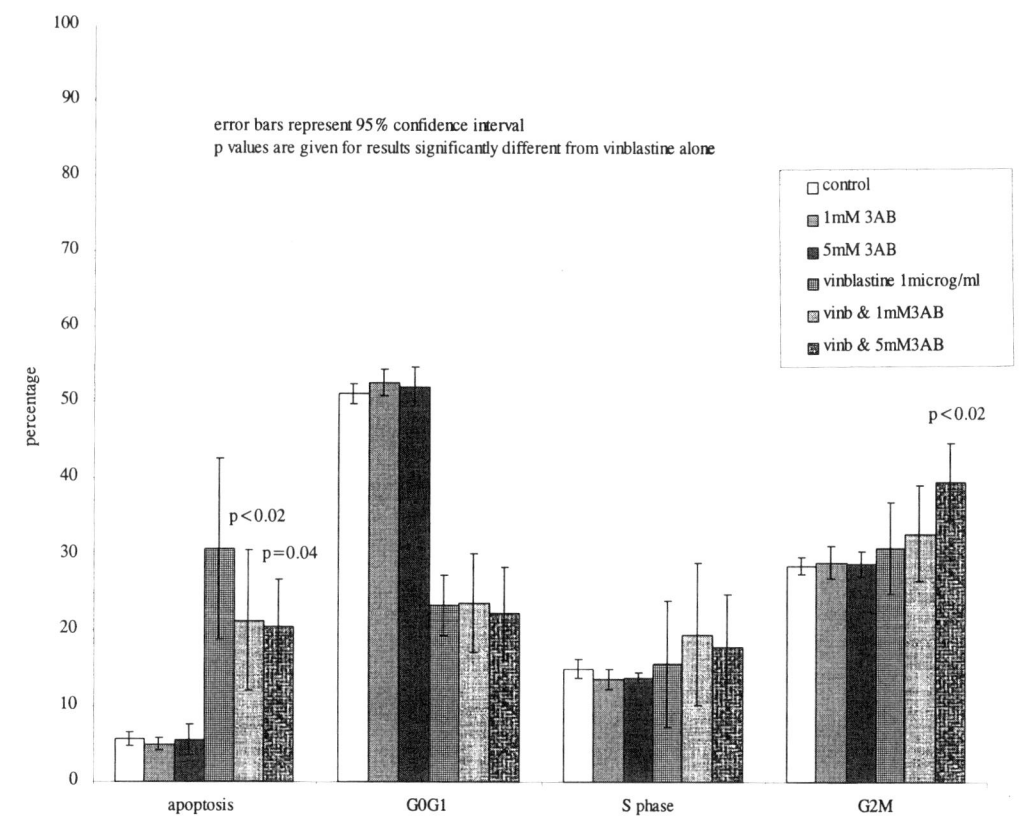

Figure 5. Effects of 3AB on vinblastine-treated HL60 cells at 24 hours. Results are from 4 independent experiments.

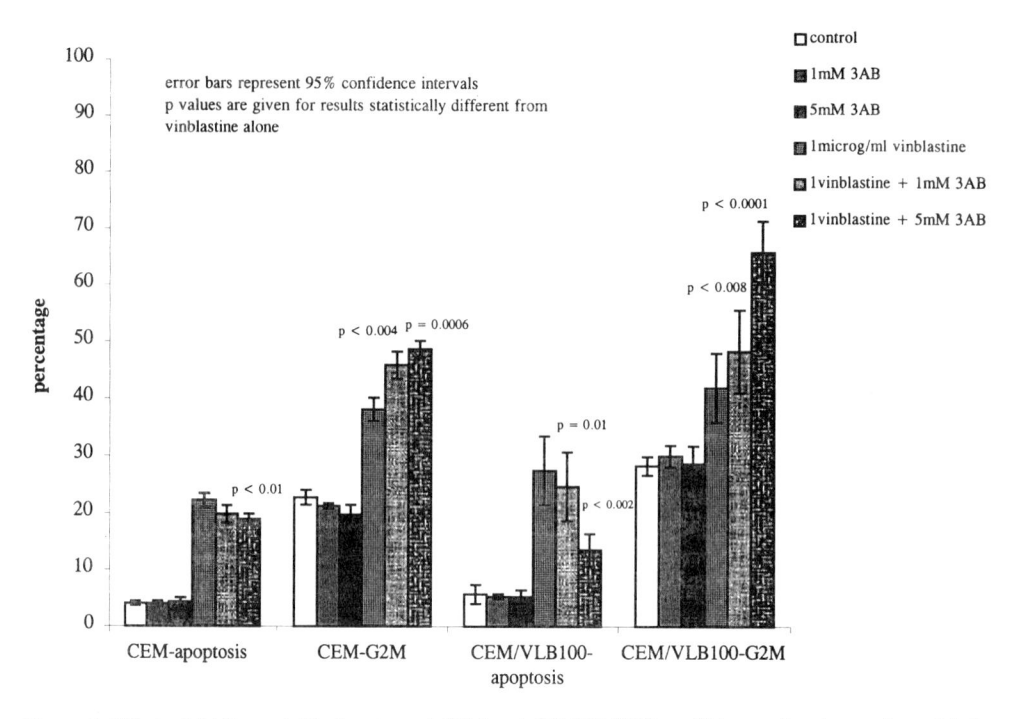

Figure 6. Effect of 3AB on vinblastine-treated CEM and CEM/VLB100 at 48 hours. Results are from 4 independent experiments.

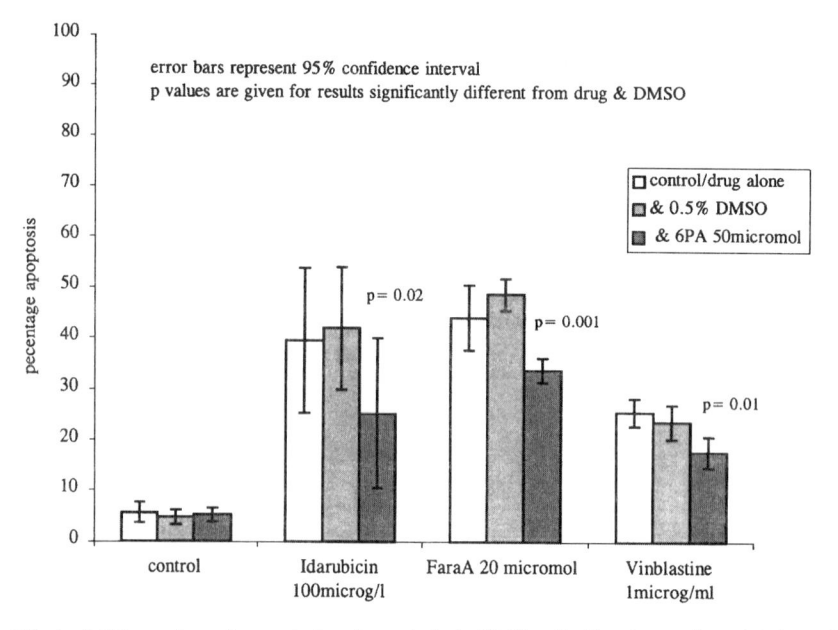

Figure 7. Effect of 6PA on chemotherapy-induced apoptosis in HL60 cells. Results are from 4 independent experiments.

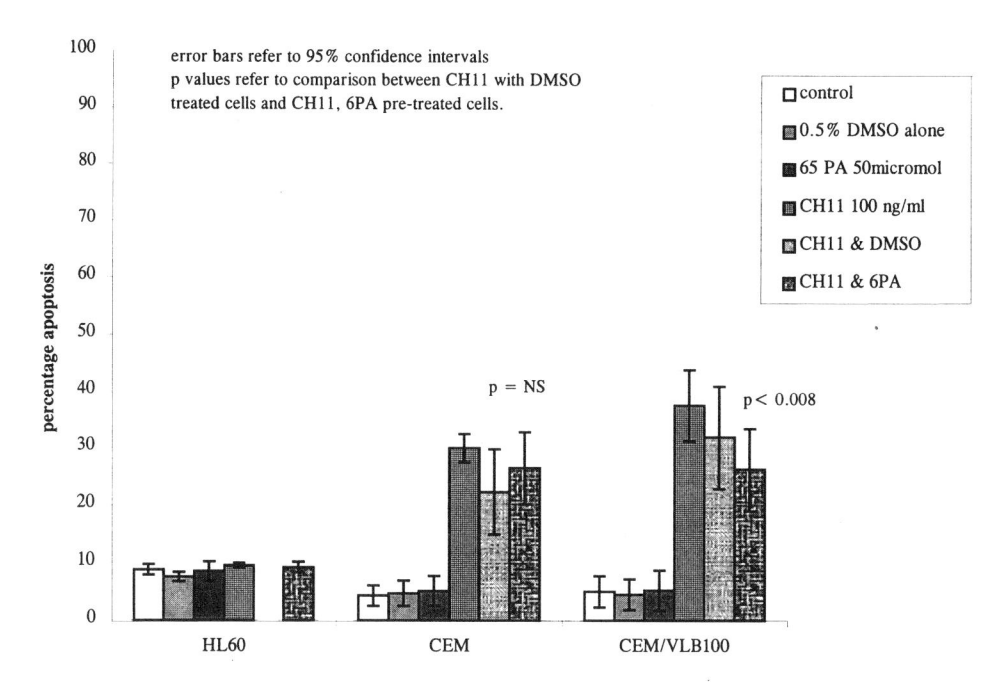

[Figure 8 chart: bar graph showing percentage apoptosis for HL60, CEM, and CEM/VLB100 cell lines with conditions: control, 0.5% DMSO alone, 65 PA 50micromol, CH11 100 ng/ml, CH11 & DMSO, CH11 & 6PA. Annotations: "error bars refer to 95% confidence intervals; p values refer to comparison between CH11 with DMSO treated cells and CH11, 6PA pre-treated cells." p = NS for CEM; p < 0.008 for CEM/VLB100.]

Figure 8. Effect of 6PA on CH11-treated cells. Results are from 4 independent experiments.

hibitor, 3AB, increases resistance rather than sensitivity to apoptosis induced by the DNA-damaging chemotherapeutic agents, etoposide, idarubicin and F-ara-A to varying degrees. 3AB has previously been shown to inhibit doxorubicin-induced HL-60 cell death, as determined by trypan blue exclusion although DNA strand break frequency was not altered,[37] suggesting that in this cell line, PARP is not involved in anthracycline-induced DNA damage repair. A conflicting report from Farzaneh and co-workers concluded that 3AB retarded repair of strand breaks induced by γ-irradiation in this cell line.[38] In CEM parental cells, however, apart from a slight reduction in F-ara-A induced apoptosis, little modulation of resistance was seen, suggesting that this effect is cell line specific; this concurs with an earlier report by Kubota and co-workers in etoposide-treated human leukaemia cells.[39] Tanaka describes apoptosis inducers in HL-60 cells that are PARP-inhibitor responsive and insensitive; the latter include teniposide and camptothecin. This report also described down-regulation of PARP activity, which occurred following DMSO, and retinoic acid induced differentiation of HL-60 cells and resulted in insensitivity to apoptosis inducers.[40]

Concerns have been expressed with respect to the specificity of 3AB and its possible effects on other metabolic pathways at the millimolar concentrations required to produce an effect on sensitivity to apoptosis induction.[41] We therefore confirmed our results in HL-60 cells with a more specific and potent inhibitor of PARP, 6PA which is active at micromolar concentrations.[42,43]

It has been shown that in etoposide[44] and doxorubicin-treated[37] HL-60 cells, cell death was preceded by a reduction in NAD and ATP levels. As PARP uses NAD as a substrate, it has been suggested that the protective effect of PARP inhibitors might be explained by prevention of ATP and therefore critical energy depletion.[45] However, nutritional depletion of NAD to undetectable levels in U937 and HL-60 cells rendered them completely resistant to apoptosis induced by tumour necrosis factor (TNF) or ultraviolet light.[46]

Initial reports suggested that PARP knockout mice developed normally but that about 30% of older mice developed epidermal hyperplasia. Mutant derived embryonic fibroblasts were able to repair DNA damage efficiently.[47] These observations negate an essential role for PARP in cell death or DNA repair. Further, Leist and colleagues showed that the susceptibility of liver cells from PARP knockout mice to CD95 or TNF was not modified.[48] In contrast, de Murcia reported that PARP knockout mice were particularly sensitive to treatment with an alkylating agent or γ-irradiation.[49] Results from experiments with knockout mice may have more relevance in elucidating a physiological role for PARP than understanding its function and the consequences of inhibition in human transformed or leukaemic cells.

Apoptosis, including that induced by chemotherapeutic agents, results in cleavage of PARP.[50] The protease identified as responsible for PARP cleavage is apopain or CPP32.[51-54] It has been proposed that the central function of CPP32 and its homologues is to cleave proteins, including PARP, which are essential for cellular repair.[55] We have shown that treatment with a PARP inhibitor increases resistance to vinblastine, a cytotoxic agent with a primary mode of action that does not involve DNA damage and also reduces apoptosis induced by the fas-ligating monoclonal antibody, CH11. In addition to the work of Tanaka,[40] these data are consistent with a more general role for PARP in the apoptotic pathway, possibly in signal transduction, although the exact point at which PARP might operate is unclear. Rosenthal has shown that poly(ADP-ribosyl)ation of nuclear proteins occurs early in the apoptotic pathway;[56] this suggests that modulation of PARP activity could potentially influence commitment to undergo apoptosis. PARP activity has recently been implicated in the regulation of p53 expression; PARP deficient cell lines exhibited a significant reduction in baseline p53 expression and activity.[57] This again suggests a role for PARP as a modulator in the apoptotic pathway, although clearly other mechanisms must operate in HL-60 cells that do not express functional p53.[58] Further work is required to clarify any potential role for PARP in the regulation of cell cycle checkpoints,[59] both p53 dependent and independent.

ACKNOWLEDGMENTS

Deborah Richardson was a Leukaemia Research Fund Clinical Training Fellow, 1996–1997 and is grateful for their support. The following have generously given their support and advice: Sunira Patel, Tim Milne, Dr. Marion Macey and Dr. Denise Syndercombe-Court. I also wish to thank my medical colleagues and friends, for their patience, encouragement and forbearance, in particular, Drs. Steve Johnson, Juliet Mills, Vinod Parameswaran and Louise Hendry.

REFERENCES

1. Sugimura T, Miwa M. Poly(ADP-ribose): historical perspective. Mol Cell Biochem. 1994, 138,5–12.
2. Brochu G, Duchaine C, Thibeault L, Lagueux J, Shah GM, Poirier GG. Mode of action of poly(ADP-ribose) glycohydrolase. Biochim Biophys Acta. 1994, 1219(2),342–50.
3. Naegeli H, Loetscher P, Althaus FR. Poly ADP-ribosylation of proteins. Processivity of a post-translational modification. J Biol Chem. 1989, 264(24),14382–5.

4. Lindahl T, Satoh MS, Poirier GG, Klungland A. Post-translational modification of poly(ADP-ribose) polymerase induced by DNA strand breaks. Trends Biochem Sci. 1995, 20(10),405–11.
5. de Murcia G, Schreiber V, Molinete M, Saulier B, Poch O, Masson M, Niedergang C, Menissier de Murcia J. Structure and function of poly(ADP-ribose) polymerase. Mol Cell Biochem. 1994, 138(1–2),15–24.
6. Ikejima M, Noguchi S, Yamashita R, Ogura T, Sugimura T, Gill D, Miwa M. The zinc fingers of human poly(ADP-ribose) polymerase are differentially required for the recognition of DNA breaks and nicks and the consequent enzyme activation. J Biol Chem. 1990, 265(35),21907–21913.
7. Buki KG, Bauer PI, Hakam A, Kun E. Identification of domains of poly(ADP-ribose) polymerase for protein binding and self-association. J Biol Chem. 1995, 270(7),3370–7.
8. Simonin F, Poch O, Delarue M, de Murcia G. Identification of potential active-site residues in the human poly(ADP-ribose) polymerase. J Biol Chem. 1993, 268(12),8529–35.
9. Shall S. The function of poly(ADP-ribosylation) in DNA breakage and rejoining. Mol Cell Biochem. 1994, 138,71–75.
10. Satoh MS, Poirier GG, Lindahl T. Dual function for poly(ADP-ribose) synthesis in response to DNA strand breakage. Biochemistry. 1994, 33(23),7099–106.
11. de Murcia G, Menissier de Murcia J. Poly(ADP-ribose) polymerase: a molecular nick-sensor. Trends Biochem Sci. 1994, 19(4),172–6.
12. Berger NA. Poly(ADP-ribose) in the cellular response to DNA damage. Radiation Res. 1985, 101(1),4–15.
13. Cleaver J, Morgan W. Poly(ADP-ribose)polymerase: a perplexing participant in cellular responses to DNA breakage. Mutation Res. 1991, 257,1–18.
14. Bramson J, Prévost J, Malapetsa A, Noë A, Poirier G, DesNoyers S, Alaoui-Jamali M, Panasci L. Poly(ADP-ribose) polymerase can bind melphalan damaged DNA. Cancer Res. 1993, 53,5370–5373.
15. Smulson M, Schein P, Mullins D, Sudhakar S. A putative role for nicotinamide adenine dinucleotide-promoted nuclear protein modificaton in the antitumour activity of N-methyl-N-nitrosurea. Cancer Res 1977, 37,3006–3012.
16. Creissen D, Shall S. Regulation of DNA ligase activity by poly(ADP-ribose). Nature. 1982, 296(271–272).
17. Purnell M, Whish W. Novel inhibitors of Poly(ADP-ribose) synthetase. Biochem J. 1980, 185,775–777.
18. Rankin P, Jacobson E, Benjamin R, Moss J, Jacobson M. Quantitative studies of inhibitors of ADP-ribosylation in vitro and in vivo. J Biol Chem. 1989, 264(8),4312–4317.
19. Banasik M, Komura H, Shimoyama M, Ueda K. Specific inhibitors of poly(ADP-ribose) synthetase and mono(ADP-ribosyl) transferase. J Biol Chem. 1992, 267(3),1569–1575.
20. Sestili P, Spadoni G, Balsamini C, Scovassi I, Cattabeni F, Duranti E, Cantoni O, Higgins D, Thomson C. Structural requirements for inhibitors of poly(ADP-ribose) polymerase. J Cancer Res Clin Oncol. 1990, 116,615–622.
21. Durkacz BW, Omidiji O, Gray DA, Shall S. (ADP-ribose)n participates in DNA excision repair. Nature. 1980, 283(5747),593–6.
22. Ding R, Pommier Y, Kang V, Smulson M. Depletion of poly(ADP-ribose) polymerase by antisense RNA expression results in a delay in DNA strand break rejoining. J Biol Chem. 1991, 267(18),12804–12812.
23. Satoh MS, Lindahl T. Role of poly(ADP-ribose) formation in DNA repair. Nature. 1992, 356(6367),356–8.
24. Nduka N, Skidmore J, Shall S. The enhancement of cytotoxicity of N-methyl-N-nitrosurea and of γ-radiation by inhibitors of poly(ADP-ribose) polymerase. Eur J Biochem. 1980, 105,525–530.
25. Brown D, Horsman M, Hirst D, Brown J. Enhancement of melphalan cytotoxicity in vivo and in vitro by inhibitors of poly (ADP-ribose) polymers. Int J Radiation Oncology. 1984, 10,1665–1668.
26. August E, Cooper D, Prusoff W. Inhibition of poly(adenosine diphosphate-ribose) polymerase by thymidine and thymidine analogues in L1210 cells and its relationship to the potentiation of the antitumour activity of 1,3-bis(2-chloroethyl)-1-nitrosurea but not of 3'-[3-(2-chloroethyl)-3-nitrosoureido]-3'-deoxythymidine. Cancer Res. 1991, 51,1586–1590.
27. Boulton S, Pemberton L, Porteous J, Curtin N, Griffin R, Golding B, Durkacz B. Potentiation of temozolomide-induced cytotoxicity: a comparative study of the biological effects of poly(ADP-ribose) polymerase inhibitors. Br J Cancer. 1995, 1995(72),849–856.
28. Sebolt-Leopold J, Scavone S. Enhancement of alkylating agent activity in vitro by PD 128763, a potent poly(ADP-ribose) synthetase inhibitor. Int J Radiation Oncology Biol Phys. 1992, 22,619–621.
29. Huet J, Laval F. Potentiation of cell killing by inhibitors of poly(adenosine diphosphate-ribose) synthesis in bleomycin-treated Chinese hamster ovary cells. Cancer Res. 1985, 45(3),987–91.
30. Hoshino J, Koeppel C, Westhäuser E. 3-aminobenzamide enhances dexamethasone-mediated mouse thymocyte depletion in vivo: implication for a role of poly ADP-rbosylation in the negative selection of immature thymocytes. Biochim Biophys Acta. 1994, 1201,516–522.
31. Witmer M, Aboul-Ela N, Jacobson M, Stamato T. Increased sensitivity to DNA-alkylating agents in CHO mutants with decreased poly(ADP-ribose) polymerase activity. Mutation Res. 1994, 314,249–260.

32. Judson I, Threadgill M. Poly(ADP-ribosylation) as target for cancer chemotherapy. Lancet. 1993, 342(8872),632.
33. Griffin RJ, Curtin NJ, Newell DR, Golding BT, Durkacz BW, Calvert AH. The role of inhibitors of poly(ADP-ribose) polymerase as resistance-modifying agents in cancer therapy. Biochimie. 1995, 77(6),408–22.
34. Beck WT, Mueller TJ, Tanzer LR. Altered surface membrane glycoproteins in vinca alkaloid-resistant human leukemic lymphoblasts. Cancer Res. 1979, 39(6),2070–6.
35. Kartner N, Riordan JR, Ling V. Cell surface p-glycoprotein is associated with multidrug resistance in mammalian cell lines. Science. 1983, 221,1285–8.
36. Darzynkiewicz Z, Bruno S, Del Bino G, Gorczyca W, Hotz MA, Lassota P, Traganos F. Features of apoptotic cells measured by flow cytometry. Cytometry. 1992, 13,795–808.
37. Tanizawa A, Kubota M, Takimoto T, Akiyama Y, Seto S, Kiriyama Y, Mikawa H. Prevention of adriamycin-induced interphase death by 3-aminobenzamide and nicotinamide in a human promyelocytic leukemia cell line. Biochem Biophys Res Commun. 1987, 144(2),1031–1036.
38. Farzaneh F, Feon S, Lebby R, Brill D, David J-C, Shall S. DNA repair in human promyelocytic cell line, HL-60. Nucleic Acids Res. 1987, 15(8),3503–3513.
39. Kubota M, Tanizawa A, Hashimoto H, Shimizu T, Takimoto T, Kitoh T, Akiyama Y, Mikawa H. Cell type dependent activation of poly (ADP-ribose) synthesis following treatment with etoposide. Leuk Res. 1990, 14(4),371–5.
40. Tanaka Y, Yoshihara K, Tohno Y, Kojima K, Kameoka M, Kamiya T. Inhibition and down-regulation of poly(ADP-ribose) polymerase results in a marked resistance of HL-60 cells to various apoptosis-inducers. Cell Mol Biol (Noisy-Le-Grand). 1995, 41(6),771–81.
41. Milam KM, Cleaver JE. Inhibitors of poly(adenosine diphosphate-ribose) synthesis: effect on other metabolic processes. Science. 1984, 223(4636),589–91.
42. Weltin D, Picard V, Aupeix K, Varin M, Oth D, Marchal J, Dufour P, Bischoff P. Immunosuppressive activities of 6(5H)-phenanthridinone, a new poly(ADP-ribose)polymerase inhibitor. Int J Immunopharmacol. 1995, 17(4),265–71.
43. Weltin D, Marchal J, Dufour P, Potworowski E, Oth D, Bischoff P. Effect of 6(5H)-phenanthridinone, an inhibitor of poly(ADP-ribose) polymerase, on cultured tumor cells. Oncol Res. 1994, 6(9),399–403.
44. Tanizawa A, Kubota M, Hashimoto H, Shimizu T, Takimoto T, Kitoh T, Akiyama Y, Mikawa H. VP-16-induced nucleotide pool changes and poly(ADP-ribose) synthesis: the role of VP-16 in interphase death. Exp Cell Res. 1989, 185(1),237–46.
45. Martin DS, Schwartz GK. Chemotherapeutically induced DNA damage, ATP depletion, and the apoptotic biochemical cascade. Oncol Res. 1997, 9(1),1–5.
46. Wright S, Wei Q, Kinder D, Larrick J. Biochemical pathways of apoptosis: nicotinamide adenine dinucleotide-deficient cells are resistant to tumour necrosis factor or ultraviolet light activation of the 24-kD apoptotic protease ans DNA fragmentation. J Exp Med. 1996, 183,463–471.
47. Wang ZQ, Auer B, Stingl L, Berghammer H, Haidacher D, Schweiger M, Wagner EF. Mice lacking ADPRT and poly(ADP-ribosyl)ation develop normally but are susceptible to skin disease. Genes Dev. 1995, 9(5),509–20.
48. Leist M, Single B, Kunstle G, Volbracht C, Hentze H, Nicotera P. Apoptosis in the absence of poly-(ADP-ribose) polymerase. Biochem Biophys Res Commun. 1997, 233(2),518–22.
49. de Murcia JM, Niedergang C, Trucco C, Ricoul M, Dutrillaux B, Mark M, Oliver FJ, Masson M, Dierich A, LeMeur M, Walztinger C, Chambon P, de Murcia G. Requirement of poly(ADP-ribose) polymerase in recovery from DNA damage in mice and in cells. Proc Natl Acad Sci USA. 1997, 94(14),7303–7.
50. Kaufmann SH, Desnoyers S, Ottaviano Y, Davidson NE, Poirier GG. Specific proteolytic cleavage of poly(ADP-ribose) polymerase: an early marker of chemotherapy-induced apoptosis. Cancer Res. 1993, 53(17),3976–85.
51. Lazebnik YA, Kaufmann SH, Desnoyers S, Poirier GG, Earnshaw WC. Cleavage of poly(ADP-ribose) polymerase by a proteinase with properties like ICE. Nature. 1994, 371(6495),346–7.
52. Schlegel J, Peters I, Orrenius S, Miller DK, Thornberry NA, Yamin TT, Nicholson DW. CPP32/apopain is a key interleukin 1 beta converting enzyme-like protease involved in Fas-mediated apoptosis. J Biol Chem. 1996, 271(4),1841–4.
53. Tewari M, Quan LT, K OR, Desnoyers S, Zeng Z, Beidler DR, Poirier GG, Salvesen GS, Dixit VM. Yama/CPP32 beta, a mammalian homolog of CED-3, is a CrmA-inhibitable protease that cleaves the death substrate poly(ADP-ribose) polymerase. Cell. 1995, 81(5),801–9.
54. Nicholson DW, Ali A, Thornberry NA, Vaillancourt JP, Ding CK, Gallant M, Gareau Y, Griffin PR, Labelle M, Lazebnik YA, et al. Identification and inhibition of the ICE/CED-3 protease necessary for mammalian apoptosis [see comments]. Nature. 1995, 376(6535),37–43.

55. Casciola-Rosen L, Nicholson DW, Chong T, Rowan KR, Thornberry NA, Miller DK, Rosen A. Apopain/CPP32 cleaves proteins that are essential for cellular repair: a fundamental principle of apoptotic death. J Exp Med. 1996, 183(5),1957–64.
56. Rosenthal DS, Ding R, Simbulan-Rosenthal CM, Vaillancourt JP, Nicholson DW, Smulson M. Intact cell evidence for the early synthesis, and subsequent late apopain-mediated suppression, of poly(ADP-ribose) during apoptosis. Exp Cell Res. 1997, 232(2),313–21.
57. Whitacre CM, Hashimoto H, Tsai ML, Chatterjee S, Berger SJ, Berger NA. Involvement of NAD-poly(ADP-ribose) metabolism in p53 regulation and its consequences. Cancer Res. 1995, 55(17),3697–701.
58. Wolf D, Rotter V. Major deletions in the gene encoding the p53 tumor antigen cause lack of p53 expression in HL-60 cells. Proc Natl Acad Sci USA. 1985, 82,790–794.
59. Masutani M, Nozaki T, Wakabayashi K, Sugimura T. Role of poly(ADP-ribose) polymerase in cell-cycle checkpoint mechanisms following gamma-irradiation. Biochimie. 1995, 77(6),462–5.

30

APOPTOTIC FRACTION IN CHILDHOOD ALL ASSESSED BY DNA *IN SITU* LABELLING IS PLOIDY INDEPENDENT

Allen F. Pyesmany, Lynne M. Ball, Margaret Yhap, M. Henry, Krista Laybolt, D. Christie Riddell, and Dick van Velzen

Department of Clinical Haemato-Oncology
Dalhousie University
IWK Grace Health Centre
5850 University Avenue, B3J 3G9
Halifax, Nova Scotia, Canada

Key words: apoptosis, DNA ploidy, in situ labelling, childhood ALL.

1. ABSTRACT

1.1. Background

Apoptotic cell fraction and presence or degree of aneuploidy may both affect treatment outcome in childhood acute lymphoblastic leukaemia (ALL), which is largely defined by drug resistance. Independence of the variables is at present not established. Until the development of in situ labelling of cells committed to the apoptotic pathway, the fraction of cells in apoptosis could not be determined objectively.

1.2. Aim

To determine the relationship between apoptotic cell fraction and karyotype in childhood ALL using in situ labelling.

1.3. Methods

1.3.1. Study Groups and Samples. Diagnostic, pretreatment bone marrow trephine and aspirate samples of 24 consecutive, unselected cases of childhood ALL were included in the study: Normal karyotype (n=11, 5M,6F), high hyperdiploid aneuploidy (DNA index >1.5, n=7, 1M,6F), complex karyotypic anomalies (n=6, 5M,1F).

1.3.2. Apoptotic Cell Labelling. In situ labelling of the 3'-OH ends of the apoptosis specific DNA (Klenow) fragment (Frag-EL, CalBiochem, USA).

1.3.3. Quantitation. Apoptotic cell fraction was established using 10 systematically random fields of >20 nuclei. Results were tabled per group. After calculations of means, differences between groups were assessed using t-test.

1.4. Results

Apoptotic cell fraction, ranging from <1 to 95%, did not differ statistically significant between the three study groups.

1.5. Conclusion

Apoptotic cell fraction in childhood leukaemia is independent of ploidy status and euploid karyotypic anomalies.

2. INTRODUCTION

The mechanisms determining leukaemic cell entry into the apoptotic pathway are presently not completely elucidated.[1–3] It is however appreciated that the accumulation of minor DNA damage in the pre-replication phases of the cell cycle and during S-phase may accumulate to reach supra-critical levels by the time post replication DNA excision repair is to take place.[4,5]

Although the precise mechanisms by which the cell assesses the extent of DNA damage are not clarified, it is perceived that there is a mechanism within cells to assess the viability of a cell depending on the extent of the DNA genome damage. If too excessive, then after a "decision" in which the cell is classified as "unrepairable", apoptosis is initiated.[6,7]

It would seem possible that within a population of leukaemic lesions, a relation might exist in which in lesions with high apoptotic cell fraction usually also show a high degree of aneuploidy.[8] Strongly abnormal karyotypes may reflect intrinsic DNA instability and/or vulnerability and as such, lesions of this character might accrue a more than average amount of DNA damage resulting in greater cell fraction that will then be entered into the apoptotic process.[9]

Thus, the apoptotic process might well be related to prognosis by affecting resistance to drug treatment and as such be related to treatment outcome in childhood ALL.[4,7]

Especially in childhood malignancy it is now true to say that at present there is no longer any natural evolution of disease and prognosis is best defined as outcome of treatment as most children will receive combination therapy. Therefore the study of the relationship between the absolute apoptotic cell fraction and treatment outcome may be of interest.

If the apoptotic cell fraction is dependent on or strongly influenced by ploidy status,[6] then the determination of an independent apoptotic cell fraction in childhood ALL may not increase the precision of any prediction of prognosis as apoptosis is no longer an additional independent variable with potential prognostic power.[1,4,5]

It is at this time accepted that, in childhood ALL, high hyperdiploid aneuploidy is not uncommonly associated with a better outcome under standardized treatment than that encountered with complex karyotypic abnormalities which include balanced translocations and cases with barely or undetectable deviations from the normal complement of 2n DNA.[10]

We therefore aimed to determine the relationship between apoptotic cell fraction and karyotype class in childhood ALL.

3. MATERIALS AND METHODS

3.1. Study Groups

Diagnostic pretreatment bone marrow trephine biopsy material and bone marrow aspirate samples of 32 consecutive, unselected cases of childhood ALL, in whom karyotypic analysis was successful, were included in the study. All children were seen in a single tertiary referral centre between the 1st of January, 1994 and the 31st of December, 1997. The cases were classified according to three groups of karyotypical abnormality:

  a. Normal karyotype. This group consisted of 15 cases of which 7 were male and 8 were female with an age distribution ranging from 8 months to 12 years.
  b. High hyperdiploid aneuploidy. These cases had a DNA index of >1.5. There were 7 patients in this group of which 1 was male and the other 6 were female. Their age ranged from 3 to 12 years.
  c. Complex karyotypic anomalies. This group comprised 10 patients of whom 7 were male and 3 were female with an age range of 1 year 7 months to 7 years of age.

3.2. Proliferation Fraction Assessment

This was carried out using immunocytochemical detection of the Ki-67 antigen in cycling nuclei through the use of a monoclonal antibody (MM1, NovaCastra, UK) directed against a cDNA defined subsegment of the Ki-67 antigen. $5\mu m$ paraffin sections of routinely formaldehyde fixed and paraffin processed pretreatment diagnostic bone marrow trephine biopsies were used.

3.3. Apoptotic Fraction Assessment

A commercially available DNA probe and kit were used (Frag-EL, CalBiochem, USA) to detect by in situ labelling the 3'-OH ends of DNA fragments excised from the genome by apoptosis specific endonucleases. Probe bound to the Klenow fragments can be detected by its horse-radish peroxidase label. This then allows for the detection of nuclei in which apoptosis is active by appropriate chromogen labelling. This technique was carried out on 10 μm paraffin section taken immediately subsequent to the 5 μm section used for Ki-67 antigen detection. Methyl green counterstaining allows for the identification of various cell types in the trephine biopsy sample.

3.4. Quantitation

A computer assisted image analysis system (Quantimet 570C) was used to systematically sample sections of the trephine biopsies with a rectangular sampling frame. Ten systematically random samples of a minimum of 20 nuclei each were selected. The counting frame used 2 forbidden and 2 inclusion edges on opposite sides of the rectangle to correct for nuclear size bias. Such nuclear size bias associated affects were expected due to the fact that with cell proliferation nuclei are appreciated to potentially increase in nuclear volume whereas with the apoptotic process nuclear size reduction is expected to progress gradually.

Progressive mean calculations were used to assess and confirm appropriate sample size and these additionally were used to confirm that in all cases after 10 samples a mean was reached that was within 10% of the final value.

3.5. Statistical Analysis

Results were tabled per group. After calculation of the mean, any differences between groups, means and ranges were assessed for probability of non difference using t-test.

4. RESULTS

The results are summarised in Table 1 and Figure 1. and further illustrated in Figures 2 and 3. The apoptotic cell fraction shows a surprisingly wide range: from <1 to 95%, especially in the light of the usual paucity of apoptotic bodies in bone marrow samples of childhood ALL.

The apoptotic cell fraction did not differ significantly between study groups. As is evident in Figure 2, a suggestion is found in the group of bone marrow samples with complex abnormalities of the karyotype, of a somewhat bimodal distribution of the value of the apoptotic cell fraction. Approximately half of the cases have a high while the other half show a relatively low apoptotic cell fraction. Possibly, but less clearly, a similar distribution of values is seen in the other groups but the fact that this is less clearly defined may in part be due to the limited number of cases within the group of high hyperdiploid aneuploidy.

5. DISCUSSION

That the apoptotic cell fraction does not show systematic differences between lesions with considerable differences in the degree of karyotypic anomaly or even with absence of abnormalities, is somewhat surprising.

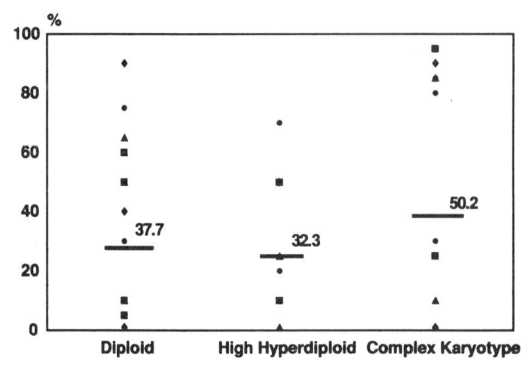

Figure 1. Diagrammatic representation of distribution of apoptotic cell fraction related to the degree of karyotypic abnormality. Note that although a number of patients with complex karyotypic defects have high apoptotic cell fractions, the average value for this parameter between groups does not differ significantly. However, the distribution of values for the group of patients with complex karyotypic abnormalities is suggestive of bimodal distribution (see text).

Table 1. Karyotype abnormality and apoptotic cell fraction in childhood ALL % Frag-EL positive nuclei

Diploid	High hyper-diploid aneuploid	Complex karyotype
10	20	80
10	25	85
5	10	25
1	5070	90
30	1	30
65	50	1
10		95
90		1
75		85
50		10
50		
40		
10		
60		
60		

It would have been expected that with high degrees of karyotypic anomaly, if these were to reflect intrinsic DNA instability, a high apoptotic cell fraction would be observed as many of the cells would gradually and progressively accumulate supra-critical levels of DNA damage.

This would result in the preclusion of DNA excision repair by initiating the alternative apoptotic cell process. However, this appears not to be the case and both high and low ranges of apoptotic cell fraction values can be found within all three groups of karyotypic anomaly.

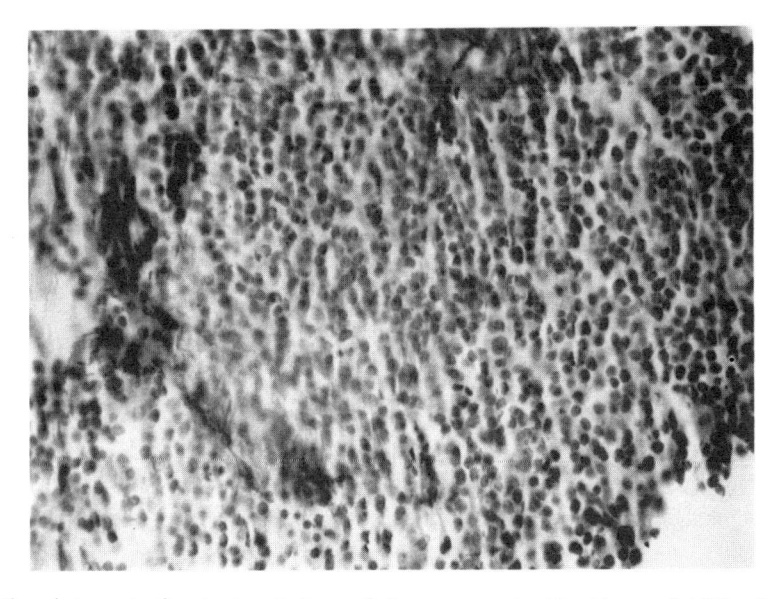

Figure 2. Microphotograph of pretreatment, diagnostic bone marrow trephine biopsy of childhood patient with ALL. Section stained by routine immunocytochemistry for the peroxidase label of the Frag-EL (CalBiochem, USA) probe for apoptosis specific DNA fragments. Note relatively high fraction of positive nuclei (>70%), with homogenous distribution throughout the marrow section shown. 10 μm paraffin section, Fast green counter stain, microscopical magnification 400 x.

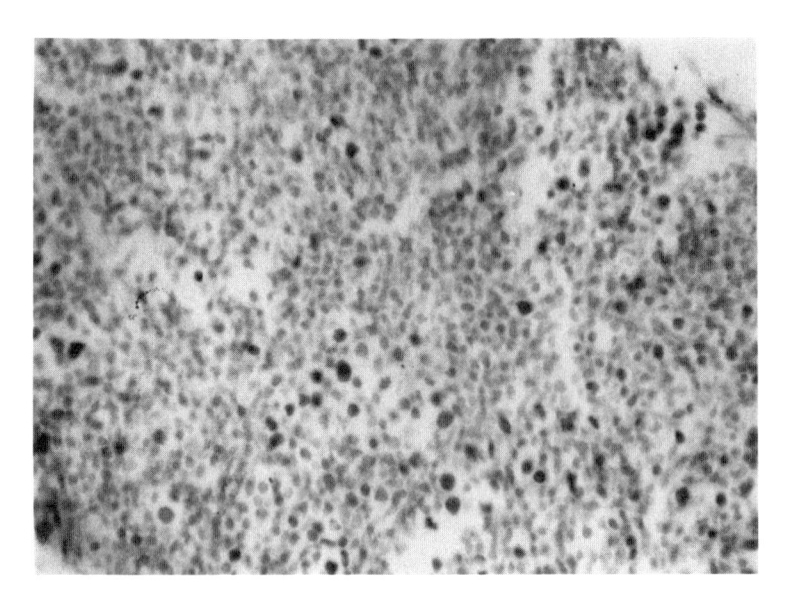

Figure 3. Microphotograph of pretreatment, diagnostic bone marrow trephine biopsy of childhood patient with ALL. Section stained by routine immunocytochemistry for the peroxidase label of the Frag-EL (CalBiochem, USA) probe for apoptosis specific DNA fragments. Note low fraction of positive nuclei (< 1%), with homogenous distribution throughout the marrow section shown. 10μm paraffin section, Fast green counter stain, microscopical magnification 400 x.

Thus the apoptotic cell fraction appears to be, at least predominantly, an independent cell biological variable that can be studied for its additional power to predict prognosis in addition to that of ploidy status.

One possible explanation for this phenomenon is that high apoptotic fractions are related to impaired DNA excision repair rather than intrinsic instability. As such, lesions with a defect of the DNA excision repair may show high apoptotic cell fractions and this mutation dependent deficiency may develop independent of other mechanisms that result in aneuploidy. If so, this mechanism would additionally support prospective studies of independent power of prognosis.

If the ability to maintain or even increase levels of DNA excision repair remains even in cases of primary unstable genome, apoptotic cell fractions may remain relatively low.

Especially under treatment with DNA directed drug moieties, an initially high apoptotic cell fraction, if it were truly to reflect deficiencies of DNA excision repair, might prove to be a powerful predictor of prognosis. This parameter may technically be determined very rapidly after bone marrow sampling without the need for short term culture and complex analysis.

In summary, the apoptotic cell fraction in childhood acute lymphoblastic leukaemia is independent of ploidy status and euploid karyotypic anomalies and as such warrants prospective studies of its independent power to predict prognosis under chemotherapeutic treatment.

ACKNOWLEDGMENTS

The authors would like to acknowledge the expert help and expertise of Mrs. C. Isenor without whom this study would not have been possible as well as the expert help and efforts of Mrs. L. Lee Maugham, without whom the manuscript would not have come to completion.

REFERENCES

1. Wyllie AH. Apoptosis and regulation of cell numbers in normal and neoplastic tissues: an overview. Cancer Met Rev, 1992, 11:95–103.
2. Hicsonmez G, Erdemli E, Tekelioglu M, Tuncer AM, et al. Morphological evidence of apoptosis in childhood acute myeloblastic leukaemia treated with high dose methyl prednisolone. Leuk Lymphoma, 1996, 22:91–6.
3. Thiele J, Zirbes TK, Lorenzen J, Kvasnicka HM, et al. Haemopoietic turnover index in reactive and neoplastic bone marrow lesions quantification by apoptosis and PCNA labelling. Ann Haematol, 1997, 75:33–9.
4. Cotter TG, Lennon SV, Glynn JG, Martin SJ. Cell death via apoptosis and its relationship to growth, development, and differentiation of both tumour and normal cells. Anticancer Res, 1990, 1:1153–60.
5. Moul JW, Bettencourt MC, Sesterhenn IA, Mostofi FK, McLeod DG, Srivastava S, Bauer JJ. Protein expression of p53, bcl-2, and Ki-67 (MIB-1) as prognostic biomarkers in patients with surgically treated, clinically localized prostate cancer. Surgery, 1996, 120:159–67.
6. Sarraf CE, Bowen ID. Proportions of mitotic and apoptotic cells in a range of untreated experimental tumours. Cell Tissue Kinet, 1988, 21:45–9.
7. Du M, Singh N, Husseuin A, Isaacson PG, Pan L. Positive correlation between apoptotic and proliferative indices in gastrointestinal lymphomas of mucosa-associated lymphoid tissue (MALT). J Pathol, 1996, 178:379–84.
8. Baxter GD, Collins RJ, Harmon BV, Kumar S, et al. Cell death by apoptosis in acute leukaemia. J Pathol, 1989, 158:123–9.
9. Coustan-Smith E, Kitenaka A, Pui CH, McNinch L, et al. Clinical relevance of Bcl2 overexpression in childhood acute lymphoblastic leukaemia. Blood, 1996, 87:1140–6.
10. Secker-Walker LM, Swansbury GJ, Hardisty RM. Cytogenetics of acute lymphoblastic leukaemia in children as a factor in the prediction of long term survival. Br J Haematol, 1982, 52:389–99.

31

PCNA BEARING STRUCTURES ARE RETAINED IN APOPTOTIC PHASE OF CHILDHOOD ALL CELL CYCLE

Lynne M. Ball, Christopher L. Lannon, Margaret Yhap, Allen F. Pyesmany, M. Henry, Krista Laybolt, D. Christie Riddell, and Dick van Velzen

Department of Pathology
Dalhousie University
IWK Grace Health Centre
5850 University Ave.
B3J 3G9, Halifax, N.S., Canada

Keywords: PCNA, apoptosis, cell cycle, childhood ALL, drug resistance.

1. ABSTRACT

1.1. Background

Drug resistance to DNA directed therapy may depend on proliferative as well as apoptotic cell fraction. PCNA/Ki67 ratio excess, possibly reflecting DNA excision repair, is of additional interest to drug resistance in MTT testing.

The cell cycle phase/antigen expression pattern in childhood acute lymphoblastic leukemia (ALL) is not known.

1.2. Aims

To study the relationship between nuclear expression of PCNA, Ki-67 and Frag-EL positivity in childhood ALL.

1.3. Methods

1.3.1. Study Groups. Diagnostic bone marrow trephine biopsies of 32 consecutive unselected cases of childhood ALL were included in the study.

1.3.2. Immunohistochemistry. Commercially available Moab PCNA (PC10, DAKO, USA), Ki-67 (MM1, NovaCastra, UK) were used to label cycling cells in routinely processed 5μm paraffin sections.

1.3.3. In-Situ Labelling of Apoptotic Cells. The 3'-OH ends of apoptosis specific DNA fragments were labelled in-situ on subsequent 10μm sections (Frag-EL, CalBiochem, USA).

1.3.4. Quantitation. After blinding and randomisation, 10 systematic random fields of >20 nuclei and nuclear size bias correction was used to determine positive nuclei fraction.

1.4. Results

While the sum of apoptotic and proliferative cell fraction (Ki-67 + Frag-EL%) equalled 100% in 5/32 cases, PCNA expression into at least the early phases of apoptosis ([%PCNA-%K-67]>[100-%Frag-EL] was found in 17/32 cases.

1.5. Conclusions

PCNA/Ki67 ratio excess may not reflect DNA excision repair activity but rather slow degradation of antigen bearing structures limiting relevance to drug resistance study.

2. INTRODUCTION

The overall effect of any DNA directed cancer therapeutic drug regimen may be influenced by both the proliferative activity of the lesion and the agent of treatment selected. The underlying mechanism linking these two factors is considered to be that while in S-phase, DNA through uncoiling is more vulnerable to direct interaction with intercalating and or alkylating as well as cross linking agents. The precise relationship between proliferation fraction as assessed by Ki67 labelling studies[1,2] and treatment outcome has not been unequivocally established.[3-8]

As there is post replication DNA excision repair, in addition to the drug concentration, the total length of the S-phase may also be related to the drug effect as during S-phase there is presumably no excision repair. With long S-phases and long duration of uncoiled state a larger number of cells may accumulate supra critical DNA damage resulting in shunting of such cells to the apoptotic pathway on post replication surveillance of the total damage to the genome.

The post replication DNA excision repair and DNA resynthesis is dependent on structures bearing PCNA antigens. These antigens, first described by Bravo et al., in 1987[9] form part of the delta DNA polymerase complex and have been studied in normal and abnormal cell proliferation of tumours based on the ability to demonstrate the nuclear expression of these antigens in formalin fixed and paraffin embedded tissues.[10] Excessive DNA excision repair may to some degree explain observed high ratios for PCNA / Ki-67 expression in proliferating childhood leukemic cells.[11-14] Previously reported as potentially reflecting immortalization, more recent investigations suggest a possibility of high levels of repair activity being present in at least some neoplastic conditions. These may be the same lesions which have been incidentally observed as spontaneously containing high levels of internuclear free DNA fragments associated with DNA excision repair activity. It is possible that in such conditions the apoptotic cell fraction, i.e., the fraction of cells within the lesion which at any time is committed to the apoptotic pathway, may also be higher.[15-18] Considerable numbers of studies have investigated the gene regulation aspects of apoptosis in (childhood) leukaemia.[19-28] However, at this stage no information is available on any studies in which the ratio of PCNA / Ki-67 expression has been analysed in relation to simultaneously established apoptotic cell fraction.

We thus aimed to study the relationship between nuclear expression of these cell cycle DNA excision repair related antigen bearing structures and the apoptotic fraction in childhood ALL.

3. MATERIALS AND METHODS

3.1. Study Groups

Thirty two consecutive unselected cases of childhood ALL, diagnosed in a single tertiary referral centre between the dates of January 1, 1994 and December 31, 1997 were included in the study.

3.2. Cell Proliferation Analysis

Using commercially available monoclonal antibodies against PCNA (PC10, DAKO, USA) and a cDNA defined segment of the Ki-67 antigen (MM1, NovaCastra, UK) were used for immunocytochemical labelling of nuclear expression of the cell cycling related antigens in routinely formaldehyde fixed paraffin processed pretreatment diagnostic bone marrow trephine biopsies specimens. 5 μm paraffin sections were used for this purpose.

3.3. Apoptotic Cell Fraction Analysis

Using a commercially available probe and kit for apoptosis specific endonuclease derived DNA fragments, the resulting 3'-OH ends of the Klenow fragments were labelled in situ using a 10μm section taken immediately after the previous 5 μm section. Making use of horseradish peroxidase labelling and DAB, any positive nuclei were identified. Counterstaining with methyl green allowed for the identification of histological cell types.

3.4. Quantitation

Specimens were blinded and randomised and in each specimen 10 systematically random fields defined by a rectangular grid were chosen to include at least 20 nuclei per sample. Using 2 forbidden and 2 inclusion sides opposite to each other, nuclear size bias possibly resulting from nuclear size increase in proliferation and nuclear size decrease in apoptosis, was avoided. Progressive mean calculations were carried out to confirm that the samples were sufficient to obtain a mean after 10 samples that was within 10% of the final mean in all cases.

3.5. Analysis

For all cases a diagram was prepared with proportional marking for Ki-67 PCNA and Frag-EL positivity.

4. RESULTS

The results of the study are summarized in Table 1 and Figure 1. And further illustrated in Figure 2–4. The sum of apoptotic and proliferative cell fraction, as identified by the percentages of Frag-EL and Ki-67 positive nuclei equalled 100% in 5/32 studied cases. As a result of this and other calculations PCNA antigen expression or retention into at least the early phase of apoptosis (see Figure 1) was found in 17/32 cases. These cases were identified as those in which the percentage of PCNA combined with the percentage of Frag-EL positive nuclei was greater than 100%.

5. DISCUSSION

The extension of PCNA antigen expression into what clearly must be the apoptotic cell disassembly phase has surprisingly not been reported prior to this study even though a

Table 1. PCNA expression related to cell cycling and apoptosis in childhood acute lymphoblastic leukemia

Case	% Ki-67	% Frag-EL	% PCNA	ACCPF
1	5	20	10	5.5
2	5	10	15	5.5
3	1	5	10	5.5
4*	10	1	30	10
5*	15	30	40	21
6	15	65	20	43
7	1	10	5	5.5
8*	10	90	40	100
9*	20	75	60	80
10	30	50	65	50
11	35	50	35	70
12	20	40	50	33
13	5	10	20	5.5
14	25	60	55	62
15	10	60	60	25
16	10	20	20	12.5
17	25	25	30	33
18	15	10	60	16
19	20	50	20	40
20	5	70	35	16.6
21	15	1	20	15.1
22	20	50	35	40
23	10	85	30	66
24	25	80	50	100
25	20	25	50	27
26	15	90	65	100
27	10	30	30	14
28	1	1	10	1
29	5	95	50	100
30	50	1	50	50.5
31	20	85	50	100
32	15	10	35	17

ACCPF = Apoptosis corrected cell proliferation fraction
*Illustrated in Figure 1.

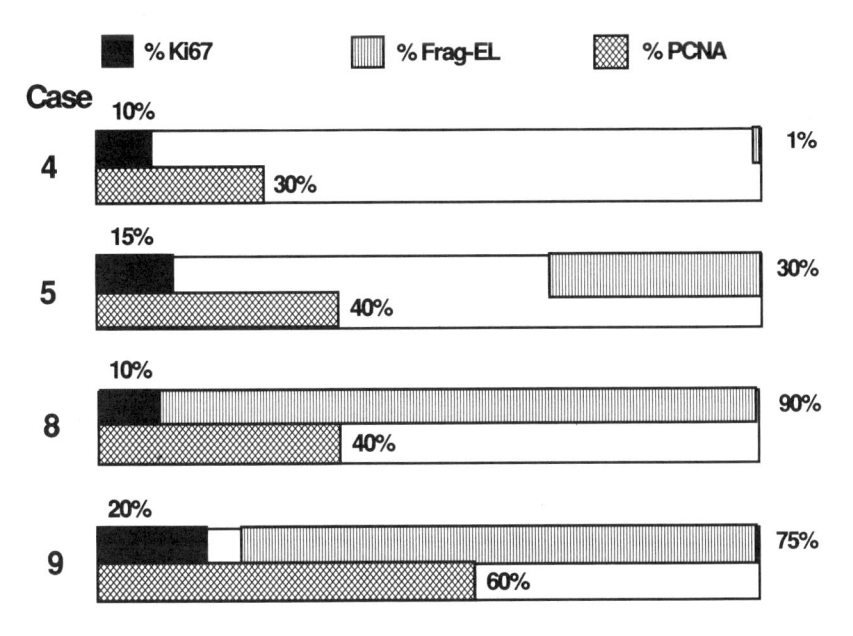

PCNA Bearing Structures Are Retained in Apoptotic Phase

Figure 1. Diagrammatic representation of the results of fraction analysis for PCNA and Ki67 expression combined with results of fraction analysis of nuclei positive for apoptosis derived DNA fragments (Frag-EL). Case numbers on left correspond to case numbers in Table 1. Note that in general PCNA/Ki67 ratio ranges from 3–4/1. Whereas in case 4 and 5, no overlap with Frag-EL positivity exists, in case 8 and 9, PCNA expression must for mathematical reasons exist while cells are already undergoing apoptosis. Case 8 shows the phenomenon of permanent cycling, i.e. the sum of the Ki67 and Frag-EL fraction is 100% and no cells exist outside of the proliferative phase of cell cycling.

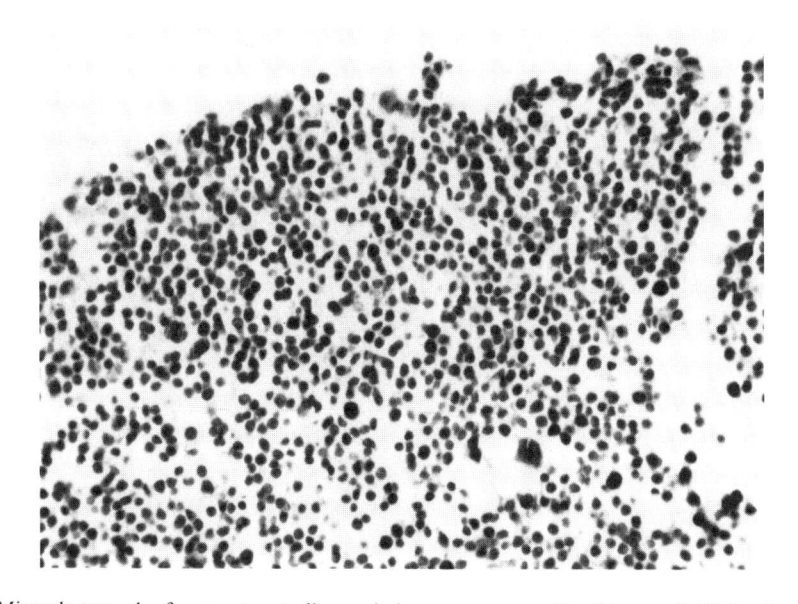

Figure 2. Microphotograph of pretreatment, diagnostic bone marrow trephine biopsy of childhood patient with ALL. Section stained by routine immunocytochemistry for the PCNA antigen (PC10, DAKO, USA). Note relatively high fraction of positive nuclei (>70%), with homogenous distribution throughout the marrow section shown. 5 μm paraffin section, Haematoxylin counter stain, microscopical magnification 400 x.

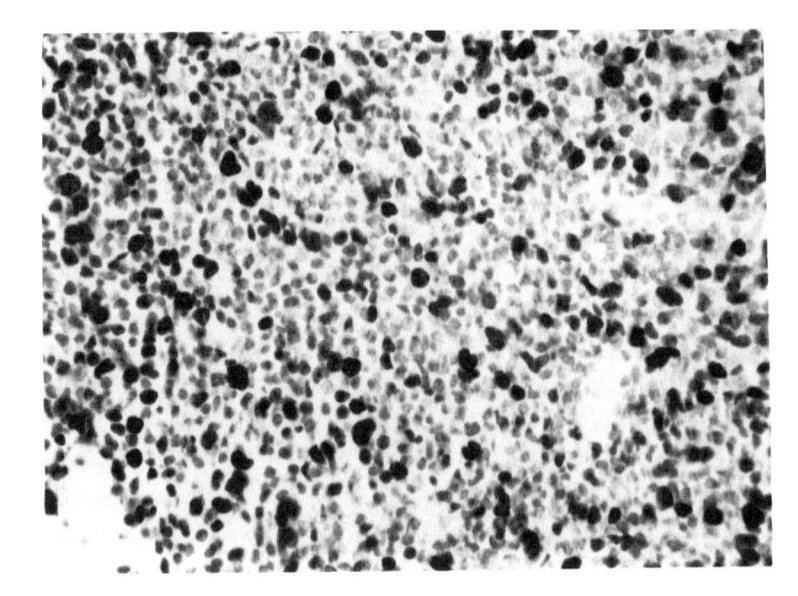

Figure 3. Microphotograph of pretreatment, diagnostic bone marrow trephine biopsy of childhood patient with ALL. Section stained by routine immunocytochemistry for the Ki67 antigen (MM1, NovaCastra, UK). Note relatively high fraction of positive nuclei (15%), with homogenous, slightly clustered distribution throughout the marrow section shown. 5 μm paraffin section, Haematoxylin counter stain, microscopical magnification 400 x.

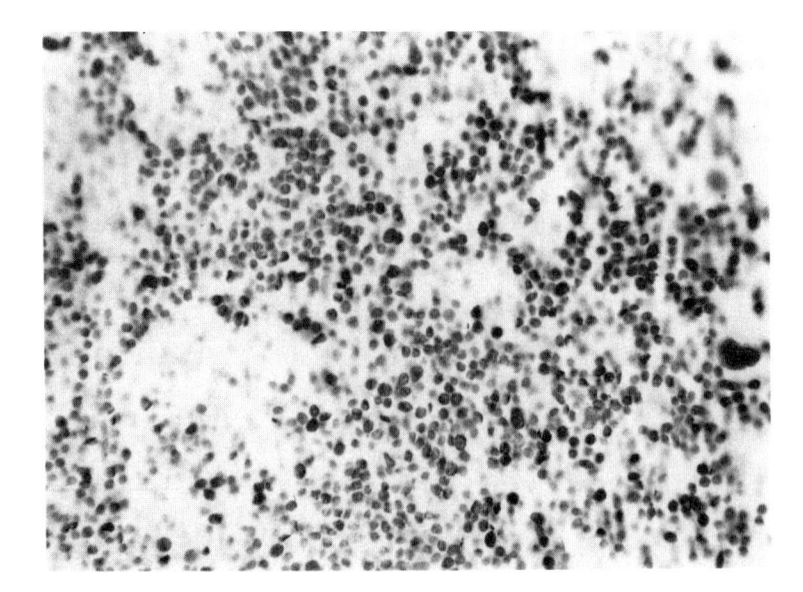

Figure 4. Microphotograph of pretreatment, diagnostic bone marrow trephine biopsy of childhood patient with ALL. Section stained by routine immunocytochemistry for the peroxidase label of the Frag-EL (CalBiochem, USA) probe for the apoptosis specific DNA fragments. Note relatively high fraction of positive nuclei (ca. 15%), with homogenous, but slightly clustered distribution throughout the marrow section shown. 10 μm paraffin section, Fast green counter stain, microscopical magnification 400 x.

comparable study was reported in 1997 in adult bone marrow.[29] At this stage the retained proteins bearing the PCNA and PC10 antigens in all probability become dissociated from any functional role normally carried out as part of the cell cycling process. This finding may then well (at least in part) provide an explanation for the regularly observed abnormally high ratios of PCNA and Ki-67 positivity within childhood ALL lesions.[10–14]

There are therefore two possible alternative contributors to such abnormal ratios. The first one may be excessive levels of post replication DNA excision repair activity due to an intrinsically unstable genome within some leukaemic cell proliferations. This would require the presence of PCNA bearing structures not related to cell cycling and thus there would be an additional fraction of cells expressing PCNA independent of S-phase and its associated markers such as the Ki67 antigen. A further argument for this hypothesis is found in the also observed spontaneous occurrence of high levels of intranuclear free DNA fragments found in comet tail analysis.

An alternative hypothesis may now be proposed as the non functional persistence of such antigen bearing structures, either fully intact or partially degraded during at least the first phases of apoptotic cell involution. A functional role for PCNA bearing structures in apoptosis, in view of the fact that in our study, 15 out of 32 cases PCNA expression was not observed during the apoptotic cell phase, seems unlikely.

In summary, we conclude from our findings that excessively high PCNA to Ki-67 expression ratios may not always reflect DNA excision repair activity related to intrinsically unstable genome. Rather, in many cases, this may represent slow degradation of antigen bearing structures during the initial stages of the apoptotic cell phase.

In the analysis of drug resistance studies, especially in vitro, this possibility must be taken into account when interpreting cell cycling activity using antigens of the PCNA group.

ACKNOWLEDGMENTS

The authors would like to acknowledge the expert and technical expertise of Mrs. C. Isenor without whose work this study would not have been possible. We also wish to thank Mrs Linda-Lee Maughan for typing this manuscript.

REFERENCES

1. Emanuels AG, Burger MPM, Hollema H, Koudstaal J. Quantitation of Proliferation-Associated Markers Ag-NOR and Ki-67 does not contribute to the prediction of lymph node metastases in squamous cell carcinoma of the vulva. Hum Pathol 1996, 27(8):807–11.
2. Gerdes J, Lemke H, Baisch H, Wacker HH, Schwab U, Stein H. 1984. Cell cycle analysis of a cell proliferation-associated human nuclear antigen defined by the monoclonal antibody Ki-67. J Immunol, 1984, 133(4):1710–5.
3. Marshal RD, Lester S, Corless C, Richie JP, Chandra R, Propert KJ, Dutta A. Expression of cell cycle-regulated proteins in prostate cancer. Cancer Res 1996, 56(18): 4159–63.
4. Boon ME, Howard CV, van Velzen D. PCNA independence of Ki-67 expression in HPV infection. Cell Biol Intl, 1993, 17(11):1001–4.
5. Gerdes J, Schwab U, Lemke H, Stein H. Production of a mouse monoclonal antibody reactive with a human nuclear antigen associated with cell proliferation. Int J Cancer, 1993, 31(1):13–20.
6. Bubendorf L, Sauter G, Moch H, Schmid HP, Gasser TC, Jordan P, Mihatsch MJ. Ki67 Labelling index: an independent predictor of progression in prostate cancer treated by radical prostectomy. J Pathol, 1996, 178:437–41.

7. Linden MD, el-Naggar AK, Nathanson SD, Jacobson G, Zarbo RJ. Lack of correlation between flow cytometric and immunohistologic proliferation measurements of tumours. Mod Pathol, 1996, 9(6):682–9.
8. Moul JW, Bettencourt MC, Sesterhenn IA, Mostofi FK, McLeod DG, Srivastava S, Bauer JJ. Protein expression of p53, bcl-2, and Ki-67 (MIB-1) as prognostic biomarkers in patients with surgically treated, clinically localized prostate cancer. Surgery, 1996, 120:159–67.
9. Bravo R, Frank R, Blundel PA, McDonald-Bravo H. PCNA is the auxillary protein of DNA polymerase delta. Nature, 1987, 326:515.
10. Hall PA, Levison DA, Woods AL, Yu CC, et al. PCNA immunolocalisation in paraffin sections: an index of cell proliferation with evidence of deregulated expression in some neoplasms. 1990, J Pathol, 162:285–94.
11. Ball LM, Pope J, Howard CV, Eccles P, van Velzen D. PCNA - Ki67 dissocoation in childhood acute lymphoblastic leukaemia. An immunofluorescent laser confocal scanning microscopical study. Cell Biol Int, 1994, 18:69–74.
12. Tsurusawa M, Ito M, Zha Z, Kawai S, Takasaki Y, Fujimoto J. Cell cycle associated expressions of proliferating cell nuclear antigen and Ki67 reactive antigen of bone marrow blast cells in childhood acute leukaemia. Leukaemia, 1992, 6:669–74.
13. Ito M, Tsurusawa M, Zha Z, Kawai S, Takasaki Y, Fujimoto J. Cell proliferation in childhood acute leukaemia. Comparison of Ki67 and Proliferating Cell Nuclear Antigen immunocytochemical and DNA flowcytometric analysis. Cancer, 1992, 69:2176–82.
14. Keim D, Hailat N, Hodge D, Hannash SM. Proliferatin cell nuclear antigen expression in childhood acute leukaemia. Blood, 1990, 76:985–90.
15. Sarraf CE, Bowen ID. Proportions of mitotic and apoptotic cells in a range of untreated experimental tumours. Cell Tissue Kinet, 1988, 21:45–9.
16. Du M, Singh N, Husseuin A, Isaacson PG, Pan L. Positive correlation between apoptotic and proliferative indices in gastrointestinal lymphomas of mucosa-associated lymphoid tissue (MALT). J Pathol, 1996, 178:379–84.
17. Cotter TG, Lennon SV, Glynn JG, Martin SJ. Cell death via apoptosis and its relationship to growth, development, and differentiation of both tumour and normal cells. Anticancer Res, 1990, 1:1153–60.
18. Wyllie AH. Apoptosis and regulation of cell numbers in normal and neoplastic tissues: an overview. Cancer Met Rev, 1992, 11:95–103.
19. Liptay S, Seriu T, Bartram CR, Schmid RM. Germline configuration of nfkb2, c-rel and bc13 in childhood acute lymphoblastic leukaemia (ALL). Leukaemia, 1977, 11:1364–6.
20. Salomons GS, Brady HG, Verwijs-Janssen M, van den Bergh JD, et al. The Bax alpha: Bcl-2 ratio modulates the response to dexamethasone in leukaemic cells and is highly variable in childhood leukaemia. Intern J Cancer, 1997, 71:959–65.
21. Uckun FM, Yang Z, Sather H, Steinherz P, et al. Cellular expression of anti-apoptotic Bcl2 oncoprotein in newly diagnosed childhood acute lymphoblastic leukaemia: a Childrens Cancer Group study. Blood, 1997, 89:3769–77.
22. Findley HW, Gu L, Yeager AM, Zhou M. Expression and regulation of Bcl2, Bcl-xl and Bax correlates with p53 status and sensitivity to apoptosis in childhood acute lymphoblastic leukaemia. Blood, 1997, 89:2986–93.
23. Tsangaris GT, Moschovi M, Mikraki V, et al. Study of apoptosis in peripheral blood of patients with acute lymphoblastic leukaemia during induction therapy. Anticancer Res, 1996, 16:3133–40.
24. Hicsonmez G, Erdemli E, Tekelioglu M, Tuncer AM, et al. Morphological evidence of apoptosis in childhood acute myeloblastic leukaemia treated with high dose methyl prednisolone. Leuk Lymphoma, 1996, 22:91–6.
25. Tsangaris GT, Tzortzatou-Stathopoulou F. Development of a quantitative method for the study of apoptosis in peripheral blood. In Vivo, 1996, 10:435–43.
26. Coustan-Smith E, Kitenaka A, Pui CH, McNinch L, et al. Clinical relevance of Bcl2 overexpression in childhood acute lymphoblastic leukaemia. Blood, 1996, 87:1140–6.
27. Debatin KM, Krammer PH. Resistance to Apo1(CD95) induced apoptosis in T-ALL is determined by Bcl2 independent ati-apoptotic program. Leukaemia, 1995, 9:815–20.
28. Baxter GD, Collins RJ, Harmon BV, Kumar S, et al. Cell death by apoptosis in acute leukaemia. J Pathol, 1989, 158:123–9.
29. Thiele J, Zirbes TK, Lorenzen J, Kvasnicka HM, et al. Haemopoietic turnover index in reactive and neoplastic bone marrow lesions quantification by apoptosis and PCNA labelling. Ann Haematol, 1997, 75:33–9.

32

APOPTOSIS CORRECTED PROLIFERATION FRACTION IN CHILDHOOD ALL IS RELATED TO KARYOTYPE

Lynne M. Ball, Allen F. Pyesmany, Margaret Yhap, Christopher L. Lannon, M. Henry, Krista Laybolt, D. Christie Riddell, and Dick van Velzen

Department of Pathology
Dalhousie University
IWK Grace Health Centre
5850 University Avenue, B3J 3G9
Halifax, Nova Scotia, Canada

Keywords: Apoptosis, karyotype, childhood ALL, cell proliferation, drug response.

1. ABSTRACT

1.1. Background

Tumour doubling time, a parameter in drug sensitivity testing, reflects both cell proliferation and apoptosis. Variable apoptosis fractions may explain the poor correlation of S-fraction and drug response. DNA aneuploidy (reflecting intrinsic DNA instability) may, by increasing apoptosis, affect drug response.

1.2. Aim

To assess the relationship between apoptosis corrected proliferation fraction and DNA ploidy in childhood acute lymphoblastic leukemia (ALL).

1.3. Methods

1.3.1. Study Groups. Thirty two consecutive, unselected diagnostic cases of childhood ALL were included in the study.

1.3.2. Karyotype. A normal karyotype was found in 15 cases (7M, 8F, age 8m-12yrs); high hyperdiploid aneuploidy (DNA index > 1.5) was found in 7 patients (1M, 7F, age 3–12yrs) whereas complex karyotypic anomalies, but with 2n or near 2n DNA were present in 10 patients (7M, 3F, age 1y7m-16 yrs).

1.3.3. Proliferation Fraction Assessment. Immunocytochemical demonstration of S-phase associated nuclear expression of the Ki-67 antigen (MM1, NovaCastra, UK).

1.3.4. Apoptosis Fraction Assessment. Binding of a horse radish peroxidase labelled DNA probe for the 3'-OH ends of apoptosis derived Klenow fragments (Frag-EL, CalBiochem, USA).

1.3.5. Quantitation. Computer assisted image analysis (Quantimet 570C), of 10 systematically random fields of a minimum of 20 nuclei each. A nuclear size bias correcting counting frame and rule were used to correct for cell proliferation associated nuclear volume increase and for the expected nuclear volume reduction resulting from apoptosis.

1.4. Results

Corrected for apoptosis, proliferation fraction was highest (mean 57.5%, range 1–100) in poor prognosis, complex karyotype anomalies. Good prognosis, high hyper diploidy showed significantly lower proliferation rates (mean 24.7%, range 12–40) ($p<0.01$, t-test).

1.5. Conclusion

Apoptosis corrected cell proliferation rate in childhood ALL is not independent of karyotype abnormality which may partly explain a relation to therapy response and prognosis.

2. INTRODUCTION

The net mass growth of a tumour is often defined in terms of tumour doubling time. This measure results from the balance of cell increase by cell proliferative activity and cell loss from the proliferating or the mature, non-dividing, end cell pool through apoptotic loss.

The apoptotic cells are no longer available to contribute to the proliferating pool. The calculation of cell proliferation fractions were based on the fraction of all cells with more than 2n DNA as assessed by flow cytometry or on the fraction of all cells expressing nuclear antigens associated with the S-phase of cell cycling. This measure may thus be extensively confounded by variable fractions of apoptotic cells within the same population.[1–4]

Previously this potential effect had been considered negligible due to the very low frequency of apoptotic nuclear bodies. To some extent dependent on the total duration of the apoptotic process and especially if the time required for apoptosis may vary, this may have been an omission that has left a considerable degree of confounding effect in play.

As studies of a possible relationship between cell proliferation fraction and treatment did not provide unequivocal results, in contrast to what one would expect, a considerable degree of confounding by apoptosis may have occurred.[5]

The absence of any relationship between cell proliferation fraction and treatment outcome especially in childhood ALL was puzzling. This is because most of the therapeutic regimens in childhood ALL involve one or more DNA directed cytostatic agents and very often combinations of intercalators and alkylators are used in one form or another.

Another parameter that has at least theoretical relationships to prognosis and outcome in DNA directed drug treatment is intrinsic DNA instability or the inability to correct, through post replication DNA excision repair, any damage which will have occurred as a result of chemotherapy, background radiation or the effects of tissue free radicals.

With an expectancy of a relationship based on either the progressive accumulation of defects due to the inability to repair minor DNA defects, or on the possible presence of intrinsic DNA instability as the cause of the aneuploid karyotypic abnormality, DNA aneuploidy has been studied for a relationship to prognosis under therapy. It is now reasonably well established that high hyperdiploid aneuploidy in childhood ALL has an association with a more favourable prognosis and a better response to therapy.[6] As progressive accumulation of DNA abnormality may at one time or another reach supra-critical levels and thus drive a cell into apoptosis, a relationship between DNA aneuploidy and apoptosis or apoptosis corrected proliferation fraction may be hypothesised.[7-11]

An explorative single centre study has reported the value of assessing karyotypic effects on cell proliferation rates in T-cell leukaemia and has found that differentiation state is related to outcome, and that in the lesions expressing late stages of differentiation, the karyotype was more likely to be normal.[12]

As such, we decided to study the relationship between apoptosis corrected proliferation fraction and DNA ploidy in childhood ALL.

3. MATERIALS AND METHOD

3.1. Study Groups

Thirty two consecutive unselected diagnostic cases of childhood ALL all seen in the tertiary referral centre between 1 January 1994 and 31 December 1997, were included in the study. Patient ages varied from 8 months to 16 years of age.

3.2. Results of Karyotype Analysis

Based on the results of karyotypic analysis and flow cytometric/image cytometry analysis patients were divided into the following groups. There were 15 patients with a normal karyotype (diploid, 2n DNA in flow cytometry). Of these 7 were male, 8 were female. They ranged in age from 8 months to 12 years. There were 7 patients with high hyperdiploid aneuploidy (DNA index >1.5). One of these was male, 6 were female with an age range of 3 to 12 years. Of the 10 patients with complex karyotypic anomalies, 7 were male and 3 were female. They ranged in age from 1 year 7 months to 6 years of age.

3.3. Proliferation Fraction Assessment

Immuno-cytochemical analysis of the cell proliferation fraction in tissue was carried out using monoclonal antibody MM1 as supplied by NovaCastra, UK which detects a cDNA defined subsegment of the Ki-67 antigen and is applied to routinely formaldehyde fixed and paraffin processed 5μm sections. A pressure cooker antigen retrieval system was used.

3.4. Apoptosis Fraction Assessment

Cells undergoing apoptosis were detected in 10 μm tissue sections taken parallel to the previous 5 μm sections and from the same pretreatment diagnostic bone marrow trephine biopsies using a commercially available probe and kit (Frag-EL, CalBiochem, USA). The system is based on DNA in situ labelling of specific DNA fragments excised from the genomic DNA by apoptosis specific endonucleases. The probe binds to the exposed 3'-OH ends of the Klenow fragments which is subsequently labelled by horseradish peroxidase and DAB. Counterstaining with methyl green allows for histological confirmation of cell types.

3.5. Quantitation

Measurement of the nuclear fraction positive for Ki-67 or for Frag-EL was carried out using 10 systematically random samples of a minimum of 20 nuclei and a rectangular counting frame with 2 forbidden and 2 including sides on opposite sides of the frame. This was used to correct for nuclear size bias which may have resulted from the nuclear size increase expected during cell proliferation and nuclear size decrease as the result of the apoptotic process. Progressive mean method was used to ensure that the mean after 10 samples was within 10% of the final mean in all cases. The analysis made use of a computer assisted image analysis system (Quantimet 570C).

3.6. Statistical Analysis

Differences between groups were assessed using t-test for the difference of the mean and standard deviations using SPSS statistical packet.

4. RESULTS

The results of the study are summarized in Table 1–3 and Figure 1.

Table 1. Karyotype abnormality, apoptosis and cell proliferation fraction in childhood ALL—diploid lesions

% Ki-67	% Frag-EL	ACCPF
5	10	5.5
5	10	5.5
1	5	1
10	1	10
15	30	21
15	65	43
5	10	5.5
10	90	100
20	75	80
30	50	60
35	50	70
20	40	33
5	10	5.5
25	60	62
10	60	25

ACCPF = Apoptosis corrected cell proliferation fraction

Table 2. Karyotype abnormality, apoptosis and cell proliferation fraction in childhood ALL—high hyperdiploid lesions

% Ki-67	% Frag-EL	ACCPF
10	20	12.5
25	25	33
15	10	16
20	50	40
5	70	16.6
15	1	15
20	50	40

ACCPF = Apoptosis corrected cell proliferation fraction.

Although there is extensive overlap between the values of diploid and complex karyotypic lesions, lesions with high hyperdiploid karyotype had significantly lower apoptosis corrected cell proliferation fractions: mean 24.7% with a range of 12–40%. (Probability of non difference <0.01, t-test.) The apoptosis corrected cell proliferation fraction was highest (mean 57.5%, range 1–100%) in lesions with poor prognosis complex karyotypic anomalies.

5. DISCUSSION

The apoptotic cell fraction in these lesions is of a surprising wide range and generally far exceeds the presence and frequency of detectable apoptotic cell bodies. This may reflect a relatively short existence of such bodies as a very late and final phase of the apoptotic process with a considerably longer time required for the preceding stages in which cells may morphologically differ very little from the other cells.

The effect of capping in $5\mu m$ sections will make the gradual reduction of nuclear volume probably undetectable until very late stages, especially as or when chromatin concentration is maintained. It is thus logical that such variable and high fractions of apoptotic cells would have confounded the interpretation of the fractions of cells labelling positive for any cell proliferation associated nuclear marker or the interpretation of a fraction of cells containing more than 2n DNA in flow cytometric studies.

Table 3. Karyotype abnormality, apoptosis and cell proliferation fraction in childhood ALL—complex karyotype lesions

% Ki-67	% Frag-EL	ACCPF
10	85	66
25	80	100
20	25	27
15	90	100
10	30	14
1	1	1
5	95	100
50	1	50
20	85	100
15	10	17

ACCPF = Apoptosis corrected cell proliferation fraction

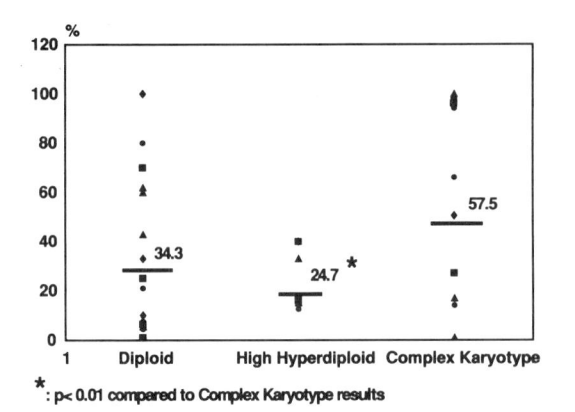

Figure 1. Apoptosis corrected cell proliferation fraction and ploidy status in childhood ALL. Diagram of distribution of apoptosis corrected cell proliferation fraction for each of the three study groups as defined by the degree of karyotypic abnormality. Note the significantly increased mean ACCPF in complex karyotype abnormality with a considerable number of cases showing permanent cycling (ACCPF = 100%). Note also the very low maximal values for ACCPF in cases of high hyperdiploid aneuploidy which are known to be associated with a better long term survival.

*: p< 0.01 compared to Complex Karyotype results

The correction for apoptosis in this study shows a clear effect in that the poor prognosis complex karyotypic anomaly group now has, although the range varies widely, an on average a much higher mean apoptosis corrected cell proliferation fraction than the group in which good prognosis is usually expected to occur more frequently, i.e., the group with high diploid aneuploidy. In this group the mean apoptosis corrected cell proliferation rate

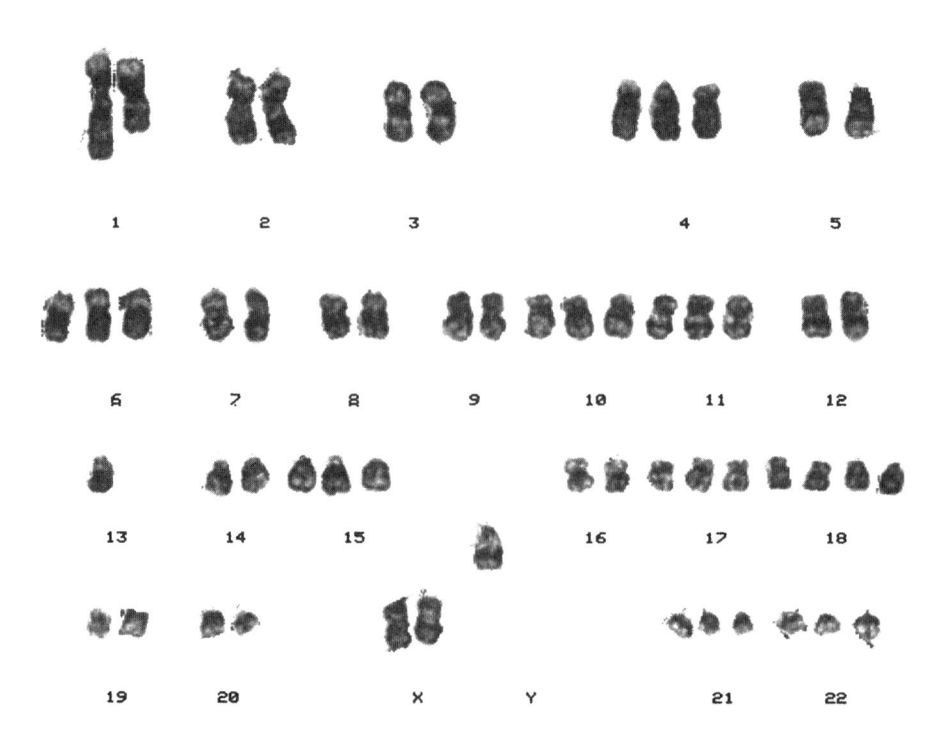

Figure 2. Complex karyotype. Microphotograph of results of karyotype analysis on a case of 56 chromosome karyotype in a male patient with leukaemia. This patient subsequently relapsed and died from infection during subsequent re-induction. Note in addition to disomy X, with a partially defective Y chromosome, a large number of trisomies in addition to partial deletion of the q-arm of chromosome 1 and further small defects.

is not only lower at 24.7% but the range is considerably restricted to values between 12% and 40%. This group differs in the apoptosis corrected proliferation fraction values from the poor prognosis complex karyotypic group at a probability of non difference <0.01 (t-test). It is thus now likely that this correction for the apoptotic cell fraction provides a cell proliferation fraction that is more biologically representative and thus may be reconsidered for study of its value as a prognostic indicator.

In summary, apoptosis corrected cell proliferation rate in childhood ALL is not independent of the karyotype abnormality and a relationship to therapy response and prognosis may very well find its basis in high proliferation rates in the poor prognosis group after correction for apoptosis.

ACKNOWLEDGMENTS

The authors wish to acknowledge the expert technical help of Mrs. C. Isenor without whose expert technical handling of the diagnostic bone marrow specimens a retrospective analysis of cell proliferation associated immunocytochemistry and molecular biological DNA studies would not have been possible. We are also grateful to Mrs Linda-Lee Maughan for typing this manuscript.

REFERENCES

1. Sarraf CE, Bowen ID. Proportions of mitotic and apoptotic cells in a range of untreated experimental tumours. Cell Tissue Kinet, 1988; 21:45–9.
2. Du M, Singh N, Husseuin A, Isaacson PG, Pan L. Positive correlation between apoptotic and proliferative indices in gastrointestinal lymphomas of mucosa-associated lymphoid tissue (MALT). J Pathol 1996; 178:379–84.
3. Cotter TG, Lennon SV, Glynn JG, Martin SJ. Cell death via apoptosis and its relationship to growth, development, and differentiation of both tumour and normal cells. Anticancer Res 1990; 1:1153–60.
4. Wyllie AH. Apoptosis and regulation of cell numbers in normal and neoplastic tissues: an overview. Cancer Met Rev 1992; 11:95–103.
5. Moul JW, Bettencourt MC, Sesterhenn IA, Mostofi FK, McLeod DG, Srivastava S, Bauer JJ. Protein expression of p53, bcl-2, and Ki-67 (MIB-1) as prognostic biomarkers in patients with surgically treated, clinically localized prostate cancer. Surgery 1996; 120:159–67.
6. Secker-Walker LM, Swansbury GJ, Hardisty RM. Cytogenetics of acute lymphoblastic leukaemia in children as a factor in the prediction of long term survival. Br J Haematol, 1982, 52:389–99.
7. Hicsonmez G, Erdemli E, Tekelioglu M, Tuncer AM, et al. Morphological evidence of apoptosis in childhood acute myeloblastic leukaemia treated with high dose methyl prednisolone. Leuk Lymphoma 1996, 22:91–6.
8. Tsangaris GT, Tzortzatou-Stathopoulou F. Development of a quantitative method for the study of apoptosis in peripheral blood. In Vivo, 1996, 10:435–43.
9. Coustan-Smith E, Kitenaka A, Pui CH, McNinch L, et al. Clinical relevance of Bcl2 overexpression in childhood acute lymphoblastic leukaemia. Blood, 1996, 87:1140–6.
10. Baxter GD, Collins RJ, Harmon BV, Kumar S, et al. Cell death by apoptosis in acute leukaemia. J Pathol, 1989, 158:123–9.
11. Thiele J, Zirbes TK, Lorenzen J, Kvasnicka HM, et al. Haemopoietic turnover index in reactive and neoplastic bone marrow lesions quantification by apoptosis and PCNA labelling. Ann Haematol, 1997, 75:33–9.
12. Cascavilla N, Musto P, Derina G, Ladogana S, et al. Are early and late T-acute lymphoblastic leukaemia different diseases. A Single Centre Study of 34 patients. Leuk Lymphoma, 1996, 21:437–42.

33

PROLIFERATION AND APOPTOSIS DOES NOT AFFECT PRESENTING WHITE CELL COUNT IN CHILDHOOD ALL

Allen F. Pyesmany, Lynne M. Ball, Margaret Yhap, M. Henry, Krista Laybolt, D. Christie Riddell, and Dick van Velzen

Department of Clinical Haemato-Oncology
Dalhousie University
IWK Grace Health Centre
5850 University Avenue, B3J 3G9
Halifax, Nova Scotia, Canada

Keywords: White cell count, ALL, cell proliferation, apoptosis, treatment, acute leukaemia.

1. ABSTRACT

1.1. Background

Treatment response/drug resistance in childhood acute lymphoblastic leukaemia (ALL) is related to presenting white cell count. This relationship might be explained by high proliferation fraction or by absence of significant apoptosis, but is presently unknown.

1.2. Aims

To study the relationship between proliferation and apoptosis in childhood ALL.

1.3. Methods

1.3.1. Study Groups. Thirty consecutive, unselected cases of childhood ALL (15M,15F). White cell count varied from 1–200 at presentation.

Drug Resistance in Leukemia and Lymphoma III, edited by Kaspers *et al.*
Kluwer Academic / Plenum Publishers, New York, 1999.

1.3.2. Proliferation/Apoptosis Fraction. Immunocytochemical detection of Ki-67 (MM1, NovaCastra, UK) on 5μm paraffin slides, Immunocytochemical detection of apoptosis specific DNA (Klenow) fragments by labelling of 3'-OH ends in 10μm paraffin sections (Frag-EL, CalBiochem, USA).

1.3.3. Quantitation. Image analysis (Quantimet 570C) using nuclear size bias correcting counting frame and rule. Calculation of proliferation (%Ki-67) fraction and of apoptosis corrected proliferation fraction (%Ki-67/100 - %apoptosis)

1.4. Results

Using both linear, logarithmic regression as well as power analysis, no relationship between variables was detected.

1.5. Conclusion

Presenting white cell count is not related to apoptotic or cell proliferative activity or to net tumour growth defined by the balance between these two processes. The relationship to treatment resistance still requires explanation.

2. INTRODUCTION

Of all the clinical prognosticators in childhood ALL, apart from gender and age at presentation, the presenting white cell count has remained one of the strongest predictors of prognosis, i.e., treatment response or drug resistance. The mechanism of this relationship is at present unclear but does in essence not reflect the phenomenon of high blood viscosity and sludging related to extremely high white cell counts.

It has been assumed that high proliferation fractions with short cell cycle time are responsible for such high numbers of peripheral circulating "blast" cells but this may not necessarily be the case. Early release into the peripheral circulation of immature blasts, otherwise contained within the bone marrow, may be a predominant independent factor at the root of this phenomenon.[1–5] However, due to technical limitations, this aspect at this stage cannot be investigated.

An additional potential factor may be the proliferation rates of white cells in the peripheral blood compartment. Active proliferation of circulating lymphoid cells is normally not encountered. Presently very little is known with respect to proliferative activity of circulating malignant cells, especially with respect to the variability thereof and a possible relationship to presenting white cell count has not been assessed.[6]

Finally, absence of apoptosis or reduced / inhibited apoptosis, may result in forced expulsion from the overcrowding bone marrow compartment into the peripheral circulation of blasts which would otherwise not be allowed to commence circulation. This event might hypothetically occur even in the presence of relatively moderate proliferation rates.[5,7–10]

Before commencing a systematic study of the hypothetically important variables as described above, a short orienting study into the relationship between proliferation apoptosis and presenting white cell count is of relevance.[11,12]

Table 1. Summary of results of study into relationship between presenting white cell count, cell proliferation and apoptosis in childhood ALL

Case	WCC 10^6/l	%Ki67	%Frag-EL	ACCPF
1	2.3	5	10	5.5
2	10.1	5	10	5.5
3	15.1	1	5	1
4	6.2	10	1	10
5	74	15	30	21
6	131.4	15	65	43
7	3	1	10	5.5
8	7.6	10	90	100
9	6.7	20	75	80
10	200	30	50	60
11	3.9	35	50	58
12	5.2	20	40	33
13	16.6	5	10	5.5
14	2.4	25	60	61.1
15	31.5	10	60	25
16	3.1	25	25	33.3
17	6.8	15	10	16
18	4	20	50	40
19	6.2	5	70	16.6
20	26.6	15	1	15.1
21	1.2	20	50	40
22	98.5	10	85	66
23	1.7	25	80	100
24	39.2	20	25	27
25	101.4	15	90	100
26	9.9	1	1	1
27	13.5	5	95	100
28	77.9	50	1	50
29	31.1	20	85	100
30	32.4	15	10	17

WCC: Presenting white cell count. %Ki67: Percentage of cells with nuclei labelling positive for cell cycling associated nuclear antigen Ki67. %Frag-EL: Percentage of cells with nuclei labelling positive for apoptosis derived DNA fragments. ACCPF: Apoptosis corrected cell proliferation fraction (%Ki67 / [100% - % Frag-EL]).

3. MATERIALS AND METHODS

3.1. Study Groups

Thirty consecutive, unselected cases of childhood ALL for whom the presenting white cell count was known and for whom appropriate representative tissue material of pretreatment diagnostic bone marrow trephine biopsy was available, were included in the study. There were 15 males and 15 females who ranged in age between 8 months and 16 years of age.

3.2. White Cell Count

These varied from 1–200.10^6/l at presentation (see Table 1).

3.3. Proliferation/Apoptosis Fraction Assessment

Proliferation fraction was assessed by immunocytochemical detection of the Ki-67 antigen using the MM1 monoclonal antibody as supplied by NovaCastra, UK and making use of 5μm paraffin slides of routinely formaldehyde fixed and processed bone marrow trephine biopsy tissue. Apoptosis detection was carried out by DNA in situ labelling of the 3'-OH ends of the DNA fragments released from tumour cell genomic DNA by apoptosis specific endonucleases.

The procedure made use of the commercially available Frag-EL probe and kit as supplied by CalBiochem, USA and was applied to 10 μm paraffin sections taken adjacent to the previous 5μm section used for proliferation assessment and from the same pretreatment diagnostic bone marrow trephine biopsy.

3.4. Quantitation

Quantitation of both parameters was carried out using computer assisted image analysis (Quantimet 570C). 10 systematically random selected fields, containing a minimum of 20 nuclei per field, were used to assure representativity of the results. A nuclear counting frame of rectangular shape with 2 forbidden and 2 including edges on opposite sides, was used to correct for nuclear size associated bias in view of the potential nuclear size increase in proliferation and nuclear size decrease with later phases of apoptosis. Based on the mean of 10 samples, with progressive mean analysis and confirmation of sufficient sample size (mean of 10 samples within 10% of final mean) the %Ki-67 positive cells was analysed for proliferation fraction, the %Frag-EL positive cells for apoptosis fraction and from these two values an Apoptosis Corrected Cell Proliferation Fraction (ACCPF) was calculated (%Ki-67 positive nuclei divided by 100 - % Frag-EL positive nuclei).

3.5. Statistical Analysis

The relationship between Ki-67 positive cell fraction, Frag-EL positive cell fraction and apoptosis corrected cell proliferation fraction and presenting white cell count was analysed using linear and logarithmic regression using SPSS statistical package.

4. RESULTS

The results of the study are summarized in Table 1 and in Figures 1–3 and further illustrated in Figure 4–6. As is evident from the data no relationship between presenting white cell count and any of the three variables studied could be detected.

5. DISCUSSION

In light of the considerable potential number of mechanisms by which either apoptosis defects and / or proliferation variables could have related to the presenting white cell count, the absence of any relationship even after correction of proliferation fraction or the fraction of cells committed to the apoptotic pathway no longer available for proliferation, is surprising.

Figure 1. Relationship of WCC to % Ki67 in childhood ALL. As is evident, even though the number of observations at the high end range of both parameters is limited, there is no clear relationship between the two parameters studied. WCC: Presenting white cell count % Ki67: Percentage of cells with nuclei labelling positive for cell cycling associated nuclear antigen Ki67.

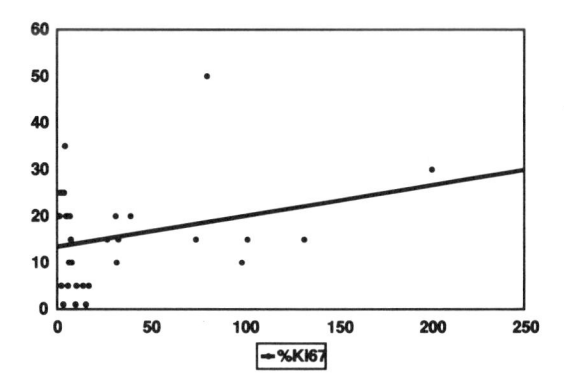

Figure 2. Relationship of WCC to % Frag-EL in childhood ALL. As is evident, even though the number of observations at the high end range of both parameters is limited, there is no clear relationship between the two parameters studied. WCC: Presenting white cell count. %Frag-EL: Percentage of cells with nuclei labelling positive for apoptosis derived DNA fragments.

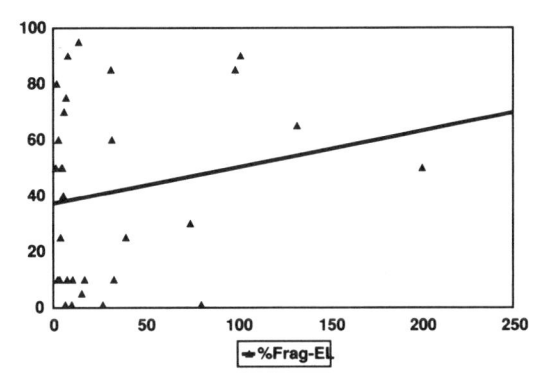

Figure 3. Relationship of WCC to ACCPF in childhood ALL. As is evident, even though the number of observations at the high end range of both parameters is limited, there is no clear relationship between the two parameters studied. WCC: Presenting white cell count. ACCPF: Apoptosis corrected cell proliferation fraction (%Ki67 / [100% - % Frag-EL]).

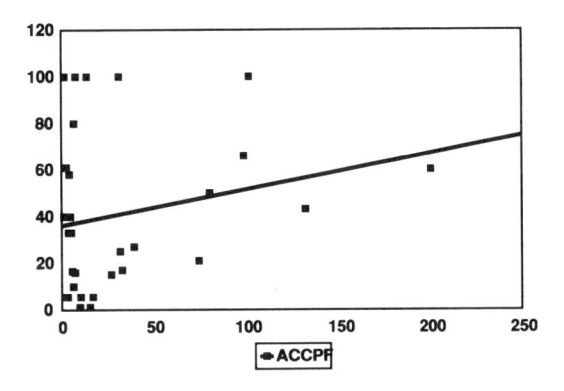

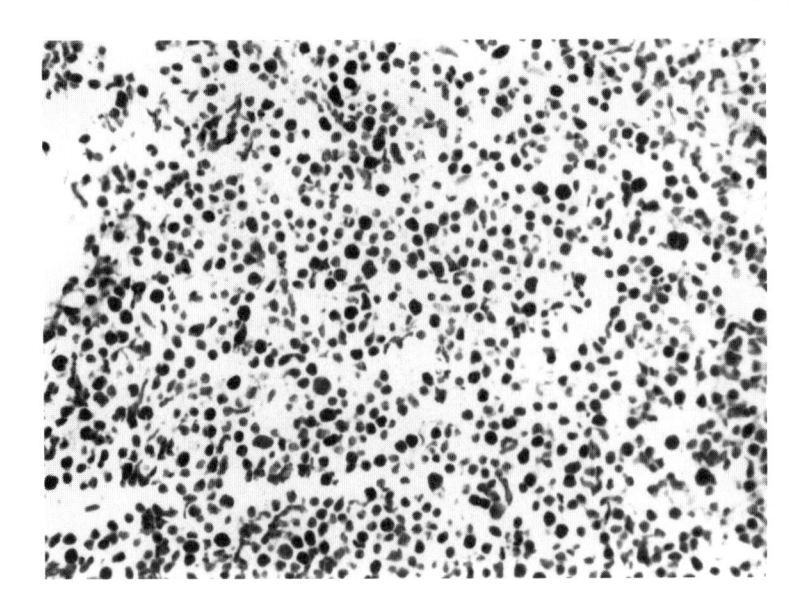

Figure 4. Microphotograph of of pretreatment, diagnostic bone marrow trephine biopsy of childhood patient with ALL. Section stained by routine immunocytochemistry for the PCNA antigen (PC10, DAKO, USA). Note relatively high fraction of positive nuclei (>50%), with homogenous distribution throughout the marrow section shown. 5 μm paraffin section, Haematoxylin counterstain, microscopical magnification 400 x.

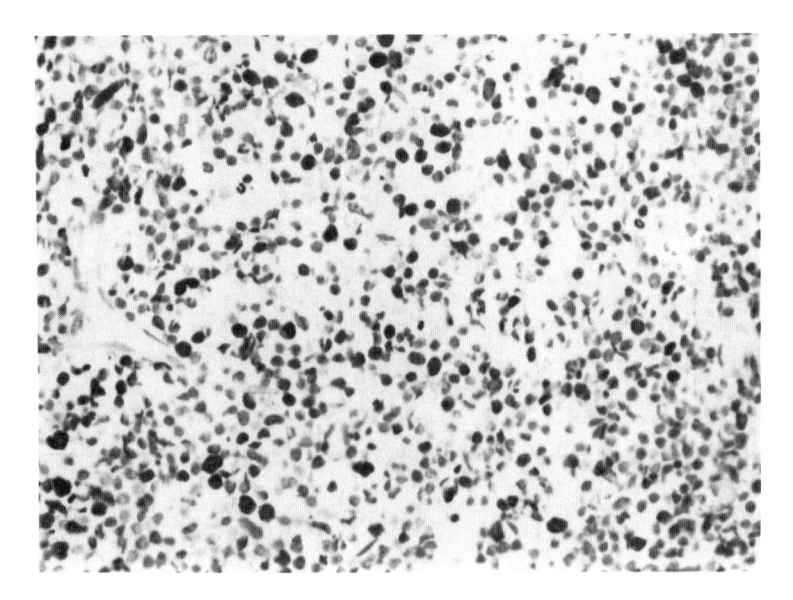

Figure 5. Microphotograph of pretreatment, diagnostic bone marrow trephine biopsy of childhood patient with ALL. Section stained by routine immunocytochemistry for the Ki67 antigen (MM1, NovaCastra, UK). Note intermediate fraction of positive nuclei (ca 10%), with homogenous distribution throughout the marrow section shown. 5 μm paraffin section, Haematoxylin counter stain, microscopical magnification 400 x.

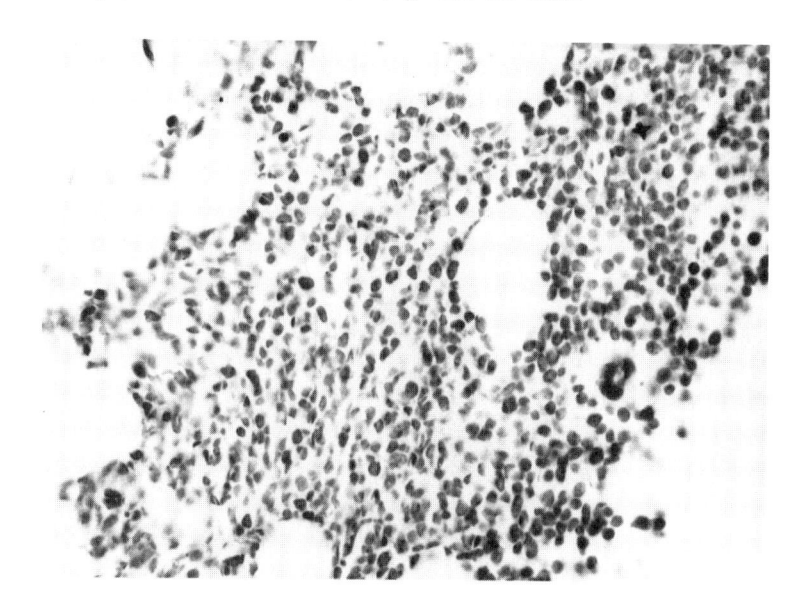

Figure 6. Microphotograph of pretreatment, diagnostic bone marrow trephine biopsy of childhood patient with ALL. Section stained by routine immunocytochemistry for the presence of Frag-EL probe (CalBiochem, USA) bound to apoptosis derived DNA fragments. Note relatively high fraction of positive nuclei (>40%), with homogenous distribution throughout the marrow section shown. 10 μm paraffin section, Fast green counter stain, microscopical magnification 400 x.

This finding indicates that the cell biological parameters that determine release from the bone marrow compartment to the peripheral circulation as well as potential variability of the capability for leukaemic cells to actively proliferate in the circulating blood compartment may be the main determinants of the presenting white cell count.

How this variable, i.e. the presenting white cell count, then affects short and long term outcome i.e., the response or resistance to drug treatment, is at this stage difficult to explain and would require further study. It can however at this stage not be excluded that additional variables exist which have not been included in the considerations of this paper.

One of such potential factors may be the secretion by many normal bone marrow cavity produced cells of a locally bound differentiation inhibitor which is secreted by cells partly in a soluble form but partly with a molecular extension that allows the cells expressing this molecule on the cell surface, to adhere to the local micro environment providing a local differentiation regulating effect. The absence of such control in the peripheral blood compartment or the independence through mutation of the neoplastic cell line of this factor may provide further foci for study of this particular issue.

From the findings we concluded that:

- The presenting white cell count in childhood ALL is not related to apoptotic or cell proliferative activity and thus to net tumour growth as it is defined by the balance between these two processes.
- The relationship between presenting white cell count and prognosis under treatment in childhood ALL still requires further explanation and warrants investigation.

ACKNOWLEDGMENTS

The authors wish to acknowledge the expert technical handling of Mrs. C. Isenor without whom the ability to carry out complex immunocytochemical and molecular biological studies in routine diagnostic specimens would not have been possible. We would also like to acknowledge the help of Mrs. Linda Lee Maughan in the preparation of this manuscript.

REFERENCES

1. Liptay S, Seriu T, Bartram CR, Schmid RM. Germline configuration of nfkb2, c-rel and bc13 in childhood acute lymphoblastic leukaemia (ALL). Leukaemia, 1977, 11:1364–6.
2. Salomons GS, Brady HG, Verwijs-Janssen M, van den Bergh JD, et al. The Bax alpha: Bcl-2 ratio modulates the response to dexamethasone in leukaemic cells and is highly variable in childhood leukaemia. Intern J Cancer 1997, 71:959–65.
3. Uckun FM, Yang Z, Sather H, Steinherz P, et al. Cellular expression of anti-apoptotic Bcl2 oncoprotein in newly diagnosed childhood acute lymphoblastic leukaemia: a Childrens Cancer Group study. Blood, 1997, 89:3769–77.
4. Tsangaris GT, Moschovi M, Mikraki V, et al. Study of apoptosis in peripheral blood of patients with acute lymphoblastic leukaemia during induction therapy. Anticancer Res 1996, 16:3133–40.
5. Coustan-Smith E, Kitenaka A, Pui CH, McNinch L, et al. Clinical relevance of Bcl2 overexpression in childhood acute lymphoblastic leukaemia. Blood, 1996, 87:1140–6.
6. Thiele J, Zirbes TK, Lorenzen J, Kvasnicka HM, et al. Haemopoietic turnover index in reactive and neoplastic bone marrow lesions quantification by apoptosis and PCNA labelling. Ann Haematol, 1997, 75:33–9.
7. Wyllie AH. Apoptosis and regulation of cell numbers in normal and neoplastic tissues: an overview. Cancer Met Rev 1992, 11:95–103.
8. Hicsonmez G, Erdemli E, Tekelioglu M, Tuncer AM, et al. Morphological evidence of apoptosis in childhood acute myeloblastic leukaemia treated with high dose methyl prednisolone. Leuk Lymphoma, 1996, 22:91–6.
9. Debatin KM, Krammer PH. Resistance to Apo1(CD95) induced apoptosis in T-ALL is determined by Bcl2 independent ati-apoptotic program. Leukaemia, 1995, 9:815–20.
10. Baxter GD, Collins RJ, Harmon BV, Kumar S, et al. Cell death by apoptosis in acute leukaemia. J Pathol, 1989, 158:123–9.
11. Findley HW, Gu L, Yeager AM, Zhou M. Expression and regulation of Bcl2, Bcl-xl and Bax correlates with p53 status and sensitivity to apoptosis in childhood acute lymphoblastic leukaemia. Blood, 1997, 89:2986–93.
12. Tsangaris GT, Tzortzatou-Stathopoulou F. Development of a quantitative method for the study of apoptosis in peripheral blood. In Vivo, 1996, 10:435–43.

34

APOPTOSIS BY ANTHRACYCLINES AT THERAPEUTIC CONCENTRATIONS IN MDR1+ HUMAN LEUKEMIC CELLS

Barbara Chiodini, Renato Bassan, and Tiziano Barbui

Division of Hematology
Ospedali Riuniti
Bergamo, Italy

Keywords: Apoptosis, Anthracyclines, MDR1.

1. ABSTRACT

Induction of apoptosis by daunorubicin (DNR) and idarubicin (IDA) was evaluated cytofluorometrically in CEM and CEM-MDR1+ leukemic cells exposed to drug concentrations similar to peak plasma levels obtainable *in vivo* (DNR 200–400 ng/ml, IDA 50–100 ng/ml, 30' incubation), and differentiating apoptosis from necrosis (FITC-annexin V+/propidium iodide- and + cells, respectively). Firstly, to set experimental conditions, apoptosis was evaluated in CEM cells at 3, 6, 12, 18, 24, 48, 72, and 96 hours from end of drug incubation, the maximal increase being noted at 24–48 hours. Net apoptosis rates were determined after subtraction of the spontaneous activity observed in untreated cells. The apoptotic effect from varying drug type and concentration was compared at 24 hours in CEM-MDR1+ cells, with and without co-incubation with MDR1 functional downregulator cyclosporin A (CSA) used at therapeutic concentration (1500 ng/ml). The results indicated that, at drug concentrations likely to be approached *in vivo* as a short-lasting peak level (IDA 100–200 ng/ml) with increased-dose IDA (>12–15 mg/m^2), pro-apoptotic effects by IDA+CSA in CEM-MDR1+ cells were significantly greater than by DNR+CSA, and corresponded to the levels observed with IDA 50 ng/ml without CSA in control CEM cells. This *in vitro* study demonstrates that it is possible to determine in the same sample cell fluorescence related to anthracyclines, apoptotic cells (FITC-annexin V positive), and necrotic cells (propidium iodide positive), and confirms that cytofluorimetric evaluation of apoptosis can reliably predict the effects of anthracyines in function of drug type, concentration and, in MDR1+ cells, concurrent MDR1 inhibition. Extension of this assay to the clinical ground may be warranted.

2. INTRODUCTION

The anthracyclines exert a strong antileukemic action in acute leukemia (acute myeloid and lymphoid leukemia, AML and ALL), as inhibitors of nuclear topoisomerase-II. Therapeutic blockade of this enzyme can switch on apoptosis, a common pathway through which most anticancer drugs eventually seem to kill tumoral cells *in vivo* (1). Following the administration of equimyelotoxic doses of daunorubicin (DNR 45 mg/m^2) and idarubicin (IDA 10–12 mg/m^2), peak plasma levels of about 200 ng/ml and 50 ng/ml are reached, respectively, lasting for only a few minutes and leading to a proportional entry of the drugs into neoplastic cells (2). Anthracycline liver metabolism is responsible for the subsequent release of alcohol metabolites daunorubicinol and idarubicinol (IDAol). Because IDAol is cytotoxic, it may contribute to the therapeutic activity of IDA (3).

IDA appears more effective than DNR in AML (4,5), and is partially capable to circumvent P-glycoprotein-related (P-170-type, MDR1) multidrug resistance (6,7). We previously demonstrated that, in MDR1+ CEM-VBL cells cultured *in vitro*, IDA with or without IDAol and with or without the MDR1 functional inhibitor cyclosporin A (CSA) exerted a greater antiproliferative effect than comparable therapeutic concentrations of DNR with or without DNRol and with or without CSA, and that CSA modulation, in the case of IDA, was evident only during the early phase of drug-cell interaction (8). In that study, the standard MTT assay and the annexin V binding assay were used in association to document the growth inhibition and pro-apoptotic effects of drugs and drugs combinations, respectively.

In the present study we expand and complement these early observations, by investigating cytofluorometrically the exact timing and rates of apoptotic cell changes inducible in CEM and MDR1+ CEM-VBL cells by the exposure to increasing concentrations of IDA and DNR (+/-CSA), and trying to differentiate in the same cell sample the information relative to anthracycline cell uptake (direct red fluorescence), apoptosis (green fluorescence by fluoresceinated annexin V bound to membrane phosphatidylserine), and cellular necrosis (red fluorescence by propidium iodide).

3. MATERIALS AND METHODS

3.1. *In Vitro* Cell Lines

Human T-lymphoblastic CEM and P-170-positive CEM-VBL cells (courtesy of Dr. L. Capolongo, Centro Ricerche Pharmacia, Nerviano, Italy) were grown in RPMI 1640 medium supplemented with 10% fetal calf serum, L-glutamine, pennicillin and streptomycin in humidified 5% CO_2 at 37 °C. CEM-VBL cells immunophenotype was MDR1-associated antigen MRK16 100% positive, CD19- HLA-DR- CD34- CD2- CD3- CD8- CD13- CD11b- (<5% positive cells), and cytoplasmic CD3+ CD5+ CD4+ (50%-100% positive cells). CEM-VBL cells were MDR1 antigen+/efflux+, as demonstrated by the 99.6% extrusion rate of $DiOC_2$ as compared with CEM cells (9).

3.2. Anthracyclines

DNR, IDA and IDAol (idarubicinol) were obtained from Pharmacia-Upjohn Group (courtesy of Dr M. Grandi, Milan, Italy). 10 μg/ml stock solutions were stored at -80 °C. The working solutions were prepared by dilution in cell culture medium and were patterned after the mean peak plasma levels reported *in vivo*, with drug incubation lasting 30' in each test (2,3,10). IDAol incubation time was prolonged to 90'. Functional blokade of MDR1 mechanism in CEM-VBL cells was attempted with CSA diluted in absolute ethanol <0.1% and RPMI 1640 medium to a final concentration of 1500 ng/ml (11). CSA was added 90' before anthracycline drugs and mantained in the medium until cell washing and evaluation of results.

3.3. Apoptosis and Necrosis

Cells undergoing apoptosis express phosphatidylserine on the cell membrane, to which annexin V binds specifically. Purified, fluorescein isothiocyanate (FITC)-labelled annexin V can be used for the cytofluorimetric enumeration of apoptotic cells (12) (Bender MedSystems-Prodotti Gianni, Milan, Italy). FITC-annexin V 2.5 μg/ml was added to cellular suspensions according to the manufacturer's technical recommendations. Necrotic cells were identified by their staining with propidium iodide 20 μg/ml (10 μl of this solution was added before FACScan analysis), that enters into dead cells because of membrane permeabilization.

3.4. Flow Cytometry

FITC-annexin V staining, propidium iodide staining, and anthracycline incorporation studies were performed according to standard methods (12,13) on a FACScan flow cytometer (Becton Dickinson, San Jose, CA, USA) equipped with an argon excitation laser light (488 nm wavelength) and 530/30 nm (FL1) and 585/42 nm (FL2) band pass filters. Cellular fluorescence of 1×10^6 cells/ml was determined after washing and resuspending of FSC-SSC gated cells, excluding cellular debris, using FL1 filter (FITC-annexin V) and FL2 filter (anthracyclinic drugs, propidium iodide) with use of the appropriate negative controls and fluorescence manual compensation to eliminate any fluorescence overlap between fluorescence by anthracycline, FITC-annexin V, and propidium iodide. Results of annexin V and propidium iodide fluorescence were expressed as per cent positive cells.

4. RESULTS

4.1. Quantitation and Timing of Apoptosis/Annexin V Binding

In the first series of experiments we evaluated the induction of apoptosis by anthracyclines in CEM cell. Apoptosis was expressed as the percent increase of FITC-annexin V positive cells after drug incubation. Figure 1a shows the results from three distinct determinations, following exposure to DNR 400 ng/ml fixed dose. In this test, DNR induced a sharp increase of annexin V binding (i.e. apoptosis) from approximately the 9th hour, and maximal apoptotic rates at 24–36 hours (≥50%-75%), while the subsequent smaller and slower incremental effects corresponded to the spontaneous changes observed in untreated control cells. We next analyzed the effects of both IDA and DNR at several concentrations, comparing apoptotic cell rates at 24 and 48 hours. In this test (Figure 1b), annexin V positivity increased proportionally to the drug concentration, without any substantial difference between the results at 24 or 48 hours, even if values at 48 hours as well as IDA-related activity were generally higher. To assess whether these pharma-

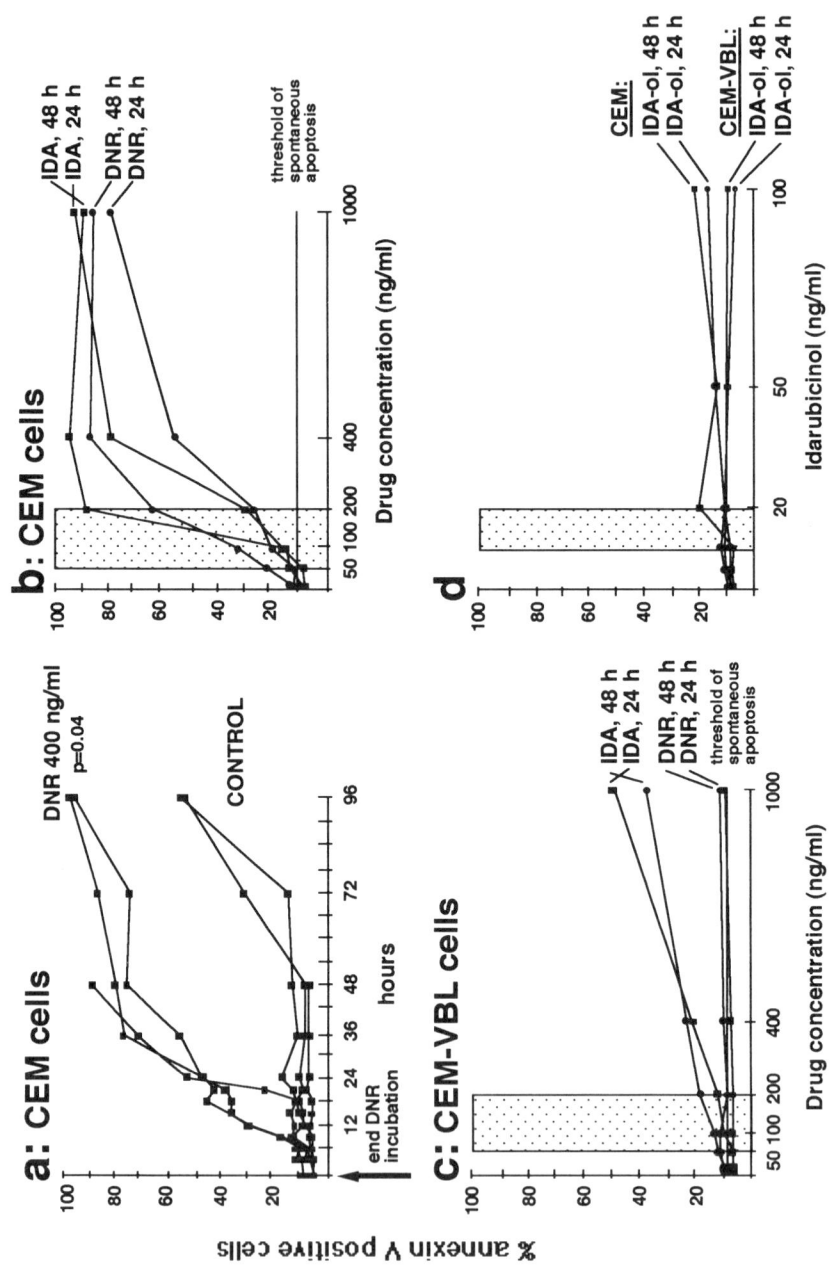

Figure 1. a) Annexin V positivity of CEM cells after 30' incubation with DNR at final concentration 400 ng/ml vs spontaneous activity of untreated control cells. b) Pro-apoptotic effects at 24–48 hours of varying concentrations of IDA and DNR in CEM cells. c) Pro-apoptotic effects at 24–48 hours of varying concentrations of IDA and DNR in CEM-VBL cells. d) Pro-apoptotic effects at 24–48 hours of varying concentrations of IDAol in CEM and CEM-VBL cells. The shadowed area is indicative of the clinically relevant ranges.

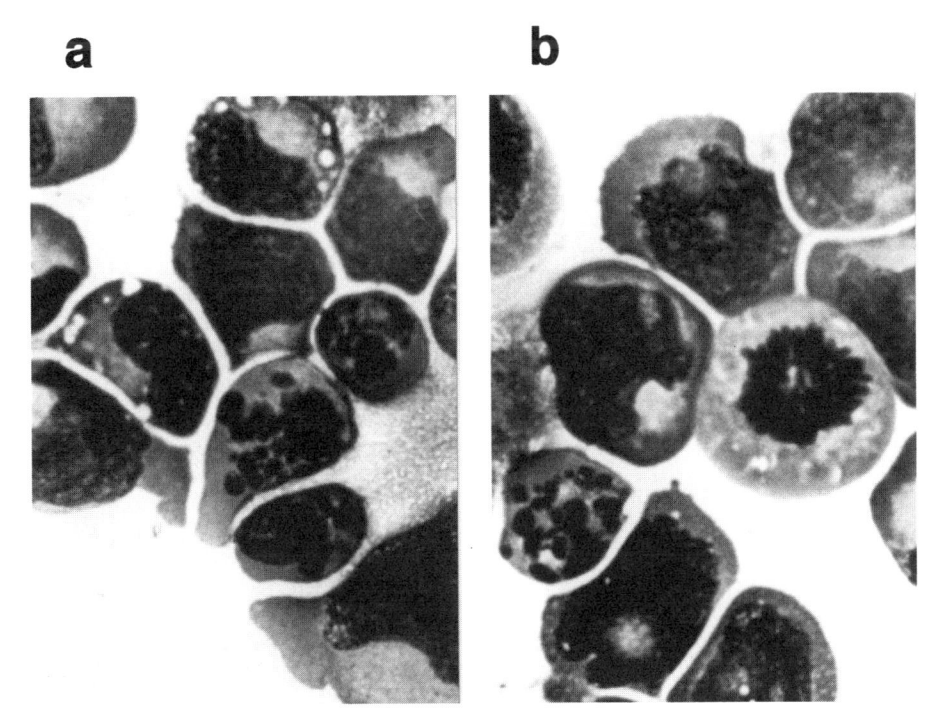

Figure 2. Morphologic pro-apoptotic effects induced by anthracyclines in CEM (a) and CEM-VBL cells (b). CEM-VBL cells partially escape drug-induced apoptosis: less apoptotic figures are observed and the mitogenic activity is mantained. May Grunwald Giemsa staining of cytospin preparation, final magnification 1000x.

cologic effects could be counterbalanced by MDR1 expression in CEM-VBL cells, as one would expect, the test was repeated using as target cells the multidrug resistant mutant cell line. In this case, a net reduction of pro-apoptotic drug activity was evident (Figure 1c), although still dependent on drug concentration and more marked for DNR. Finally, the pro-apoptotic role of IDAol was evaluated. In this test (Figure 1d), a modest effect was noted in CEM cells but not in CEM-VBL cells, with IDAol concentrations ≥50 ng/ml. DNR alcohol metabolite was not studied because noncytotoxic.

The morphologic changes observed in CEM and CEM-VBL cells exposed to anthracyclines were found to correlate well with annexin V positivity and, in particular, although some CEM-VBL cells were shown to acquire typical apoptotic characteristics (cell shrinking and nuclear fragmentation), their ability to proliferate was partially preserved while it was almost totally abolished in drug sensitive CEM cells. This different behavior is illustrated in Figure 2.

4.2. Apoptosis and Necrosis

In a second step our aim was to differentiate apoptosis from necrosis, and to define better the spontaneous rate and course over time of the two phenomena in untreated drug-sensitive cells. Since spontaneous apoptosis increased abnormally after 48 hours in CEM cells (Figure 1a), results were evaluated 24 hours following incubation with FITC-annexin V. Initially, binding of annexin V and cell staining by propidium iodide were evaluated separately (Figure 3a and b). In this assay, two different cell populations were identified

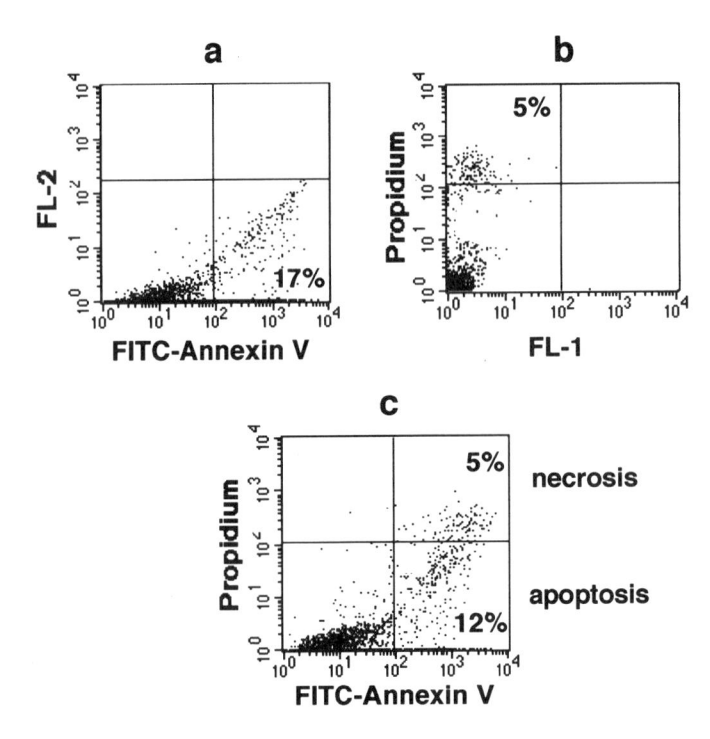

Figure 3. a) and b) Spontaneous expression of isolated FITC-annexin V and propidium iodide positivity by untreated CEM cells. c) Simultaneous expression of FITC-annexin V and/or propidium iodide positivity by untreated CEM cells.

with a basal prevalence of apoptotic over necrotic cells. Interestingly, in the simultaneous evaluation (Figure 3c), annexin V positivity could still be discriminated from propidium iodide positivity but most if not all necrotic cells were concurrently annexin V positive, so that the amount of annexin V+/propidium- cells (12%) plus that of propidium+ cells (5%) was the same as that of annexin V+ cells in the single evaluation test (17%), because of the forced inclusion in this latter category of propidium positive ones.

4.3. Alterations Induced by Anthracyclines

Whether anthracycline drugs were capable of inducing a change in apoptotic and necrotic cells rates in CEM cells was the matter of the following test. In view of fluorescence results previously obtained incubating cells with FITC-annexin V and/or propidium iodide, it was mandatory to maintain the cellular fluorescence by anthracyclines in the lower left area of the flow-cytometric dot plot system illustrated in Figure 3, outside the FL-1 and FL-2 regions prominently associated with annexin V and propidium iodide fluorescence, respectively. Representative dot plot results of FL-1 vs FL-2 scatters after exposure to either anthracycline are reported in Figure 4a-c, showing a 1–2 log intensity increase in the FL-2 channel fluorescence output due to anthracycline cellular uptake, but still significantly below the strong red fluorecence peak characteristic of propidium labeled cells and clearly separated from the FL-1 region associated with FITC-annexin V binding.

The effects of DNR and IDA employed at the above dosage on apoptosis (and necrosis) of CEM cells evaluated at 24 hours are illustrated in Figure 5a and b. By compari-

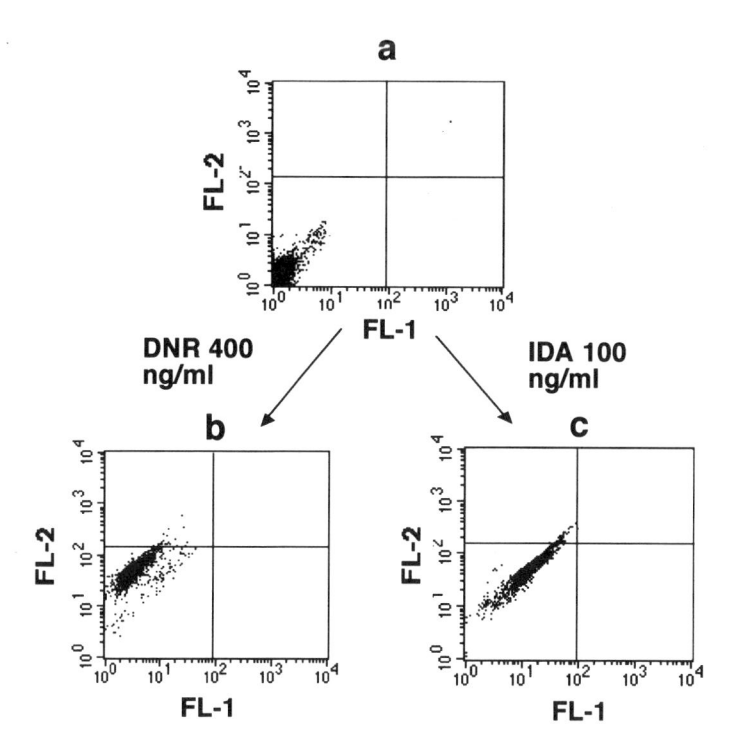

Figure 4. Increased FL-2 fluorescence of CEM cells (a) after exposure to DNR 400 ng/ml (b) and IDA 100 ng/ml (c).

son with the results in untreated cells, and in function of anthracycline cell uptake, both apoptosis and cellular death rates were increased.

The changes developing over 48 hours in apoptotic (annexin V+/propidium iodide-) and necrotic (annexin V+/propidium iodide+) cell rates after incubation of CEM cells with DNR or IDA are depicted in Figure 6a. These results underlined the strict relationship between induction of apoptosis by drugs and the subsequent appearance of necrotic cell fea-

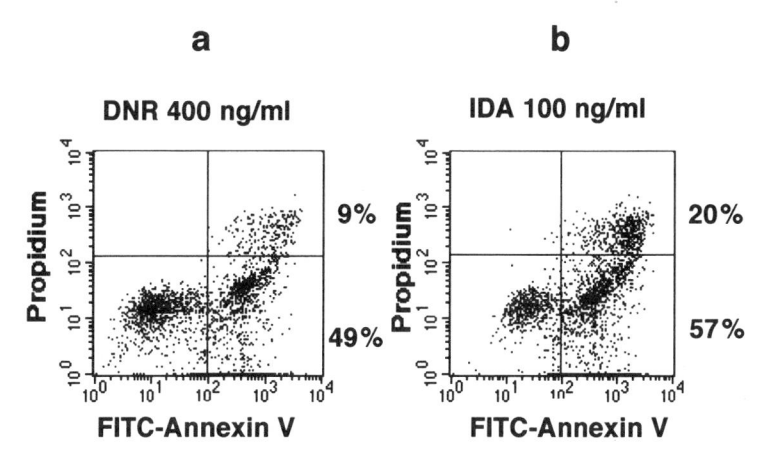

Figure 5. Dot plot analysis of apoptosis and necrosis by CEM cells exposed to DNR 400 ng/ml (a) and IDA 100 ng/ml (b).

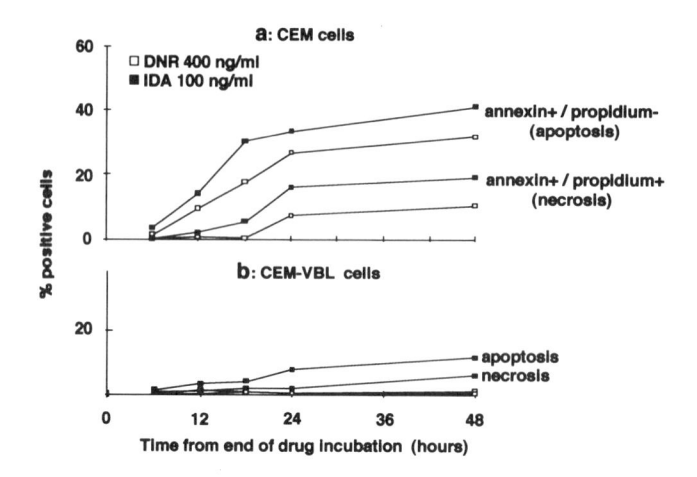

Figure 6. a) Time-course of apoptosis and necrosis by DNR 400 ng/ml and IDA 100 ng/ml in CEM cells. b) Same test in CEM-VBL cells.

tures in a fraction of annexin V positive apoptotic cells, presumably as final step of drug-induced cellular damage. This conclusion is supported also by the evaluation, in this test, of net results after subtraction of spontaneous annexin V and propidium iodide positivity values observed in untreated control cells. With DNR, the lag-phase between increased apoptosis and the appearance of necrotic cells was about 6 hours, and probably a similar or even faster temporal relationship occurred with IDA if one looks at the results after 6–12 hours.

4.4. Results in MDR1+ CEM Cells and Modulability by CSA

The test performed in CEM cells (Figure 6a) was repeated in CEM-VBL cells (Figure 6b). In this instance, apoptosis by IDA was reduced and it was almost completely undetectable with DNR. The induction of apoptosis at 24 hours by increasing concentrations of DNR and IDA is displayed in Figure 7a, reporting net values for comparative purposes

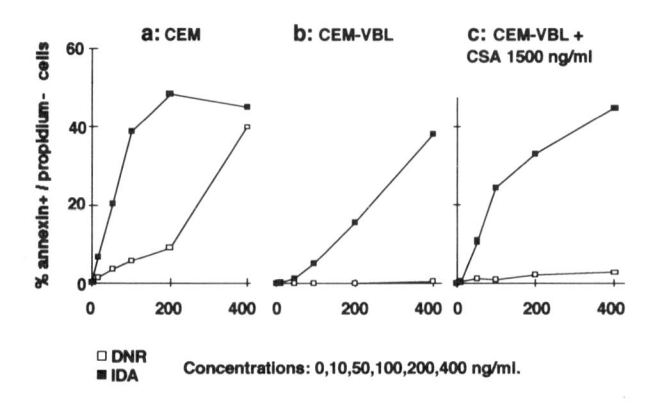

Figure 7. a) Pro-apoptotic effects by increasing concentrations of DNR and IDA on CEM cells. b) Same test in CEM-VBL cells. c) Same test in CEM-VBL cells plus MDR1 inhibitor CSA 1500 ng/ml.

Table 1. Comparative results of net FITC-annexin V positivity (apoptosis) induced by DNR and IDA with or without CSA 1500 ng/ml in CEM and CEM-VBL cells

Drug concentration (ng/ml)	CEM cells[a] DNR	CEM cells[a] IDA	CEM-VBL cells[a] DNR	CEM-VBL cells[a] IDA	CEM-VBL cells[a] DNR+CSA	CEM-VBL cells[a] IDA+CSA
10	1.1±1	6.7±2.9	0±0	0.2±0.1	0.4±0.6	0.6±0.4
50	3.6±1.7	20.1±9.5	0.1±0.1	1.2±0.7	1±0.8	10.7±6[1]
100	5.8±0.7	38.7±4.3	0±0	5.3±1.2	0.9±0.8	24.5±5.7[2]
200	9.3±2.7	48.7±4.7	0±0	15.6±4.3	2±0.8	32.9±4.4[3]
400	39.9±1.9	45.2±6.4	0.3±0.3	38±5.8	2.9±0.4	45±2.9

[1] p = 0.053 vs IDA 50, p = 0.069 vs DNR 200 + CSA
[2] p = 0.005 vs IDA 100, p = 0.002 vs DNR 200 + CSA
[3] p = 0.008 vs IDA 200, p = 0.0001 vs DNR 200 + CSA
[a] Mean ± SD

with CEM cells (Figure 6a). In CEM cells, IDA was more active, particularly at lower drug concentrations, so that the proportion of cells induced into apoptosis by IDA 100 ng/ml was similar to that obtained with DNR 400 ng/ml. In CEM-VBL cells (Figure 7b), this difference was even more striking since DNR exerted no pro-apoptotic effect while IDA was nearly as active as DNR in CEM cells, since the graphics of apoptosis by DNR in CEM cells and by IDA in CEM-VBL cells were superimposable.

The final test was aimed to detect and quantitate the changes induced by the addition of the MDR1 functional inhibitor CSA, used at a final concentration that can be achieved in a clinical study and that has a minimal impact on spontaneous apoptosis (increased by 3.5% at 36 hours in control tests). In this assay, once more considering only net apoptosis rates (proportions of annexin V+/propidium iodide- cells after subtraction of spontaneous activities in untreated control cells), apoptosis by DNR was only slightly increased by CSA, even using the higher DNR concentration, while IDA-related effects became more evident and, using IDA 100–200 ng/ml plus CSA, were similar to those observed in CEM cells with IDA 50–100 ng/ml (Figure 7a). Whether the results obtained in CEM-VBL cells were analyzed comparing DNR and IDA or the same IDA concentrations with or without CSA (Table 1), any statistically significant difference was consistently in favor of the IDA-CSA combination.

5. DISCUSSION

Since it has become widely available for clinical studies, initially for AML and lately for ALL too, the new anthracycline-type drug IDA attracted justified attention for its improved therapeutic index over DNR, due to an augmented cytotoxic power in reason of peculiar pharmacodynamic characteristics and to lower cardiac toxicity. The results from the first controlled clinical trials confirmed IDA to be associated with more and sometimes longer remissions in AML (4,5). Interest was subsequently raised by the concurrent description of MDR1 functional overexpression in AML as an unfavorable independent prognostic sign in several clinical series, and by the the lower vulnerability to MDR1 of IDA demonstrated by *in vitro* studies in MDR1+ human leukemic cells of both myeloid and lymphoid lineage (6,7). More recently, we were pushed to investigate further this diversity in the light of the first published results of clinical trials incorporating MDR1 blockade by CSA, quinidine, or PSC 833 compound as an adjunct to treatment or retreatment regimens for acute leukemias. While the conceptual lay-out and the preliminary clinical results from these and other similar ongoing studies have been presented (11,14–16), we raise a question about the choice of the optimal drug(s) to be administered along with MDR1 modifiers to patients with multidrug resistant leukemias.

In our studies we compared the pro-apoptotic effects *in vitro* by DNR and IDA employed at pharmacologically relevant concentrations, and used as MDR1 inhibitor CSA at an intermediate *in vitro* dosage (1500 ng/ml) that is achievable in patients who receive continuous infusion CSA 16/mg/kg/d, and that seems able to affect at some extent the MDR1 functional activity of leukemic cells (11). CSA was chosen because an easily accessible and low-priced drug and because of its well known acute and chronic toxicity profile. Moreover, CSA can be directly cytotoxic to leukemic cells of all lineages (17) and, in the intravenous formulation, it is coupled with the oily vehicle cremophor EL which can exert additional anti-MDR1 activity (18).

We previously demonstrated that DNR and IDA behave differently when used *in vitro* against CEM-VBL cells in the presence of CSA (8). Differing from DNR, the intracellular accumulation of IDA by CEM-VBL cells can be increased by CSA only during the 30' drug incubation period but it is unaffected 12 hours later. This difference is most probably explained by IDA's greater lipophilicity that probably allows, upon partial blockade of MDR1 functional activity by CSA, a very quick formation of irreversible drug-topoisomerase II-DNA ternary complexes, that are no longer influenced by membrane transport mechanisms and are eventually capable to induce cellular activation of programmed cell death programs.

In this study we assessed in greater detail the inducibility of apoptosis by DNR and IDA in CEM-VBL cells, with or without CSA. The single-step cytofluorimetric assay allowed detection of anthracycline-induced apoptosis as well as end-stage cellular necrosis, and was highly sensitive to the modifications of drug type, concentration, MDR1 expression, coincubation with CSA, and time. The results pointed once more to the superiority of IDA over DNR especially when the multidrug resistance mechanism was expressed by CEM-VBL cells. FITC-annexin V binding was confirmed as an easy and sensitive apoptosis test that correlates well with morphologic cell changes and DNA fragmentation test, and it was possible to differentiate apoptotic cells from necrotic cells, the latter characterized by a positive labeling with propidium iodide, without any overlap fluorescence with antracycline cellular load. Since necrosis appeared somewhat later than apoptosis in most assays and varied proportionally to the former, it is likely that apoptotic cells eventually turned into necrotic ones, given that *in vitro* they cannot be cleared by scavenger cells sensitized by apoptosic signals as it normally occurs in tissues *in vivo*.

The evaluation of net apoptotic cell rates at 24 hours and after subtraction of spontaneous values of untreated control cells was in our opinion the best way to assess drug-related effects, since spontaneous apoptosis and necrosis were subject to relatively ample fluctuations and the evaluation at 48–96 hours was hampered by a substantial increase of both annexin V binding and propidium iodide labeling by control cells.

If induction of apoptosis is the major way through which anthracyclines and other topoisomerase II inhibitors suppress the neoplastic cell growth, then this sensitive, simple and rapid cytofluorimetric assay can make it possible to detect this primary therapeutic effect *in vitro* at the single-cell level, facilitating comparative studies between drugs and drug/MDR1 inhibitor combinations. If apoptosis is the common final pathway of drug-induced cellular damage, then this assay could be highly sensitive to drug resistance by other mechanisms (MRP, LRP, GST, atMDR, and of course dysrupted apoptosis regulation). Our studies demonstrates that, in CEM and MDR1+ CEM-VBL cells, apoptosis is variably increased in correlation with the use of IDA, DNR, their concentrations, and the additional use of CSA. We have preliminary data obtained in other leukemic cell lines that show a heterogeneous behavior, in terms of spontaneous apoptotic threshold, time-course to apoptotic response, and drug-induced apoptosis. Eventualy, different drug-induced apoptotic profiles could reveal new aspects of drug sensitivity in acute leukemias expressing any one or more drug resistance mechanism(s) and help to design more effective clinical trials.

If we think that our observations are potentially useful to the management of MDR1 positive leukemias, IDA seems to have more chances than DNR not only as a drug but even, or even better, if downregulation of MDR1 molecular machinery is attempted, in our case with CSA. On the other hand, if the results from our apoptosis studies are consistent, as it seems, with an increase of pro-apoptotic and clinical activities in function of IDA dosage (19), then reducing the durability of CSA infusion (<12 hours) on days of an increased-dose IDA administration would be, for toxicity reasons, not only mandatory but even possible by virtue of IDA's short-lasting sensitivity to cellular uptake regulation by CSA (8). An augmented-dose IDA plus short-course CSA multidrug blockade regimen is an attractive option for a new phase I trial in refractory and high-risk leukemias.

REFERENCES

1. Hannun YA. Apoptosis and the dilemma of cancer chemotherapy. Blood 89: 1845–1853, 1997.
2. Speth PAJ, Minderman H, Haanen C: Idarubicin v daunorubicin: preclinical and clinical pharmacokinetic studies. Semin Oncol 16: 2–9, 1989 (suppl 2).
3. Ames MA, Spreafico F: Selected pharmacologic characteristics of idarubicin and idarubicinol. Leukemia 6: 70–75, 1992 (suppl 1).
4. Wheatley K: Meta-analysis of randomized trials of idarubicin (IDAR) or mitozantrone (MITO) versus daunorubicin (DNR) as induction therapy for acute myeloid leukemia (AML). Blood 86: 434a, 1995 (suppl 1, abstr).
5. Bassan R, Barbui T: Remission induction therapy for adults with acute myelogenous leukemia: towards the ICE age? Haematologica 80: 82–90, 1995.
6. Ross D, Tong Y, Cornblatt B: Idarubicin (IDA) is less vulnerable to transport-mediated multidrug resistance (MDR) than its metabolite idarubicinol (IDAol) or daunorubicin (DNR). Blood 82: 257a, 1993 (suppl 1, abstr 1015).
7. Berman E, McBride M: Comparative cellular pharmacology of daunorubicin and idarubicin in human multidrug-resistant leukemia cells. Blood 79: 3267–3273, 1992.
8. Chiodini B, Bassan R, Borleri G, Lerede T, Barbui T. Idarubicin activity against multidrug resistant (mdr-1+) cells is increased by cyclosporin A. In: Hiddemann W et al (eds.) Acute Leukemias VII. Springer, Berlin 1998, pp. 475–482.
9. Leith CP, Chen I-M, Kopecky KJ, et al: Correlation of multidrug resistance (MDR1) protein expression with functional dye/drug efflux in acute myeloid leukemia by multiparameter flow cytometry: identification of discordant MDR⁻/efflux⁺ and MDR⁺/efflux⁻ cases. Blood 86: 2329–2342, 1995.
10. Reid JM, Pendergrass TW, Krailo MD, Hammond GD, Ames MM: Plasma pharmacokinetics and cerebrospinal fluid concentrations of idarubicin and idarubicinol in pediatric leukemia patients. A Childrens Cancer Study Group report. Cancer Res 50: 6525–6528, 1990.
11. List AF, Speier C, Greer J, et al: Phase I/II trial of cyclosporine as a chemotherapy-resistance modifier in acute leukemia. J Clin Oncol 11: 1652–1660, 1993.
12. Koopman G, Reutelingsperger CPM, Kuijten GAM, et al: Annexin V for flow cytometric detection of phosphatidylserine expression on B cells undergoing apoptosis. Blood 84: 1415–1420, 1994.
13. Kokenberg E, Sonneveld P, Delwel R, et al: In vivo uptake of daunorubicin by acute myeloid leukemia (AML) cells measured by flow cytometry. Leukemia 2: 511–517, 1988.
14. List AF: The role of multidrug resistance and its pharmacological modulation in acute myeloid leukemia. Leukemia 10: S46-S51, 1996 (suppl 2).

15. Solary E, Caillot D, Chauffert B, et al: Feasibility of using quinine, a potential multidrug resistance-reversing agent, in combination with mitoxantrone and cytarabine for the treatment of acute leukemia. J Clin Oncol 10: 1730–1736, 1992.
16. Kornblau SM, Estey E, Madden T, et al: Phase I study of mitoxantrone plus etoposide with multidrug blockade by SDZ PSC-833 in relapsed or refractory acute myelogenous leukemia. J Clin Oncol 15: 1796–1802, 1997.
17. Ito C, Ribeiro RC, Behm FG, Raimondi SC, Pui C-H, Campana C. Cyclosporin A induces apoptosis in childhood acute lymphoblastic leukemia cells. Blood 91: 1001–1007, 1998.
18. Ross DD, Wooten PJ, Tong Y, et al: Synergistic reversal of multidrug-resistance phenotype in acute myeloid leukemia by cyclosporin A and cremophor EL. Blood 83: 1337–1347, 1994.
19. Weiss M, Maslak P, Megherian L, Scheinberg D. A phase I trial of a single high dose of idarubicin combined with high dose cytarabine (ARA-C) as induction therapy in relapsed and refractory adult patients with acute lymphoblastic leukemia (ALL). Blood 86: 786a, 1995 (suppl 1, abstr 3131).

BCL-2 EXPRESSION IN CHILDHOOD LEUKEMIA VERSUS SPONTANEOUS APOPTOSIS, DRUG INDUCED APOPTOSIS, AND IN VITRO DRUG RESISTANCE

E. G. Haarman,[1] G. J. L. Kaspers,[1] R. Pieters,[1] C. H. van Zantwijk,[1] G. J. Broekema,[1] K. Hählen,[2] and A. J. P. Veerman[1]

[1]Department of Pediatric Hematology/Oncology
University Hospital Vrije Universiteit
De Boelelaan 1117, 1081 HV Amsterdam, The Netherlands
[2]Department of Pediatric Hematology/Oncology
Sophia Children Hospital, 60 Dr. Molewaterplein
3015 GJ Rotterdam, The Netherlands

Keywords: Bcl-2, apoptosis, drug resistance, leukemia, childhood.

1. ABSTRACT

The antileukemic activity of cytotoxic drugs is increasingly thought to be the result of induction of apoptosis. Several proto-oncogenes have been related to the regulation of this process. In this study we evaluated the relation between bcl-2 expression, spontaneous and dexamethasone (DXM) induced apoptosis, and in vitro resistance to DXM, prednisolone (PRD) and cytarabine (ARA) determined using the total cell kill colorimetric methyl-thiazol-tetrazolium salt (MTT) assay, in childhood acute lymphoblastic leukemia (ALL). Drug resistance was expressed as the LC50 value, the drug concentration lethal to 50% of the cells. Fourty-six samples taken at initial diagnosis (iALL) and 31 samples taken at relapse (rALL) were incubated in culture medium, with and without DXM. Bcl-2 expression and apoptosis were measured flowcytometrically, the latter using DNA histogram analysis. Bcl-2 expression was 1.4 fold higher in rALL than in iALL (p=0.008). Both spontaneous and DXM induced apoptosis increased significantly from 0 to 48 hours (in up to 71%, 81% of the cells respectively). Bcl-2 expression was inversely correlated with the extent of spontaneous apoptosis after 24 hours in iALL (r=-0.40, p=0.05). Relapsed samples, but not samples obtained at presentation, expressing high levels of bcl-2 displayed increased resistance to drug induced apoptosis (r=-0.63, p= 0.02). In iALL high bcl-2 expression appeared to be related to low LC50 values of ARA. No correlations were found for DXM or PRD. In conclusion, DXM excerts its cytotoxic effect at least partly by means of induction of apoptosis. Bcl-2 inhibits drug induced apoptosis in rALL. However in iALL bcl-2 expression is not associated with increased in vitro drug resistance, nor with increased resistance to drug induced apoptosis.

2. INTRODUCTION

Over a decade ago bcl-2 was discovered in the study of the t(14;18) chromosome translocation present in B-cell leukemia and a high percentage of follicular lymphoma's.[1–3] Bcl-2 protein is a 26 Kd-integral membrane protein broadly distributed within the cell, predominantly localized to the perinuclear endoplasmatic reticulum or to the mitochondrial membranes.[4-6]

Subsequent studies have shown that bcl-2 confers a survival advantage to various types of cells by inhibiting apoptosis or "programmed cell-death", an active form of cellular suicide.[7–9] The cytotoxic effects of various chemotherapeutic drugs, including the glucocorticoids, are increasingly related to the induction of apoptosis.[10] Various studies have shown an association between increased resistance to chemotherapeutic agents and decreased capacity to undergo apoptosis.[11–13] Therefore bcl-2 may be considered as a general drug resistance related protein, and may in that respect, have an unfavorable prognostic value.[14–16] In support of this it was found in adult acute myeloid leukemia that high levels of bcl-2 correlated with high white bloodcell count (WBC) and poor prognosis.[17–18] Conversely, cytokine- or anti-sense mediated reduction of bcl-2 expression increases the sensitivity of various tumor cell-lines to several cytotoxic drugs.[19–20]

However in childhood acute lymphoblastic leukemia (ALL) the role of bcl-2 is not yet clear. Few studies have been performed on patient samples, including relatively low numbers of patients (especially in case of relapsed (rALL) patients). Though the various authors agree that bcl-2 expression in leukemic blasts is the rule in childhood ALL, conflicting results were found with regard to the relation between bcl-2 expression and clinical response to chemotherapy.[21–23] Whereas one study could not demonstrate any correlation between the level of expression of bcl-2 and prognosis,[21] another study demonstrated a correlation with poor initial response to chemotherapy.[22] In contrast Coustan-Smith and colleges found that high bcl-2 levels were associated with improved survival and the absence of chromosomal abnormalities.[23]

For the above outlined reasons we decided to evaluate bcl-2 expression in samples obtained from children suffering from iALL and rALL. Findings were correlated with the degree of spontaneous apoptosis and drug induced apoptosis determined by means of propidium iodide (PI)-staining, and in vitro drug resistance using the total cell kill colorimetric methyl-thiazol-tetrazolium salt (MTT) assay.

3. MATERIALS AND METHODS

3.1. Leukemic Samples

Bone marrow and/or peripheral blood samples taken for routine diagnostic procedures were obtained from 77 children suffering from ALL. Forty-six samples were taken at initial diagnosis (iALL) and 31 at relapse (rALL).

Mononuclear samples were separated by Ficoll density gradient centrifugation (Ficoll Paque, density 1.077g/ml; Pharmacia, Sweden) and washed twice in RPMI 1640

(Gibco, UK) containing 2% fetal calf serum with 10 min periods of centrifugation at 300 g. Microscopic slides of citospun cells were prepared by centrifugation of 50 μl aliquots with 0.5×10^6 cells/ml at 50 g for 7 minutes. After May-Grünwald-Giemsa staining of cytospins we routinely counted 200 cells by light microscopy to determine the proportion of lymphoblasts. When less than 90% of the mononuclear fraction were blasts, samples were purified using immunomagnetic beads as described earlier.[24]

3.2. Flowcytometric Analysis of Bcl-2 Expression

After centrifugation, cells were fixed using 100 μl paraformaldehyde 1% with 5 minutes incubation at 4 °C. Then cells were washed using PBS (containing bovine serum albumin and sodium azide), and subsequently incubated with 100 μl Triton X-100 0.05% at 4°C during 5 minutes. Next after washing the cells twice, 20 μl cell suspension and 20 μl of specific anti-antibody recognizing bcl-2 (mouse monoclonal antibody, Cambridge research, Sanbio, DM 11.925) were incubated at 4°C for 30 minutes. After washing with PBS, 50 μl of conjugate (fluoresceine isothiocyanate (FITC)-conjugated rabbit anti-mouse F(ab')$_2$, DAKOPATTS, F313) or non-specific isotype matched immunoglobin as negative control was added to the cell pallet followed by 30 minutes incubation at 4°C. Then cells were washed twice and 300 μl of PBS (without bovine serum albumin) was added to the pallet. Subsequently the percentage of protein-positive cells (dot-blot) as well as the fluorescence index (FI; intensity of staining related to that of the control) were measured.

3.3. Drugs

The drugs used in the present study were prednisolone (PRD), Dexamethasone (DXM) and cytarabine (ARA), which were obtained from our hospital pharmacy. DXM and ARA were obtained as solutions ready for use. PRD was dissolved in saline. All drugs were further dissolved in RPMI 1640. The following drug concentration ranges were used for the MTT-assay (μg/ml): PRD 0.05 to 2000, ARA 0.002 to 2.5 and DXM 0.0002 to 6. The cells that were used for apoptosis-measurements were incubated with 2 concentrations of DXM: 1 and 10 μg/ml.

3.4. Apoptosis-Measurements

After isolation of leukemic cells as described above, a suspension was prepared of 2×10^6 cells/ml. The suspension was divided in several flasks, 3 for control measurements (at t = 0, t = 24 and t = 48 hours) and 6 for each drug to be tested (2 concentrations, 3 different time-points conform control measurements). Each flask contained 50 μl of drug solution and 200 μl of cell suspension. Cells were continuously incubated with drug and apoptosis measurements were performed at the above mentioned time-points.

Cells were centrifuged and 300 μl of hypotoneous propidium iodide (PI) solution was added. This solution was prepared as follows: 5 mg PI, 100 mg Rnase, 100 μl Triton-X and 100 mg sodium-citrate. Next, PI fluorescence of 5000 cells (or better: nuclei) for each sample was analyzed using a FACScan (BD), and a DNA histogram was plotted. The cells in the sub-G_0/G_1 peak (sub-diploid cells) were considered apoptotic cells. This was confirmed in our laboratory by DNA gel electrophoresis and by morphologic examination (data not shown). The percentage of apoptotic cells can thus be determined.

3.5. Drug Resistance Assay

In vitro drug cytotoxicity was determined using the MTT assay. The assay conditions were essentially the same as previously described.[24] Briefly, aliquots of 80 μl cell suspension were added to 96-well microculture plates containing 20 µl aliquots of drug solutions. Leukemic cells were exposed to 6 concentrations of each drug in duplicate for 4 days. Control leukemic cells were cultured in the absence of drugs. At day 4 we determined the number of viable control cells by trypan blue dye exclusion. May-Grünwald-Giemsa stained cytospins of control cells showed that all samples contained ≥70% blasts after 4 days culturing, which is required for reliable test-results.[24] Next, we added 10 µl of 5 mg/ml MTT (Sigma) to each well. The microculture plates were shaken gently for 1 minute and incubated for 6 hours. The yellow tetrazolium salt MTT is reduced to dark colored formazan by viable cells only. Formazan crystals were dissolved in 100 µl acidified isopropanol. The optical density (OD) was measured at 565 nm with an EL-312 microplate reader (Biotek Instruments Inc., Winooski, USA). The OD is linearly related to the number of viable cells. After correction for the optical density of the culture medium, leukemic cell survival (LCS) was calculated as follows:

$$LCS = (OD_{drug\text{-}exposed\ well}) / (mean\ OD_{control\ wells}) \times 100\%.$$

The LC_{50} value, the drug concentration lethal to 50% of the blasts, was calculated from the obtained dose-response curves and used as measure for the in vitro drug cytotoxicity.

3.6. Statistics

The relationship between two variables was tested by the Spearman's rank correlation test. A p-value smaller than 5% was considered to be statistically significant (2-tailed test). The Mann-Whitney U test was used for analysis of unpaired observations.

4. RESULTS

4.1. BCL-2 Expression in Childhood Leukemia

All leukemic samples were positive for bcl-2. The FI of bcl-2 differed up to ten-fold within iALL, and up to 4-fold in rALL (Figure 1.) Bcl-2 expression was significantly higher in rALL than in iALL (median in presentation samples=9.4, median in relapsed samples=12.7; p=0.008).

4.2. Spontaneous Apoptosis, Drug Induced Apoptosis and in Vitro Drug Resistance

Spontaneous and DXM induced apoptosis were time-dependent in both leukemia sub-groups (in up to 71% and 81% of the cells respectively, Tables 1 and 2.). Untreated samples tend to show less spontaneous apoptosis then relapsed patients. However large interindividual differences existed within each leukemia subgroup. Statistically significant correlations were found between spontaneous and drug induced apoptosis in both samples taken at initial diagnosis and at relapse (Tables 3 and 4).

When correlating spontaneous apoptosis with in vitro drug resistance we only found a weak correlation between the extent of spontaneous apoptosis at $t = 0$ and in vitro drug resistance for ARA in iALL ($r = -0.37$, $p = 0.04$). When correlating DXM induced apoptosis with in vitro drug resistance we found that iALL samples that are more sensitive to DXM induced apoptosis displayed lower LC50 values for DXM and PRD ($r = -0.43$, $p = 0.02$, $n = 29$; rho = -0.38, $p = 0.03$, $n = 31$). No such correlations were found in rALL.

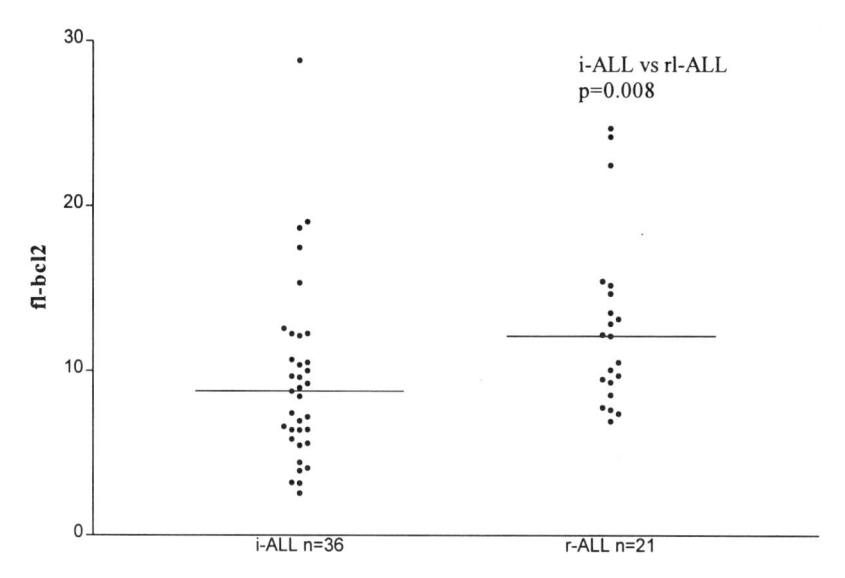

Figure 1. Fluorescence index of bcl-2 expression (Fl-bcl-2) in childhood leukemia subgroups. Horizontal lines represent median values.

4.3. Bcl-2 Expression versus Spontaneous Apoptosis, Drug Induced Apoptosis and in Vitro Drug Resistance

In iALL, but not in rALL, a weak but significant inverse correlation was found between the rate of spontaneous apoptosis after 24 hours incubation and bcl-2 expression in iALL (rho = -0.40, p = 0.05, n = 24). However in these samples no correlations were found between bcl-2 expression and drug induced apoptosis. Moreover bcl-2 expression was inversely correlated with the LC50 values of ARA (r = -0.37, p = 0.046, n = 30).

In contrast, relapsed samples that displayed high levels of bcl-2 expression were more resistant to DXM induced apoptosis measured after 24 hours and 48 hours incubation (Figure 2; r = -0.53, p = 0.02, n = 16 and r = -0.63, p = 0.02, n = 14). In rALL we did not find statistically significant correlations between bcl-2 and in vitro drug resistance.

5. DISCUSSION

Bcl2, due to its anti-apoptotic properties has been implicated as an unfavorable prognostic factor and potential target for therapeutic intervention in both hematologic and solid malignancies.[17,20,25–27] However its role in childhood leukemia remains unclear.[21–23]

Table 1. Spontaneous apoptosis in initial and relapsed acute lymphoblastic leukemia. Indicated are the median (and range) percentages of leukemic cells in apoptosis

	iALL (n=35)	rALL (n=26)
t=0 hours	1 (0-22)	1 (0-21)
t=24 hours	16 (0-60)	21 (1-64)
t=48 hours	24 (1-66)	41 (6-71)

Table 2. Dexamethasone induced apoptosis in initial and relapsed acute lymphoblastic leukemia. Indicated are the median (and range) percentages of leukemic cells in apoptosis

	iALL (n=34)	rALL (n=26)
t=24 hours concentration		
low	19 (3-82)	23 (2-84)
high	23 (3-77)	20 (0-82)
t=48 hours concentration		
low	43 (2-88)	40 (14-83)
high	39 (2-90)	42 (9-86)

In the present study we confirmed that in childhood ALL bcl-2 levels are highly variable, as has also been shown by Salomons et al.[28] and Coustan-Smith et al.[23] In rALL we found an elevated level of bcl-2 as compared to samples taken at relapse, confirming the data obtained by Maung et al.[22] This suggests the implication of bcl-2 in the increased drug resistance as found in relapsed ALL.[28] In support of this we found that bcl-2 expression was inversely correlated with the extent of DXM induced apoptosis in rALL. However no significant correlations were found with in vitro DXM resistance, but the numbers were small.

In iALL however increased bcl-2 expression was not related to the extent of drug induced apoptosis. In contrast high bcl-2 expression appeared to be related to a low LC50 value of ARA, i.e., cells which expressed high levels of bcl-2 were more sensitive to the cytotoxic effects of ARAC.

In our study we also demonstrated a statistically significant correlation between spontaneous apoptosis and drug induced apoptosis in both iALL and rALL. This is probably due to the fact that values obtained for drug induced apoptosis were not corrected for spontaneous apoptosis Part of the apoptotic cells found after incubation with DXM would also have entered the apoptotic cycle without having been exposed to this drug. Correction for this phenomenon was unfortunately not possible due to the nature of the study.

The lack of association between higher bcl-2 expression and resistance to cytotoxic drugs as measured by the MTT assay may be explained by the fact that other proteins like bax may offset the anti-apoptotic effects of bcl-2. The bcl-2/bax ratio appears to be central in the molecular regulation of apoptosis.[16,29] Other proteins that may also be involved are: bcl-x_s, bcl-x_l, mcl-1, bak and bag.[19]

Another explanation might be that not the level of expression of these proteins at the start drug exposure is predictive for the cytotoxic response, but rather the up- and down regulation in response to apoptotic stimuli. Findley et al. showed in pediatric leukemic cell lines expressing the wild-type p53 that cell-lines sensitive to γ-radiation down regu-

Table 3. Correlation between spontaneous and drug induced apoptosis in iALL at different time points and after incubation with different concentrations DXM. Indicated are the Spearman's correlation coefficients (r), the 2-tailed p-values (p) and the number of observations (n)

	dex low t=24	dex high t=24	dex low t=48	dex high t=48
ctr t=0	r=0.046 p=0.80 n=34	r=0.14 p=0.44 n=34	r=0.17 p=0.34 n=33	r=0.21 p=0.24 n=33
ctr t=24	r=0.51 p=0.002 n=34	r=0.54 p=0.001 n=34	r=0.36 p=0.043 n=32	r=0.406 p=0.043 n=32
ctr t=48	r=0.50 p=0.004 n=32	r=0.64 p.001 n=32	r=0.71 p.001 n=32	r=0.78 p.001 n=33

Table 4. Correlation between spontaneous and drug induced apoptosis in rALL at different time points and after incubation with different concentrations DXM. Indicated are the Spearman's correlation coefficients (r), the 2-tailed p-values (p) and the number of observations (n)

	dex low t=24	dex high t=24	dex low t=48	dex high t=48
ctr t=0	r=0.019 p=0.929 n=24	r=0.009 p=0.97 n=24	r=-0.012 p=0.96 n=22	r=-0.029 p=0.90 n=22
ctr t=24	r=0.844 p.001 n=26	r=0.671 p.001 n=26	r=0.371 p=0.074 n=24	r=0.461 p=0.023 n=24
ctr t=48	r=0.729 p.001 n=24	r=0.55 p=0.005 n=24	r=0.57 p=0.004 n=24	r=0.69 p.001 n=24

lated bcl-2 and upregulated bax, whereas resistant cell lines did not alter the bcl-2 or bax expression.[30]

A third explanation is that also other mechanisms contribute to drugresistance. For example in case of glucocorticoids, a low number of glucocorticoid receptors or structural defects of these and increased DNA-methylation which inhibits binding of the activated receptor to the DNA have been shown to contribute to glucocorticoid resistance.[31]

A point of interest in respect of the (lack of) prognostic value of bcl-2 is that bcl-2 displays not only anti-apoptotic, but also anti-proliferative effects.[32] Low bcl-2 expression may therefore be associated with a high proliferative rate and therefore result in a poor prognosis.

In conclusion, DXM excerts its cytotoxic effect at least partly by means of induction of apoptosis. Bcl2 inhibits drug induced apoptosis in rALL. However in iALL bcl-2 expression is not associated with increased in vitro drug resistance, nor with increased resistance to drug induced apoptosis. A limitation to our pilot-data is that bcl-2 expression was evaluated only at the start of culture and that therefore the up- and downregulation of bcl-2 in response to drug exposure was not studied. Moreover it has become clear that other apoptotic regulating gene products interact with bcl-2. These factors will be included in future studies.

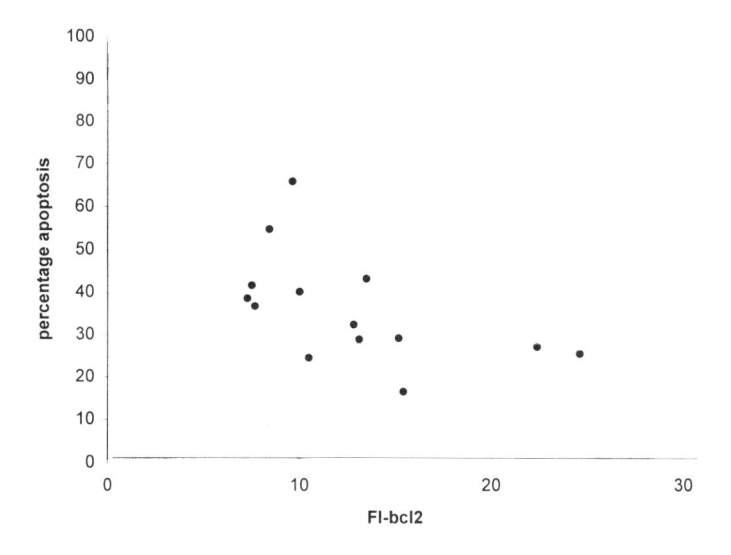

Figure 2. Relation between fluorescence index (Fl)-bcl-2 and dexamethasone induced apoptosis after 48 hours in rALL (r = -0.63, p = 0.016, n = 14).

ACKNOWLEDGMENTS

This work is supported by The Dutch Cancer Society (grant VU 97-1564)

REFERENCES

1. Yunis JJ, Oken MM, Kaplan ME, Ensrud KM, Howe RR, Theologides A. Distinctive chromosomal abnormalities in histologic subtypes of non-Hodgkin's lymphoma. New England Journal of Medicine 1982, 307: 1231–1236
2. Tsujimoto Y. Overexpression of the human bcl-2 gene product results in growth enhancement of Ebstein-Barr virus immortalized B cells. Proc Nat Acad Sci USA 1984, 86: 1958–1962
3. Cleary ML, Smith SD, Sklar J. Cloning and structural analysis of cDNA for Bcl-2 and a hybrid bcl-2/immunoglobulin transcript resulting from the t(14;18) translocation. Cell 1986, 47: 19–28
4. Chen-Levy Z, Nourse J, Cleary ML. The bcl-2 candidate proto-oncogene product is a 24-kilodalton integral-membrane protein highly expressed in lymphoid cell lines and lymphomas carrying the t(14:18) translocation. Mol Cell Biol 1989, 9: 701–710
5. Hockenbery DM, Zutter M, Hickey W, Nahm M, Korsmeyer S. Bcl-2 protein is topographically restricted in tissues characterized by apoptotic cell death. Proc Natl Ac Sci USA 1991, 16: 8479–8483
6. Lu QL, Elia G, Lucas S, Thomas JA. Bcl-2 proto-oncogene expression in Ebstein-Barr virus associated nasopharyngeal carcinoma. Cancer 1993, 53: 29–35
7. Nunez G, London L, Hockenbery D, Alexander M, McKearn JP, Korsmeyer SJ. Deregulated Bcl-2 gene-expression selectively prolongs survival of growth factor-deprived hemopoietic cell lines. J Immumol 1991, 144: 3602–3610
8. Bissonette RP, Echeverri F, Mahboubi A, Green DR. Apoptotic cell death induced by c-myc is inhibited by bcl-2. Nature 1992, 359: 552–554
9. Fanidi A, Harrington EA, Evan GI. Cooperative interaction between c-myc and bcl-2 proto-oncogenes. Nature 1992, 359: 554–556
10. Hickman JA. Apoptosis induced by anti-cancer drugs. Cancer Metast Rev 1992, 11: 121–139
11. Dive C, Hickman JA. Drug-target interactions: Only first step in the commitment to programmed cell death? Br J Cancer 1991, 64: 192–196
12. O'Connor PM, Wassermann K, Sarang M, Magrath I, Bohr VA, Kohn KW. Relation between DNA cross-links, cell-cycle, and apoptosis in Burkitt's lymphoma cell lines differing in sensitivity to nitrogen mustard. Cancer Res 1991, 51: 6550–6557
13. Lowe SW, Ruley HE, Jacks T, Housman DE. p53-dependent apoptosis modulates the cytotoxicity of anti-cancer agents. Cell 1993, 74: 957–967
14. Miyashita T, Reed JC. Bcl-2 oncoprotein blocks chemotherapy-induced apoptosis in a human leukemia cell line. Blood 1990, 81: 151–157
15. Sentman CL, Shutter JR, Hockenbery D, Kanagawa O, Korsmeyer SJ. Bcl-2 inhibits multiple forms of apoptosis but not negative selection in thymocytes. Cell 1991, 67: 879–888
16. Smets LA, Van Den Berg J, Acton D, Top B, Van Rooij H, Verweij-Janssen. Bcl-2 expression and mitochondrial activity in leukemic cells with different sensitivity to glucocorticoid-induced apoptosis. Blood 1994, 84: 1613–1619
17. Campos L, Rouault JP, Sabido O, Oriol P, Roubi N, Vasselon C, Archimbaud E, Magaud JP, Guyotot D. High expression of bcl-2 protein in acute myeloid leukemia cells is associated with poor respons to chemotherapy. Blood 1993, 81: 3091–3096
18. Porwit-MacDonald A, Ivory K, Wilkinson S, Wheatley K, Wong L, Janossy G. Bcl-2 protein expression in normal human bone marrow precursors and in acute myelogenous leukemia. Leukemia 1995, 9: 1191–1198
19. Reed JC. Bcl2: prevention of apoptosis as a mechanism of drug resistance. Hematol Oncol Clin North Am 1995, 9: 451–473
20. Lotem J, Sachs L. Control of sensitivity to induction of apoptosis in myeloid leukemic cells by differentation and bcl-2 dependent and independent pathways. Cell Growth Differ 1994, 5: 321-327
21. Gala JL, Vermeylen C, Cornu G, Ferrant A, Michaux JL, Philippe M, Martiat P. High expression of bcl-2 is the rule in acute lymphoblastic leukemia, except in Burkitt subtype at presentation, and is not correlated with the prognosis. Ann Hematol 1994, 69: 17–24

22. Maung ZT, Maclean ER, Reid MM, Pearson AD, Proctor SJ, Hamilton PJ, Hall AG. The relationship between bcl-2 expression and response to chemotherapy in acute leukaemia. Br J Haematol 1994, 88: 105–109
23. Coustan-Smith E, Kitanaka A, Pui CH, McNinch L, Evans WE, Raimondi SC, Behm FG, Arico M, Campana D. Clinical relevance of bcl-2 over-expression in childhood acute lymphoblastic leukemia. Blood 1996, 87: 1140–1146
24. Kaspers GJL, Veerman AJP, Pieters R, Broekema GJ, Huismans DR, Kazemier KM, Loonen AH, Rottier MMA, Van Zantwijk CH, Hahlen K, Van Wering ER. Mononuclear cells contaminating leukemic samples tested for cellular drug resistance using the methyl-thiazol-tetrazolium assay. Br J Cancer 1994, 10: 1047–1052
25. Castle VP, Heidelberger KP, Bromberg J, Ou X, Dole M, Nunez G. Expression of the apoptosis-surpressing gen bcl-2 in neuroblastoma is associated with unfavorable histology and N-myc amplification. Am J Path 1993, 143: 1543–1550
26. McDonnell TJ, Troncoso P, Brisbay SM, Logothetis C, Ching LWK, Hsieh JT, Tu SM, Campbell ML. Expression of the protooncogene bcl-2 in the prostate and its association with emergence of androgen-independent prostate cancer. Cancer Res 1992, 52: 6940–6944
27. Reed JC., Kitada S, Takayama S, Miyashita T. Regulation of chemoresistance by the bcl-2 oncoprotein in non-Hodgkin's lymphoma and lymphoblastic leukemia cell lines. Ann Oncol 1994, 5: 61–65
28. Klumper E, Pieters R, Veerman AJP, Huismans DR, Loonen AH, Hählen K, Kaspers GJL, Van Wering ER, Hartmann R, Henze G. In vitro cellular drug resistance in children with relapsed/refractory acute lymphoblastic leukemia. Blood 1995, 86: 3681–3688
29. Salomons GS, Brady HJM, Verwijs-Janssen M, Van Den Berg JD, Hart AAM, Van Den Berg H, Behrendt H, Hählen K, Smets L. The Baxα: bcl-2 ratio modulates the respons to dexamethasone in leukemic cells and is highly variable in childhood acute leukemia. Int J Cancer 1997, 71: 959–965
30. Findley HW, Gu l, Yeager AM, Zhou M. Expression and regulation of bcl-2, bcl-xl and bax correlate with p53 status and sensitivity to apoptosis in childhood acute lymphoblastic leukemia. Blood 1997, 89: 2986–2993
31. Kaspers GJL, Pieters R, Klumper E, De Waal FC, Veerman AJP. Glucocorticoid resistance in childhood leukemia. Leuk & Lymphoma 1994, 13: 187–201
32. Schena M, Larsson LG, Gottardi D, Gaidano G, Carlsson M, Nilsson K, Caligaris-Cappio F. Growth and differentiation-associated expression of bcl-2 in B-chronic lymphocytic leukemia cells. Blood 1992, 11: 2981–2989

36

COMPARISON OF BCL-2 AND BAX PROTEIN EXPRESSION WITH *IN VITRO* SENSITIVITY TO ARA-C AND 6TG IN AML

S. E. Balkham, J. M. Sargent, A. W. Elgie, C. J. Williamson, and C. G. Taylor

Haematology Research
Pembury Hospital
Kent TN2 4QJ, United Kingdom

Keywords: AML, drug resistance, BCL-2, BAX, ara-C, 6TG.

1. ABSTRACT

Activity of BCL-2 protein may be antagonised by BAX protein expression, thereby affecting cellular sensitivity to chemotherapeutic drugs. We analysed the BCL-2 protein expression of blast cells from 19 patients by flow cytometry and immunocytochemistry. This was compared to *in vitro* sensitivity to the anthracyclines and antimetabolites using the MTT assay. We found a significant correlation between BCL-2 expression and *in vitro* response to two antimetabolite drugs. One of 7 patients (14%) whose cells were sensitive to ara-C expressed BCL-2 compared to 4/4 patients (100%) whose cells were resistant to ara-C *in vitro* ($p = 0.05$). Furthermore, none of the three patients whose cells were sensitive to 6-TG expressed BCL-2 compared to 6/9 patients (67%) whose cells were resistant *in vitro* ($p = 0.045$). We found no other correlation between BCL-2 expression and any other chemotherapeutic drug analysed.

The ratio of BCL-2 to BAX may be more relevant clinically, therefore cells from a further 9 patients were analysed for both proteins. Whilst there was no overall relationship between BCL-2/BAX ratios and sensitivity to ara-C and 6TG, individual patients could be identified whose blast cells were resistant to ara-C and had high BCL-2/BAX ratios. Further analysis of the significance of these ratios to drug resistance may be of future prognostic value.

2. INTRODUCTION

Defects in triggering the apoptotic pathway could lead to poor responses to chemotherapy in patients with AML. Apoptosis (programmed cell death) is now recognised as being a tightly regulated process which is thought to be subdivided into three different stages: induction, triggering and execution.[1] The BCL-2 family includes both anti- and pro- apoptotic effectors. At least fourteen homologs of BCL-2 protein have now been identified,[2] which are capable of either enhancing or suppressing apoptosis.

Recent work has identified that BAX protein acts as a trigger or amplifier of cell death as opposed to a protector and that BCL-2 appears to regulate BAX.[3] By suppressing BAX activity its function is down regulated and neutralized, hence cells are protected from cell death. It is therefore likely that expression of BCL 2/BAX protein ratios may be important factors in the regulation of apoptosis.

To investigate whether the sensitivity of ara-C and 6TG is altered due to overexpression of BCL-2 protein we analysed BCL-2 protein levels by flow cytometry and immunocytochemistry and examined the relationship between our results and both *in vitro* drug resistance using the MTT assay and *in vivo* clinical response after therapy. We also tested nine of the same samples for BAX protein levels by flow cytometry to assess whether there was any significant relationship between either BAX protein expression alone or BCL-2/BAX ratios and *in vitro* drug resistance to ara-C and 6TG.

3. METHODS

3.1. Patients

Peripheral blood and bone marrow samples from 28 patients with AML were analysed, 22 with *de novo* AML and 6 with AML 2^0 to MDS. The samples were collected into citrate phosphate dextrose. Blast cells were harvested by density gradient centrifugation using lymphocyte separation medium. A final cell preparation in RPMI 1640 culture medium with 10% FCS and antibiotics was prepared. Samples were examined morphologically using May Grünwald Giemsa stain to identify percentage of blast cells present. The initial number of viable and dead cells in each sample was determined using the trypan blue dye exclusion test. All samples contained >80% blasts and > 90% viable cells.

Cytospins of final cell preparations were also prepared, air dried and stored at -20°C for immunocytochemical staining. Cells were cryopreserved for flow cytometry.

3.2. MTT Assay

Patients blast cells were incubated with epirubicin, idarubicin, daunorubicin, doxorubicin, mitoxantrone, ara-C, etoposide and 6TG to test their individual responses. A 48h continuous drug exposure at 37°C, 5% CO_2 was followed by the addition of MTT for 4hrs. Results (formazan OD) were expressed as the percentage of the control and the LC_{50} (concentration of drug required to kill 50% of cells) was calculated.

3.3. Immunocytochemistry

The Alkaline Phosphatase (AP) staining procedure was used, and slides were analysed within two months of cytospin preparation. Slides were scored for percentage positivity and staining intensity using a scale from 0 for negative and 4+ for strong positive.

For statistical analysis a cut off point of 20% was used to distinguish between positive and negative results.

3.4. Flow Cytometry Analysis of BCL-2 and BAX Protein

Cryopreserved samples were rapidly thawed, permeabilized and stained either directly with FITC conjugated BCL-2 monoclonal antibody or indirectly using FITC conjugated anti-mouse IgG after a BAX monoclonal antibody.

400µl of a 1×10^5/ml cell suspension in PBS were permeabilized using 4% paraformaldehyde solution and 50µl of triton X. Cells were then washed twice in cold PBS. The pelleted cells were then incubated for thirty minutes at 4^0C with primary antibody or isotype negative control. After washing, and FITC staining if required, the cells were resuspended in 300µl of PBS and immediately analysed on the flow cytometer. BCL-2 was measured as percentage positivity.

BCL-2 and BAX results were expressed as the ratio of the mean fluorescence associated with the test over that of the isotype control. A further ratio of BCL-2 to BAX protein expression was also calculated by dividing the ratio for BCL-2 by the ratio for BAX.

3.5. Statistics

Spearmans rank correlation coefficient was used to measure any associations between these apoptotic related proteins and the LC_{50} values for cytotoxic drugs. 2×2 contingency analysis was used to look for differences between categories of protein expression and clinical parameters. Mann Whitney U was used to assess differences between groups of patients.

4. RESULTS

4.1. Correlation of BCL-2 with *in Vitro* Drug Sensitivity

We found a significant correlation between BCL-2 expression, as assessed by immunocytochemistry, and *in vitro* response of two antimetabolite drugs, ara-C and 6TG. 1/7 patients (14%) whose cells were sensitive to ara-C expressed BCL-2 compared to 4/4 patients (100%) whose cells were resistant to ara-C (Figure 1; p = 0.05). Furthermore, none of the 3 patients whose cells were sensitive to 6TG expressed BCL-2 compared to 6/9 patients (67%) whose cells were resistant *in vitro* (Figure 2; p = 0.05). We found no other correlation between BCL-2 expression and any other chemotherapeutic drug analysed.

4.2. Correlation of BAX Expression with *in Vitro* Drug Sensitivity

There was no overall relationship between BAX expression, as measured by flow cytometry (median ratio 2.4, range 1.3–2.8) and *in vitro* sensitivity to ara-C and 6TG.

4.3. Correlation of BCL-2/BAX Ratios with *in Vitro* Drug Sensitivity

Likewise, there was no overall correlation between *in vitro* sensitivity to ara-C and 6TG exposure and BCL-2/BAX ratios (range 8.6–30.8, median = 13.5, n = 8). However it was possible to identify individual patients demonstrating high BCL-2/BAX ratios and who appeared resistant to ara-C.

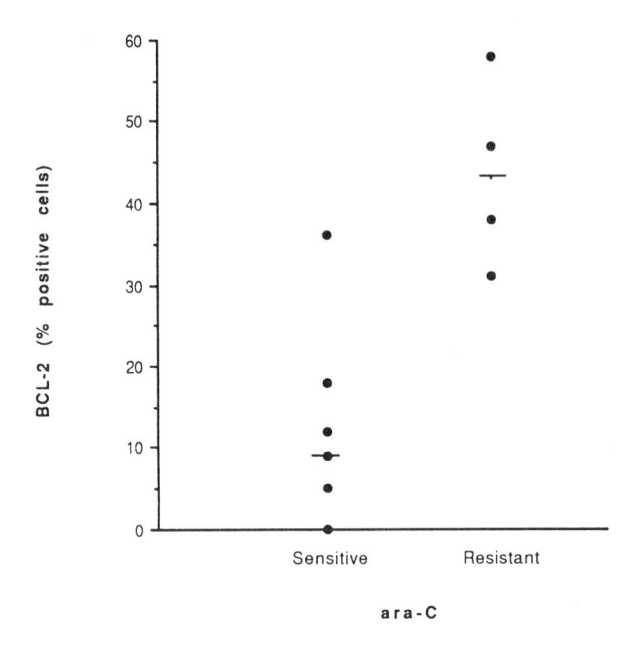

Figure 1. Relationship between BCL-2 expression and sensitivity to ara-C.

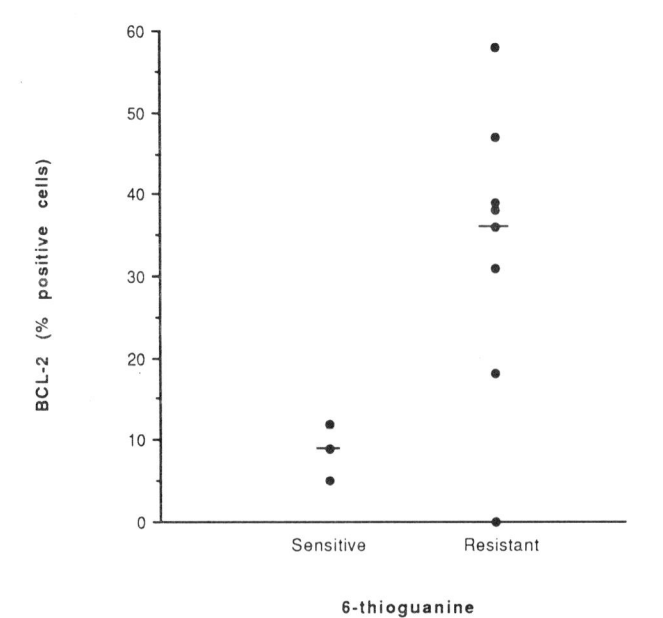

Figure 2. Relationship between BCL-2 expression and sensitivity to 6TG.

4.4. Correlation of BCL-2 with Clinical Parameters

BCL-2 expression, as measured by either immunocytochemistry or flow cytometry did not appear to correlate with *in vivo* response after a 3 drug regimen. Surprisingly, in our study we found that untreated patients expressed higher BCL-2 levels than those who had been treated previously (median 38% compared to 5%, p = 0.05).

5. DISCUSSION

Current thinking on how cytotoxic drugs kill cells is largely centred around the malignant cell's capacity to enter the apoptotic pathway and then execute the process. It may be therefore, that expression of BCL-2 and BAX proteins either alone or simultaneously could influence this process.

We have found that blast cells that were resistant *in vitro* to ara C or 6TG had higher levels of BCL-2 protein as measured by immunocytochemistry although we found no significant relationship between BCL-2 expression and chemosensitivity for other drugs tested. Our results therefore suggest that treatment with ara-C and 6TG may be improved by modulation of BCL-2 expression. It is possible that different classes of drugs could trigger the apoptotic response by a variety of mechanisms. It is also highly probable that expression of BCL-2 protein alone is unlikely to be the only clinical indicator of patients responses to treatment as it is becoming increasingly apparent that BCL-2 overexpression alone does not necessarily equate with poor prognosis in patients with AML. Indeed, we found that untreated patients expressed higher BCL-2 levels than those who had been previously treated. However, Banker *et al* reported apoptosis in the presence and absence of BCL-2 overexpression.[4] These findings suggest that evidence of BCL-2 expression alone may not be sufficient to alter the pathway of apoptotic execution. To support this theory, Brouset *et al* found that although the apoptosis regulatory BAX protein was frequently expressed in their patients, only 53% expressed BCL-2 positivity.[5] It has been postulated therefore that patients with higher BAX expression should demonstrate an improved response to chemotherapy.[6] However, in our study we found no overall correlation between *in vitro* sensitivity to ara-C and 6TG and BAX expression.

It is probably more likely therefore that combined ratios of BCL-2/BAX protein may be more significant than the individual protein ratios alone as recent studies also indicate that higher BCL-2/BAX ratios correlated with chemoresistance whereas low ratios correlated with chemosensitivity.[7] Despite no correlation overall between BCL-2/BAX ratios and *in vitro* sensitivity to ara-C and 6TG in this study, individual samples could be identified showing *in vitro* resistance to ara-C and high BCL-2/BAX ratios. BCL-2/BAX ratios may therefore be critical in determining whether cells are resistant or sensitive to treatment.[4]

It is clear from the above results that several issues still need to be addressed. Before *in vitro* apoptotic assays are used to predict treatment outcome in patients with AML to different therapeutic agents it will be important that clear and distinct laboratory identification of apoptosis is universally defined. Although apoptosis has been experimentally described by identification of DNA fragmentation (DNA laddering) a recent study suggests that these features may not necessarily be components of apoptosis[6] but simply signs of degradation. Other features may be more relevant, such as changes in the cell membrane which can be demonstrated, for example, by increased Annexin V binding.[4]

Although the small number of samples tested limit the conclusions we can draw we intend to continue further studies of BCL-2 and BAX ratio expression in relation to drug resistance.

ACKNOWLEDGMENTS

We are grateful for the support of the Kent Leukaemia and Cancer Equipment Fund.

REFERENCES

1. Green D, Martin S. The killer and the executioner: How apoptosis controls malignancy. Current Opinion in Immunology, 1995, 7, 694–703.
2. Reed JC. BCL-2 and the regulation of programmed cell death. J Cell Biol, 1994, 124, 1–6.
3. Reed JC. BCL-2: Prevention of apoptosis as a mechanism of drug resistance. Hematol/Oncol Clin, 1995, 9, 451–473.
4. Banker D, Groudine M. Measurement of spontaneous and therapeutic agent induced apoptosis with BCL-2 protein expression in acute myeloid leukaemia, Blood, 1997, 89, 243–255.
5. Brousset P, Benharroch D. Frequent expression of the cell death - inducing gene *bax* in Reed-Sternberg cells in Hodgkin's Disease. Blood, 1996, 87, 2470–2478.
6. Pepper C, Bentley P. Regulation of clinical chemoresistance by BCL-2 and BAX oncoproteins in B-cell chronic lymphocytic leukaemia. Br J Haematol, 1996, 95, 513–517.
7. Pepper C, Hoy T. BCL-2/BAX ratios in chronic lymphoctic leukaemia and their correlation with in vitro apoptosis and clinical resistance. Br J Cancer, 1997, 76, 935–938.

SYNTHETIC CYCLIN DEPENDENT KINASE INHIBITORS

New Generation of Potent Anti-Cancer Drugs

Marián Hajdúch,[1,*] Libor Havlíèek,[2] Jaroslav Veselý,[3] Radko Novotný,[4] Vladimír Mihál,[1] and Miroslav Strnad[5]

[1]Laboratory of Experimental Medicine, Department of Paediatrics
 Faculty of Medicine and Faculty Hospital in Olomouc
 Puškinova 6, 775 20 Olomouc, Czech Republic
[2]Institute of Toxicology and Forensic Chemistry, 1st Faculty of Medicine
 Charles University, 110 00 Prague 1, Czech Republic
[3]Institute of Pathophysiology, Faculty of Medicine
 Palacký University, Hnìvotínská 3, 775 15 Olomouc, Czech Republic
[4]Department of Microscopic Methods, Faculty of Medicine
 Palacký University, I.P. Pavlova 6, 775 20 Olomouc
[5]Laboratory of Growth Regulators
 Institute of Experimental Botany
 Šlechtitelù 21, 772 00 Olomouc, Czech Republic

Keywords: cell cycle; cyclin dependent kinase; olomoucine, roscovitine, flavopiridol, butyrolactone I.

1. ABSTRACT

The unsatisfactory results of current anti-cancer therapies require the active search for new drugs, new treatment strategies and a deeper understanding of the host-tumour relationship. From this point of view, the drugs with a capacity to substitute the functions of altered tumour suppressor genes are of prominent interest. Since one of the main functions of oncosuppressors is to mediate cell cycle arrest via modification of cyclin dependent kinases

---

[*] Corresponding author. Tel.: +420-68-585 4473, Fax: +420-68-585 2505, e-mail: marian@risc.upol.cz

Drug Resistance in Leukemia and Lymphoma III, edited by Kaspers *et al.*
Kluwer Academic / Plenum Publishers, New York, 1999.

(CDKs) activity, the compounds with ability to substitute altered functions of these genes in neoplastic cells are of prominent interest. Synthetic inhibitors of cyclin dependent kinases (CDKIs) are typical representatives of such drugs. Olomoucine (OC), flavopiridol (FP), butyrolactone I (BL) and their derivatives selectively inhibit CDKs and thus constrain tumor cell proliferation under *in vitro* and/or *in vivo* conditions. We originally discovered OC and its inhibitory activity toward CDK1 family of CDKs, and recently reported the induction of apoptosis and tumor regression following OC application. Moreover, the OC family of synthetic CDKIs has the capacity to directly inhibit CDK7, the principal enzyme required for activating other CDKs, and thus these compounds are the first known CDK7 inhibitors. Its unique mechanism of action and potent anti-cancer activity under both *in vitro* and *in vivo* conditions provide a unique tool to inhibit tumour cell proliferation, and to selectively induce apoptosis in neoplastic tissues. The mechanisms of anti-cancer activities of FP, BL, OC and related synthetic CDKIs are compared and discussed in this paper.

2. INTRODUCTION

Transformation of a normal human cell to a cancer cell is a multistep process that is likely to involve loss of growth restraining functions (such as tumour suppressors), and gain of growth promoting functions (such as dominantly acting oncogenes). These alterations frequently result in unconstrained cellular proliferation and aberrant cell cycle regulation. The majority of alterations in human cancer cells were located in the G1/S transition of the cell cycle[1,2] (Figure 1). The retinoblastoma (RB) and p53 proteins are key regulators in the passage of cells through G1.[1,2] The p53 protein has the hallmarks of a transcription factor; it has a sequence specific DNA binding domain, and its amino-terminus has a transcriptional activation domain.[3,4] DNA damage is the main inducer of the rise in p53 protein level, and the consequent transcription of p53 dependent genes, e.g., bax, GADD45,[5] p21^{WAF1},[5,6] etc. These proteins promote DNA repair via blockade of the cell cycle machinery (p21^{WAF1}),[5] DNA synthesis (p21^{WAF1}),[5] directly participate in the repair of DNA (GADD45),[5] and induce apoptosis (bax) when the DNA damage is too severe to be correctly repaired.

The most important function inhibition of cyclin dependent kinases and cell cycle in response to DNA damage is played by a family of natural cyclin dependent kinase inhibitors (Figure 1). These inhibitors are proteins that bind to and inhibit the activity of CDKs.[1,2,7] One of the first of these to be identified was p21^{WAF1} which is broad inhibitor of CDKs.[5,9] In addition to CDKs inhibitory activity, the carboxy terminus of p21^{WAF1} potently inhibits DNA replication by inactivation of PCNA, an auxiliary subunit of δ-DNA polymerase.[5,10] Thus so far, seven CDK inhibitors (CDKIs) have been identified, p27 and p57 are similar to p21^{WAF1} at the amino terminus and have broad specificity for CDKs.[7] p16, p15, p18, and p19 are CDKIs that form a second family with a more restricted CDKs specificity, which is mainly directed toward CDK4/6 kinases.[7] With exception of p21^{WAF1}, majority of intrinsic CDKIs were found frequently mutated/deleted in various primary tumor cells.[7] However, although p21^{WAF1} is commonly deleted in cancer cell lines, its deletion/mutation in primary tumours is an extremely rare event.[7] It suggests the importance of p21^{WAF1} for cancer cell under *in vivo* conditions, probably due to mediation of tumor resistance to chemotherapy, radiotherapy and/or nutrition deprivation. This hypothesis receives indirect evidence from recently published communication of Bunz et al.,[10] indicating that drug sensitivity of cancer cells is associated with lack of p21^{WAF1}, which results in uncoupling of mitotic and DNA synthetic phases of the cell cycle.

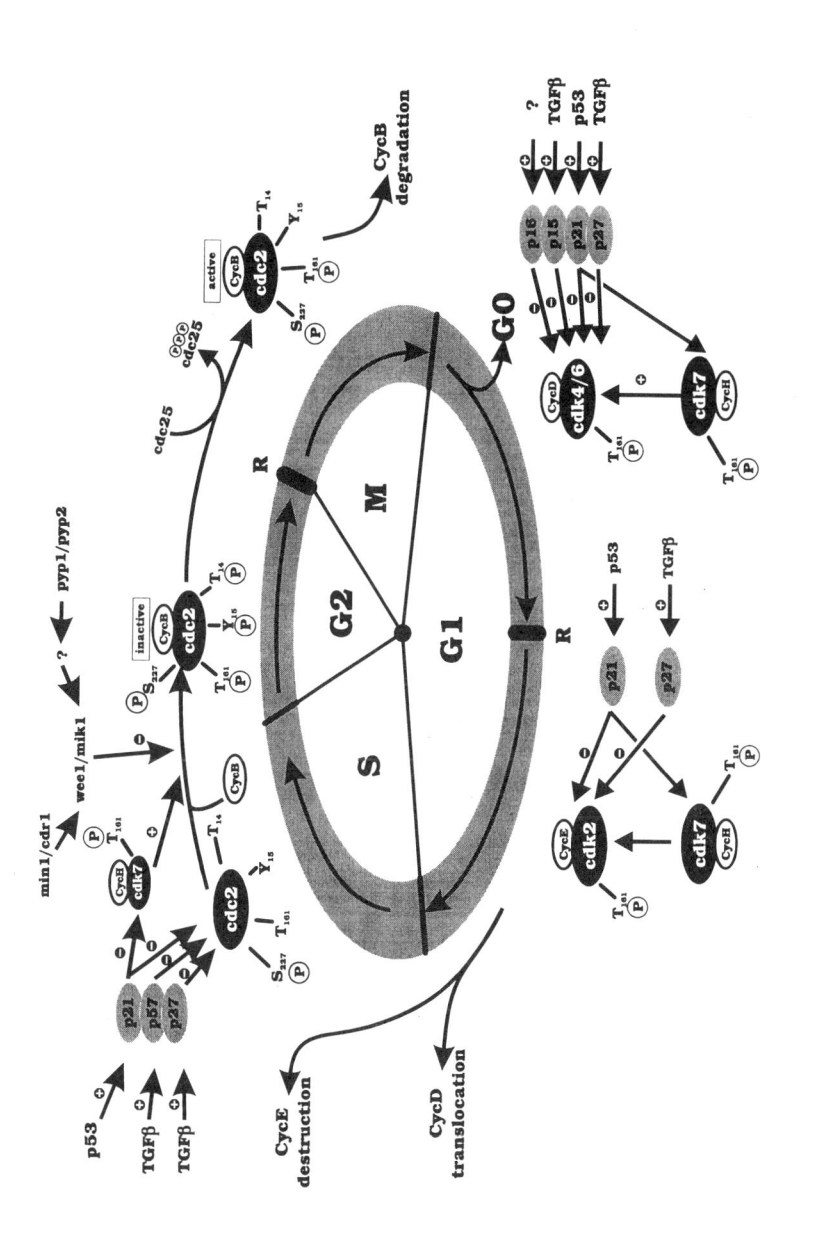

Figure 1. Multiple steps of the cell cycle regulation.

In addition to intrinsic CDKIs, the activity of cyclin-CDK complexes is regulated by phosphorylation processes. Phosphorylation dependent activation/inhibition of enzyme activity was precisely studied on the model of mitotic CDK1 kinase (Figure 1), although identical or similar mechanisms were already confirmed in other CDKs. Upon association of CDK1 with corresponding cyclin, the complex is activated by phosphorylation on T161 by CDK7 kinase.[11,12] Since the mitotic activation of CDK1 requires precise timing, the premature enzymatic activity is prevented by inhibitory phosphorylation on T14/Y15 by wee1/mik1 gene products.[12] Wee1 is, however, itself negatively regulated by nim1 protein kinase, and by unidentified protein kinase at mitosis.[12] T161, T14, Y15 phosphorylated inactive complex is cumulated in G2, and upon entry into M phase of the cell cycle, it undergoes activating dephosphorylation on T14 and Y15, which results in release of active T161 phosphorylated CDK1/cyclin B complexes.[12] Dephosphorylation is mediated by isoenzymes of CDC25 phosphatase[12] (Figure 1).

The disruption of the p53 dependent cell cycle checkpoint is commonly associated with human neoplasia,[4,14] and these cells fail to induce G1 arrest via p21[WAF1] dependent inhibition of CDKs. Growing knowledge about the mechanisms of cell cycle regulation in malignant versus non-malignant cells leads to the design of new drugs and therapeutic strategies to control CDKs activity in tumor cells via restoring or mimicking the functions of inactivated suppressor proteins on G1/S checkpoint. These include the gene transfer of wild type tumor suppressor genes,[15,16] reactivation of mutant p53 by wild-type carboxy-terminal peptide,[17] antisense therapy directed against selected CDKs, the identification of small peptides on carboxy-terminal domain of p21[WAF1] which display capacity to inhibit CDK4 activity;[18] the discovery of butyrolactone I, flavopiridol, olomoucine and related compounds (Figure 1), the inhibitors of CDK1, CDK2 and/or CDK4 respectively. These substances have already been shown to inhibit tumor proliferation and induce cell death under *in vitro* and/or *in vivo* conditions. The biological activities and structure/effectiveness relations are described and discussed in following chapters.

3. FLAVOPIRIDOL

Flavopiridol (Figure 2), (-)-cis-5,7-dihydroxyphenyl-2-(2-chlorophenyl)-8-[4-(3-hydroxy-1-methyl)piperidinyl]-4H-1-benzopyran-4-one hydrochloride hemihydrate (L868275), is a compound which belongs to the family of polyhydroxylated flavones together with other flavonoid structures with cytotoxic and anti-cancer activity, e.g., quercitin and genistein.[19,20,21] Flavones are known to exhibit biological activity via inhibition of various protein kinases, mainly protein kinase C. However, one of the flavonoid compounds, namely flavopiridol (FP), has been described to selectively inhibit CDKs.[19,20,21,22] The compound was derived from a product originally obtained from the indian plant *Dysoxylum binectariferum* and its production is currently fully synthetic. The ability of FP to inhibit tumour cell proliferation *in vitro* in therapeutically attractive concentrations (an average 50% tumour growth inhibition concentration = 3 µM in NCI screen[23]) has initiated an active search for molecular target(s) of this drug. The anti-cancer activity of FP is associated with both G1/S and G2/M arrests.[22,23,24,25] Consequently, it has been demonstrated that the inhibition of CDK1, CDK2 and CDK4 (Table 1) is responsible for the cell cycle block following the treatment of tumour cells with FP.[22,23,24] The inhibitory concentrations of FP toward individual CDKs compared to the other synthetic CDKIs are listed in Table 1. Interestingly, exposition of tumour cells to FP induces transient increase in CDK4 activity (3 hours post treatment), which is followed by rapid decrease thereafter.[4] This down-regulation of CDK4 enzymatic activity appears to be due to

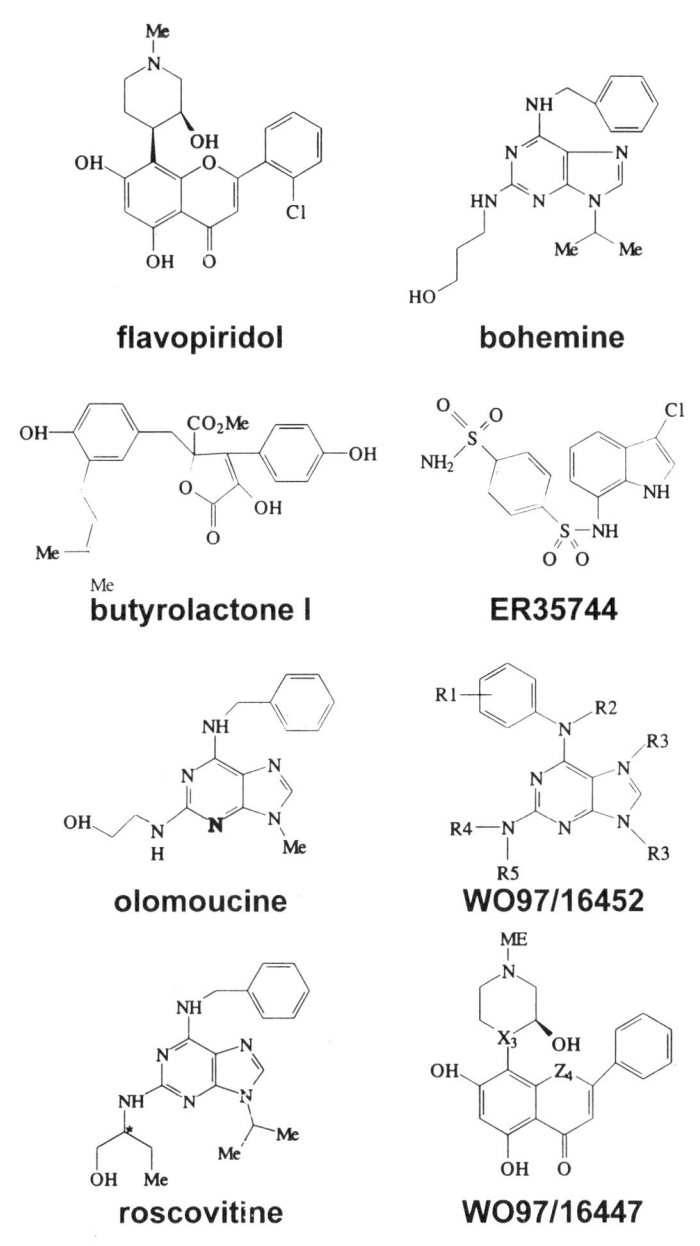

Figure 2. Chemical structures of synthetic cyclin dependent kinase inhibitors.

both the direct enzyme inhibition with FP and the decrease in cyclin D levels, since the quantity of CDK4 remained unchanged.[24] The appearance of hypophosphorylated isoforms of RB proteins was consistently reported with the down regulation of key cyclin dependent kinases by FP.[22,24] This data is consistent with FP induced G1/S block. In addition to the antiproliferative capacity of the inhibitor, induction of apoptosis in CEM (human T-lymphoblasts) cell line has been reported.[22] More importantly, the cell lines with altered p53 gene are hyper-sensitive to FP.[22] The ability of tumour cell lines to develop drug resistance to FP and related com-

Table 1. Survey of kinase inhibitory activities of known synthetic cyclin dependent kinase inhibitors. Note that kinase inhibitory activities of individual CDKIs are not fully comparable due to various amounts of cold ATP used in kinase assays

	Kinase inhibitory activity (IC50; µM)							
	cdc2/cyclinB	cdk2/cyclinE	cdk4	cdk7	erk1	PKC	PKA	EGFR
Olomoucine	7.0	3.0	>250	11.3	50	1000	>2000	400
Roscovitine	0.65	0.7	>250	1.4	34	100	>1000	100
Bohemine	1.0	ND	>250	1.8	ND	ND	ND	ND
Butyrolakton I	0.6	0.8	ND	ND	94	160	260	>590
Flavopiridol	0.03	0.17	0.1	ND	19	14	>50	22

Erk1-extracellular receptor kinase 1; PKC-protein kinase C; PKA-protein kinase A; EGFR-epidermal growth factor receptor kinase; ND-not yet determined.

pounds was also studied. It was demonstrated that drug resistance is associated with increase in CDK1 protein levels in cells resistant to FP.[22]

The structural basis for specificity of FP toward CDKs was determined in a X-ray crystalographic study.[26] It has been proved that the binding of the aromatic portion of the inhibitor to the adenine binding pocket of CDK2, and the position of the phenyl group of FP enables the inhibitor to make contacts with the enzyme not observed in the ATP complex structure.[26]

Following the *in vitro* studies, anti-cancer activity and toxicity of FP was analysed under *in vivo* conditions. The drug inhibited growth of nude mouse transplanted human xenografts of lung, breast, colon, stomach and brain tumours.[23,27] The major dose-limiting toxicities were haematological and gastrointestinal[27]. Phase I clinical trial with FP was recently completed at NCI.[23,27] The drug was being applied in 72 hour continual intravenous infusion every 2 weeks. The study included patients with different advanced solid tumours: renal, colon, prostate, non-Hodgkin's lymphoma, breast, etc. Maximum tolerated dose (MTD) obtained was 50 mg/m^2/day and the dose limiting toxicity was secretory diarrhea.[23] Following the diarrhea prophylaxis with loperamide, maximum tolerated dose increased to 78 mg/m^2/day, and the dose limiting toxicity was symptomatic hypotension of unknown origin.[23] Nonetheless, the steady state plasma concentrations of the drug reached median value of 344 nM, which was described to effectively inhibit CDKs and proliferation of breast and lung carcinomas *in vitro*.[23] In agreement with pharmacokinetics, FP induced several partial/minimum responses in tumour patients.[23] Recently published paper of Parker et al., describe that cells from hematopoietic neoplasms appear to be very susceptible to FP induced apoptosis and therefore clinical trials in hematopoietic neoplasms should be of high priority.[25]

4. BUTYROLACTONE I

Butyrolactone I (Figure 2), α-oxo-β-(p-hydroxyphenyl)-γ-(p-hydroxy-m-3,3-dimethylallylbenzyl)-γ-methoxycarbonyl-γ-butyro-lactone, was first identified within the screening of CDK1 and CDK2 kinase inhibitors from cultured mediums of *Aspergillus* species F-25799.[28] The compound competitively inhibits CDK1/cyclinB and CDK2/cyclinA complexes *in vitro*.[28,29] BL shows only minimal inhibitory activity in other protein kinase assays (Table 1). The compound displays a capacity to inhibit proliferation of several non-small- and small-cell lung cancer cell lines[30] with IC$_{50}$ values in the order of 50 μg/ml. No cross-resistance of several drug-resistant cell lines, including those with multidrug resistance phenotype and five cisplatin-resistant cell lines to BL was observed. The compound inhibited the blockade of S-phase entry, the G2/M transition,[30,31] RB phosphorylation,[31] DNA synthesis and decreased intracellular CDK1 levels.[30] However, further experiments have to be performed to demonstrate anti-tumor activity of BL *in vivo*.

5. CYTOKININE DERIVED CYCLIN DEPENDENT KINASE INHIBITORS

Cytokinine compounds were first recognized by their ability to induce cell division in certain plant tissues, and, are known to evoke a diversity of responses in plants.[32] These compounds are characterized as N^6-substituted adenines which at least in plants occur as nucleosides, nucleotides, 3,7,9,O-glucosides and conjugates with amino acids.[33] Besides the free compounds, cytokinins also occur as nucleoside components in tRNA of plants, animals and microorganisms.[34] Cytokinin residues incorporated in tRNA are always located at position 37 to the 3′-end of the tRNAs anti-codon that read codons starting with U[35]. Specific location of cytokinin nucleosides in the tRNAs and their distribution among the tRNA species indicates a specific role of cytokinins in tRNA function. The basic cytokinin moiety in yeast and animal tRNAs is N^6-(^{2}-isopentanyl)adenosine (iPA).[35] The release of free IPA upon turnover of tRNA is expected in plants and microorganisms, however, it has never been detected in animals. On the contrary, in mammalian tissue culture systems iPA inhibited cell proliferation in a variety of cell lines.[36] It was shown that iPA constrain the growth of Ehrlich ascitic carcinoma, mouse L1210 leukemia, human myeloid leukemias,[37] but not sarcoma 180, adenocarcinoma 735, Walker 256 carcinosarcoma[36] and human lymphatic leukemias.[37] Cultured lymphocytes stimulated by phytohemaglutinin were also inhibited by iPA.[38] Corresponding to cytokinin activity in plants, the lower concentrations of iPA (10^{-7}M) stimulated lymphocyte proliferation in the same assay.[39] Since iPA showed moderate anti-tumour effects in mice, it was considered to enter preclinical tests. The main toxicity of IPA in animals was hepatic damage, pancreatic atrophy, it inhibited proliferation of gastrointestinal and lymphoid tissues and induced granulocytosis. In a child with acute promyelocytic leukemia, the drug induced repeatedly complete, albeit short-lasting bone marrow remission.[40]

The anti-tumour activities of iPA and its stimulatory activity in plant tissue cultures promoted the synthesis of other cytokinins.[37] Unfortunately, among cytokinins synthesized so far only N^6-benzyladenosine has been passed through a variety of cell culture assays and pre-clinical trials.[41] The majority of these experiments were performed in the seventies without continuation in later decades. However, 20 years later, being stimulated by the progress in the cell cycle research and the old results of reporting cytokinin anti-cancer activity, we decided to study whether or not these compounds influence the molecular mechanisms of the cell division cycle. The most interesting question was whether or not these hormones interact with known regulatory proteins of the mammalian cell cycle (cyclin-dependent kinases, cyclins, etc.), since the plant homologues had not yet been discovered at that time. The wild range of plant hormones were screened for the modulation of CDK1/cyclin B complex activity by one member of our team (J.V.) in Dr. L. Meijer (CNRS, France) laboratory, and surprisingly, he discovered that 2-(2-hydroxyethylamino)-6-benzylamino-9-methylpurine selectively inhibits CDK1 and homologous kinases at micromolar concentrations[42] (Figure 2, Table 1). The compound was named olomoucine in honour of the city of Olomouc, where the majority of our team works. OC is a derivative of 6-benzylaminopurine, the cytokinin most frequently used in plant *in vitro* systems. OC was originally developed by Letham's group[43] and was used frequently by plant biologists to inhibit cytokinin glucosylation on the purine ring. OC selectively inhibits CDK1/cyclin B kinase, a key mitotic factor, which is highly conserved and strongly implicated in the basic mechanisms of the cell cycle control in all eukaryotes.[44] The compound failed to inhibit other cellular kinases, such as protein kinase C, cAMP- and cGMP kinases, etc.[42] In the mean time we have synthesized a number of compounds with a higher potency than OC to inhibit CDK1. One of them was named roscovitine (ROSC), 2-(R)-(1-ethyl-2-hydroxyethylamino)-6-benzylamino-9-isopropylpurine.[45] OC derived synthetic CDKIs behave as a competitive inhibitors for ATP binding to CDK1.[42] In collaboration with Drs. De Azevedo and Kim from University of California the crystal structures of both the OC and ROSC were determined.[46,47] It showed that the purine portion of the inhibitors bind to the adenine binding pocket of CDK2. The position of the benzyl ring group of the inhibitors bind to the adenine pocket of CDK2. The position of the benzyl ring group of the inhibitor enables the compounds to make contacts with the enzyme not observed in the ATP-complex structure.[46,47] Thus, the analysis of the position of this benzyl ring explain the specificity of roscovitine in inhibiting CDK2. The knowledge of the CDK2-iPA/OC/ROSC complex crystal structure allowed us to design more potent CDKIs. Since that time we have synthesized hundreds of biologically active compounds with more than 10 to 30-fold increase in CDK1 inhibitory capacity. The structure-activity relationships of CDK inhibition showed that the 1,3 and 7 positions of the purine ring must remain free, probably for a direct interaction, in which it behaves as a hydrogen bond acceptor.[48] On the contrary, OC, ROSC and other C^2, N^6, N^9-trisubstituted adenines exerted a high CDK1 inhibitory capacity. Removal or change of the side chain at position 2 or the hydrophobic group at position 9 dramatically decreased the inhibitory activity of both OC and ROSC.[48]

When the enzyme targets of the cytokinine derived CDKIs were identified, it was suggested that OC and related C2, N^6, C9 - substituted adenines should exhibit an anti-mitotic and anti-cancer activities. The cellular effects of OC were investigated in a large variety of plant and animal models. This compound inhibits the G1/S transition of unicellular algae (dinoflagellate and diatom). It blocks *Fuccus* zygote cleavage and development of *Laminaria* gametophytes.[49] Stimulated *Petunia* mesophyl protoplasts are arrested in G1 by OC. By arresting cleavage it blocks development of *Calanus* copepod larvae. It reversibly inhibits the serotonin-induced prophase/metaphase transition of clam oocytes; furthermore, it triggers the release of these oocytes from their meiotic metaphase I arrest, and induces nuclei formation.[49] OC slows down the prophase/metaphase transition in cleaving sea urchin embryos, but does not affect the duration of the metaphase/anaphase and anaphase/telophase transitions. It also inhibits prophase/metaphase transition triggered by various agonists.[49] *Xenopus* oocyte maturation, the *in vivo* and *in vitro* phosphorylation of elongation factor EF-1 are inhibited by OC and ROSC.[45,49] Mouse oocyte maturation is delayed by this compound, whereas parthenogenetic release from metaphase II arrest is facilitated. Growth of tumor cells is inhibited by OC and ROSC, and both compounds showed capacity to inhibit cell cycle at G1/S and G2/M transitions.[42,45,49,50,51] OC is able to potentiate mitoxantrone induced apoptosis of tumor cells.[52] However, on the other hand, OC inhibited apoptosis in differentiated neuronal cells upon withdrawal of neuronal growth factor, and thus showed differential activity against differentiated and malignant tissues.[53] Although OC is a relatively weak CDK inhibitor, we and the others have demonstrated sufficient efficacy of this drug to induce apoptosis[50,51,54] (Figure 3) and tumor regression following *in vivo* application in several animal tumor models and in the case of spontaneous dog malignant melanoma.[54] Recently, it was reported that OC and ROSC induce apoptosis in tumor cells, which is accompanied with decrease in cellular CDK1 levels.[50]

Synthetic Cyclin Dependent Kinase Inhibitors

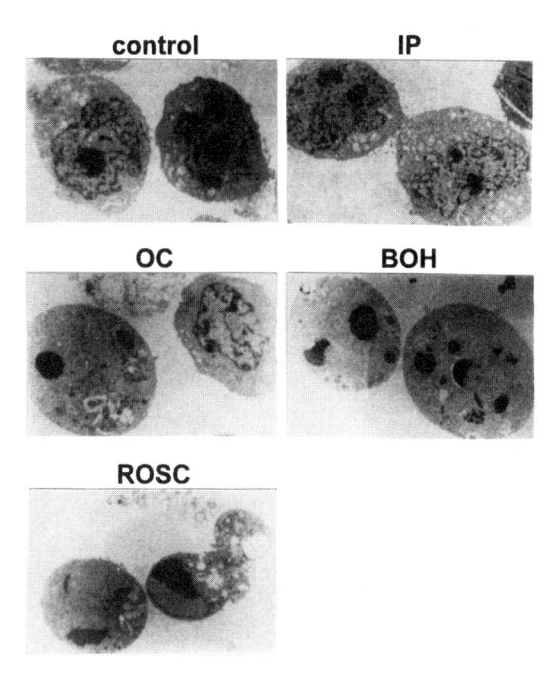

Figure 3. Olomoucine derived synthetic cyclin dependent kinase inhibitors induce apoptosis in CEM cell line 6 hours after exposition to 70 μM concentrations of individual compounds (electron microscopy, 5.000x). Typical morphological hallmarks of apoptosis—chromatin condensation and nuclear fragmentation—were detected in OC/BOH/ROSC, but not in control or IP (ineffective homologue) treated cells.

During the study of a new generation of cytokinins with CDK1 kinase inhibitory activity we have identified the mechanism of anti-cancer activity of these compounds.[51] The study was performed on structurally related, albeit in CDKs inhibition ineffective compound isopentenyladenine (IP) and potent CDKs inhibitors: OC, ROSC and a new compound, which was named bohemine (BOH) - 2-[(3-hydroxypropyl)amino]-6-benzylamino-9-isopropylpurine (Figure 2). Although these drugs failed to down regulate CDK4 activity *in vitro* as we have reported previously, CDK4 has been inhibited under *in vivo* conditions due to direct inhibition of CDK7 (Table 1), and, correspondingly, CDK7-mediated activating phosphorylation of CDK4 on T161. The OC derived synthetic CDKIs induced apoptosis in many tumor and leukaemic cell lines *in vitro* at 1–30 μM concentrations, while the non-malignant cells survived concentrations above 250 μM. Compound induced apoptosis (Figure 3) was independent of nucleo/proteosynthesis *de novo*, however, it was inhibited by YVAD peptide, a specific inhibitor of ICE proteases, and ocadaic acid, an inhibitor of cellular phosphatases. The activation of ICE proteases during apoptosis was further confirmed by lamin B and RB proteins cleavage.[51] To analyze the mechanism of drug resistance to CDKIs, CEM T-lymphoblasts were treated with gradually increasing subtoxic doses of BOH and drug resistant sub-lines were prepared. These cultures demonstrated unique mechanisms of resistance: 1)decreased proliferation, 2)induction of cellular senescence, 3)inhibition of CDK1 and CDK7 expression, 4)restoration of p21^{WAF1} expression, 5)decrease in DNA-polymerase, and 6)DNA-telomerase activities.[51] Using the mouse model of P388D1 leukemia and B16 melanoma we demonstrated ability of OC and BOH, but not ROSC and IP to increase medium survival time, or eventually to cure the animals with transplanted tumors.[51] This observation showed that there is no direct correlation between *in vitro* and *in vivo* effectiveness of various synthetic CDKIs, since the ROSC is more potent inhibitor of CDK1 *in vitro* than OC/BOH, however it did not show corresponding *in vivo* activity. Nonetheless, more experiments have to be done to substantiate these conclusions. In agreement with these observations, our pilot pharmacokinetics and metabolic experiments clearly demonstrated the rapid clearance of BOH from the organism (Veselý, J., unpublished results) and thus indicated that optimization of drug application schema could dramatically improve *in vivo* anti-cancer activity.

In addition to experimental animal tumors, we have reported the induction of apoptosis in the case of spontaneous dog melanoma following OC application.[54] The drug was being applied intravenously in a single dose of 8 mg/kg/day for 7 days in succession. Repeated bioptic examinations of metastatic cervical lymph nodes showed rapid induction of apoptosis in tumor cells as soon as on the 3rd day of treatment. Standard clinical and laboratory examinations failed to demonstrate the side effects of the therapy. There were no detectable manifestations of myelosuppression, hepatotoxicity, nephrotoxicity and neurotoxicity. However, transient anemia developed following bleeding from a devitalized tumor mass. For this reason, the dog underwent surgery to minimize tumor load as well as to eliminate the source of bleeding. Two kilograms of primary tumor were extirpated in the course of surgery including cervical node metastases. Unfortunately, the dog died soon after surgery due to respiratory depression. Histological examinations of the tumor tissue showed marked apoptosis of melanoma cells in both the primary tumor and metastases. The induction of programmed cell death of cancer cells by OC resulted in rapid eradication of at least 50% of the tumor cells. The remaining melanoma cells retained excellent *in vitro* sensitivity to OC when compared to drugs currently used in clinical practice.[54]

In conclusion, it should be stressed that OC and related compounds expressed higher anti-cancer activity than initially realized. Our current effort is to initiate phase I clinical study with the most promising representative(s) of this family of compounds. It seems possible that the ability of OC and related compounds to inhibit CDK7 activity, induce apoptosis, and thus constrain tumor cell proliferation, together with its capacity to cross the mechanisms of multidrug resistance, may provide a significant therapeutic benefit for cancer patients in the future.

ACKNOWLEDGMENT

This project was supported, in parts, from the Grant Agency of Czech Republic (204/96/K047), Ministry of Education of Czech Republic (VS96154), the Cancer Research Foundation in Olomouc, League Against Cancer Prague and from the profit of Terry Fox Run organized by Canadian Embassy in Prague. The technical assistance of Anna Janošťáková, Mária Šafážová, editrorial help of Richard Kožínek and Kasmine Jess are greatly appreciated.

REFERENCES

1. Strauss, M., Lukáš, J., Bártek, J.: Unrestricted cell cycling and cancer. Nature Med. 1995, 1, 1245–1246
2. Bártek, J., Lukáš, J., Strauss M.: A common pathway to tumor growth: deregulation of Rb-dependent restriction point control (Review). Oncol. Rep., 1996, 3, 237–240.
3. Levine A., J., Momand, J., Finlay, C.A.: The p53 tumour supressor gene. Nature, 1991, 351, 453–456
4. Hollstein, M., Sidransky, D., Vogelstein, B., Harris, C.C.: p53 mutations in human cancers. Science, 1991, 253, 49–53.
5. Gartel, A.L., Serfas M.S., Tyner, A.L.: p21 - Negative regulator of the cell cycle. P.S.E.M.B., 1996, 213, 138–149

6. El-Deiry, W.S., Harper, J.W., O'Connor, P.M.: WAF1/CIP1 is induced in p53-mediated G1 arrest and apoptosis. Cancer Res., 1994, 54, 1169–1174
7. Grana, X., Reddy, E.P.: Cell cycle control in mammalian cells: role of cyclins, cyclin dependent kinases (CDKs), growth suppressor genes and cyclin-dependent kinase inhibitors (CDKIs). Blood, 1995, 11, 211–219
8. Xiong, Y., Hannon, G.J., Zhang, H., Casso, D., Kobayashi, R., Beach, D.: p21 is a universal inhibitor of cyclin kinases. Nature, 1993, 336, 701–704
9. Luo, Y., Hurwitz, J., Massague, J.: Cell-cycle inhibition by independent CDK and PCNA binding domains in p21^{Cip1}. Nature, 1995, 375, 159–161
10. Waldman, T., Lengauer, C., Bunz, F., Kinzler, K., Vogelstein, B.: The role of p21 in cell cycle control and drug sensitivity. Cell Cycle Therapeutics. The Conference held on November 6–7, 1997, Washington, DC, USA. Book of Abstracts. Published by International Business Communications (225 Turnpike Road, Southborough, MA 01772–1749, USA)
11. Solomon, J.M., Harper, J.W., Shuttleworth, J.: CAK, the p34 cdc2 activating kinase, contains a protein identical or closely related to p40MO15. EMBO J., 1993, 12, 3133–3142
12. Pines J., Hunter, T.: Cyclin-dependent kinases: an embarrassment of riches. In: Hames, B.D., Glover, D.M. (Eds.): Cell cycle control, Oxford University Press, New York, 1997, 144–176
13. Taubert, H., Meye, A., Wurl, P.: Prognosis is associated with p53 mutation type foe soft tissue sarcoma patients. Cancer Res., 1996, 56, 4134–4136
14. Strang, P., Nordstrom, B., Nilsson, S., Bergstrom R., Tribukait, B.: Mutant p53 protein as a predictor of survival in endometrial carcinoma. Eur. J. Cancer, 32A, 598–602
15. Asgari, K., Sesterhenn, I.A., McLeod, D.G., Cowan, K., Moul J.W., Seth, P., Srivastava, S.: Inhibition of the growth of pre-established subcutaneous tumor nodules of human prostate cancer cells by single injection of the recombinant adenovirus p53 expression vector. Int. J. Cancer, 1997, 71, 377–382
16. Sandig, V., Brand, K., Herwig, S., Lukas, J., Bartek, J., Strauss, M.: Adenovirally transferred p16$^{INK4/CDKN2}$ and p53 genes cooperate to induce apoptotic tumor cell death. Nature Med., 1997, 3, 313–319
17. Selivanova, G., Iotsova, V., Okan, I., Fritsche, M., Strom, M., Groner, B., Graftstrom, R.C., Wiman, K.G.: Restoration of the growth suppression function of mutant p53 by a synthetic peptide derived from the p53 C-terminal domain. Nature Med., 1997, 3, 632–638
18. Ball, K.L., Lain, S., Fahraeus, R., Smythe, C., Lane, D.P.: Cell-cycle arrest and inhibition of Cdk4 activity by small peptides based on the carboxy-terminal domain of p21^{WAF1}. Curr. Biol., 1996, 7, 71–80
19. Worland, P.J., Kaur, G., Stetler-Stevenson, M., Sebers, S., Sartor, O., Sausville, E.A.: Alteration of the phosphorylation state of p34^{cdc2} kinase by the flavone L86–8275 in breast carcinoma cells (correlation with decreased H1 kinase activity). Biochem. Pharmacol., 1993, 46, 1831–1840
20. Kaur, G., Stetler-Stevenson, M., Sebers, S., Worland, P., Sedlacek, H., Myers, Ch., Czech, J., Naik, R., Sausville, E.: Growth inhibition with reversible cell cycle arrest of carcinoma cells by flavone L86–8275. J. Natl. Cancer Inst., 1992, 84, 1736–1740
21. Losiewicz, M.D., Carlson, B.A., Kaur, G., Sausville, E.A., Worland, P.J.: Potent inhibition of cdc2 kinase activity by the flavonoid L86–8275. Biochem. Biophys. Res. Commun., 1994, 201, 589–595
22. Webster, K.: Targeting the cell cycle. In: Cell Cycle Therapeutics. The Conference held on November 6–7, 1997, Washington, DC, USA. Book of Abstracts. Published by International Business Communications (225 Turnpike Road, Southborough, MA 01772–1749, USA)
23. Sausville, E.: Flavopiridol and UCN-01: Cell cycle modulators in clinical trial. In: Cell Cycle Therapeutics. The Conference held on November 6–7, 1997, Washington, DC, USA. Book of Abstracts. Published by International Business Communications (225 Turnpike Road, Southborough, MA 01772–1749, USA)
24. Carlson, B.A., Dubay, M.M., Sausville, E.A., Brizuela, L., Worland, P.J.: Flavopiridol induces G$_1$ arrest with inhibition of cyclin-dependent kinase (CDK) 2 and CDK 4 in human breast carcinoma cells. Cancer Res., 1996, 56, 2973 2978
25. Parker, B.W., Kaur, G., Nieves-Neira, W., Taimi, M., Kolhagen, G., Shimizu, T., Losiewicz, M.D., Pommier, Y., Sausville, E.A., Senderowicz, A.M.: Early induction of apoptosis in hematopoietic cell lines after exposure to flavopiridol. Blood, 1998, 91, 458–465
26. Azevedo (Jr.), W.F., Mueller-Dieckmann, H.J., Schulze-Gahmen, U., Worland, P.J., Sausville, E., Kim, S.H.: Structural basis for specificity and potency of a flavonoid inhibitor of human CDK2, a cell cycle kinase. Proc. Natl. Acad. Sci., 1996, 93, 2735–2740
27. Christian, M.C., Pluda, J.M., Ho, P.T.C., Arbuck, S.G., Murgo, A.J. and Sausville, E.A.: Promising new agents under development by the division of cancer treatment, diagnosis, and centers of the National Cancer Institute. Semin. Oncol., 1997, 2, 219–240

28. Kitagawa, M., Okabe, T., Ogino, H., Matsumoto, H., Suzuki-Takahashi, I., Kokubo, T., Higashi, H., Saitoh, S., Taya, Y., Yasuda, H., Ohba, Y., Nishimura, S., Tanaka, N., Okuyama, A.: Butyrolactone I, a selective inhibitor of cdk2 and cdc2 kinase. Oncogene, 1993, 8, 2425–2432
29. Someya, A., Tanaka, N., Okuyama, A.: Inhibition of cell cycle oscillation of DNA replication by a selective inhibitor of the cdc2 kinase family, butyrolactone I, in Xenopus egg extracts. Biochem. Biophys. Res. Commun., 1994, 198, 536–545
30. Nishio K., Ishida, T., Arioka, H., Kurokawa, H., Fukuoka, K., Nomoto, T., Fukumoto, H., Yokote, H., Saijo, N.: Antitumor effects of butyrolactone I, a selective cdc2 kinase inhibitor, on human lung cancer cell lines. Anticancer Res., 1996, 16, 3387–3395
31. Kitagawa, M., Higashi, H., Suzuki-Takahashi, I., Okabe, T., Ogino, H., Taya, Y., Nishimura, S., Okuyama, A.: A cyclin-dependent kinase inhibitor, butyrolactone I, inhibits phosphorylation of RB protein and cell cycle progression. Oncogene, 1994, 9, 2549–2557
32. Skoog, F., Armstrong, D.J.:Cytokinins. Annu. Rev.Plant Physiol., 1970, 21, 359–384
33. Shaw, G.: Chemistry of adenine cytokinins. In: Mok, D.W.S., Mok, M.C. (Eds): Cytokinins, Chemistry, Activity and Function, 15–34, CRC Press, Boca Raton
34. McGaw, B. A., Burch, L. R.: Cytokinin biosynthesis and metabolism. In: Davies, P.J. (Ed.): Plant Hormones, Physiology, Biochemistry and Molecular Biology, 98–117. Kluwer Academic Publishers, Dordrecht
35. Sprinzl, M., Dank, N., Nock, S., Schon, A.: Compilation of tRNA sequences and sequences of tRNA genes. Nucl. Acid. Res. 9, 2127–2171
36. Slak, D., Simpson, C.L., Minich, E.: Toxicological and antiproliferative effects of N^6-(^{2}-isopentenyl)adenosine, a natural component of mammalian transfer RNA. Cancer Res. 1970, 30,1429–1439
37. Grace, J.T., Hakal, M.T., Hall, R.M., Blakeslee, J.: N^6-Substituted adenine derivatives as growth inhibitors of human leukemic myeloblasts and S-180 cells. Proc. Am. Assoc. Cancer Res. 1967, 8, 23–27
38. Gallo, R.C., Whang-Peng, J., Perry, S.: Isopentenyl-adenosine stimulates and inhibits mitosis of lymphocytes treated with phytohemagglutinin. Science 1969, 165, 400–402
39. Suk, D., Simpson, C.L., Minich, E.: Antitumor and toxicologic effects of N^6-(^{2}-isopentenyl)adenosine (iPA). Proc. Am. Assoc. Cancer, Res., 1968, 9, 69–74
40. Jones, R., Grace, J.T., Mittelman, A., and Woodruff, M.W.: Human pharmacology and initial clinical trail of isopentenyl adenosine (iPA). Proc. Am. Assoc. Cancer Res., 1968, 9, 35
41. Mittelman, A., Evans, J.T., Chheda, G.B.: Cytokinins as chemotherapeutic agents. Ann. N. Y. Acad. Sci., 1972, 15, 225–23
42. Veselý, J., Havlíček, L., Strnad, M., Blow, J.J., Donella.Deana, A., Pinna, L., Letham, D.S., Kato, J., Detivaud, L., Leclerc, S., Meijer, L.: Inhibition of cyclin-dependent kinases by purine analoques. Eur. J. Biochem., 1994, 224, 771–786
43. Parker, C.W., Wilson, M., Letham, D.S., Cowley, D.E., MacLeod, J.K.: Inhibitors of two new enzymes which metabolize cytokinins. Phytochem.,1986, 25, 303–310
44. Norbury, C., Nurse, P.: Animal cell cycles and their control. Ann. Rev. Biochem., 1992, 61, 441–470
45. Meijer, L., Borgne, A., Mulner, O., Chong, J.P.J., Blow, J.J., Inagaki, N., Inagaki, M., Delcros J.-G., Moulinoux, J.-P.: Biochemical and cellular effects of roscovitine, a potent and selective inhibitor of the cyclin-dependent kinases cdc2, cdk2 and cdk5. Eur. J. Biochem., 1997, 243, 527–536
46. Schulze-Gahmen, U., Brandsen, J., Jones, H. D., Morgan, D.O., Meijer, L., Veselý, J., Kim, S.-H.: Multiple modes of ligand recognition: Crystal structures of cyclin-dependent protein kinase 2 in complex with ATP and two inhibitors, olomoucine and isopentenyladenine. Proteins: Structure, function, and genetics, 1995, 22, 378–391
47. De Azavedo, W.F., Leclerc, S., Meijer, L., Havlíček, L., Strnad, M., Kim, S.-H.: Inhibition of cyclin-dependent kinases by purine analogues. Crystal structure of human cdk2 complexed with roscovitine. Eur. J. Biochem., 1997, 243, 518–526
48. Havlíček, L., Hanuš, J., Veselý, J., Leclerc, S., Meijer, L., Shaw, G., Strnad, M.: Cytokinin-derived cyclin-dependent kinase inhibitors: synthesis and cdc2 inhibitory activity of olomoucine and related compounds. J. Med. Chem., 1997, 40, 1997, 408–412
49. Abraham, R.T., Acquarone, M., Andersen, A., Asensi, A., Belle, R., Berger, F., Bergounioux, C., Brunn, G., Buquet-Fagot, C., Fagot, D., Glab, N., Goudeau, H., Goudeau, M., Guerrier, P., Houghton, P., Hendriks, H., Kloareg, B., Lippai, M., Marie, D., Maro, B., Meijer, L., Mester, J., Mulner-Lorillon, O., Poulet, S.A., Schierenberg, E., Schutte, D., Vaulot, D., Verlhac, M.H.: Cellular effects of olomoucine, an inhibitor of cyclin-dependent kinases. Biol. Cell, 1995, 83, 105–120
50. Schutte B., Nieland L., van Engeland M., Henfling M. E. R., Meijer L., Ramaekers C. S.: The effect of the cyclin-dependent kinase inhibitor olomoucine on cell cycle kinetics. Exp. Cell Res., 1998, 236, 4–15
51. Hajdúch M., Nosková V., Havlíček L., Feketová G., Gojová L., Michálek T., Novotný R., Kryštof V., Kotala V., Veselý J., Strnad M., Mihál V.: Olomoucine-derived synthetic cdk inhibitors: the mechanism of

apoptotic death of tumor cells and *in vivo* antitumor activity. *In*: In: Cell Cycle Therapeutics. The Conference held on November 6–7, 1997, Washington, DC, USA. *Book of Abstracts*. Published by International Business Communications (225 Turnpike Road, Southborough, MA 01772–1749, USA)

52. Ongkeko, W., Ferguson, D.J.P., Harris, A.L., Norbury, C.: Inactivation of cdc2 increases the level of apoptosis induced by DNA damage. J. Cell Sci., 1995, 108, 2897–2904
53. Markus, M.A., Kahle, P.J., Winkler, A., Hortsmann, S., Anneser, J.M., Borasio, G.D.: Survival-promoting activity of inhibitors of cyclin-dependent kinases on primary neurons correlates with inhibition of c-Jun kinase-1. Neurobiol. Dis., 1997, 4, 122–133
54. Hajdúch, M., Koláø, Z. Novotný, R., Hanuš, J., Mihál, V., Hlobílková, A., Nosková, V., Strnad, M.: Induction of apoptosis and regression of spontaneous dog melanoma following *in vivo* application of synthetic cyclin-dependent kinase inhibitor olomoucin. Anti-Cancer Drugs, 1997, 8, 1007–1013

FACTORS CONTRIBUTING TO THE RESISTANCE TO APOPTOSIS INDUCED BY TOPOISOMERASE I INHIBITORS IN VINCRISTINE RESISTANT CELLS

Valérie Palissot,[1] Aurélie Trussardi,[2] Marie-Claude Gorisse,[2] and Jean Dufer[1]

[1]Laboratoire de Physiologie Cellulaire
EA 2063, IFR 53, 51, rue Cognacq Jay
51100 Reims, France
[2]Institut Jean-Godinot
1, rue du général Koenig
51100 Reims, France

Keywords: Apoptosis, Resistance, Topoisomerases inhibitors, BCL-2, Pgp, MRP.

1. ABSTRACT

The activity of numerous antineoplasic drugs is correlated with their capacity to induce the apoptotic process. In this study, apoptosis induced by the topoisomerase I (Topo I) inhibitors camptothecin (CPT) and the CPT-11 active metabolite SN-38 was evaluated on HL-60 cells and their multidrug resistant variant HL-60-Vincristine cells. Both CPT and SN-38 induced high levels of apoptosis in sensitive cells but very low levels in MDR cells. The role of the different genes and proteins usually implicated in the drug resistance phenomenon was studied. The Pgp independence of the two drugs was suggested by the lack of modulation of anti-Topo I effects with verapamil. Moreover CPT and SN-38 induced a strong decrease of mdr1 mRNA in MDR treated cells. MRP mRNA expression was very low in drug sensitive and resistant cells and decreased during treatments in both cell lines. However, MRP protein was not detected in control and MDR cells suggesting that this pump was probably not implicated in this resistance phenomenon. Topo I and BCL-2 proteins displayed a higher expression in MDR cells but only Topo I proteins decreased during treatments in the two cell lines. These data suggest that in addition to the classical multidrug resistance phenotype, dysregulation of proteins associated with DNA replication and apoptotic process could contribute to acquired resistance to a large panel of drugs, including those which are not considered as substrates for Pgp.

2. INTRODUCTION

The treatment of cancer comes up against cellular resistance to antineoplasic drugs. Known resistance mechanisms include decreased cellular drug accumulation due to over-expression of P-glycoprotein (Pgp), the product of mdr1 gene or to MRP over-expressed protein. These drugs transporters act as efflux pump to numerous chemotherapeutic agents (anthracyclin-vinca alcaloïds) and to gluthatione drug conjugates. Others mechanisms contributing to resistance could include modulations of the level of the drug targets or of the apoptotic process.[1] To overcome the resistance problem, MDR unrelated drugs have been proved such as camptothecin and its derivative Irinotecan. These topoisomerase I inhibitors induce cellular apoptosis and some of these have been proposed as an alternative treatment in human colon cancer.[2] In order to elucidate the effects of topoisomerase I inhibitors on multidrug resistant cells, we have used these drugs on sensitive and resistant human promyelocytic leukemic HL-60 cells. Our investigation was to find out whether these topoisomerase I inhibitors (camptothecin: CPT and the irinotecan active metabolite: SN-38) could induce normal apoptosis in MDR cells.

3. MATERIAL AND METHODS

3.1. Chemicals

Camptothecin (CPT), was obtained from Sigma chemical Co (St-Louis, MO). SN-38 was kindly provided by Rhône Poulenc Rorer (Vitry sur seine, France). All were dissolved in DMSO. Vincristine was purchased from Lilly France (Saint-Cloud) under the pharmaceutical form Oncovin. Cell culture media and fetal calf serum were from Gibco/BRL (Grand Island, NY). Stock preparations from all reagents were stored at -20°C. All were diluted to appropriate final concentrations in RPMI 1640 medium.

3.2. Cell Culture and Drug Treatment

The human promyelocytic leukemia cell line HL-60 was obtained from ECACC (Salisbury, UK). Multidrug-resistant cells HL-60 VCR were kindly provided by Pr G. Laurent (Toulouse, France).[3] The two cell lines were grown in suspension culture in RPMI 1640 medium supplemented with 10% heat-inactivated fetal bovine serum, 1% L-glutamine at 2 mM, 100 units/ml Penicillin G, and 100 mg/ml Streptomycin. All cultures were maintained under a fully humidified atmosphere of 95% air-5% CO_2 at 37°C. Cultures were passaged twice weekly. Exponentially growing cells were used in all experiments. Cell viability was assessed by the ability to exclude trypan blue (0.5 % w/v, Sigma). Cells were seeded at 2.10^5 cells /ml in medium with the topoisomerases I inhibitors CPT and SN-38 at 1 µM or with various concentrations of VCR. CPT and SN-38 stock solutions were diluted to ensure a final concentration of less than 0.03% and 0.1% for DMSO for CPT and SN-38 respectively. These concentrations did not induce apoptosis or differentiation in HL-60 cells.

3.3. DNA Gel Electrophoresis

10^6 cells were incubated at 50°C for 2 hours in 20 µl of lysis buffer (150mM NaCl, 10 mM Tris-HCl, 10 mM EDTA, pH8), containing 0,5 mg/ml Proteinase K, and 0.5 % SDS. DNA was then incubated during 1hour at 37° C with 0.1 mg/ml of RNase, (DNase free) prior to electrophoresis on 2 % (w/v) agarose gel overnight at 24V.

3.4. Flow Cytometry Analysis for Apoptosis Quantification

Cells were fixed with 70 % ethanol, washed in phosphate buffered saline, and stained in phosphate buffered saline containing 0.1 mM EDTA, 0.1% Triton X-100, 50 µg/ml propidium iodide, and 25 µg/ml RNase A (Boerhinger Mannheim, Germany).[4] Cells were analysed with an Ortho 50H cytometer (Ortho Instruments, Westwood, MA) equiped with 300mW argon laser emitting at 488 nm. An MCA 3000 computer (Bruker, Wissembourg, France) allowed list-mode acquisition and analysis of at least 20,000 cells.

3.5. Reverse Transcription Polymerase Chain Reaction (RT-PCR)

Total cellular RNA was extracted by Trizol method and cDNA was synthesized with 1 µg of total RNA. mdr1 RT PCR was performed as previously described.[5] mrp RT PCR was performed with 1 µg RNA and 5 µM of random hexamer in solution containing 67 mM $MgCl_2$, 670 mM Tris, HCl (pH) 8.8 , 166 mM $(NH_4)_2 SO_4$, 0.25 mM each of dNTPs, and 200 units of reverse transcriptase for 30 min at 42 °C. PCR was carried out for 32 cycles in 100 µl solution of 1.5 mM $MgCl_2$, 0.25 mM of each dNTPs, cDNA derived from 1 µg of RNA and 1.5 units of Taq DNA polymerases, 0.6 µM mrp primers and 0.3 µM β2m primers. Each cycle of PCR consisted of 45 s of denaturation at 94°C, 45 s of annealing at 61 °C and 90 s of extension at 72 °C. Primer DNA sequences were previously described[6]

3.6. Flow Cytometry Analysis for Pgp Quantification

Expression of Pgp was determined with specific monoclonal antibody and isotype control, using a FACscan (Coulter, Hyaleah, CA). 5.10^5 cells each of HL-60 or HL-60 VCR, treated or not with CPT and SN-38, were incubated with 8.4 µg/ml of MRK16 (Valbiotech, Paris France) or IgG2a isotypic control at room temperature for 30 min. Cells were washed with PBS/10%FCS twice and counterstained with FITC-labeled goat anti mouse IgG2a antibody (Dako, Copenhagen, DK). Cells were washed with PBS/10 % FCS and 10,000 cells were analysed.

3.7. Immunocytochemistry of MRP Protein

Tumor cell line preparations (30,000 cells) were centrifuged, rapidly air-dried and fixed in cold acetone during 20 minutes. Slides were washed with PBS and incubated in saturation buffer (PBS, BSA 1%, FCS 20%) for 30 minutes at room temperature before overnight incubation with MRPm6 antibody (0.4 µg/ml, Monosan, Uden, NL) at 4°C. Cells were washed twice with TBS and stained using the APAAP kit (Dako, Copenhagen, DK) following the manufacturer's instructions. Lack of the primary antibody and the MRP positive A549 line were used as negative and positive control, respectively.

3.8. BCL-2 Protein Immunoblotting

Total protein were isolated using approximately 10^7 cells lysed by quick freezing at -80° C and thawing at 37°C in 100μl lysing buffer (0.125 M Tris-HCl [pH 6.8]; 10% glycerol; 2 % SDS, 100 mM dithiotreitol) containing proteinase inhibitors, including leupeptin, aprotinin, bestatin, benzamidin. Protein concentrations were then determined by Bradford assay using BioRad protein Assay Kit (Richmond, CA). Protein samples (20 μg/lane) were separated on 12% SDS-polyacrylamide gradient gels, then transfered onto a nitrocellulose membrane (Amersham, Arlington Heights, IL,) in transfer buffer (3 g/l Tris-base, 14.4 g/l glycin, 20 % methanol). Membrane were blocked in TBS-Tween 0.1% containing 10% dry milk at room temperature for 90 min. Membranes were immunoblotted with the anti BCL-2 mouse monoclonal antibody 124 (Dako) at 0.5 μg/ml. Proteins were visualized using a peroxidase-conjugated goat anti-mouse secondary antibody (Jackson, Westgrove, PA) at 1:20 000 in PBS containing 1% of BSA, and the ECL detection kit (Amersham).

3.9. Topoisomerase I Immunoblotting

Nuclear proteins were extracted from 10^7 cells as previously described.[7] Protein samples (20 μg/lane) were separated on 8% SDS-polyacrylamide gradient gels, then treated as described above. Primary antibody used for immunoblotting was mouse polyclonal antibody kindly provided by Dr I. Bronstein (University of York) at 1:100.

4. RESULTS

4.1. Expression of Pgp and MRP

Pgp and MRP expressions were analysed in drug sensitive HL-60 cell line and its resistant subline HL-60 VCR both at the protein level by flow cytometry with MRK16 antibody and immunocytochemistry with anti MRP subclone 6, and at the mRNA level by RT-PCR. Pgp was not detected in HL-60 cells but was overexpressed in HL60 VCR cells as shown at mRNA (Figure 1) and protein levels (Figure 2). After treatments with CPT or SN-38, the mdr1 expression decreased as well as Pgp expression after 24 hours treatments. MRP mRNA was detected in the two cell types at equivalent very low levels (Figure 3) but protein expression could not be observed (data not shown).

4.2. Apoptosis Time Course in HL-60 and HL-60/VCR Treated with CPT and SN-38

Apoptotic DNA fragmentation was observed on electrophoresis agarose gels (Figure 4) and measured by flow cytometry (Figure 5). Following exposure to 1μM CPT and SN38, sensitive HL-60 cells rapidly undergo apoptosis in vitro. The number of sensitive HL60 apoptotic cells increased with the time of treatments. MDR-HL60 VCR cells display a partial resistance to apoptosis induced by CPT and SN-38 as compared with their sensitive counterpart. The maximal percentage of drug resistant apoptotic cells (approximately 25%) was obtained after 6hrs of treatment and did not increase further during 24 hrs induction with the same drugs concentrations. As HL-60 VCR cells overexpress Pgp, the effects of the Pgp modulator Verapamil at 30μM (a concentration that blocks Pgp) on

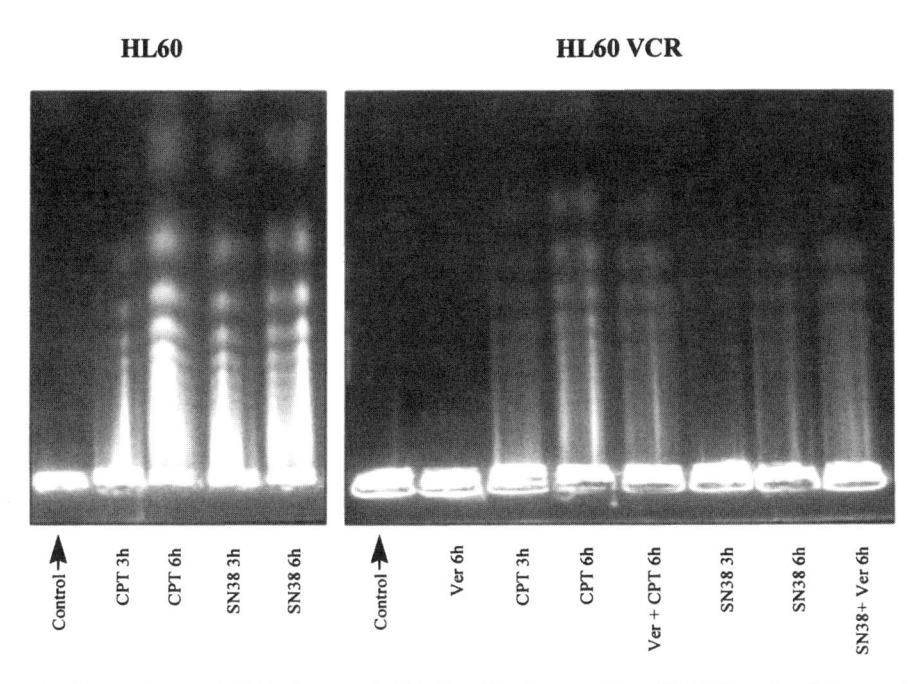

Figure 1. Internucleosomal DNA cleavage in HL-60 cells. Drug-sensitive (HL60-S) and multidrug-resistant (HL60-VCR) cells were incubated for 3 to 6 h with the topoisomerase I inhibitors, camptothecin (CPT) or SN-38 both at 1 µM, in the presence or absence of verapamil 30 µM (Ver). DNA cleavage was evaluated by conventional agarose gel electrophoresis on cellular extracts from 10^6 cells.

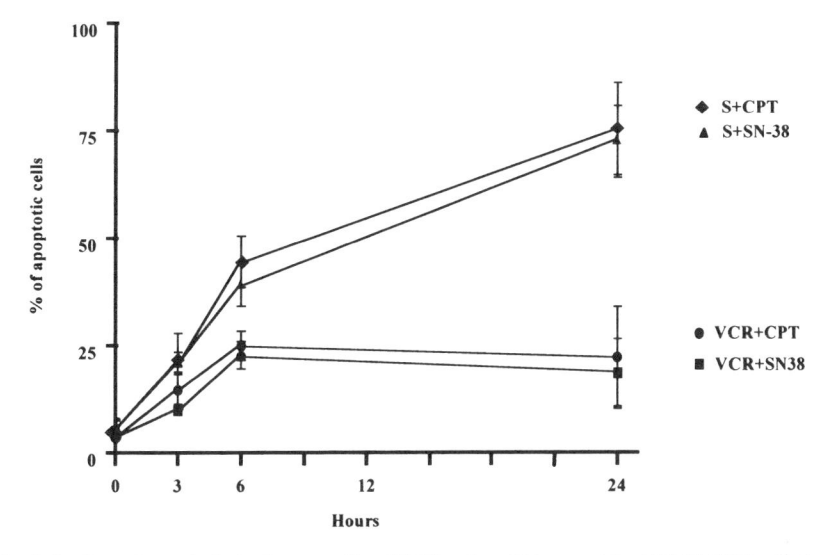

Figure 2. Induction of apoptosis in drug-sensitive HL60 and multidrug-resistant HL60-VCR cells by CPT and SN-38. Both drugs were used at 1 µM concentration. Apoptosis was quantified by flow cytometry.

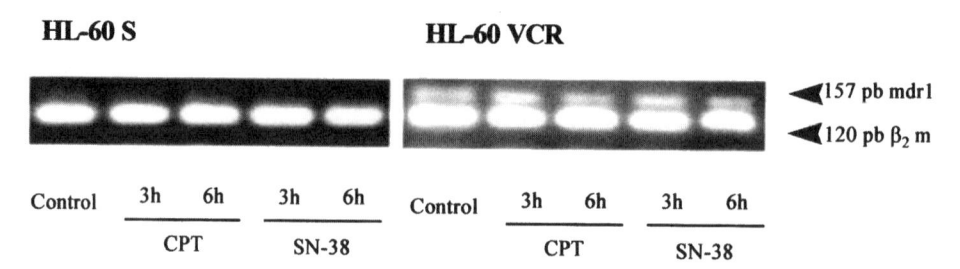

Figure 3. mdr 1 mRNA expression in HL-60 and HL-60 VCR cells. RT-PCR analysis using specific primers of mdr1 was performed on 1μg mRNA of drug-sensitive HL60 and multidrug-resistant HL60-VCR cells. Cells were treated for 3 to 6 h with CPT (1 μM), or SN-38 (1 μM).

the apoptosis induced in these cells by CPT or SN-38 were studied. Apoptotic cell death was analysed by flow cytometry and DNA gel electrophoresis. After 6 hours of treatments with 1 μM CPT and SN-38, the percentages of apoptotic cells were 25% ± 5.3 and 23.4% ± 4.9 respectively. Verapamil alone induced 3.8 % ± 1.4 apoptotic cells as compared to 4.6% ± 0.7 in control cells. When used in combinaison with the topoisomerases I inhibitors, verapamil did not modulate the apoptosis induction. The apoptotic cell percentages respectively 24.4% ± 5.4 and 26.3% ± 5.6 for CPT+Ver and SN-38+ Ver.

4.3. Expression of Topoisomerase I Protein (Topo I) in HL60 and HL-60/VCR Cells

In order to look if resistance could be due to change in expression of the topoisomerase I target, the basal level of this protein was evaluated in HL-60 and HL-60 VCR cells by immunoblotting. Results appear on Figure 6. The topoisomerase I protein was overexpressed in HL-60 VCR cells. Inductions of apoptosis by topoisomerase inhibitors decrease this protein level in HL-60 cells after 6h treatment with CPT and as soon as 3h with SN-38. HL-60 VCR topo I protein level was strongly decreased only after 6h treatment with SN-38.

4.4. Expression of BCL-2 Protein in HL-60 and HL-60/VCR Cells

In order to investigate the role of bcl-2 protein in the development of the apoptosis resistance observed in MDR HL60-VCR cells, its expression level was examined by im-

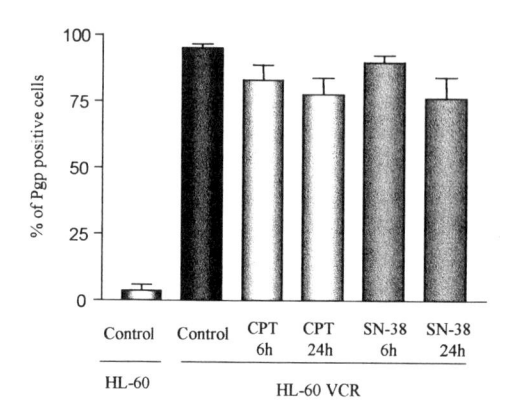

Figure 4. Flow cytometry detection of Pgp in HL-60 and HL-60 VCR cells. Expression of Pgp was analysed by flow cytometry using monoclonal antibody against Pgp in drug-sensitive HL60 and multidrug-resistant HL60-VCR cells. Cells were treated for 6 to 24 h with CPT (1 μM), or SN-38 (1 μM).

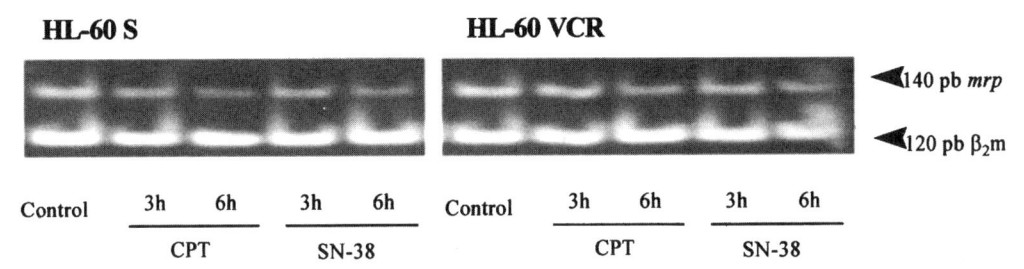

Figure 5. MRP mRNA expression in HL-60 and HL-60 VCR cells. RT-PCR analysis using specific primers of MRP was performed on 1µg mRNA of drug-sensitive HL60 and multidrug-resistant HL60-VCR cells. Cells were treated for 3 to 6 h with CPT (1 µM), or SN-38 (1 µM).

munoblotting with anti-BCL-2 mouse MAb. As shown in Figure 7, BCL-2 is up-regulated in HL60/VCR cells as compared to HL60 control cells. This BCL-2 protein expression was not modified by inductions of apoptosis with CPT and SN38, either after 3 or 6 hours of treatment.

5. DISCUSSION

The failure of current approaches to the management of malignant cells calls for the development of novel therapeutic strategies. These may include Pgp unrelated drugs as topoisomerase I inhibitors CPT and derivatives. In this regard, the present study reports that CPT and SN38 are two drugs that are potent apoptosis inducers in drug sensitive HL-60 leukemic cells. On the contrary, apoptosis is induced only partially in MDR HL-60 selected with vincristine. Moreover, our results show that this relative insensivity of HL-60 VCR to these two Topo I inhibitors does not seem to be associated, neither with P-gp overexpression as verapamil was unable to modulate this phenomenon, nor with MRP expression. It has been suggested that mechanisms that underlie apoptosis could be modified in drug resistant HL60 cells.[8,9] However, these observations seem to be dependent on the cell lines and drugs used. For example, MCF7-Adr or HL-60-Taxol MDR cell lines appear resistant to chemotherapeutic drugs or Fas apoptotic stimuli[8,10] whereas CEM-VLB appear more sensitive to apoptosis induced by dexamethasone or acivicin.[11,12] However, CPT and SN-38, which appeared not transported by Pgp or MRP, can decrease their mRNA levels

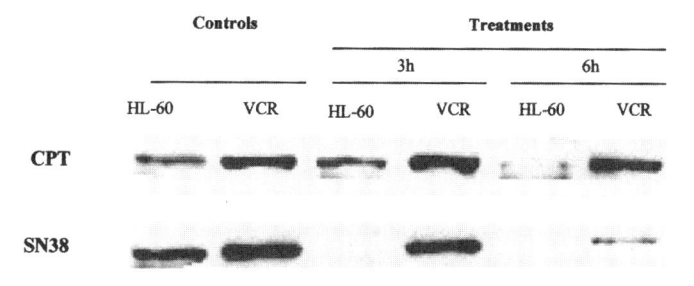

Figure 6. Expression of Topo I protein in HL-60 and HL-60 VCR cells. Topo I protein expression was quantified by immunoblotting on nuclear extract from drug-sensitive (S) and drug-resistant (VCR) HL60 cells treated or not with CPT (1 µM), or SN-38 (1 µM) for 3 to 6 h.

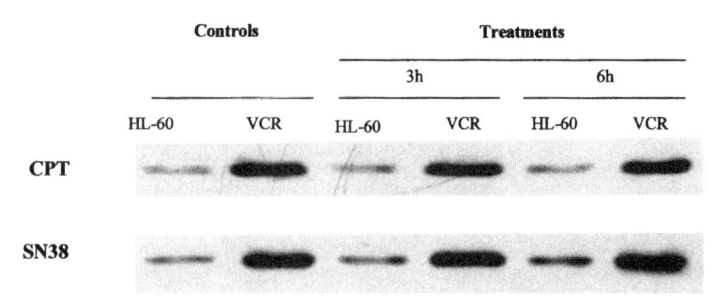

Figure 7. Expression of BCL-2 protein in HL-60 and HL-60 VCR cells. BCL-2 protein expression was quantified by immunoblotting on cellular extract from drug-sensitive (S) and drug-resistant (VCR) HL-60 cells treated or not with CPT (1 µM), or SN-38 (1 µM) for 3 to 6 h.

as commonly observed with transcription inhibitors, suggesting a possible modulation of resistance mechanisms. Another mechanism of resistance could reside in an increase of chemotherapeutic drug target.[1] HL-60 VCR cells appear to overexpress Topo I proteins. However, treatments of these cells by CPT or SN-38 result in decreases of Topo I without any increase in apoptotic cell numbers. Therefore, this modulation in drug target expression could be implicated only partially in the regulatory mechanism of apoptosis in HL-60 VCR cells. Another source of resistance to apoptosis in HL-60 VCR cells could be related to the BCL-2 protein overexpression observed in MDR cells as compared to their sensitive counterparts. As suggested, BCL-2 protein could mediate protection from apoptosis by antagonization of the mitochondrial dysfonction preceding nuclear apoptosis induced by chemotherapeutic agents.[13] However, variations of BCL2 expression differ strongly among the different cell lines tested so far and is either increased (our data), or unchanged,[8,9] or even decreased.[10] These discrepancies could be attributed either to the techniques used to assess BCL-2 expression,[8] or to the drug used to select MDR cells. In this work, we show that overexpression of BCL-2 protein could not be modulated with Topo I inhibitors and could therefore explain the partial resistance observed.

In conclusion, drug resistance in tumor cells appears as a highly multifactorial phenomenon. Therefore, the identification and characterization of apoptosis regulation in the resistant cells might be potentially useful for developing new therapeutic strategies cancers resistant to chemotherapeutic treatments.

ACKNOWLEDGMENTS

We thank I. Bronstein (YORK) for mouse polyclonal Topo I antibody. G. Laurent (Toulouse) for HL-60 VCR cells, A. Kolkes, and F. Belloc for expert advices. This work was supported by a grant from the Comité Départemental des Ardennes de la Ligue Contre le Cancer. V. Palissot was supported by grant from the Association de recherche sur le Cancer (ARC).

REFERENCES

1. Lehnert M. Clinical multidrug resistance in cancer: a multifactorial problem. Eur. J. Cancer, 1996, 321, 912–920.

2. Chen AY, Chiang Y, Milan P, Monroe EW, Mansukh CW, Leroy FL. Camptothecin overcomes MDR1- mediated resistance in human KB carcinoma cells. Cancer Res, 1991, 51, 6039–6044.
3. Bailly J.D., Muller C., Jaffrezou J.P., Demur C., Cassar G., Bordier C., Laurent G. Lack of correlation between expression and function of P-glycoprotein in acute myeloid leukemia cell lines. Leukemia, 1995, 9, 799–807.
4. Darzynkiewicz Z, Bruno S, Del Bino G, Gorczyca W, Hotz MA, Lassota P, Traganos F. Features of apoptotic cells measured by flow cytometry. Cytometry, 1992, 13, 795–808.
5. Chevillard S, Pouillart P, Beldjord C, Asselin B, Beuzeboc P, Magdelénat H, Vielh P. Sequential assessment of multidrug phenotype and measurement of S-phase fraction as predictive markers of breast cancer response to neoadjuvant chemotherapy. Cancer, 1996, 77, 292–300.
6. Bordow SB, Haber M, Madafiglio J, Cheung B, Marshall GM, Norris MD. Expression of the multidrug resistance- associated protein (MRP) gene correlates with amplification and overexpression of the N-myc oncogene in chilhood neuroblastoma. Cancer Res., 1994, 54, 5036–5040.
7. Morceau F, Aries A, Lalhil R, Devy L, Jardillier JC, Jeannesson P, Trentesaux C. Evidence for distinct regulation processes in the aclacinomycin and doxorubicin mediated differentiation of human erythroleukemic cells. Biochem. Pharmacol., 1996, 51, 839–845.
8. Kim C.H., Gollapudi S., Lee T., Gupta S. Altered expression of the genes regulating apoptosis in multidrug resistant human myeloid leukemia cell lines overexpressing MDR1 or MRP gene. Int. J. Oncol., 1997, 11, 945–950
9. Blagosklonny M.V., Alvarez M., Fojo A., Neckers L.M. BCL-2 protein downregulation is not required for differentiation of multidrug resistant HL-60 leukemia cells. Leuk. Res., 1996, 20, 101–107.
10. Ogretmen B., Safa A.R. Down regulation of apoptosis related bcl-2 but not bcl-x_L or bax proteins in multidrug resistant MCF-7/ Adr human breast cancer cells. Int. J. Cancer,1996, 67, 608–614.
11. Graber R., Losa A. Changes in the activities of the signal transduction and transport membrane enzymes in CEM lymphoblastoid cells by glucocorticoid-induced apoptosis. Anal.Cell.Pathol., 1995, 8, 159–176.
12. Graber R, Losa A. Apoptosis in human lymphoblastoid cells induced by Acivicin, a specific γ-glutamyl-transferase inhibitor. Int. J. Cancer, 1995, 62, 443–448.
13. Decaudin D., Geley S., Hirsh T., Castedo M., Marchetti P., Macho A., Kofler R., Kroemer G. Bcl-2 and Bcl-Xl antagonize the mitochondrial dysfunction preceding nuclear apoptosis induced by chemotherapeutic agents. Cancer Res., 1997, 57, 62–67.

39

TWO DISTINCT MODES OF ONCOPROTEIN EXPRESSION DURING APOPTOSIS RESISTANCE IN VINCRISTINE AND DAUNORUBICIN MULTIDRUG-RESISTANT HL60 CELLS

Rajae Belhoussine, Hamid Morjani, Reynald Gillet, Valérie Palissot, and Michel Manfait

Université de Reims
IFR 53, UPRES EA2063, UFR de Pharmacie
51 rue Cognacq Jay
51096 Reims cedex, France

Keywords: daunorubicin, apoptosis, cytosolic pH, mitochondrial potential, oncoproteins, resistance.

1. ABSTRACT

Apoptosis is a genetically regulated cell death process which results in a variety of morphological changes like chromatin condensation and DNA fragmentation. The decision between survival or death in response to an apoptotic stimulus is determined and regulated in part by oncoproteins which include proteins of the Bcl-2 family (bcl-2, bax, bcl-x_L) and bcr-abl. We investigated the effect of these proteins on the induction of this phenomenon in human promyelocytic leukemic HL60 cells and two multidrug resistant homologues selected respectively with vincristine (HL60/VCR) and daunorubicin (HL60R/DNR). We show that sensitive cells at 1 µm and HL60/VCR cells at DNR IC_{50} were able to undergo apoptosis while HL60R/DNR did not even at much higher concentration of DNR. However, treatment with synthetic C_2-ceramide did not sensitize HL60/DNR cells to apoptosis. Cell death through apoptosis or necrosis was accompanied by acidification of the cytosol without mitochondrial membrane depolarization. Western blotting analysis shows that bax is expressed at slightly elevated level in HL60S/VCR in comparison with the other cells lines. Bcl-2 is overexpressed in HL60/VCR but not in

HL60R/DNR. However, this cell line displayed a higher expression of bcl-x$_L$. Interestingly, bcr-abl, a dysregulated tyrosine kinase was detected only in HL60R/DNR cells. DNR at the IC$_{50}$, has no effect on expression of the oncoproteins. These data suggest that in addition of the multidrug resistance phenotype, bcr-abl translocation and bcl-x$_L$ overexpression could also account for the development of resistance to cell death induced by anthracyclines in leukemic cells

2. INTRODUCTION

Apoptosis represents a major regulatory mechanism in development growth and differentiation (1). This process in conceptualised as an inducible pre-programmed pathway of sequential biochemical events that are only partially known, leading to cell shrinkage, loss of cell-cell contact, chromatin condensation and finally activated of calcium-dependant endonucleases that cleave DNA at selective inter-nucleosomal linker sites (2).

Several drugs used in cancer therapy have been shown to affect divers intracellular targets in conferring a lethal effect through apoptosis in cancer cells (3). The anthracycline daunorubicin is widely used in the treatment of many neoplastic diseases, especially acute myeloid leukaemia (AML). Its cytotoxic effect is the result of free radicals and oxy-radicals stemming from quinone-generated redox activity (4), intercalation between DNA bases leading to distortion of double helix and/or stabilisation of complex formed between DNA and topoisomerase II (5). More recently, Fisher and co-workers have shown that anticancer treatment may kill through apoptosis by activating a metabolic pathway (3). Other authors have shown that daunorubicin induces activation of a neutral sphingomyelinase that hydrolyses sphingomyelin to produce ceramide (6). This latter can modulate a number of biological mechanisms such activation of a serine threonine proteine kinase, ceramide activated protein kinase (CAPK) (7), activation of phosphatase (8) and apoptosis (9). The cell death pathway induced by ceramide may be regulated by different factors including proteins of the Bcl-2 family. Some of these proteins have anti-apoptotic properties like bcl-2, bcl-x$_L$, mcl-1(10). Other proteins such as bax, bcl-x$_S$ and bad, behave as pro-apoptotic proteins (11). These proteins have the capacity to form homodimers or heterodimers with some of their homologues (12). The relative ratios of pro- and anti-apoptotique family proteins determine the ultimate sensitivity or resistance of cells to a variety of apoptotic signals.

Several theories could explain the anti-apoptotic effect of oncoproteins including protection of cells from reactive oxygen species (ROS). This protection is accompanied by hyper-polarisation of the resting cell membrane potential which implicate high level Na+/k+ ATPase pump activity (13,14), protein transport, cystein protease activation and mitochondrial permeability transition (15). More recently, Minn et coll. have shown that three dimensional structure of bcl-x$_L$ was similar to the structure of the pore forming domains of bacterial toxins. This results suggests that bcl-x$_L$ form an ion-conducting channel and maintain cell survival by regulating the permeability of intracellular membranes (16). In others works, it has been shown that genetic rearrangement in the mdr-1 expressing cells lead to a reciprocal translocation between the long arms of chromosome 9 and 22. In at least 95% of chronic myeloid leukemia cases, this fusion result in hybrid gene whose bcr-abl protein product have elevated abl tyrosine kinase activity and induces high resistance to apoptosis (17).

In this study, we investigated the effect of bcl-2, bax, bcl-x$_L$ and bcr-abl on the regulation of apoptotic process induced by daunorubicin in sensitive HL60 cells and two multidrug resistant homologues selected respectively with vincristine (HL60R/VCR) and daunorubicin (HL60R/DNR). We show that daunorubicin resistant cell line, which expresses high level of P-glycoprotein, exhibits an apoptosis-resistance phenotype which is accompanied by the bcr-abl translocation and bcl-x$_L$ overexpression. Selection of resistant cells with vincristine leads to the overexpression of bcl-2 protein. Bcl-2 overexpression did not protect cells from apoptotic effect of daunorubicin. We conclude that bcl-2 and bcl-x$_L$ provide differential protection from apoptosis induced by anticancer drugs and that bcl-x$_L$ in addition to bcr-abl translocation provide better protection than bcl-2.

3. MATERIALS AND METHODS

3.1. Chemicals

Daunorubicin (DNR) and Carbonyl-cyanide m-chlorophenylhydrazone (CCCP) were obtained from Sigma (St-Louis, MO). Carboxy-SNARF-1-AM (acetoxymethyl ester form) and JC-1 were provided by molecular probes (Eugene, OR). Bcl-x$_L$ was provided from Interchim (Mont luçon, France). Bcl-2 monoclonal antibody was from Sigma, bax and bcr-abl polyclonal antibodies were provided from Santa Cruz Biotechnology (Santa Cruz, CA). MRK16 monoclonal antibody was purchased from Valbiotech (Paris, France). Fas monoclonal antibody was provided by Immunotech (Marseille, France)

3.2. Cell Culture

The human promyelocytic leukemia cell lines HL60 (18) were cultured in RPMI 1640 medium with 2 mM ultraglutamin supplemented with 10% heat-inactivated fetal calf serum and antibiotics. Cells were maintained at 37°C in a humidified atmosphere containing 5% CO2. Resistant HL60 cells were maintained in the presence of 1 µM vincristine for HL60R/VCR and 200 nM daunorubicin for HL60R/DNR. HL60S/DNR and HL60R/DNR were provided by Dr F.Belloc (University of Bordeaux, France).

3.3. Cytotoxic Effect of Daunorubicin, MTT Assay

HL60 cells were maintained at 37°C in absence of DNR in a 96 multi-well dish (10^4 cells/well). After one day, DNR at concentrations ranging from 0.05 µM to 5 µM was added to sensitive HL60 cells (HL60KS/VCR and HL60S/DNR), and from 1 µM to 40 µM for both VCR and DNR resistant cells (HL60R/VCR and (HL60R/DNR). After a period of 1hr, cells were washed and incubated for 2 days in fresh medium before MTT assay measurements. Cell viability was afterwards determined by addition of 20 µl of 2.5 mg/ml MTT for 3 hours at 37°C. Then, the medium was discarded and 200 µl of DMSO were added to each well. Optical densities were measured at 540 nm using a "Series 750 microplates reader" (Cambridge Technology, Watertown, MA). Cell growth values were calculated by rationing optical densities of treated and control cells (19).

3.4. Flow Cytometry Analysis of Fas and P-gp Expression

For flow cytometric determination of cell-surface P-glycoprotein and fas, all sensitive and resistant HL 60 cells were washed and incubated for 30 min at 4°C in presence of 10 µg/ml of both Mabs MRK16 and fas. Mab MRK16 recognizes an external epitope of

Pgp. After washing with ice cold phosphate buffer solution (PBS) containing 1% BSA (Sigma), cells were incubated for 30 min at 4°C with F(ab') fragment of goat anti-mouse IgG fluorescein-conjugate (Sigma) used at working dilution of 1:50 and washed. fas antibody is coupled to FITC. Cells were immediately analyzed with a FACScan flow cytometer (Becton-Dickinson, Mountain View, CA, USA). The excitation was an argon ion laser emitting at 488 nm. Fluorescence emission was collected after passage through a 530 nm band pass filter. Data were collected and analyzed on a Hewlett-Packard model 310 computer interfaced with the FACScan. The green fluorescence, related to P-glycoprotein and fas expression, was measured on a logarithmic scale.

3.5. Confocal Laser Scanning Microspectrofluorometry for Measurements of Nuclear DNR Concentration, Cytosolic pH, and Polarization of Mitochondrial Membrane

This technique was applied to the acquisition and analysis of X-Y emission spectra from a confocal section within a single living cancer cells treated with fluorescent probes. The new microspectrofluorometer M51 (Dilor, Lille, France) is coupled with an ionised argon laser 2065 (Spectra Physics, les ULIS, France). For our measurements, 2 µW laser beam emitting at 457.9 nm (daunorubicin), 488 nm (JC-1) and 514 nm (Carboxy-SNARF-1-AM) was used. The optical microscope (Olympus BH-2, Tokyo, Japan) is equipped with 100X phase contrast water-immersion objective (Olympus). Collection of the fluorescence emission in the 500–700 nm range for all probes were obtained through the same optics. The thickness of the optical section was controlled by opening a square pinhole from 50 to 1200 µm. For intracellular measurements, the pinhole size was fixed to a diameter of 200 µm. The fluorescence emission was spectrally dispersed by diffraction grating (300 grooves mm^{-1}) and was analyzed with an air-peltier-cooled CCD detector (Wright, Stonehouse, UK) supplied by an 1125 X 298 pixel sensor element. Spectral scan images were obtained by a line illumination system which employs a two-dimensional detector and a system of two synchronized scanning mirrors that provides the spectra accumulation of hundreds of point on the sample simultaneously on real confocal mode for each point. The laser beam being moved by the first scanning mirror along the X axis in the plane of the cell. The emitted light from the line is time-encoded on the first scanning mirror and transmitted to the pinhole diaphragm for confocal filtration. After passing through the diaphragm, the signal is decoded by the second scanning mirror vibrating in phase with first one. The motorized stage displaced the sample in the Y-axis after each line illumination with a minimum step size of 0.1 µm. Then, (50x50) spectra were recorded at different locations of the cell and a whole spectral images is generated by the line by line scanning system (20, 21).

3.5.1. Determination of Nuclear Concentration of Daunorubicin. The fluorescence emission spectrum originating from nuclei of HL60 cells treated with DNR F(λ), can be expressed as a sum of the spectral contributions of free DNR, DNA-bound DNR and signal of nuclear autofluorescence (22)

$$F(\lambda) = C_f.F_f(\lambda) + C_b.F_b(\lambda) + C_n.F_n(\lambda)$$

where F_f and F_b are the fluorescence spectra of free and bound drug referred to a unitary concentration. Taking this concentration into account, C_f and C_b represent intranuclear concentrations of free and bound drug, respectively; C_n is the contribution of auto-fluorescence responsible for the intrinsic nuclear spectrum F_n. In aqueous solution, each of these contributions has a characteristic spectral shape. The fluorescence yield in the free form was 40 times higher than that of the bound-DNA form. These spectral contributions lead to the concentrations of free and DNA-bound DNR. The sum of the values obtained gives the total nuclear concentration of DNR (22–25).

3.5.2. Measurement of Cytosolic pH in HL60 Cells. We have measured pH of the cytosol after drug treatment. Treatment with DNR was followed by 45 min incubation with 4µM of Carboxy-SNARF-1-AM at 37°C. All areas of the cytoplasm demonstrated an isotropic distribution of the probe. Emission intensity ratios I_{580nm}/I_{640nm} of cytosolic spectra were determined in 30 cells. To obtain quantitative relationship between emission ratios and pH, Carboxy-SNARF1-AM stained cell line was exposed to buffer at known pH containing 20µM of nigericin, 150 mM KCl and 50 mM sodium phosphate. Treatment with nigericin equilibrates all internal compartments of the cell to the pH of incubating buffer. The I_{580nm}/I_{640nm} were determined and appear to be sensitive between pH 6 and pH 9. The pH curve appears similar to that obtained by the following equation:

$$pH = pKa + \log10 ((Ra - Ri)/(Ri - Rb)) \times (Fa(\lambda 2)/Fb(\lambda 2))$$

$$Ri = I_{580nm}/I_{640nm},$$

$\lambda 1$: 580nm, $\lambda 2$: 640nm, Ra and Rb were respectively ratios in acidic and basic buffer.

$$Fa(\lambda 2)/Fb(\lambda 2)$$

is the normalization factor.

3.5.3. Measurement of Mitochondrial Membrane Depolarisation. Analysis of mitochondrial membrane potential was developed using the lipophilic cationic probes JC-1 and spectral imaging analysis. The green fluorescence JC-1 monomer (emits at 530 nm after excitation at 488nm) excites at low concentration or at low membrane potential. Depending on the potential membrane, JC-1 is able to form so-called red fluorescent J-aggregates (excitation, 488nm; emission 590nm) at higher concentration or higher potentials. Thus, the color of the dye changes reversibly from green to greenish orange as the mitochondrial membrane become more polarized. Therefore, the I_{590nm}/I_{530nm} emission ratio value allows the observation of mitochondrial dysfunction. Cells treated with CCCP at 50 µM for 10 min to disrupt the membrane potential were used as positive control. Residual potential as % of control was expressed as following:

$$(R \text{ treated} / R \text{ control}) \times 100, R : I_{590nm}/I_{530nm}.$$

3.6. Agarose Gel Electrophoresis for DNA Fragmentation

Oligonucleosomal fragmentation of genomic DNA was determined as follows. DNR-treated and untreated Cells (1×10^6) were lysed in 200 µl of lysis buffer (150 mM NaCl, 10mM Tris-HCl, 10 mM EDTA [pH 8], 0.5% sodium dodecyl sulfate and 0.5 mg/ml proteinase K (Boehringer, Mannhein, Allmagne) and incubated at 50°C for at least 10 hours. DNA was extracted with 60 µl of 3M sodium acetate and 400 µl of cold ethanol

(99.5%) mixed and kept on ice at least for 30 min for ethanol precipitation. DNA pellets were centrifuged at 14.500 r.p.m for 15 min at 4°C and discarded. Pellets were washed twice in cold 70% ethanol and centrifuged at 14.500 r.p.m at 5 min. DNA pellets were dissolved in 25 µl of TE buffer (Tris-EDTA), RNase was added and then incubated at 37°C for 1 hour. DNA from each sample was electrophoresed at 60 V for 1hr through a 2% agarose gel in TBE buffer. DNA bands were visualized under UV light after staining with ethidium bromide. A was used as molecular size marker.

3.7. Western Blot

Aliquot of 5×10^6 cells were washed once with phosphate-buffered saline (PBS), pelleted and extracted in lysis buffer which contain 0.125 M Tris-HCl [pH 6,8], 10% glycerol, 2% SDS, 100 mM dithiotreitol, proteinase inhibitors, including 10µg/ml leupeptin, 2µg/ml aprotinin, 2 µg/ml pepstatin A and 0.5 mM phenylmethylsulphonylfluoride (PMSF) by quick freezing at -80°C and thawing at 37°C. Cells extracts were then centrifuged at 10 000g for 10 min at 4°C. The supernatant was recovered and its protein concentration was then determined by Bradford assay using Bio-Rad protein assay kit (Richmond, CA). For western blot, 20–30 µg total cell proteins were separated on 12% SDS-polyacrylamide gradient gels and then transferred for 2 hrs at 60 V, 4°C onto a nitrocellulose membrane (Amersham, Arlington Heights, IL) in transfer buffer (3g/l Tris-base, 14,4 g/l glycin, 20% methanol). Membranes were blocked in TBS-Tween 0.1% containing 10% dry milk at room temperature for 1h and then used for western bolt analysis. Primary antibodies used for immunodetection are: an anti-bcl-2 diluted at 1/500, anti-bax at 0.5 µg/ml, Bcl-x$_L$ at 1.2 µg/ml and anti-bcr-abl at 1 µg/ml, followed by 1 hr incubation with their specific anti-mouse (bcl-2) or anti-rabbit (anti-bax, anti-bcl-x$_L$, and bcr-abl) peroxidase conjugated second antibodies. Proteins were visualized using the ECL chemoluminescent detection kit (Amersham).

4. RESULTS

4.1. Phenotypic Characterization

Mdr1 gene overexpression and P-gp overproduction was determined by using MRK16 antibody and flow cytometric analysis. Results show that both resistant cell lines were positive for MRK16 antibody (Figure 1). The fluorescence signals in resistant cell lines (solid line) are different from that of sensitive HL60 cells. This results are representative of high expression of P-gp in resistant cells. When compared with sensitive HL60 cell lines, HL60R/DNR and HL60R/VCR were characterized by several typical features of the MDR phenotype: cross-resistance pattern to different cytotoxic drugs (anthracycline and vinca-alcaloid). The results of MTT essay after 1hr incubation in the presence of daunorubicin at the IC$_{50}$, and daunorubicin nuclear accumulation at these concentrations are summarized in Table 1. Results show that both resistant cell lines displayed highest degree of resistance to daunorubicin in comparison with sensitive cells. The concentrations which induce 50% of growth inhibition (IC$_{50}$) were 30 µM for HL60R/DNR and 10 µM for HL60R/VCR, 0.06 µM and 0.2 µM in their sensitive corresponding cells. When exposed to their respective DNR IC$_{50}$, both resistant cells displayed increased accumulation of daunorubicin (507 µM for HL60R/VCR and 1053 µM for HL60R/DNR) than their corresponding sensitive cells (375 µM for HL60S/VCR and 916 µM for HL60S/DNR) demonstrating their intracellular tolerance to the drug.

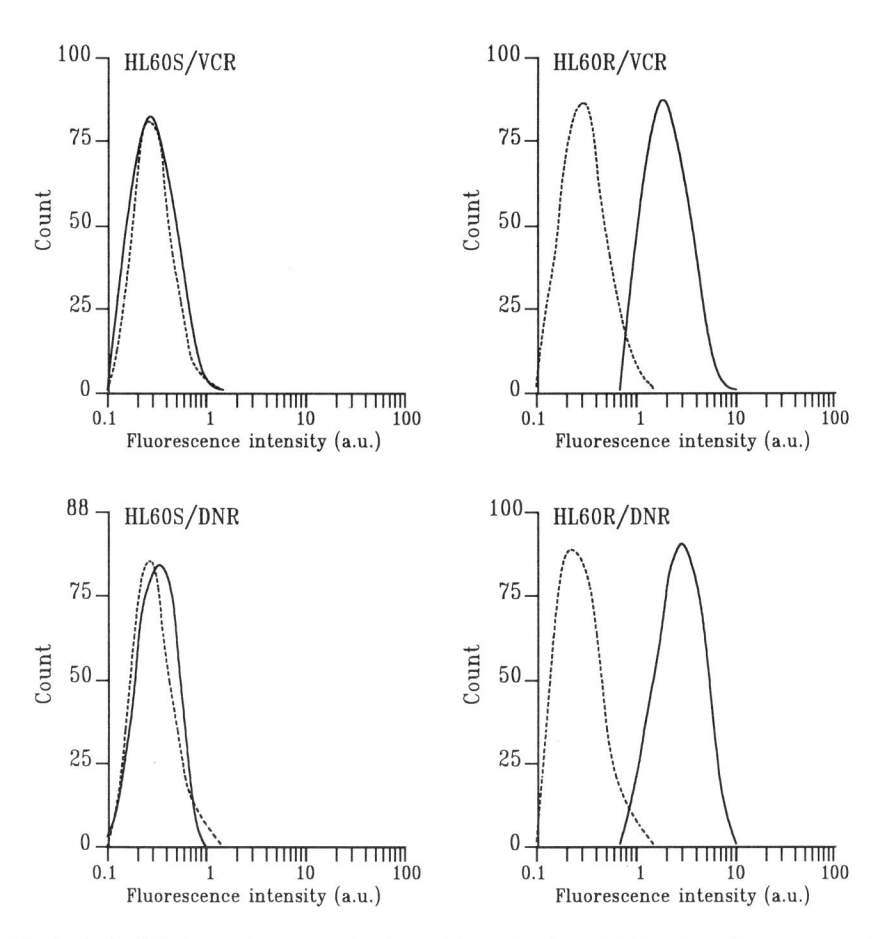

Figure 1. Analysis of P-glycoprotein expression in sensitive and resistant HL60 cells by flow cytometry (dashed line, isotype control; solid line, assay with MRK16 antibody recognized with a fragment of goat anti-mouse IgG fluorescein-conjugate). In the two sensitive cells, the two histograms overlap, indicating a lack of P-gp. In HL60/VCR and HL60/DNR cells, the histogram patterns of the assay using MRK16 and the isotype control are representative of cells with high expression of P-gp.

Table 1. Cytotoxic effect of DNR and its nuclear accumulation in HL60 cell at the IC$_{50}$.

	HL60S	HL60/VCR	HL60SP3	HL60/DNR
DNR IC$_{50\,(mM)}$	0.2	10	0.06	30
DNR nuclear accumulation $_{(mM)}$	375	507	916	1053

Cells were incubated for 1hr with DNR, washed with fresh medium free of drug and incubated for 2 days at 37°C before MTT test. Results are mean of three independent experiments. Each one performed in octaplates. Nuclear accumulation of DNR was evaluated by microspectrofluorometry. Results are means of 3 independent experiments, each one performed on 20–30 cell nuclei.

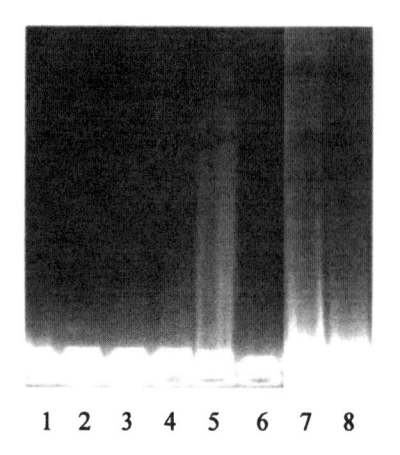

Figure 2. Internucleosomal DNA fragmentation induced by DNR in sensitive and resistant HL60 cells. DNA that was extracted from cells incubated for 1 hr with different concentrations of DNR, followed by 6hr incubation at 37°C, was fractionated on 2% agarose gels as described in "material and methods". DNR induced DNA fragmentation in sensitive and HL60/VCR cells (lane 5, 7, 8) whereas, no fragmentation of DNA was observed in HL60/DNR (lane 6).

4.2. Daunorubicin Induced DNA Fragmentation in Sensitive and HL60R/VCR But Not in HL60/DNR

In order to assess the nature of cell death induced by DNR. Sensitive cells treated for 1h with 1 μM of DNR, HL60R/VCR and HL60R/DNR treated with IC_{50} of DNR, washed and incubated for 6hrs at 37°C were examined by submitting the DNA to agarose gel electrophoresis. Figure 2 shows that treatment of sensitive and VCR resistant HL60 cells with appropriate concentration of DNR resulted in apoptotic DNA degradation detected by the typical DNA ladder consisting of 180pb fragment by agarose gel electrophoresis. In contrast, HL60R/DNR cells do not commit apoptosis even at much higher concentration. Thus, it appears that DNR has two different transduction signals to lead to cell death in HL60R/VCR and HL60R/DNR.

4.3. Fas-Antigen Expression

Recently, fas antigen has been recognized to mediate apoptosis (26). Since it was found that resistance to apoptosis was correlated with a loss of surface fas-protein expression (27). The role of fas-antigen in the regulation of this process was examined in sensitive and resistant HL60 cells. Flow-cytometry analysis (Figure 3) shows that all HL60 cells were positive for fas antibody and that the two sensitive HL60 cell lines (3.85 and 2.75) have slightly elevated level of this antigen in comparison with their resistant counterparts (3.5 and 2.35).

4.4. Expression of Oncoproteins Regulating Apoptotic Cell Death

We measured the protein expression of some oncogenes implicated in the regulation of apoptosis. Western blot analysis of the expression of bcl-2 and related proteins is shown in Figure 4. We show that HL60R/DNR display significant overexpression of bcl-x_L whereas, no expression was detectable in sensitive and HL60R/VCR cells. The bcl-2 protein is overexpressed in HL60R/VCR in comparison with HL60S/CVR cells. However, the expression of this protein is reduced in HL60R/DNR compared with HL60S/DNR. Since the function of bcl-2 and bcl-x_L involves heterodimerization with homologous proteins such as bax (12), we examined the level of its expression. We found that bax protein is expressed at slightly elevated level in HL60S/VCR in comparison with the other cell lines.

To explain the resistance to apoptosis observed in HL60R/DNR, we used western blot (Figure 4) to detect the expression of bcr-abl protein. Results allowed to detect a band

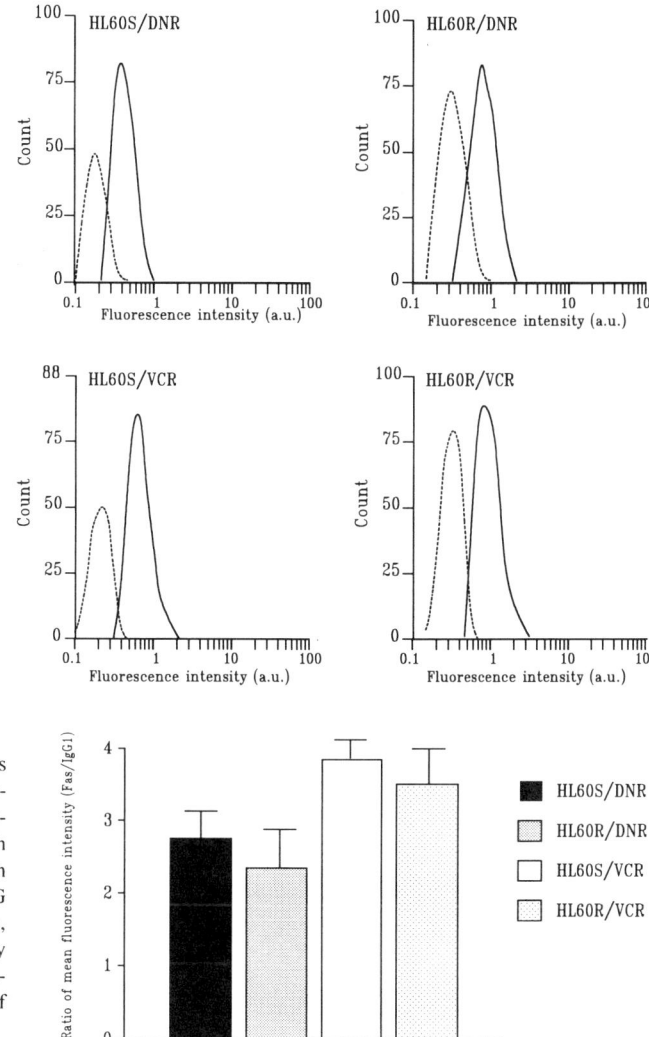

Figure 3. Flow cytometric analysis of fas expression in sensitive and resistant HL60 cells: (dashed line, isotype control; solid line, assay with anti-fas antibody recognized with fragment of goat anti-mouse IgG fluorescein-conjugate). In all cases, the histogram patterns of the assay using anti-fas antibody and the isotype control are representative of cells with overexpression of fas.

of the expected size 210 kD for the bcr-abl protein in only HL60R/DNR cells, whereas sensitive and HL60/VCR cells were negatives.

4.5. Effect of DNR on the Expression of Oncoproteins

To confirm the role of oncoproteins in modulating chemoresistance, we measured their expression by western blot after 1hr incubation with IC_{50} of DNR, followed by 6hrs at 37°C in medium free of drug. Result is shown in Figure 5. By the technique used, It appears that DNR has no effect on the expression of oncoproteins after 6hrs.

4.6. Effect of Exogenous Ceramide on the Induction of DNA Fragmentation

The HL60R/DNR cell line has shown high resistance to apoptosis in comparison with HL60R/VCR and sensitive HL60 cells. To determine whether an exogenous ceramide

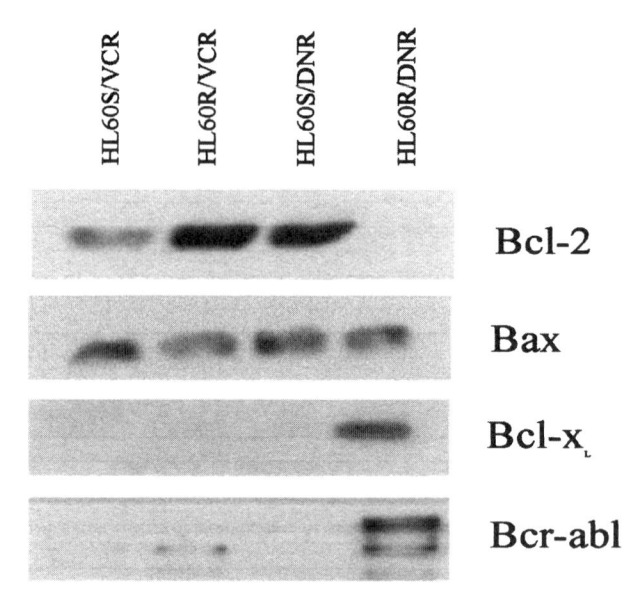

Figure 4. Western blot analysis of bcl-2, bax and bcl-x_L as well as bcr-abl in sensitive and resistant HL60 cells. A total of 50 μg (bax, bcl-xL, bcr-abl) and 20 μg (bcl-2) of soluble protein per track were loaded. Proteins were identified by specific rabbit or mouse peroxidase conjugated second antibody (see material and methods).

could sensitize these cells to apoptosis, we treated the cells with 50 μM of synthetic cell-permeant C2-ceramide for 6 hrs. As shown in Figure 6, synthetic ceramide caused significant DNA fragmentation in sensitive and HL60R/VCR but no fragmentation was observed in HL60R/DNR. Thus bcl-x_L and bcr-abl translocation appear to block exogenous ceramide -induced cytotoxicity.

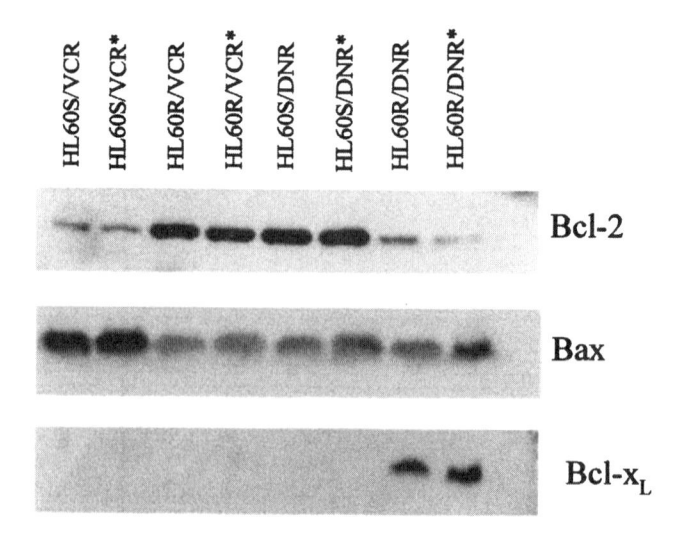

Figure 5. Effect of daunorubicin on the oncoprotein expression. Cells were incubated with appropriate inhibitory concentration of daunorubicin washed and incubated for 6 hrs at 37°C in medium free of drug before western blot analysis (*: treatment with DNR).

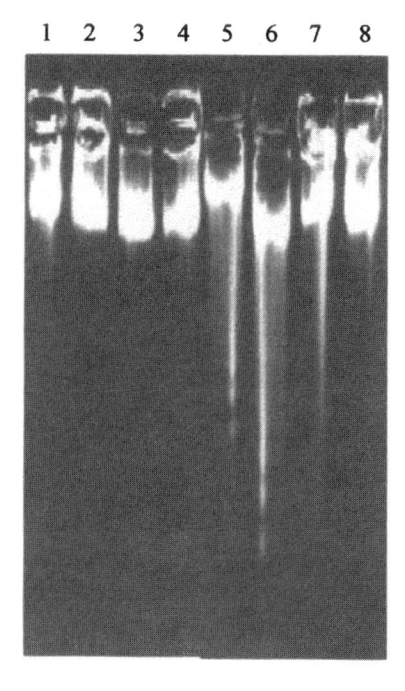

1: HL60S/VCR control
2: HL60R/VCR control
3: HL60S/DNR control
4: HL60R/DNR control
5: 1 + C2-ceramide
6: 2 + C2-ceramide
7: 3 + C2 ceramide
8: 4 +C2 ceramide

Figure 6. Autoradiograph of a gel containing DNA samples from control and synthetic C2-ceramide treated cells. Exogenous C2-ceramide induces apoptosis in sensitive HL60 cells and HL60R/VCR, whereas no fragmentation was observed in HL60R/DNR.

4.7. Effect of DNR Treatment on Cytosolic pH

Since acidification is essential to the process of DNA degradation that takes place during apoptosis or cell necrosis, We have measured pH of the cytosol after drug treatment. Treatment with DNR was followed by 45 min incubation with 4μM of Carboxy-SNARF-1-AM at 37°C.

The results are summarized in Figure 7. Data show that DNR lead to an acidification of the cytosol at different times of incubation. The cytosolic pH in HL60S/VCR was lowered from 7.26 to about 7.02 after 1hr and 6.94 after 6hrs. In HL60S/DNR, it decreased from 7.32 to 7.21 after 1 hr and 6.94 after 6hrs. In HL60R/VCR resistant cells, pH decreased from 7.59 to about 6.97 after 1hr and 7.16 after 6hrs. HL60R/DNR cells do not undergo apoptosis even at much higher concentration. Necrosis of these cells was accompanied by a decease of pH from 7.57 to 7.10 after 1hr and 7.01 after 6hrs.

4.8. Mitochondrial Membrane Evolution during Apoptosis

Figure 8 represents mitochondrial potential of treated cells as compared with control. Only CCCP treatment induces depolarization of mitochondrial membrane. DNR lead to programmed cell death in HL60 cells without affecting mitochondrial permeability.

For control cells, all spectra from the cellular compartment displayed a majority yellow-orange band at 590nm which corresponds to polarisation of mitochondrial membrane. After treatment by CCCP during 10 min followed by 6 μM incubation for 45 min, all spec-

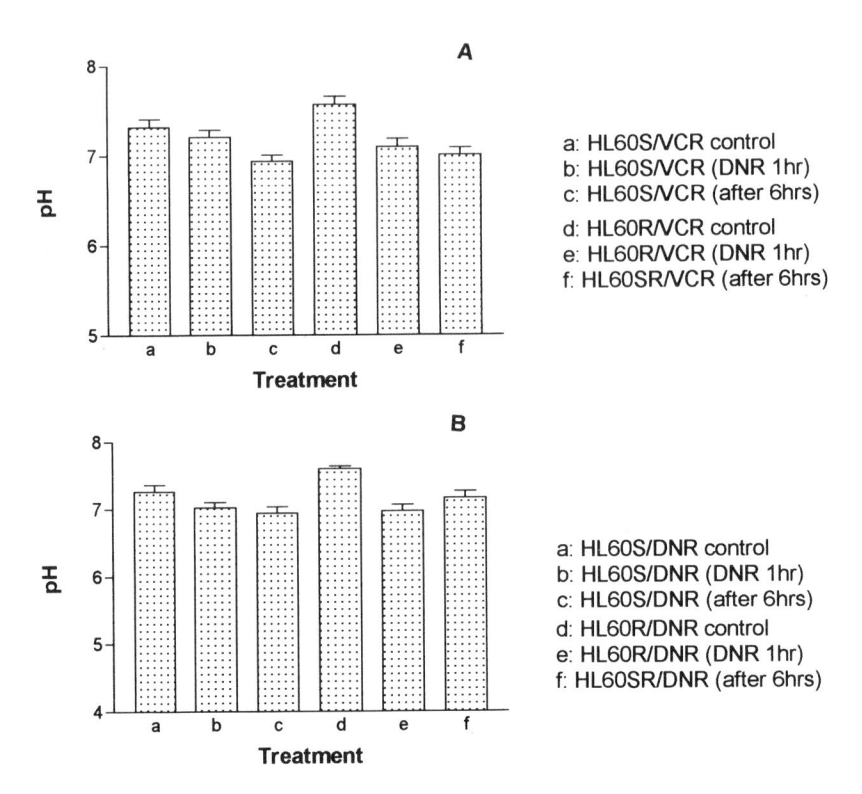

Figure 7. Effect of DNR on cytosolic pH. Cells were incubated with DNR IC$_{50}$ for 1 hr washed and incubated at 37°C for 6hrs. Carboxy-SNARF-1-AM was added 45 min before microspectrofluorometric measurements. We show that acidification of cytosolic pH is an early event in apoptosis induced by DNR.

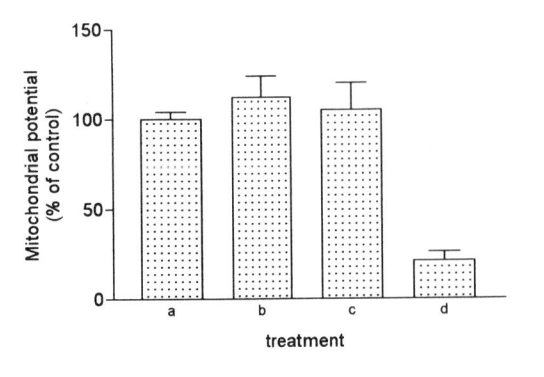

Figure 8. Mitochondrial potential (% of control) values of treated HL60cells as compared with control cells (100%). a: control, b: DNR for 1hr, c: DNR for 6 hrs and d: positive control (CCCP).

tra displayed a majority green band at 530nm which characterizes depolarized mitochondrial membrane (Data not shown).

5. DISCUSSION

5.1. Daunorubicin Induced Different Cell Death in Sensitive and Resistant HL60 Cells

When treated with daunorubicin at 1µM (sensitive cells) and IC$_{50}$ (resistant cells), sensitive HL60 cells and vincristine resistant ones were able to undergo apoptosis. However, HL60R/DNR resistant cell line was unable to do so, even at much higher concentrations. Allouche and co-workers have shown that daunorubicin induces apoptosis in sensitive HL60 cell lines by triggering a sphingomyelin hydrolysis after 10–15 min with a concomitant ceramide generation (28). When exposed to exogenous ceramide, sensitive HL60 cells and vincristine resistant ones undergo apoptosis with levels similar to that obtained with daunorubicin treatment, whereas, HL60R/DNR resist to apoptosis induced by ceramide. Selection of resistant HL60 cell lines in the presence of anthracyclines or vinca-alcaloides leads to the overexpression of two distinct oncoproteins. In HL60R/VCR, we show that the cells displayed high level of bcl-2 oncoprotein, whereas, in daunorubicin selected ones, high level of bcl-x$_L$ was observed. Overexpression of bcl-2 is known to block apoptosis induced by a variety of stimuli (29–32). Its overexpression in HL60R/VCR do not protect cells from apoptotic effect of DNR. HL60R/DNR were found to contain decreased level of this protein. In other works, it has been shown that bcl-x$_L$ oncoprotein is a stronger protector against apoptosis than bcl-2 (33, 34). Using site-specific mutagenesis, Cheng et al. have shown that the amino-acid residues critical for protection of cells by bcl-x$_L$ are clustered within the bcl-2 homology region 1 and 2 (BH1 and BH2 regions), and that the residues necessary for bcl-x$_L$ function are not identical to those required for bcl-2 function (35). We conclude that bcl-2 and bcl-x$_L$ provide differential protection from apoptosis induced by anthracyclines and that bcl-x$_L$ provides better protection from apoptosis than bcl-2 protein.

5.2. Overexpression of Bcl-x$_L$ Is Accompanied by Bcr-Abl Translocation

Drug resistance observed in cells from patients in the chronic phase of CML is associated with an increased survival stimulus afforded to the leukemic cells via the suppression of apoptosis (36, 37). The principal cytogenetic characteristic of CML is the formation of the Philadelphia chromosome bearing the chimeric bcr-abl gene, which encodes a constitutively activated abl protein tyrosine kinase (38). By using several techniques, we found that highly apoptosis-resistant HL60R/DNR cell line was accompanied by bcr-abl translocation. This is in agreement with previous results showing that bcr-abl confer an apoptosis-resistance phenotype (39) and that activation of this protein is accompanied with up regulation of bcl-x$_L$ (40). However the normal activity of abl tyrosine kinase was never reported to induce resistance to apoptosis. In this case, sensitive HL60 cells and HL60R/VCR ones did not show the bcr-abl translocation.

The fas cell-surface antigen has been described to mediate apoptosis after ligand binding or crosslinking with agonist antibodies (41). Mc Gahon and collaborators have reported that v-abl can inhibit fas-meditated apoptosis (42). We thus investigated the expression level and efficiency of fas as mediator of apoptosis. When compared with the two sensitive cell lines (HL60S/VCR and HL60S/DNR), fas antigen was found to be expressed approximately at the same level in their resistant cell lines (HL60R/VCR and HL60R/DNR). Indeed, sensitive HL60 cells which are a good responder to other stimuli (drugs, serum deprivation, ceramide) exhibited a low level of fas espression and reduced responce to fas antibodies (43). Therefore, expression of fas could not account in itself for apoptosis resistance or sensitivity in our models. We have analysed the expression of oncoproteins during treatment with DNR, we found that this drug did not induce variations in oncoproteins expression after 6hrs. It seems to act essentially on cytosolic acidification and ceramide production.

5.3. Acidification of Cytosolic pH Is Essential for Cell Death

Treatment of sensitive and resistant HL60 cells with daunorubicin lead to intracellular acidification after 1hr incubation. This phenomenon was accompanied by programmed cell death in sensitive and HL60R/VCR cells and necrosis of HL60R/DNR. Intracellular acidification was observed in the case of apoptosis induced by several agents like anti-fas, cycloheximide, ceramide and by short-wavelength UV light exposure (44). It has been suggested that apoptosis represents an aborted mitosis (45) and that alkalinisation is a necessary concomitant of mitosis (46). This lead to suggest that in an analogue manner, acidification may be essential for cell death through apoptosis or necrosis. In this case, Gottlieb and co-workers have shown that treatment with cell-permeable bases like chloroquine and imidazol decreased both characteristic nuclear changes and DNA fragmentation in cells undergoing apoptosis (44). Thus, cytosolic pH acidification is an essential and early event to the process of genome destruction. This feature is consistent with idea that the acidic endonucleases participate in DNA cleavage during apoptosis. In addition to acidic endonucleases, other proteins which operate at low pH may be activated and participate in apoptosis or necrosis. These include acidic sphingomyelinase which hydrolyses sphingomyelin (47) and cytoskeletal regulatory protein that is activated by H^+ and whose ability to depolymerize filamentous actinmay be essential for the cytoskeletal changes that occur in apoptotic cells (48).

5.4. Depolarization of Mitochondrial Membrane Is Not Required for Genome Destruction in HL60cells

One of the first common manifestation of the apoptotic process is a disruption of mitochondrial membrane function, including a dissipation of the $\Delta\Psi m$ and/or the mitochondrial release of protease activators. This mitochondrial alteration marks the point of no return of the apoptotic process. This phenomenon is due to the opening of the mitochondrial permeability transition pores. These pore are protein complexes formed at the contact sites between the mitochondrial inner and outer membranes, and whose opening/closing characteristics are influenced by multiple parameters (49). More recently, Kroemer and coworkers, Zamzami and coworkers have shown that transfection of cells with bcl-2 or bcl-x_L inhibits the early mitochondrial changes associated with apoptosis (50). In the case of the induction of apoptosis by anthracyclines, acidification of the cytosol appear essential for DNA fragmentation whereas, mitochondrial potential membrane decrease is not required for this phenomenon.

ACKNOWLEDGMENTS

We thanks G. Simon for his contribution to the flow cytometry analyses and F. Belloc for his kind gift of HL60S/DNR and HL60R/DNR cells.

REFERENCES

1. Raff MC. Social controls on cell survival and cell death. Nature 1992 356: 397–400.
2. Vaux DL. Toward an understanding of the molecular mechanisms of physiological cell death. Proc Natl Acad Sci USA 1993 90:786–789.
3. Fisher DE. Apoptosis in cancer therapy: crossing the threshold. Cell 1994 78: 539–542.
4. Sinha BK, Mimnaugh EG. Free radicals and anticancer drug resistance: oxygen free radicals in the mechanisms of drug cytotoxicity and resistance by certain tumors. Free Radic Biol Med 1990 8:567–581.
5. Cornarotti M, Tinelli S, Willmore E, Zunino F, Fisher LM, Austin CA, Capranico G. Drug sensitivity and sequence specificity of human recombinant DNA topoisomerases Iialpha (p170) and IIbeta (p180). Mol Pharmacol 1996 50: 1463–1471.
6. Jaffrézou JP, Levade T, Bettaieb A, Andrieu N, Bezombes C, Maestre N, Vermeersch S, Rousse A, Laurent G. Daunorubicin-induced apoptosis: triggering of ceramide generation through sphingomyelin hydrolysis. EMBO J 1996 15: 2417–2424.
7. Mathias S, Dressler KA, Kolesnick RN. Characterization of a ceramide-activated protein kinase: stimulation by tumor necrosis factor alpha. Proc Natl Acad Sci U S A 1991 88: 10009–10013.
8. Dobrowsky RT, Kamibayashi C, Mumby MC, Hannun YA. Ceramide activates heterotrimeric protein phosphatase 2A. J Biol Chem 1993 268: 15523–15530.
9. Obeid LM, Linardic CM, Karolak LA, Hannun YA. Programmed cell death induced by ceramide. Science 1993 259: 1769–1771.
10. Reed JC. Bcl-2 family proteins: regulators of chemoresistance in cancer. Toxicol Lett 1995 82:155–158.
11. Ottilie S, Diaz JL, Horne W, Chang J, Wang Y, Wilson G, Chang S, Weeks S, Fritz LC, Oltersdorf T. Dimerization properties of human BAD. Identification of a BH-3 domain and analysis of its binding to mutant BCL-2 and BCL-XL proteins. J Biol Chem 1997 272: 30866–30872
12. Oltvai ZN, Milliman CL, Korsmeyer SJ. Bcl-2 heterodimerizes in vivo with a conserved homolog, Bax, that accelerates programmed cell death. Cell 1993 74: 609–619.
13. Gilbert M, Knox S. Influence of Bcl-2 overexpression on Na+/K(+)-ATPase pump activity: correlation with radiation-induced programmed cell death. J Cell Physiol 1997 171 : 299–304.
14. Gilbert MS, Saad AH, Rupnow BA, Knox SJ. Association of BCL-2 with membrane hyperpolarization and radioresistance. J Cell Physiol 1996 168:114–122.
15. Zamzami N, Marchetti P, Castedo M, Hirsch T, Susin SA, Masse B, Kroemer G. Inhibitors of permeability transition interfere with the disruption of the mitochondrial transmembrane potential during apoptosis. FEBS Lett 1996 384 :53–57.
16. Minn AJ, Velez P, Schendel SL, Liang H, Muchmore SW, Fesik SW, Fill M, Thompson CB. Bcl-x(L) forms an ion channel in synthetic lipid membranes. Nature 1997 385: 353–357.
17. Chapman RS, Whetton AD, Chresta CM, Dive C. Characterization of drug resistance mediated via the suppression of apoptosis by Abelson protein tyrosine kinase. Mol Pharmacol 1995 48: 334–343.
18. Bailly JD, Muller C, Jaffrézou JP., Demur C, Cassar G, Bordier C, Laurent G, Lack of correlation between expression and function of P-glycoprotein in acute myeloid leukemia cell lines, Leukemia 1995 9: 799–807.
19. Sebille S, Morjani H, Poullain MG and Manfait M Effect of S9788, cyclosporin A and verapamil on intracellular distribution of THP-doxorubicin in multidrug-resistant K562 tumor cells, as studied by laser confocal microspectrofluorometry. Anticancer Res 1994 14:2389–2394.
20. Sharonov S, Chourpa I, Valisa P, Fleury F, Feofanov A, Manfait M. Confocal spectral imaging analysis. Eur. Microsc. Anal. 1994 32: 23–25.
21. Sharonov S, Chourpa I, Morjani H, Nabiev I, Feofanov A, Manfait M. Confocal spectral imaging analysis in studies of the spatial distribution of antitumour drugs within living cancer cells. Anal. Chim Acta. 290: 40–47, 1994.
22. Gigli M, Doglia S, Millot JM, Valentini L and Manfait M. Quantitative study of doxorubicin in living cell nuclei by microspectrofluorometry. Biochim Biophys Acta 1988 950:13–20.

23. Gigli M, Rasoanaivo T W D, Millot JM, Jeannesson P, Rizzo V, Jardillier JC., Arcamone F and Manfait M. Correlation between growth inhibition and intranuclear doxorubicin and 4'-iododoxorubicin quantitated in living K562 cells by microspectroflurometry. Cancer Res 1989 49:560–564.
24. Millot JM, Rasoanaivo TWD, Morjani H and Manfait M. Role of the aclacinomycin A - doxorubicin association in reversal of doxorubicin resistance in K562 tumour cells. Br J Cancer 1989 69: 678–684.
25. Millot J.M, Joly P, Benoist H, Manfait M, Doxorubicin nuclear distribution necessary to induce erythroid differentiation of K562 cells. J cell Pharmacol 1991 2 : 1–8.
26. Friesen C, Herr I, Krammer PH, and Debatin KM. Involvement of the CD95 (APO/Fas) recepetor/ligand system in drug-induced apoptosis in leukemia cells. Nature Medicine 1996 2 : 574–577.
27. Cai Z, Stancou R, Korner M, Chouaib S. Impairment of Fas-antigen expression in adriamycin-resistant but not TNF-resistant MCF7 tumor cells. Int J Cancer 1996 68:535–546.
28. Allouche M, Bettaieb A, Vindis C, rousse A, Grignon , C, Laurent G. Influence of bcl-2 overexpression on the ceramide pathway in daunorubicin-induced apoptosis of leukemic cells. Oncogene 1997 14, 1837–1845.
29. Boise LH, Gonzalez-Garcia M, Postema CE, Ding L, Lindsten T, Turka LA, Mao X, Nunez G, Thompson CB. bcl-x, a bcl-2-related gene that functions as a dominant regulator of apoptotic cell death. Cell 1993 74 : 597–608.
30. Shimizu S, Eguchi Y, Kosaka H, Kamiike W, Matsuda H, Tsujimoto Y. Prevention of hypoxia-induced cell death by Bcl-2 and Bcl-xL. Nature 1995 374 : 811–813.
31. Nakayama K, Nakayama K, Negishi I, Kuida K, Shinkai Y, Louie MC, Fields LE, Lucas PJ, Stewart V, Alt FW, Loh DY. Disappearance of the lymphoid system in Bcl-2 homozygous mutant chimeric mice. Science 1993 261: 1584–1588.
32. Motoyama N, Wang F, Roth KA, Sawa H, Nakayama K, Nakayama K, Negishi I, Senju S, Zhang Q, Fujii S, Loh DY. Massive cell death of immature hematopoietic cells and neurons in Bcl-x-deficient mice. Science 1995 267 : 1506–1510.
33. Gottschalk AR, Boise LH, Thompson CB, Quintans J. Identification of immunosuppressant-induced apoptosis in a murine B-cell line and its prevention by bcl-x but not bcl-2. Proc Natl Acad Sci U S A 1994 91:7350–7354.
34. Simonian PL, Grillot DA, Nunez G. Bcl-2 and Bcl-XL can differentially block chemotherapy-induced cell death. Blood 1997 90 : 1208–1216.
35. Cheng EH, Levine B, Boise LH, Thompson CB, Hardwick JM. Bax-independent inhibition of apoptosis by Bcl-XL. Nature 1996 379 : 554–556.
36. Bedi A, Zehnbauer BA, Barber JP, Sharkis SJ, Jones RJ. inhibition of apoptosis by BCR-ABL in chronic myeloid leukemia. Blood 1994 83: 2038–2044.
37. McGahon AJ, Brown DG, Martin SJ, Amarabte-Mendes GP, Cotter TG, Cohen GM, Green DR. Downregulation of Bcr-Abl in K562 cells restores susceptibility to apoptosis : characterization of the apoptotic death. Cell Death Differ 1997 95–104.
38. Daley GQ, Ben-Neriah Y. Implicating the bcr/abl gene in the pathogenesis of Philadelphia chromosome-positive human leukemia. Adv Cancer Res 1991 57:151–184.
39. McGahon A, Bissonnette R, Schmitt M, Cotter KM, Green DR, Cotter TG. BCR-ABL maintains resistance of chronic myelogenous leukemia cells to apoptotic cell death. Blood 1994 83:1179–1187.
40. Chen Q, Turner J, Watsan AJM, Dive C. v-Abl protein tyrosine kinase (PTK) mediated suppression of apoptosis is associated with the up-regulation of Bcl-XL. Oncogene. 1997 15: 2249–2254.
41. Oehm A, Behrmann I, Falk W, Pawlita M, Maier G, Klas C, Li-Weber M, Richards S, Dhein J, Trauth BC, Posting H, and Krammer PH. Purification and molecular cloning of the APO-1 cell surface antigen, a member of the tumor necrosis factor/nerve growth factor receptor superfamily. Sequence identity with the Fas antigen. J Biol Chem 1992 267:10709–10715.
42. McGahon AJ, Nishioka WK, Martin SJ, Mahboubi A, Cotter TG, Green DR. Regulation of the Fas apoptotic cell death pathway by Abl. J Biol Chem 1995 270 : 22625–22631.
43. Belloc F, Cotteret S, Labroille G, Schmit V, Jaloustre C, Dumain P, Dirrieu F, Reiffers J, Boisseau MR, Bernard P, Lacombe F. Bcr-abl translocation can occur during the induction of multidrug resistance and confers apoptosis resistance on myeloid leukemic cell lines. Cell Death Differ 1997 4:806–814.
44. Gottlieb RA, Nordberg J, Skowronski E, Babior BM. Apoptosis induced in Jurkat cells by several agents is preceded by intracellular acidification. Proc Natl Acad Sci U S A 1996 93: 654–658.
45. Evan GI, Wyllie AH, Gilbert CS, Littlewood TD, Land H, Brooks M, Waters CM, Penn LZ, Hancock DC. Induction of apoptosis in fibroblasts by c-myc protein. Cell 1992 69: 119–128.
46. Rozengurt E. Early signals in the mitogenic response. Science 1986 234: 161–166.

47. Jaffrézou JP, Chen G, Duran GE, Muller C, Bordier C, Laurent G, Sikic BI, Levade T. Inhibition of lysosomal acid sphingomyelinase by agents which reverse multidrug resistance. Biochim Biophys Acta 1995 1266: 1–8.
48. Lamb JA, Allen PG, Tuan BY, Janmey PA. Modulation of gelsolin function. Activation at low pH overrides Ca2+ requirement. J Biol Chem 1993 268: 8999–9004.
49. Kroemer G, Zamzami N, Susin SA. Mitochondrial control of apoptosis. Immunol. Today 1997 18 : 44–51.
50. Zamzami N, Marchetti P, Castedo M, Decaudin D, Macho A, Hirsch T, Susin SA, Petit PX, Mignotte B and Kroemer G. Sequential reduction of mitochondrial transmembrane potential and generation of reactive oxygen species in early programmed cell death. J Exp Med 1995 182 : 367–377.

40

GENETIC ABNORMALITIES AND DRUG RESISTANCE IN ACUTE LYMPHOBLASTIC LEUKEMIA

Ching-Hon Pui and William E. Evans

St. Jude Children's Research Hospital and The University of Tennessee
Memphis, Tennessee

ABSTRACT

Recent advances in cytogenetics and molecular genetics have made it possible to identify an array of genomic abnormalities with prognostic and therapeutic significance. Hyperdiploidy >50 chromosomes and *ETV6-CBFA2* fusions have been used to identify low-risk cases, and *BCR-ABL* and *MLL-AF4* to define high-risk leukemias. Despite their clinical utility, the risk classification system based on these findings lack absolute precision and should be complemented with other variables, the most important of which is the early blast cell response to remission induction therapy. Studies of tumor suppressor genes and proto-oncogenes in the *BCL2* family genes may unravel the mechanisms of leukemia cell progression and the development of drug resistance, leading to innovative therapies.

As the cure rates for childhood acute lymphoblastic leukemia (ALL) approach 80%,[1] precise methods of risk assessment are needed to permit better selection of treatment that is neither excessive nor inadequate for individual patients. Because one or more genetic abnormalities underlie every case of leukemia, a risk assignment system based on primary genetic abnormalities has great intuitive appeal. Even though over 90% of childhood ALL cases can be readily classified according to numerical or gross structural chromosomal abnormalities, molecular analyses are essential to identify therapeutically relevant, submicroscopic genetic lesions not visible by karyotyping.[2] This review focuses mainly on recent advances in genetic studies that have contributed to therapeutic advances or that hold promise for the future.

Hyperdiploidy >50 Chromosomes

Hyperdiploidy >50 (or a DNA index ≥1.16) is a well recognized genetic finding that is associated with a B-cell precursor phenotype, a low presenting leukocyte count, age between 1 and 9 years, and a favorable prognosis. Using an in vitro drug sensitivity assay, Kasper et al.,[3] demonstrated that hyperdiploid blasts are more sensitive to antimetabolites and L-asparaginase than are leukemic cells with other ploidy features. The exquisite drug sensitivity of these cells can be explained by their tendency to accumulate increased amounts of methotrexate and methotrexate polyglutamates (active metabolites),[4] and by their marked propensity to undergo spontaneous apoptosis.[5] However, as many as 20% of hyperdiploid >50 cases still relapse on contemporary treatment. Factors thought to confer a poor prognosis among hyperdiploid >50 cases are the presence of an isochromosome 17q, lack of trisomy of both chromosomes 4 and 10, increased survival of leukemic cells in stroma-supported culture, and a lower modal chromosomal number (i.e., 51–55 chromosomes).[5-7] Each of these associations requires confirmation in larger clinical trials.

ETV6-CBFA2 Fusion

Cases with *ETV6-CBFA2* (or *TEL-AML*) fusion represent another favorable subtype of B-cell precursor ALL, constituting 25% of cases with this phenotype and almost 60% of those with chromosomal abnormalities involving the 12p region.[8] Although the genetic lesion clearly results from the t(12;21), this translocation is essentially undetectable by cytogenetic methods because of the marked similarity of chromosomal segments involved in the rearrangement; hence, its detection requires fluorescence in situ hybridization, Southern blot analysis or reverse transcriptase – polymerase chain reaction (RT-PCR) assay. These cases are characterized by a favorable age (1 to 9 years), a nonhyperdiploid karyotype, and an increased frequency of expression of myeloid-associated antigens (CD13 and CD33).[9-13] Some investigators have suggested that the favorable prognosis and preponderance of *ETV6-CBFA2* fusions among cases of childhood ALL offset the unfavorable outcome of other myeloid-associated antigen-positive cases, resulting in an overall lack of significant difference in treatment results between myeloid antigen-positive and antigen-negative cases.[12] However, in our most recent study, myeloid-antigen expression lacked prognostic significance even after exclusion of cases with *ETV6-CBFA2* (C-H Pui, et al, unpublished data).

In a Pediatric Oncology Group study, the *ETV6-CBFA2* fusion conferred a favorable prognosis even among patients treated with antimetabolite-based therapy.[14] However, further in vitro study of blast cells with this abnormality showed that these cases accumulated lower levels of methotrexate polyglutamates than do other B-lineage cases,[15] suggesting that the improved outcome attributed to this genetic change may be due to an entirely different mechanism. This result is consistent with that of our preliminary analysis of an in vivo study in which methotrexate polyglutamate accumulation did not differ significantly between leukemic blasts with rearranged *TEL* and those with germline *TEL*, even among nonhyperdiploid cases.[13] Despite a number of studies indicating that the *ETV6-CBFA2* fusion is a favorable prognostic feature,[8-14] recent studies of relapsed ALL disclosed a frequency of this genetic abnormality, comparable to that in newly diagnosed cases.[16-19] Moreover, patients with this genetic lesion at relapse had a longer second remission than did other cases.[19] Thus, the presence of a chimeric *ETV6-CBFA2* gene may only delay (rather than decrease) relapses in childhood ALL. It is also possible that the high frequency of this genetic abnormality at relapse is the consequence of a new genetic alteration,[19] a hypothesis requiring prospective molecular analysis of leukemic cells at diagnosis and at relapse. In one of our Total Therapy studies, the cumulative risk of radiation-included malignant brain tumors was significantly higher in cases with the *ETV6-CBFA2* than in other cases (C-H Pui et al., unpublished data), raising the possibility that these patients may have a predisposition to the development of malignancy. In view of this association and the overall improvement of CNS control achieved with early intensification of intrathecal and systemic therapy,[1] use of cranial irradiation should be avoided in cases with the *ETV6-CBFA2* gene.

BCR-ABL Fusion

The t(9;22) with *BCR-ABL* fusion (Philadelphia chromosome), one of the best- characterized translocations in cancer genetics, is associated with a poor overall clinical outcome. The fusion gene product is expressed as either the P190 or P210 protein, with the former accounting for at least three-fourths of all cases bearing the Philadelphia chromosome.[20] While treatment outcome does not appear to differ between cases with the P210 or P190 product,[20] we have shown that some patients, characterized by a low presenting leukocyte count, can become long-term survivors when treated with intensive multiagent chemotherapy, obviating the need for transplantation in first remission.[21] This finding was recently confirmed by a Berlin-Frankfurt-Münster (BFM) study, in which prednisone sensitivity surpassed initial leukocyte count as a predictor of treatment outcome.[20] In that study, t(9;22)-positive cases with a good initial response to prednisone treatment had a long-term event-free survival of 40% when treated with chemotherapy alone, suggesting that delay of allogeneic transplantation until second remission may be appropriate for this subset of patients.

MLL Rearrangement

It is well recognized that *MLL* rearrangements, especially the *MLL-AF4* fusion gene resulting from the t(4;11), are associated with a dismal prognosis.[22,23] In fact, the poor overall outcome of treatment in infants with ALL has been attributed to the high frequency of *MLL* rearrangements, *MLL-AF4* fusion in particular.[24-26] We found that *MLL-AF4* fusion did not confer as poor a prognosis in children 1 to 9 years old as it does in infants or older children.[23] Currently, most investigators recommend very aggressive therapy, including allogeneic transplantation, for cases with *MLL-AF4* fusion, especially in infants and adolescents. However, most patients lack suitable donors and the results of transplantation have yet to be proven superior to those of intensive chemotherapy. Much effort has been expended in identifying effective agents for these cases. In this regard, cytarabine was found to be a highly effective gent in one in vitro study of lymphoblasts from infants,[27] and use of this agent and high-dose methotrexate were credited with an improved outcome in a small study of infant ALL.[28] These findings have formed the basis of an international treatment protocol for infant ALL, now under development (R. Pieters et al., personal communication).

E2A-PBX1 Fusion

Once associated with a poor prognosis, pre-B ALL cases carrying the *E2A-PBX1* fusion gene now have greatly improved clinical responses, comparable to those of standard-risk B-cell precursor ALL. There are no consistent prognostic features that can be used to refine risk assignment in cases with *E2A-PBX1* fusion. Two studies suggested that a reciprocal balanced translocation was associated with a poor prognosis among the t(1;19) cases,[29,30] a finding that we were unable to confirm.[31] Nonetheless, it is important to recognize a small unique subgroup of t(1;19) cases that are characterized by an early pre-B phenotype, hyperdiploidy, a lack of *E2A-PBX1* fusion, and a favorable prognosis with antimetabolite-based therapy.[31]

TUMOR SUPPRESSOR GENES

The two most well-studied tumor suppressor genes in ALL are *P53* and *MTS1/P16^{INK4a}*. *P53* can be inactivated through gene mutation or overexpression of the MDM2 oncoprotein, capable of complexing with P53 and inhibiting wild-type P53 activities. However, *P53* inactivation is relatively uncommon in childhood ALL (2% to 4% of cases) and primarily occurs in relapsed or refractory T-cell ALL.[32-35] By contrast, homozygous deletions or hypermethylation of the gene promoter region of *MTS1/P16^{INK4a}* is very common, occurring in as many as 30% of B-cell precursor ALL and 80% of T-cell ALL cases.[36-41] The clinical significance of the gene deletion is controversial. While several studies that combined both B-cell precursor and T-cell ALL cases showed a correlation between an adverse prognosis and this genetic abnormality,[39-41] we and others were not able to confirm this relationship.[39-41] Recent studies showed that the product of a second alternative reading frame (ARF) of the MTS locus is a tumor suppressor,[42,43] challenging the critical role of *P16^{INK4a}* in carcinogenesis.

BCL-2 AND RELATED PROTEINS

A wide variety of stimuli can trigger apoptosis by activating downstream caspases which then cleave specific protein substrates. One such pathway is mitochondria-dependent and is governed by BCL2 and at least 12 of its homologs.[44,45] Some of these proteins are antiapoptotic (e.g., BCL-2, BCL-X$_L$) while others are proapoptotic (e.g., BAX, BAK, BIK, BID, and BAD). These proteins can either heterodimerize with each other or homodimerize with themselves.[44,45] *BCL-2* was the first anti-cell death gene to be identified and remains the best studied member of this family. While inappropriate expression of the *BCL-2* oncogene can block cell death induced by a variety of agents, we and others found that overexpression of this protein did not by itself correlate with treatment outcome in childhood ALL.[46,47] In a study of pediatric ALL cell lines, high levels of BCL-X$_L$ correlated with *P53* mutations and in vitro resistance to irradiation-induced apoptosis.[48] Moreover, among cell lines that retained wild-type P53, those exhibiting radiation-induced apoptotic responses showed upregulation of *BAX* and downregulation of *BCL-2*. In another study of several different leukemic cell lines, high *BCL-2:BAX* ratios were associated with in vitro resistance to cytotoxic agents.[49] Hence, an understanding of the interactions among these BCL-2 binding proteins should provide valuable insights into the overall control of cell fate decisions and may suggest new therapeutic means to overcome drug resistance by leukemic cells.

ACKNOWLEDGMENT

Supported in part by the following awards from the U.S. Public Health Service, National Institutes of Health, National Cancer Institute: Leukemia Program Project grant P01-CA20180, R37-CA36401 and CORE Cancer Center Support grant CA21765, by a

Center of Excellence grant from the State of Tennessee and by the American Lebanese Syrian Associated Charities (ALSAC).

REFERENCES

1. Pui, C.-H., Mahmoud, H.H., Rivera, G.K., Hancock, M.L., Sandlund, J.T., Behm, F.G., et al. Early intensification of intrathecal chemotherapy virtually eliminates central nervous system relapse in children with acute lymphoblastic leukemia. *Blood*, 92 411–415.
2. Pui, C.-H. (1997) Acute lymphoblastic leukemia. *Pediatr Clin North Am*, 44, 831–846.
3. Kaspers, G.J.L., Smets, L.A., Pieters, R., Van Zantwijk, C.H., Van Wering, E.R., and Veerman, A.J.P. (1995) Favorable prognosis of hyperdiploid common acute lymphoblastic leukemia may be explained by sensitivity to antimetabolites and other drugs: Results of an in vitro study. *Blood*, 85, 751–756.
4. Synold, T.W., Relling, M.V., Boyett, J.M., Rivera, G.K., Sandlund, J.T., Mahmoud, H., et al. (1994) Blast cell methotrexate-polyglutamate accumulation in vivo differs by lineage, ploidy, and methotrexate dose in acute lymphoblastic leukemia. *J Clin Invest*, 94, 1996–2001.
5. Kumagai, M., Manabe, A., Pui, C.-H., Behm, F.G., Raimondi, S.C., Hancock, M.L., et al. (1996) Stroma-supported culture of childhood B-lineage acute lymphoblastic leukemia cells predicts treatment outcome. *J Clin Invest*, 97, 755–760.
6. Harris, M.B., Shuster, J.J., Carroll, A., Look, A.T., Borowitz, M.J., Crist, W.M., et al. (1992), Trisomy of leukemic cell chromosomes 4 and 10 identifies children with B-progenitor cell acute lymphoblastic leukemia with a very low risk of treatment failure: A pediatric oncology group study. *Blood*, 79, 3316–3324.
7. Raimondi, S.C., Pui, C.-H., Hancock, M.L., Behm, F.G., Filatov, L., and Rivera, G.K. (1996) Heterogeneity of hyperdiploid (51–67) childhood acute lymphoblastic leukemia. *Leukemia*, 10, 213–224.
8. Raimondi, S.C., Shurtleff, S.A., Downing, J.R., Rubnitz, J., Mathew, S., Hancock, M., et al. (1997) 12p abnormalities and the *TEL* gene (*ETV6*) in childhood acute lymphoblastic leukemia. *Blood*, 90, 4559–4566.
9. McLean, T.W., Ringold, S., Neuberg, D., Stegmaier, K., Tantravahi, R., Ritz, J., et al. (1996) TEL/AML-1 dimerizes and is associated with a favorable outcome in childhood acute lymphoblastic leukemia. *Blood*, 11, 4252–4258.
10. Rubnitz, J.E., Behm, F.G., Pui, C.-H., Evans, W.E., Relling, M.V., Raimondi, S.C., et al. (1997) Genetic studies of childhood acute lymphoblastic leukemia with emphasis on *p16*, *MLL*, and *ETV6* gene abnormalities: results of St. Jude Total Therapy Study XII. *Leukemia*, 11, 1201–1206.
11. Borkhardt, A., Cazzaniga, G., Viehmann, S., Valsecchi, M.G., Ludwig, W. D., Burci, L., et al. (1997) Incidence and clinical relevance of TEL/AML1 fusion genes in children with acute lymphoblastic leukemia enrolled in the German and Italian multicenter therapy trials. *Blood*, 90, 571–577.
12. Baruchel, A., Cayuela, J.M., Ballerini, P., Landman-Parker, J., Cezard, V., Firat, H., et al. (1997) The majority of myeloid-antigen positive (My+) childhood B-cell precursor acute lymphoblastic leukemias express *TEL-AML1* fusion transcripts. *Br J Hematol*, 99, 101–106.
13. Rubnitz, J.E., Downing, J.R., Pui, C-H., Shurtleff, S.A., Raimondi, S.C., Evans, W.E., et al. (1997) *TEL* gene rearrangement in acute lymphoblastic leukemia: A new genetic marker with prognostic significance. *J Clin Oncol*, 15, 1150–1157.
14. Rubnitz, J.E., Shuster, J., Land, V.J., Link, M.P., Pullen, J., Camitta, B.M., et al. (1997) Case-control study suggests a favorable impact of *TEL* rearrangement in patients with B-lineage acute lymphoblastic leukemia treated with antimetabolite-based therapy: A pediatric oncology group study. *Blood*, 89, 1143–1146.
15. Whitehead, W.M., Payment, C., Vuchich, M-J., Cooley, L., Lauer, S.J., Mahoney, D.H., et al. (1998) The TEL-AML1 translocation and methotrexate polyglutamate (MTXPG) levels in childhood B-progenitor cell acute lymphoblastic leukemia (pro-B ALL): a pediatric oncology group study. *Proc AACR*, 39, 329.
16. Nakao, M., Yokota, S., Horiike, S., Taniwaki, M., Kashima, K., Sonoda, Y., et al. (1996) Detection and quantification of *TEL/AML1* fusion transcripts by polymerase chain reaction in childhood acute lymphoblastic leukemia. *Leukemia*, 10, 1463–1470.
17. Lanza, C., Volpe, G., Basso, G., Gottardi, E., Barisone, E., Spinelli, M., et al. (1997) Outcome and lineage involvement in t(12;21) childhood acute lymphoblastic leukaemia. *Br J Haematol*, 97, 460–462.
18. Harbott, J., Viehmann, S., Borkhardt, A., Henze, G., and Lampert, F. (1997) Incidence of TEL/AML1 fusion gene analyzed consecutively in children with acute lymphoblastic leukemia in relapse. *Blood*, 12, 4933–4937.
19. Seeger, K., Adams, H-P., Buchwald, D., Beyermann, B., Kremens, B., Niemeyer, C., et al. (1998) *TEL-AML1* fusion transcript in relapsed childhood acute lymphoblastic leukemia. *Blood*, 91, 1716–1722.

20. Schrappe, M., Aricò, M., Harbott, J., Biondi, A., Zimmermann, M., Conter, V., et al. (1998) Ph[+] childhood acute lymphoblastic leukemia: good initial steroid response allows early prediction of a favorable treatment outcome. *Blood*, **92**, 2730–2741.

21. Ribeiro, R. C., Broniscer, A., Rivera, G.K., Hancock, M.L., Raimondi, S.C., Sandlund, J.T., et al. (1997) Philadelphia chromosome-positive acute lymphoblastic leukemia in children: durable responses to chemotherapy associated with low initial white blood cell counts. *Leukemia*, **11**, 1493–1496.

22. Behm, F.G., Raimondi, S.C., Frestedt, J.L., Liu, Q., Crist, W.M., Downing, J.R., et al. (1996) Rearrangement of the *MLL* gene confers a poor prognosis in childhood acute lymphoblastic leukemia, regardless of presenting age. *Blood*, **87**, 2870–2877.

23. Pui, C.-H., Frankel, L.S., Carroll, A.J., Raimondi, S.C., Shuster, J.J., Head, D.R., et al. (1991) Clinical characteristics and treatment outcome of childhood acute lymphoblastic leukemia with the t(4;11) (q21;q23): A collaborative study of 40 cases. *Blood*, **77**, 440–447.

24. Chen, C-S., Sorensen, P.H.B., Domer, P.H., Reaman, G.H., Korsmeyer, S.J., Heerema, N.A., et al. (1993) Molecular rearrangements on chromosome 11q23 predominate in infant acute lymphoblastic leukemia and are associated with specific biologic variables and poor outcome. *Blood*, **81**, 2386–2393.

25. Pui, C.-H., Behm, F.G., Downing, J.R., Hancock, M.L., Shurtleff, S.A., Ribeiro, R.C., et al. (1994) 11q23/*MLL* rearrangement confers a poor prognosis in infants with acute lymphoblastic leukemia. *J Clin Oncol*, **12**, 909–915.

26. Rubnitz, J.E., Link, M.P., Shuster, J.J., Carroll, A.J., Hakami, N., Frankel, L.S., et al. (1994) Frequency and prognostic significance of *HRX* rearranagements in infant acute lymphoblastic leukemia: A Pediatric Oncology Group study. *Blood*, **84**, 570–573.

27. Pieters, R., den Boer, M.L., Durian, M., Janka, G. Schmiegelow, K., Kaspers, G.J.L., et al. (1998) In vitro drug resistance testing in infant acute lymphoblastic leukemia cells - implications for treatment. *Leukemia*, **12**, 1344–1348.

28. Silverman, L. B., McLean, T.W., Donnelly, M.J., Gilliland, D.G., Gelber, R.D., and Sallan, S.E. (1996) Improved outcome for infants with acute lymphoblastic leukemia (ALL) with intensification of therapy. *Blood*, **88** (Suppl 1), 668a.

29. Secker-Walker, L.M., Berger, R., Fenaux, P., Lai, J.L., Nelken, B., Garson, M., et al. (1992) Prognostic significance of the balanced t(1;19) and unbalanced der(19)t(1;19) translocations in acute lymphoblastic leukemia. *Leukemia*, **6**, 363–369.

30. Uckun, F.M., Sensel, M.G., Sather, H.N., Gaynon, P.S., Arthur, D.C., Lange, B.J., et al. (1998) Clinical significance of translocation t(1;19) in childhood acute lymphoblastic leukemia in the context of contemporary therapies: a report from the Children's Cancer Group. *J Clin Onc*, **16**, 527–535.

31. Pui, C.-H., Raimondi, S.C., Hancock, M.L., Rivera, G.K., Ribeiro, R.C., Mahmoud, H.H., et al. (1994) Immunologic, cytogenetic, and clinical characterization of childhood acute lymphoblastic leukemia with the t(1;19)(q23;p13) or its derivative. *J Clin Oncol*, **12**, 2601–2606.

32. Hsiao, M.H., Yu, A.L., Yeargin, J., Ku, D., and Haas, M. (1994) Monhereditary p53 mutations in T-Cell acute lymphoblastic leukemia are associated with the relapse phase. *Blood*, **83**, 2922–2930.

33. Diccianni, M.B., Yu, J., Hsiao, M., Mukherjee, S., Shao, L.-E., and Yu, A.L. (1994) Clinical significance of *p53* mutations in relapsed T-cell acute lymphoblastic leukemia. *Blood*, **84**, 3105–3112.

34. Marks, D.I., Kurz, B. W., Link, M.P., Ng, E., Shuster, J.J., Lauer, S.J., et al. (1996) High incidence of potential p53 inactivation in poor outcome childhood acute lymphoblastic leukemia at diagnosis. *Blood*, **87**, 1155–1161.

35. Marks, D.I., Kurz, B.W., Link, M.P., Ng, E., Shuster, J.J., Lauer, S.J., et al. (1997) Altered expression of p53 and *mdm*-2 proteins at diagnosis is associated with early treatment failure in childhood acute lymphoblastic leukemia. *J Clin Oncol*, **15**, 1158–1162.

36. Okuda, T., Shurtleff, S.A., Valentine, M.B., Raimondi, S.C., Head, D.R., Behm, F., et al. (1995) Frequent deletion of $p16^{INK4a}$/*MTS1* and $p15^{INK4b}$/*MTS2* in pediatric acute lymphoblastic leukemia. *Blood*, **85**, 2321–2330.

37. Takeuchi, S., Bartram, C.R., Seriu, T., Miller, C.W., Tobler, A., Janssen, J.W.G., et al. (1995) Analysis of a family of cyclin-dependent kinase inhibitors: p15/MTS2/INK4B, p16/MTS1/INK4A, and p18 genes in acute lymphoblastic leukemia of childhood. *Blood*, **86**, 755–760.

38. Lolascon, A., Faienza, M.F., Coppola, B., della Ragione, F., Schettini, F., and Biondi, A. (1996) Homozygous deletions of cyclin-dependent kinase inhibitor genes, $p16^{INK4A}$ and p18, in childhood T cell lineage acute lymphoblastic leukemias. *Leukemia*, **10**, 255–260.

39. Heyman, M., Rasool, O., Brandter, L.B., Liu, Y., Grandér, D., Söderhäll, S., et al. (1996) Prognostic importance of $p15^{INK4B}$ and $p16^{INK4}$ gene inactivation in childhood acute lymphocytic leukemia. *J Clin Oncol*, **14**, 1512–1520.

40. Zhou, M., Gu, L., Yeager, A.M., and Findley, H.W. (1997) Incidence and clinical significance of $CDKN2/MTS1/P16^{ink4A}$ and $MTS2/P15^{ink4B}$ gene deletions in childhood acute lymphoblastic leukemia. *Pediatr Hematol Oncol*, **14**, 141–150.
41. Kees, U.R., Burton, P.R., Lü, C., and Baker, D.L. (1997) Homozygous deletion of the *p16/MTS1* gene in pediatric acute lymphoblastic leukemia is associated with unfavorable clinical outcome. *Blood*, **89**, 4161–4166.
42. Kamijo, T., Zindy, F., Rousel, M.F., Quelle, D.E., Downing, J.R., Ashmun, R.A., et al. (1997) Tumor suppression at the mouse *INK4a* locus mediated by the alternative reading frame product $p19^{ARF}$. *Cell*, **91**, 649–659.
43. Gardie, B., Cayuela, J-M., Martini, S., and Sigaux, F. (1998) Genomic alterations of the $p19^{ARF}$ encoding exons in T-cell acute lymphoblastic leukemia. *Blood*, **91**, 1016–1020.
44. Kroemer, G. (1997) The proto-oncogene Bcl-2 and its role in regulating apoptosis. *Nature Med*, **3**, 614–620.
45. Reed, J.C. (1997) Double identity for proteins of the Bcl-2 family. *Nature*, **387**, 773–776.
46. Coustan-Smith, E., Kitanaka, A., Pui, C-H., McNinch, L., Evans, W.E., Raimondi, S.C., et al. (1996) Clinical relevance of *BCL-2* overexpression in childhood acute lymphoblastic leukemia. *Blood*, **87**, 1140–1146.
47. Uckun, F.M., Yang, Z., Sather, H., Steinherz, P., Nachman, J., Bostrom, B., et al. (1997) Cellular expression of antiapoptotic BCL-2 oncoprotein in newly diagnosed childhood acute lymphoblastic leukemia: A Children's Cancer Group study. *Blood*, **89**, 3769–3777.
48. Findley, H.W., Gu, L., Yeager, A.M., and Zhou, M. (1997) Expression and regulation of Bcl-2, Bcl-xl, and Bax correlate with p53 status and sensitivity to apoptosis in childhood acute lymphoblastic leukemia. *Blood*, **89**, 2986–2993.
49. Salomons, G.S., Brady, H.J.M., Verwijs-Janssen, M., Van Den Berg, J.D., Hart, A.A.M., Van Den Berg, H., et al. (1997) The Baxα:Bcl-2 ratio modulates the response to dexamethasone in leukaemic cells and is highly variable in childhood acute leukaemia. *Int J Cancer*, **71**, 959–965.

41

RESISTANCE TESTING AND MECHANISMS OF RESISTANCE IN CHILDHOOD LEUKEMIA

Studies from Amsterdam

R. Pieters, G. J. L. Kaspers, N. L. Ramakers-van Woerden, M. L. den Boer,
M. G. Rots, Ch. M. Zwaan, E. G. Haarman, and A. J. P. Veerman

University Hospital Vrije Universiteit
Department of Pediatric Hematology/Oncology
De Boelelaan 1117
1081 HV Amsterdam, The Netherlands

1. INTRODUCTION

The prognosis of children with leukemia has improved dramatically due to the development of effective combination chemotherapy. Nevertheless, about 25% of children with acute lymphobalstic leukemia (ALL) and 50% of children with acute myeloid leukemia (AML) die of resistant or relapsed disease. On the other hand, patients who are curable with relatively mild chemotherapy as used in the seventies, will nowadays be overtreated and suffer from unnecessary side-effects. This is due to the fact that therapy has been intensified for all patients in (successful) attempts to cure an increasing number of children.Therefore, it is of the highest importance to identify children with highly sensitive leukemia that can be cured with minimal therapy and children who need specifically intensified therapy. Our research program focusses on the relation between molecular biological characteristics, drug resistance and prognosis in pediatric oncology. Here, results from some recent and currently ongoing studies in leukemia will be described.

2. DRUG RESISTANCE TESTING

2.1. Prognostic Value of in Vitro Cellular Drug Resistance

In the late eighties we adapted short-term culture assays such as the methyl-thiazoltetrazolium (MTT) assay and the differential staining cytotoxicity assay (DiSC) assay to determine drug resistance in acute leukemia cells directly obtained from patients.[1] These assays measure the endpoint of the action of anticancer drugs, i.e. cell kill, but give no information on the mechanism of cell kill. A small retrospective study suggested that especially in vitro resistance to prednisolone was related to the outcome of children with ALL.[2] Two prospective studies followed. In the first study in collaboration with the Dutch Childhood Leukemia Study Group, in vitro resistance was determined at initial diagnosis in 152 children with ALL. Resistance to each of the drugs prednisolone, vincristine and L-asparaginase was related to the probability of event-free survival (EFS). When the results for these drugs were combined in a resistance profile, the EFS at 3 years for patients with sensitive cells was 100%, with intermediately sensitive cells 84% and with resistant cells 43%. At multivariate analysis, drug resistance appeared to be the strongest prognostic factor, independent of all other known risk factors.[3] The control leukemic cell survival and resistance to other classes of drugs were not significantly related to prognosis.

The second prognostic study started in 1992 by the German COALL Study Group in co-operation with our laboratory. Using identical cut-off points of resistance, the in vitro resistance profile was confirmed to be the strongest independent prognostic factor in ALL. Based upon these data, the new treatment protocol of the COALL Study Group that started in August 1997, includes a stratification based upon the resistance profile. In this way patients with relatively sensitive cells that have an excellent prognosis will receive therapy reduction while patients with relatively resistant cells will receive intensified treatment. Prospective studies on the prognostic value of in vitro resistance to cytosine arabinoside (AraC) and anthracyclines in childhood and adult AML are in progress. A pilot study in adult AML suggested that resistance to AraC and daunorubicin was related to survival.[4] In a large study encompriring >100 children with relapsed ALL, these relapsed cells were shown to be highly resistant to many but not all classes of drugs.[5]

2.2. Cell Biological and Clinical Characteristics versus Drug Resistance

Studies were done to evaluate whether the prognostic factors DNA ploidy, immunophenotype, age and gene rearrangements reflected differences in drug resistance. The favorable prognosis of children with hyperdiploid commonALL appeared to be related to a relatively high sensitivity to the antimetabolites 6-mercaptopurine, 6-thioguanine, and AraC and to L-asparaginase.[6]

High risk patients defined by age and immunophenotype were also found to express specific drug resistance profiles.[7,8] Infants with ALL, associated with a dismal prognosis, display a very high resistance to glucocorticoids (prednisolone and dexamethasone) and L-asparaginase but a remarkably high sensitivity to AraC.[9] This knowledge forms one of the backbones of an International treatment protocol for infants with ALL that has recently been initiated. The relation between MLL gene rearrangements (11q23 translocations such as t(4;11); MLL: mixed lineage leukemia), CD10 negative precursor B-lineage (proB) immunophenotype and drug resistance in infant ALL is currently being studied.

The t(12;21) translocation resulting in TEL/AML1 gene fusion, present in about 25% of childhood common/preB-ALL, may be associated with a good prognosis. Preliminary results indicate that TEL/AML1 positive cells are not significantly more sensitive to any of the drugs tested compared to TEL/AML1 negative common/preB-ALL cells.

The relation between other important gene abnormalities in ALL such as p16 deletions and the t(9;22) translocation and resistance is being studied.

3. MECHANISMS OF RESISTANCE

Because many drugs are used in the treatment of childhood leukemia and many factors may be responsible for resistance to each drug, it is unlikely that one mechanism is responsible for clinical resistance. The advantage of culture assays described above is that they measure the endpoint of different mechanisms of resistance, i.e., cell kill. However, to understand and modulate or circumvent resistance, studies on mechanisms in patients' cells are obligatory.

3.1. Resistance to Thiopurines

We have studied the relationship between several purine pathway enzymes and thiopurine resistance in childhood ALL. Low activities of hypoxanthine guanine phosphoribosyl transferase (HGPRT), an enzyme that forms active nucleotides from the thiopurines, were not related to thiopurine resistance in patients' ALL cells.[10] Breakdown of the active nucleotides by high activities of cytoplasmic 5'-nucleotidase and phosphatases but not ecto-5'nucleotidase might play a role in thiopurine resistance in ALL.[11,12]

3.2. Multidrug Resistance

A very recent prospective study on multidrug resistance (MDR) mechanisms showed that the MDR-1 gene encoded P-glycoprotein and the multidrug resistance associated protein (MRP) were not related to resistance to anthracyclines, epipodophyllotoxins and vinca-alkaloids in childhood ALL. However, the lung resistance protein (LRP) may contribute to a decreased anthracycline accumulation and retention in these cells.[13] The cell size appeared to be an important factor that is often overlooked when measuring these parameters. The expression of topoisomerase IIα gene was not related to resistance in ALL.[14] Prospective studies on the relevance of these MDR mechanisms in childhood AML are ongoing in our laboratory. ALL cells were significantly cross-resistant to all types of drugs, with greater cross-resistance between structurally related drugs.[15] It will be studied whether this general drug resistance can be attributed to a trigger-independent common pathway leading to programmed cell death (apoptosis).

3.3. Resistance to Methotrexate

Resistance to methotrexate (MTX) can theoretically be present at three levels: (1) membrane transport, (2) polyglutamation and (3) target enzymes. The relevance of defects at these three levels is studied in a collaborative study between our laboratory and the department of Medical Oncology, University Hospital Vrije Universiteit, Amsterdam, the Netherlands (G.J. Peters, G. Jansen). After a drug-free period, AML and T-ALL cells were found to be more resistant to MTX compared to common/preB-ALL cells as established by an in situ thymidylate synthase inhibition assay. Both impaired formation of MTX polyglutamates by a low activity of folylpolyglutamate synthetase (FPGS) and a high breakdown of these polyglutamates by a high activity of folylpolyglutamate hydrolase (FPGH) are mainly responsible for the resistance of AML cells to MTX. However, preliminary data suggest that not all types of AML are MTX resistant and currently we are analyzing this in further detail. MTX resistance in T-lineage ALL is related to a low FPGS but not to a high FPGH activity. Promising new antifolates are studied in patients' samples for their effectiveness to circumvent mechanisms of MTX resistance

3.4. Resistance to Glucocorticoids

An important area of research that has recently been started at our laboratory is glucocorticoid resistance since this plays a very important role in clinical failure to chemotherapy in ALL. The relevance of putative resistance mechanisms to prednisolone and dexamethasone and strategies to modulate or circumvent glucocorticoid resistance are being studied. Among these are the capacity of cortivazol, meta-iodobenzylguanidine (MIBG) and DNA hypomethylation as ways to modulate or circumvent this resistance. Another important topic that is subject of ongoing studies is the relation between cell death regulatory genes and drug induced apoptosis such as p53/mdm2, bax, bad, bcl-xl and bcl-xs. The role of the Fas receptor/ligand mediated cell death in anthracycline sensitivity and resistance is analyzed together with the capacity of cytokines to modulate the inhibition of cell death by changes in the Fas-mediated pathway.

ACKNOWLEDGMENTS

Many studies described here are performed in collaboration with the Dutch Childhood Leukemia Study Group, the German COALL Study Group and BFM Group and with other departments of the University Hospital Vrije Universiteit, especially Medical Oncology, Pathology and Hematology. The work on leukemia is supported by grants from the Dutch Cancer Society (VU 87-17, 89-06, 90-05, 93-641, 94-679, 95-521, 97-1564) and is currently carried out in co-operation with the following technicians: D.R. Huismans, K. Kazemier, A.H. Loonen, M.M.A. Rottier, R. Wünsche, C.H. van Zantwijk.

Adapted from a report for the ECC Newsletter, volume 7, number 1, 1998, pp 6–8.

REFERENCES

1. Pieters R, Loonen AH, Huismans DR, Broekema GJ, Dirven MWJ, Heyenbrok MW, Hählen K, Veerman AJP. In vitro drug sensitivity of cells from children with leukemia using the MTT assay with improved culture conditions. Blood 1990; 76: 2327–2336.
2. Pieters R, Huismans DR, Loonen AH, Hählen K, Van der Does-van den Berg A, Van Wering ER, Veerman AJP. Relation of cellular drug resistance to long-term clinical outcome in childhood acute lymphoblastic leukaemia. Lancet 1991; 338: 399–403.
3. Kaspers GJL, Veerman AJP, Pieters R, Van Zantwijk CH, Smets LA, Van Wering ER, Van der Does-van den Berg A. In vitro cellular drug resistance and prognosis in newly diagnosed childhood acute lymphoblastic leukemia. Blood 1997; 90: 2723–2729
4. Klumper E, Ossenkoppele GJ, Pieters R, Huismans DR, Loonen AH, Rottier MMA, Westra G, Veerman AJP. In vitro resistance to cytosine arabinoside, not to daunorubicin, is associated with the risk of relapse in de novo acute myeloid leukaemia. Br J Haematol 1996; 93: 903–910.
5. Klumper E, Pieters R, Veerman AJP, Huismans DR, Loonen AH, Hählen K, Kaspers GJL, Van Wering ER, Hartmann R, Henze G. In vitro cellular drug resistance in children with relapsed/refractory acute lymphoblastic leukaemia. Blood 1995; 86: 3861–3868
6. Kaspers GJL, Smets LA, Pieters R, Van Zantwijk CH, De Waal FC, Van Wering ER, Veerman AJP. Favorable prognosis of hyperdiploid common acute lymphoblastic leukemia may be explained by sensitivity to antimetabolites and other drugs: results of an in vitro study. Blood 1995; 85: 751–756.
7. Pieters R, Kaspers GJL, Van Wering ER, Huismans DR, Loonen AH, Hählen K, Veerman AJP. Cellular drug resistance profiles that might explain the prognostic value of immunophenotype and age in childhood acute lymphoblastic leukemia. Leukemia 1993; 7: 392–397.
8. Kaspers GJL, Pieters R, Van Zantwijk CH, Van Wering ER, Veerman AJP. Clinical and cell biological features related to cellular drug resistance of childhood acute lymphoblastic leukemia cells. Leuk Lymphoma 1995; 19: 407–416.

9. Pieters R, Den Boer ML, Durian M, Janka-Schaub GE, Schmiegelow K, Kaspers GJL, Van Wering ER, Veerman AJP. Relation between age, immunophenotype and in vitro drug resistance in 395 children with acute lymphoblastic leukemia - implications for treatment of infants. Leukemia 1998; 12: 1344–1348.
10. Pieters R, Huismans DR, Loonen AH, Peters GJ, Hählen K, Van der Does-van den Berg A, Van Wering ER, Veerman AJP. Hypoxanthine-guanine phosphoribosyl-transferase in childhood leukemia: relation with immunophenotype, in vitro drug resistance and clinical prognosis. Int J Cancer 1992; 51: 213–217.
11. Pieters R, Thompson LF, Broekema GJ, Huismans DR, Peters GJ, Pals ST, Horst E, Hählen K, Veerman AJP. Expression of 5'-nucleotidase (CD73) related to other differentiation antigens in leukemias of B-cell lineage. Blood 1991; 78: 488–492.
12. Pieters R, Huismans DR, Loonen AH, Peters GJ, Hählen K, Van der Does-van den Berg A, Van Wering ER, Veerman AJP. Relation of 5'-nucleotidase and phosphatase activities with immunophenotype, drug resistance and clinical prognosis in childhood leukemia. Leuk Res 1992; 16: 873–880.
13. Den Boer ML, Pieters R, Kazemier KM, Rottier MMA, Zwaan ChM, Kaspers GJL, Janka-Schaub GE, Henze G, Creutzig U, Scheper RJ, Veerman AJP. Relationship between major vault protein/lung resistance protein, multidrug resistance-associated protein, P-glycoprotein expression, and drug resistance in childhood leukemia. Blood 1998; 91: 2092–2098.
14. Klumper E, Giaccone G, Pieters R, Broekema G, Van Ark-Otte J, Van Wering ER, Kaspers GJL, Veerman AJP. Topoisomerase IIα gene expression in childhood acute lymphoblastic leukemia. Leukemia 1995; 9: 1653–1660.
15. Kaspers GJL, Pieters R, Van Zantwijk CH, Van Wering ER, Van der Does-van den Berg A, Veerman AJP. Prednisolone resistance in childhood acute lymphoblastic leukemia: vitro-vivo correlations and cross-resistance to other drugs. Blood 1998; 92: 1–8.

PHARMACOKINETICS OF ANTICANCER DRUGS *IN VITRO*

Alexandra Wagner,[*] Georg Hempel, H. G. Gumbinger,[*] Heribert Jürgens, and Joachim Boos

Department of Pediatric Hematology and Oncology
Department of Pharmacologie
WWU Münster, Albert-Schweitzer 33, Germany

Keywords: Pharmacokinetics, drug sensitivity assay, stability, unphysiological, pitfall.

1. ABSTRACT

It is generally assumed that drug concentration does not change significantly under cell culture conditions. Nevertheless, most of the therapeutic trials in acute leukemia that were based on *in vitro* drug sensitivity assays of patient samples have been disappointing. In order to show possible pitfalls of unphysiological alterations *in vitro* we investigated concentration versus time curves, metabolism and effects on the culture media for some antineoplastic drugs.

Oxazaphosphorines and cytarabine were incubated in RPMI and in established cell lines and measured by HPLC. HPLC also served to measure enzyme activity and levels of related amino acids at various concentrations of asparaginase, ammonia release was photometrically determined. Etoposide was monitored by HPLC relative to different contents of FCS in RPMI.

All oxazaphosphorines showed a rapid decrease of *in vitro* activity down to about 10% within 4–6 h, and 2% within 72 h. The level of cytarabine, when incubated in RPMI, was stable over 24h, and no change was seen with K562, while a rapid decrease to below 50% occurred within 6h in the presence of HL 60 and BLIN. 2 U/L of asparaginase led to asparagine depletion of the medium within 4h, while 200 U/L were associated with a preferential increase of glutamic acid and ammonia. Further, there was evidence of instability

---

[*] Corresponding author: Alexandra Wagner, Dept. of Pediatric Hematology and Oncology, Albert-Schweitzerstr. 33 D-48149 Münster. Phone: 49-251-8347706; Fax (private): 49-251-846858 E-mail: WAGNEAL@uni-muenster.de Please use the private fax number for corresponding.

Drug Resistance in Leukemia and Lymphoma III, edited by Kaspers *et al.*
Kluwer Academic / Plenum Publishers, New York, 1999.

by rapid adsorption to plastic surfaces (paclitaxel) or isomerisation (etoposide) in RPMI with low FCS content.

The instability of drugs *in vitro* is attributed to a variety of different factors: i.e. physico-chemical instability results in inactivation of oxazaphosphorines, cytarabine dissappears by cellular metabolism without saturation depending on the cell-line. Epiphenomena like adsorption and isomerisation *in vitro* are unphysiological.

Results of drug sensitivity assays should be interpreted with great caution.

2. INTRODUCTION

In vitro drug sensitivity testing of etablished cell lines and of patient samples is a major tool in the preclinical testing of chemotherapeutics. Targeted therapy concepts e.g. of childhood acute leukemia are established on the basis of drug resistance testing such as the 3-[4.5-dimethylthiazol-2-yl]-2.5-diphenyl tetrazolium bromide (MTT) assay (1). The validity of short term total "cell kill" assays like MTT was demonstrated by correlation of *in vitro* results and clinical response in leukemia (2)

Furthermore, clonogenic assays have been considered to be the gold standard for *in vitro* chemosensitivity testing. (3) Nevertheless, results of therapy trials on the basis of *in vitro* assays have been disappointing. Large discrepancies in results among different investigators have prompted cautionary reports against its widespread application in clinical practice.(4) Many aspects of the assay still require technical improvement and standardization.

It is generally assumed that drug concentration does not change significantly under cell culture conditions and the initial drug concentration is often used as if it stayed constant throughout the culture period. Pharmacokinetics of the drug are usually not monitored.

In vivo the efficacy of a given drug depends on pharmacokinetic parameters such as protein binding, distribution volume, clearance, equilibrium constants etc. The calculation of these variables is based on an open system and a steady-state configuration of the individual compartments. As the *in vitro* system is closed those variables, which have been established for most of the substances, are not applicable. Nevertheless, the concentration of the substances applied *in vitro* also changes over time, and, moreover, the medium may be subject to change in that metabolites cannot be further metabolized and accumulate. These unphysiological effects may directly influence the cytotoxic activity in the assay, which in turn might affect the results in terms of their clinical relevance.

Possible *in vitro* pitfalls will have to be evaluated for each drug such that *in vitro* studies of drug exposure will mimic the clinical situation. In order to show models of unphysiological alterations *in vitro* we investigated the concentration versus time curves, the metabolism, the isomerisation and the effects on the culture media and on established cell lines for some frequently used cytostatic drugs, namely activated oxazaphosphorines (4-OOH-cyclophosphamide, 4-OOH-perhydroxyifosfamide and mafosfamide), cytarabine, asparaginase and etoposide.

3. MATERIALS AND METHODS

3.1. Oxazaphosphorines

Activated oxazaphosphorines (cyclohexaminate of mafosfamide, 4-hydroperoxycyclophosphamide, 4-hydroperoxytrofosfamide and 4-hydroperoxyifosfamide) were kindly supported by Asta Medica, Frankfurt, Germany.

Acrolein and trans-2-hexenal as reference substances were obtained from Sigma Chemical Co., St. Louis, USA, HPLC-reagents from Merck, Darmstadt, Gemany (3-aminophenol, hydroxylaminhydrochlorid, hydrochloric acid). The HPLC system consisted of a double piston pump (LKB model 2150 Pharmacia, Sweden) and a fluorescence detector (RF-530 Shimadzu, Duisburg, Germany). For separation a reversed phase Nucleosil C 18 column (5 µm; length: 125 mm; inner diameter: 4 mm) and a 30 mm precolumn of the same packing material were used (Macherey-Nagel, Düren, Germany). RPMI-1640 medium and FCS were obtained from Gibco, BRL, Maryland, USA.

Samples containing RPMI 1640 medium and activated metabolites in various concentrations (1.25 µg/ml, 5 µg/ml and 20 µg/ml) were incubated at 37^0C for 4 days (n = 4). That time corresponds to the average duration of an MTT-assay. Metabolite concentrations were determined by HPLC at times 0h, 1h, 2h, 3h, 4h, 5h, 6h, 7h, 8h, 24h, 48h, 72h, and 96h. The acrolein formed reacts with 3-aminophenol to form 7-OH-quinoline (7-OH-QU), and both can be detected fluorometrically according to methods published elsewhere. (5)

3.2. Cytarabine

Cytosine arabinoside (cytarabine) was obtained from Sigma Chemical Co. St. Louis, USA. The HPLC equipment contained a reversed phase LiChro-Sorb RP-18 column (Merck, Darmstadt, Germany), phosphate buffer (pH = 7, Baker Chemicals) for eluation, UV detector (2141LKB, Pharmacia). K562, HL-60 and BLIN as characterised elsewhere. (6) RPMI-1640 medium and FCS were obtained from Gibco, BRL, Maryland, USA.

Various concentrations of cytosine arabinoside as used in MTT assays by several investigators (7) (0.5 µg/ml, 2.0 µg/ml and 10 µg/ml) were incubated in RPMI-1640 medium containing 20% FCS (n=4) with addition of K562, HL-60 and BLIN (0.5 Mio /ml medium) (n=5) for 2h, 6h, and 24h.

Cytosine arabinoside was measured at time 0 and after 2h, 6h, and 24h by HPLC modified after published methods. (8)

3.3. Asparaginase Activity and Amino Acid Analysis

Asparaginase pharmaceutically graded as E. coli enzyme was obtained from Medac GmbH, Hamburg, Germany, RPMI-1640 medium and fetal calf serum (FCS) from Gibco, BRL, Maryland, USA. Asparaginase was measured by Photometer Novaspec II (Pharmacia LKB, Sweden), ammonium sulfate as reference substance was obtained from Merck (Darmstadt, Germany). Concentrations of asparagine, aspartic acid, glutamine and glutamic acid were determined by RP-HPLC-System (Bromma LKB, Sweden). HPLC reagents were obtained from Merck, Darmstadt (O-phthaldialdehyde, eluant buffers, regenerant buffers, sulfosalicylic acid), Baker Chemicals, Heidelberg, Germany (acetic acid) Carl Roth GmbH (ethanol), Sigma Chemical Co., St. Louis, USA (amino acid standards).

RPMI 1640 medium containing 9% FCS was incubated with various concentrations of asparaginase (2, 200, 2000 and 10.000 U/L) for 1h, 4h, and 24h (n=4). Asparaginase-free medium was incubated and used for comparison. Ammonia release was determined photometrically after addition of Nessler's solution. Further details of the asparaginase assay were published elsewhere. (9)

Pharmacokinetics, i.e., area under data of the concentration versus time curve (0–24h), were calculated by TOPFIT version 2.0, a pharmacokinetic and pharmacodynamic data analysis system for the PC. (10) The AUD of asparaginase substrates and products was related to rising levels of asparaginase.

3.4. Etoposide

Etoposide was obtained as Vepesid® from Bristol Arzneimittel GmbH, Germany, HPLC reagents (high purity water, methanol, acetonitrile and acetic acid) from Baker Chemicals, Germany. The HPLC system consisted of a pump (Model 2248, LKB, Bromma, Sweden), a 20 µl loop (Latek, Germany), a reversed phase LiChro-Sorb RP-18 column (Merck, Germany) and an electrochemical detector (LKB, Pharmacia, Germany).

Etoposide was measured by HPLC. The potential of detection was 0.83 V. At a flow rate of 1ml/min, the retention time was 9.4 min and the limit of detection was 25 ng/ml. Since the isomers of etoposide have equivalent molar extinction coefficients, quantification of cis-etoposide was performed by the same HPLC-system at a retention time of 11.5 min. Details were described elsewhere (11).

Various concentrations of etoposide routinely used in MTT-assays (0.182µg/ml, 1.82 µg/ml and 18.2 µg/ml) were incubated in RPMI medium (+10%FCS) (n=4). Following incubation at 37°C, trans- and cis-etoposide were determined at times 0, 1, 24, 48, 72, and 96 hours.

4. RESULTS

4.1. Oxazaphosphorines

Immediately following the incubation of the activated oxazaphosphorines, concentrations started to decrease. The detectable amount was less than 50% within the first 2–3h. After 6–8 h the concentrations reached a stable level at 10–20% of the initial values. There was no relevant difference between mafosfamide, 4-OOH-cyclophosphamide, 4-OOH-ifosfamide and 4-OOH-trofosfamide (data not shown).

4.2. Cytarabine

Incubation of 10 µg/ml cytarabine with medium alone showed no decrease within 24h. By contrast, when cytarabine was incubated with HL-60 and BLIN, the initial concentration of the medium decreased rapidly, with a detectable amount of less than 50%

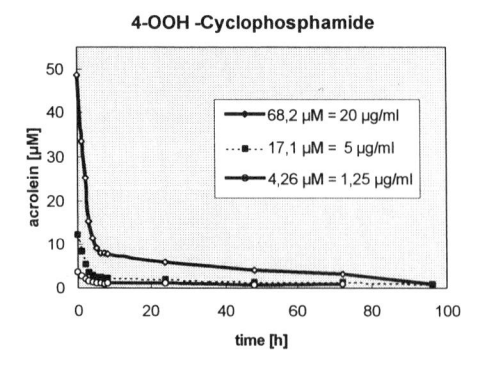

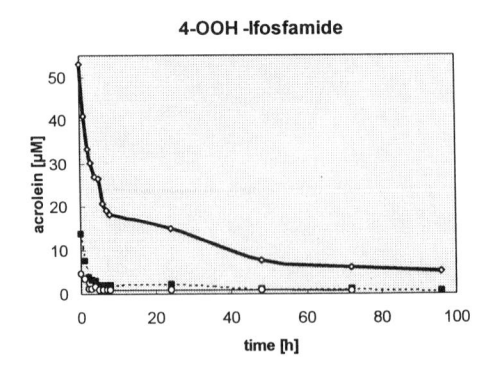

Figure 1. Loss of activated oxazaphosphorines 4-OOH cyclophosphamide und 4–00H-ifosfamide in applied concentrations. No relevant difference of mafosfamide and 4–00H-trofosfamide concerning the decrease within the first hours after incubation in RPMI-medium (data not shown).

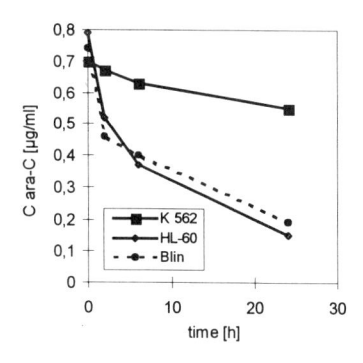

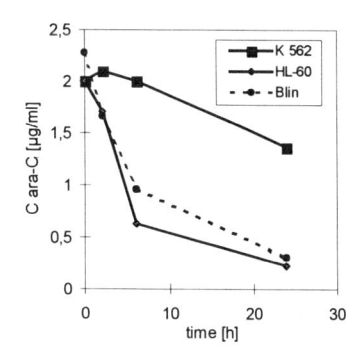

Figure 2. Cytarabine (0.5 μg/ml and 2.0 μg/ml) after incubation in RPMI + 20% FCS in dependence on applied cell culture system. Incubation of 10 μg/ml cytarabine in RPMI showed no decrease within 24h, data not shown. After incubation with HL-60 and BLIN the initial concentration decrease rapidly within 6h. Elimination of high concentrations faster and at a higher extent. In K562, after 24h 80% (0.5 μg/ml) respectively 70% (2 μg/ml) of the initial concentration were still detectable.

within 6h. After 24h, 10–20% of the applied drug could be found in the medium. With high concentrations of cytarabine, the amounts eliminated from the medium appeared to be larger and the elimination rate faster.

In the presence of K562, the disappearance of cytarabine from the medium was not observed. In the low drug concentration assay (0.5μg/ml) 80% of the initial cytarabine concentration was still detectable by HPLC after 24h. When K562 was incubated with 2 μg/ml, 70% of the drug concentration were present after 24h.

4.3. Asparaginase

Without addition of asparaginase the amino acid profile (asparagine, aspartic acid, glutamine, glutamic acid) remained constant throughout the incubation time. At the very low concentration of 2 U/l of asparaginase which is ineffective *in vivo* the medium appeared nearly asparagine-depleted after 4h. Correspondingly, higher levels of aspartic acid were found, but the effect on the glutamine-glutamic acid system was still low. At that time the rise in concentration of ammonia was also still limited. At higher concentrations of asparaginase (200 E/l) the depletion of the medium from asparagine was reached sooner (at about 1h after incubation). Glutamine was desaminated to form glutamic acid and ammonia.

After a 4h incubation time with 10.000 U/L of asp the medium was nearly glutamine-depleted showing high levels of glutamic acid (AUD$_{0-24h}$ > 30 mmol x h/L) and a subsequent dramatic increase of ammonia with AUD$_{0-24h}$.>50 mmol x h/L.

By contrast, the *in vitro* effect of asparaginase on the concentration-time curve of asparagine appeared to be nearly independent of the applied concentrations of asparaginase. The calculated AUDs of aspartic acid from hour 1 to hour 24 after incubation of asparaginase doses >200 U/L were about 10 mmol x h/L.

The activity of asparaginase itself remained constant (data not shown).

4.4. Etoposide

The concentration of trans-etoposide decreased to 50% after 96h of incubation, while the isomer cis-etoposide increased. This isomerisation was not influenced by the amount of FCS in the medium or the initial concentration applied (data not shown).

Table 1. Concentrations [μM/L] of substrates (light columns) and products (shaded columns) of ASNase at different time points related to different concentrations of ASNase (n = 4)

Time [h]	ASNase IU/L	Asparagine μM/L	Aspartic acid μM/L	Glutamine μM/L	Glutamic acid μM/L	Ammonia μM/L
0	0	294	145	1466	183	484
1	0	335	154	1494	194	452
	2	273	198	1511	199	517
	200	0,44	446	1393	222	769
	2000	*0,1	483	1251	491	1086
	10000	*0,1	492	458	1226	2086
4	0	304	149	1498	191	525
	2	89	380	1554	200	780
	200	*0,1	476	1370	419	1019
	2000	*0,1	483	384	1285	2171
	10000	*0,1	557	2,25	1475	2437
24	0	286	162	1414	194	699
	2	0,24	414	1295	189	975
	200	*0,1	463	452	1265	1983
	2000	*0,1	434	2,2	1569	2570
	10000	*0,1	444	*0,1	1579	2486

*Below limit of detection (< 0.1 μM/L)

5. DISCUSSION

The instability of drugs *in vitro* is attributed to a variety of different factors. Physico-chemical instability is related to the inactivation of oxazaphosphorines. All of the therapeutically used oxazaphosphorines (cyclophosphamide, ifosfamide and trofosfamide) are prodrugs and require cellular activation by the mixed-function oxidase system of the liver to form the corresponding 4-hydroxy-derivatives. The activating reaction is hydroxylation at ring position. The 4-OH-metabolites are unstable and therefore cannot be isolated as pure substances. In vitro tests usually use either the hydroperoxides, which hydrolise to form the 4-OH-metabolites in hydrous solutions, or mafosfamide which hydrolyses spontaneously in aqueous solution forming 4-hydroxy-cyclophosphamide.

A 50% loss of activity was apparent after 2–3h incubation of activated putatively stable 4-OH-metabolites in cell culture medium. Thus, a stable concentration x time product of the initial drug probably cannot be established. Those results are in accordance with

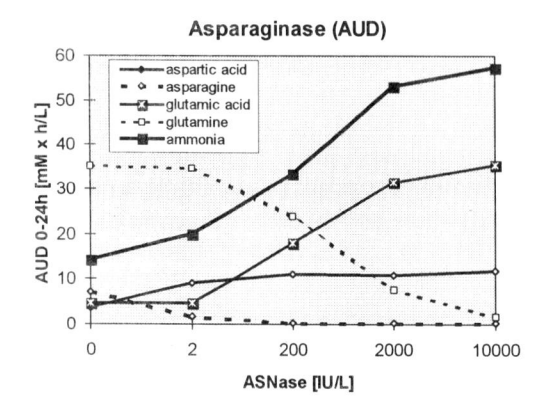

Figure 3. AUD's (area under the data of the concentration-time-curve, 0–24 h) of ASNase-substrates asparagine and glutamine and products aspartic acid, glutamic acid and ammonia [mM x h/L] after incubation with rising levels of ASNase (0–10000 IU/L). AUD was calculated by using the linear trapezoidal rule.

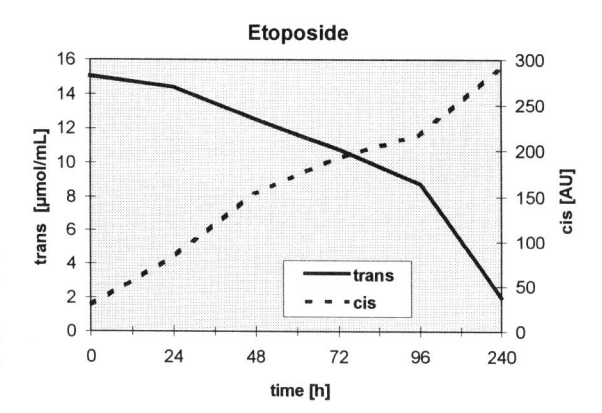

Figure 4. Decrease of trans-Etoposide (18,2 µMol/mL) and increase of cis-Etoposide (arbitrary units) after incubation in RPMI. Isomerisation not influenced by the applied initial concentration of parent etoposide or the amount of FCS (data not shown).

findings from *in vitro* stability assays of mafosfamide previously reported by other investigators. They observed *in vitro* degradation of mafosfamide within 30 minutes. As a consequence the duration of exposure to mafosfamide in pre-incubation-tests (PIT) and clinical purging of patients' bone marrow has been limited. (12)

Drug resistance in cell culture systems after 4h incubation and subsequent MTT-assay according to *Pieters et al* may thus be attributed to overly short exposure to relevant cytotoxic concentrations of the antineoplastic drug. (13)

In vitro drug sensitivity testing of ALL cells with mafosfamide for example was done in concentrations ranging from 0.098 to 100µg/ml. The leukemic samples were incubated for 4 days following one single application of mafosfamide, so that, strictly speaking, the LC 50 values of mafosfamide simply cannot be related to the 96h interval. The evidence regarding incubation times and clinically achievable concentrations as well as guidelines defining the AUC or dose scheduling of oxazaphosphorines on the basis of *in vitro* cytotoxicity assays becomes artificial.

The cellular metabolism of drugs is another example for unphysiological in vitro-effects. Obviously the stability of cytarabine depends on the particular cell culture system applied *in vitro*. Cytarabine may undergo cellular metabolism and decrease *in vitro*.

There is no general evidence of a constant level of cytarabine during the 96h incubation time. BLIN and HL-60 might appear resistant because of their high cellular turnover rate *in vitro*. *In vivo* this effect could probably be overcome by using continous infusion rather than the intravenous bolus application of cytarabine. Before the incubation the stability of the particular cytotoxic agents that will be applied should therefore be tested with each cell line.

Furthermore, the interpretation of *in vitro* results may have additional pitfalls originating from the unphysiological alteration of the culture medium by active enzymes such as asparaginase.

Asparaginase is an enzyme that is widely used in the therapy of acute lymphocytic leukemias and lymphomas. It catabolizes asparagine to form aspartic acid and ammonia. When there is no asparagine available in the plasma, malignant lymphoblastic cells, in contradistinction to normal and most malignant cells, are probably unable to synthesize asparagine by asparagine synthetase. The lack of externally available asparagine causes a block in protein synthesis and subsequent apoptotic death. (14)

In vitro, maintenance levels of asparaginase catabolize the available amount of asparagine which cannot be replenished. Besides, the inherent glutaminase activity which accounts for 3–5% of the asparaginase activity results in desamination of glutamine to glutamic acid and ammonia, which is of minor importance *in vivo*. (15)

In vitro changes in the amino acid pattern of the medium even extend beyond the asparagine depletion. The dose-response relationship between the asparaginase activity and related substrates and products exceeds the effect on asparagine. Toxic levels of asparaginase products like glutamic acid and ammonia are reached even at low concentrations of asparaginase, while the depletion of glutamine is more pronounced *in vitro* than *in vivo*.

Drug sensitivity assays of leukemic cells from children and normal peripheral blood lymphocytes using the MTT assay usually involve concentrations of asparaginase between 3 and 10000 U/l. Cells were suspended in RPMI medium containing 2mM L-glutamine and 20% FCS. The LC_{50} for peripheral leukemic cells was about 200 U/l, for bone marrow cells about 360 U/l. (16). At this dosage the area under data curves (0–24h) of ammonia and glutamic acid increased exponentially. The aspartic acid curve rose steadily up to a concentration of 200 U/l asparaginase in the incubation medium, and, after asparagine-depletion was complete, reached a plateau due to the unavailability of asparagine.

In vivo, continuously high levels of glutamic acid and ammonia are not observed because the products are metabolized by the organism. (9)

Further, a lack of substrates, namely glutamine, occurs *in vitro*. The extent of the glutamine decrease exceeds the decrease observed in patients with any dose of asparaginase, where the glutamine-depletion is largely compensated by the hepatic glutamine synthetase.

The contribution of various changes in the amino acid pattern of the medium to the cytotoxic effect remains unclear. Asselin and coworkers have recently suggested that the *in vitro* sensitivity to asparaginase of lymphoblasts from patients correlates with their short term outcome. (17)

However, clinical trials have failed to establish a clear dose response relationship. (18). Between concentrations of 0.0001 and 0.1U/ml asparaginase the *in vitro* killing of leukemia cells was independent of the concentration. At 1.0 U/ml, the MTT assay showed a further increase in cytotoxic activity, which suggests that the addition of asparaginase may be responsible for some additional *in vitro* mechanism of cell killing other than asparagine depletion. Neither glutamine nor glutamic acid, aspartic acid or ammonia were determined in these studies. The additional cytotoxic effect may be due to the unphysiological pattern of substrates and products of asparaginase.

An evaluation of the mechanism of asparaginase cytotoxicity *in vitro* based on a specified amino acid composition of the medium is warranted. The reduction of available substrates for asparaginase may cause a reduction of potentially cytotoxic products. However, one has to be aware that growth does need a certain minimum amount of amino acids. For the time being, results of *in vitro* cytotoxicity assays involving asparaginase should be interpreted with caution.

The isomerisation to form compounds of different activity is another possible mechanism of degradation under cell culture conditions. According to *Mader et al.* and coworkers the degradation of *trans*-etoposide to its isomer *cis*-etoposide is rapid under cell culture conditions. (19) By contrast, stock solutions of etoposide remain stable for several weeks. (20) Clonogenic assays showed the IC_{50} of *cis*-etoposide to be 100-fold higher than that of *trans*-etoposide. (21) Isomerisation within the extended incubation time of colony forming assays has also been observed by other investigators. (22)

According to our own results, 50 % of the parent *trans*-isomer transforms into the *cis*-isomer within 96h. Under different culture conditions *Mader et al* observed a loss of

90% of the active drug within 1 week, which corresponds to the average incubation time of clonogenic assays. They showed that the degradation is influenced by the pH-value and the ionic strenght of the medium, not by organic compounds.

In analogy to this phenomenon detailed work of our group has shown that the incubation of retinoic acids under cell culture conditions results in rapid non-enzymatic isomerisation which generates retinoid acid isomers that exert different effects due to different receptor affinities. (23)

A review of the literature reveals additional pitfalls of *in vitro* studies. There is, for example, evidence of instability of paclitaxel (taxol) by adsorption to the surface of applied cell-culture material and a saturable protein binding. (24)

After 19h of incubation in 1% methanolic aqueous solution, paclitaxel decreased to about 40% in glass tubes and to 67% in polypropylene tubes, independent of the initial concentration of 0.18 or 1.8µg/mL. The concentration of taxol declined to 73% in polystyrene tissue culture plates with Dulbeccos modified eagle medium without fetal bovine serum (FBS), while no such decline was detectable after addition of 9% FBS. Obviously, the lower extent and saturability of protein binding of taxol in FBS-containing culture medium differed from that in human plasma.

Several investigators performed clonogenic assays in order to define the dose-response relationship of paclitaxel. (25) According to results of *Song et al.* the numerous differences in the protein binding and hence the differences in pharmacologically active, free drug concentrations under the two conditions need to be considered when extrapolating *in vitro* data to an *in vivo* situation. Monitoring the actual concentration of free drug throughout the incubation time instead of working with the initial total concentration may help to overcome the problem of false conclusions from *in vitro* data. In this context, one should also consider the potential effect of solvents. *In vitro*, paclitaxel is used both in pure form dissolved in DMSO and dissolved in cremophor. Cremophor which belongs to the group of chemosensitizers most possibly exerts an additional cytotoxic effect via MDR modulation by competitive blocking of the MDR binding sites for P-glycoprotein (26) This in turn leads to the intracellular accumulation of cytotoxic agents. Those effects are observed both *in vitro* and *in vivo*, but they differ in intensity depending on the particular cell line used. According to own unpublished results, cremophor in low concentrations seems to be cytotoxic itself. In MTT-assays, cultured Ewing's sarcoma cells (VH-64) were killed by the solvent cremophor in concentrations $\geq 0.0075\%$ (corresponding to a final concentration of paclitaxel ≥ 1 µM) after 24 hour incubation. Evidently, at relevant concentrations, cremophor produced a similar inhibition effect as the active drug paclitaxel.

The lipophilic detergent Tween 80, a polyethylene glycol which is commonly used as a solvent for etoposide, probably acts by the same mechanism of MDR modulation as cremophor.(27) Previous investigations of our group using the MTT test on several neuroblastoma cell lines revealed the solvent to be as toxic as the pure substance etoposide. (28)

Other substances respond to effects of the *in vitro* situation as such. The stability of anthracyclincs e.g. clearly appears related to temperature and light conditions. Under typical in vitro conditions a significant loss of anthracyclines occurred over short incubation periods. For example, 48h incubation at 39°C of 10 µg/ml doxorubicin (DOX) in rabbit plasma results in complete disappearance of the initial fluorescence as determined by NP HPLC, whereas less than 25% of the parent drug was degraded at 4°C. (29) When samples were protected from light, degradation was slightly slowed. In anthracyclines the decrease is possibly due to an increase of apolar compounds. (30)

In conclusion, the instability of drugs under *in vitro* conditions is attributed to a variety of different factors. Physico-chemical instability may result in inactivation of oxazaphosphorines, cytosine arabinoside probably disappears by cellular metabolism depending on the cell-line, and isomerisation may be responsible for decreasing levels of trans-etoposide. Active enzymes (i.e., asparaginase) may lead to unphysiological alterations of the culture medium because enzyme products or metabolites cannot be eliminated by the *in vitro* system and may continue to exert their probably cytotoxic effects. There is evidence of some other possible mechanisms like binding to surfaces of cell culture materials and unphysiological protein binding (paclitaxel) or rapid degradation to form detoxified products due to various conditions of the culture like temperature and light (anthracyclines), all of which result in the instability of anticancer agents under *in vitro* conditions.

In summary, results of *in vitro* cytotoxicity assays may be helpful with respect to responsiveness, but should be interpreted with caution and should not immediately be translated into clinical decisions.

AKNOWLEDGMENTS

The authors wish to thank Gabriele Braun-Munzinger for editing the manuscript.

REFERENCES

1. Pieters R., Loonen A.H:, Huismans D.R., Broekema G.J., Dirven M.W.J., Heyenbrok M.W.,Hählen K., Veerman A.J.P. *In vitro* drug sensitivity of cells from children with leukemia using the MTT assay with improved culture conditions. Blood 1990, 76, 2327–2336
2. Pieters R., Kaspers G.J.L., van Wering E.R., Huismans D.R., Loonen A.H:, Hählen K., Veerman A.J.P. Cellular drug resistance profiles that might explain the prognostic value of immunophenotype and age in childhood acute lymphoblastic leukemia. Leukemia 1993, 7, 392–397
3. Weisenthal, L.M., Lippmann,M.E.: Clonogenic and nonclonogenic *in vitro* chemosensitivity assays. Cancer Treat Rep 1993 69:615–624
4. Selby, P, Buick R.N., Tannock I.A.A., A critical appraisal of the "human tumor-stem cell assay" N Engl J Med 1983, 308:129–134
5. Boos J., Küpker F., Blaschke G, Jürgens H. Trofosfamide metabolism in different species-ifosfamide is the predominant metabolite. Cancer Chemother Pharmacol 1993, 33: 71–76
6. Wörmann B, Anderson JM, Liberty JA, Gajl-Peczalska K, Brunning RD, Silbermann TL, Arthur DC, LeBien TW. Establishment of a leukemic cell modell for studying human pre-B to B cell differentiation. J Immunol 1989, 142: 110–117
7. Kaspers, G.J.L., Veerman A.J.P., Pieters R., Broekema G.J., Huismans D.R., Kazmier K.M., Loonen A.H., Rottier M.A.A., Van Zantwijk C.H., Hählen K., Van wering E.R. Mononuclear cells contaminating acute lymphoblastic leukaemic samples tested for cellular drug resistance using the methyl-thiazol-tetrazolium assay. Br J Cancer, 1994, 70:1047–1052
8. Woollard, G.A. An unusual column effect during analysis of 5-fluorocytosine by high-performance liquid chromatography. J of Chromatogr 1986, 368: 162–163
9. Boos J, Werber G, Ahlke E, Schultze-Westhoff P, Nowak-Göttl U, Würthwein G, Verspohl EJ, Ritter J, Jürgens H. Monitoring of asparaginase activities and asparagine levels in children on different asparaginase preparations. Eur J Cancer 1996, 32: 1544–50
10. Heinzel G, Woloszcak R and Thomann P. Dr. Karl Thomae GmbH, Schering AG, Gödecke AG, Stuttgart;Jena; New York G. Fischer, 1993
11. Liliemark, E., Petterson B, Peterson C., Liliemark J. High-performance liquid chromatography with fluorometric detection for monitoring of etoposide and its cis-isomer in plasma and leukaemic cells. J of chromatography B: biomedical applications 1995, 669:311–317
12. Sindermann, H, Peukert M, Hilgard P. Bone marrow purging with mafosfamide- A critical survey. Blut 1989, 59:432–441

13. Pieters, R., Loonen A.H:, Huismans D.R., Broekema G.J., Dirven M.W.J., Heyenbrok M.W.,Hählen K., Veerman A.J.P. *In vitro* drug sensitivity of cells from children with leukemia using the MTT assay with improved culture conditions. Blood, 1990, 76, 2327–2336
14. Capizzi R. L., Bertino J.R., Skeel R.T., Creasey W.A., Zanes R., Olayon C., Peterson R.G., Handschumacher R.E. L-Asparaginase: clinical, biochemical, pharmacological and immunological studies. Ann Intern Med 1971, 74, 893–904
15. Cooney DA, Handschumacher RE L-asparaginase and L-asparagine metabolism. Annu Rev Pharmacol 1970, 10, 421–440
16. Kaspers G.J.L., Pieters R., Van Zantwijk C.H., De Laat P.A.J.M., De Waal F.C., Van Wering, Veerman A.J.P. *In vitro* drug sensitivity of normal peripheral blood lymphocytes and childhood leukaemic cells from bone marrow and peripheral blood. Br J Cancer 1991, 64, 469–474
17. Asselin, BL, Ryan D, Frantz CN, Bernal SD, Leavitt P, Sallan SE and Cohen HJ. *In vitro* and *in vivo* killing of acute lymphoblastic leukemia cells by Asparaginase. Cancer Res 1989, 49, 4363–4371
18. Ertel IJ, Nesbit ME, Hammond D, Weiner J and Sather H. Effective dose of Asparaginase for induction of remission in previously treated children with acute lymphoblastic leukemia: a report from Childrens Cancer Study Group Cancer Res. 1979, 39, 3893–3896
19. Mader R.M., Steger, GG, Moser K, Rainer H., Krenmayr P.,Dittrich C. Instability of the anticancer agent etoposide under *in vitro* culture conditions, Cancer Chemother Pharmacol 1991, 27, 354–360
20. Yang L.Y., Drewinko B. Cytotoxic efficacy of reconstituted and stored antitumor agents. Cancer Res 1985, 45, 1511–1515
21. Evans W.E., Sinkule J.A:, Crom W.R., Dow L.W., Look A.T., Rivera G.Pharmacokinetics of teniposide (VM 26) and etoposide (VP 16) in children with cancer. Cancer Chemother Pharmacol 1982, 7, 147–150
22. Ludwig R., Alberts D.S., Chemical and biological stability of anticancer drugs used in a human tumor clonogenic assay. Cancer Chemother Pharmacol 1984, 12, 142–145
23. Lanvers C, Jürgens H, Blaschke G., Boos J. Non-enzymatic isomerisation of retinoic acids during incubation in RPMI 1640 medium. poster presented at 9th NCI-EORTC Symposium on New Drugs in Cancer Therapy, 1996
24. Song, D., Hsu, L.-F., Jessie, L.-S. Binding of taxol to plastic and glass containers and protein under *in vitro* conditions, J Pharm Sci 1996, 85, 29–31
25. Liebmann JE, Cook, J.A., Lipschultz C., Teague D., Fisher J., Mitchell JB. Cytotoxic studies of paclitaxel (Taxol) in human tumour cell lines. Br J Cancer 1993, 68, 1104–1109
26. Ross, D.D., Wooten P.J., Tong Y., Cornblatt B., Levy C., Sridhara R., Lee E.J., Schiffer C.A. Synergistic reversal of multidrug-resistance phenotype in acute myeloid leukemia cells by cyclosporin A and cremophor EL. Blood 1994, 83, 1337–1347
27. Dudeja P.K., Anderson, K.M., Harris J.S., Buckingham L., Coon J.S. Reversal of multidrug resistance phenotype by surfactants: relationship to membrane lipid fluidity. Arch Biochem Biophys 1995, 319, 309–315
28. Fulda S., Honer, M., Menke-Moellers,I, Berthold,F. Antiproliferative potential of cytostatic drugs on neuroblastoma cells *in vitro*. Eur J Cancer 1995, 31, 616–621
29. Beijnen JH, Wiese G, Underberg WJ Aspects of the chemical stability of Doxorubicin and seven ohter anthracyclines in acidic solution. Pharm Weekbl Sci 1985, 7, 109–116
30. Bachur NR, Gee M, Daunorubicin metabolism by rat tissue preparations. J Pharmacol Exp Ther 1971, 177, 567–572

43

DOWN SYNDROME AND ACUTE MYELOID LEUKEMIA

Lessons Learned from Experience with High-Dose Ara-C Containing Regimens

Yaddanapudi Ravindranath* and Jeffrey W. Taub

Children's Hospital of Michigan
Barbara Ann Karmanos Cancer Institute
Wayne State University
Detroit, Michigan

INTRODUCTION

Down Syndrome (DS) children have a 10- to 20-fold increase in both acute lymphocytic leukemia and acute myeloid leukemia.[1,2] Prior studies with conventional dose regimens have shown that the outcome for DS children with AML is same as those without DS.[3]

In December 1990, at the combined meeting of the International Society of Hematology and the 32nd Meeting of the American Society of Hematology in Boston, we reported that all twelve children with Down Syndrome and Acute Myeloid Leukemia (AML) treated on a high-dose Ara-C containing protocol survived, disease-free, 3+ years compared to a 33% survival in 273 patients without Down Syndrome treated on the same POG # 8498 protocol.[4,5] Since then, there has been a lively debate about: (1) who should get credit for the first observations of improved survival of Down Syndrome children treated on current regimen; (2) is the AML in Down Syndrome children really AML, and not a myelodysplastic syndrome; and (3) what is the biochemical basis for the improved response in Down Syndrome children compared to non-Down Syndrome children. I would like to set the record straight, although I am fully aware that there will be arguments and counter-arguments. Professor Sverre Lie from Oslo made an anecdotal reference to the improved outcome of Down children with AML treated on the high-dose protocols of the Nordic studies in his review on AML published in

---

*Correspondence to: Y. Ravindranath, M.D. Children's Hospital of Michigan 3901 Beaubien Boulevard Detroit MI 48201 USA

the *European Journal of Paediatrics* in 1989.[6] However, the importance of this observation was not recognized fully as Levitt, Stiller, and Chessels—in their 1990 review on Down Syndrome and acute leukemia—did not reference to these observations. In May 1990, at the American Society of Clinical Oncology meeting, Dr. B. Lampkin, in presenting the data on CCG 213 trial, made a casual observation that Down Syndrome children had a better outcome than the non-DS children, but this was not included in the abstract of the paper.[7] It was left, then, to a relative neophyte in AML to bring to focus the unique sensitivity of AML in DS children, particularly to the high-dose Ara-C containing regimens.[1,2] The publication of the results presented in the ASH abstract, however, proved somewhat difficult to publish as the manuscript was summarily rejected by *Lancet*. During the course of the next year or so, I was challenged by B. Lampkin ("what are *they* (DS children) teaching us"), and by Professor Riehm, asking me for a hypothesis for the superior outcome. In searching for this hypothesis, first, my associate Dr. Jeffrey W. Taub, pointed out the possible role of cystathionine B-synthase in the well-known susceptibility of DS children to Methotrexate. Since at the same time, our institution was participating in a POG pilot study of Methotrexate induced modulation of Ara-C metabolism, I was able to put together a hypothesis that, in effect, DS cells are primed for Ara-C toxicity on account of the altered reduced folate pools and the consequent reduction in deoxycytidine triphosphate. The results of our experience and the hypothesis were then published in 1992.[2] In the course of the next few minutes, you will see that the improved sensitivity to chemotherapy in DS children is more complex, and perhaps more generic and is linked to the well-known increase in reactive oxygen radical generation and the consequent apoptosis.[8] But, first, to our initial hypothesis on the Ara-C metabolism.

BIOCHEMICAL BASIS FOR THE ENHANCED RESPONSE TO CHEMOTHERAPY IN DS

The inter-relationships of increased activity of CBS, folate B12 metabolism and Ara-C phosphorylation are summarized in Figure 1.

1. Cytarabine Metabolism

Both deoxycytidine and Ara-C are phosphorylated by deoxycytidine kinase. Deoxycytidine kinase is subject to feedback inhibitory regulation of deoxycytidine triphosphate (dCTP). Therefore, if dCTP levels are decreased, either endogenously as it occurs in DS, or by methotrexate-mediated inhibition of deoxycytidine synthesis, or by inhibition of ribonucleotide reductase by agents such as hydroxyurea, fludarabine, or gemcytidine, deoxycytidine kinase is released from this feedback inhibition, and therefore, there is the potential for increased generation of Ara-C triphosphate.

2. Why Should There Be Decreased Deoxycytidine Triphosphate Pools in DS?

There are two potential mechanisms; (a) increased activity of CBS, by reducing the generation of tetrahydrofolate, results in a decreased synthesis of deoxythymidine triphosphatse (dTTP). Low dTTP levels release the inhibition of deoxycytidine deaminase, thereby resulting in increased deamination of dCMP, and therefore, low levels of dCTP ensue; (b) a second potential affect of increased CBS is the decreased formation of s-adenosyl-methionine which may result in a non-specific hypomethylation of several genes in-

Table 1. Down syndrome and acute myeloid leukemia

Time interval (in days) between courses of treatment on pog 8821[*]			
DAT–HDA	HDA–VP/AZ	VP/AZ–DHDA	DHDA-DAT
DS			
34	35	28	35
(14–48)	(20–45)	(18–60)	(21–79)
Non-DS			
26	26	34	28
(14–60)	(19–53)	(18–53)	(20–52)

Values are median and range.
DAT = Daunorubicin 45 mg/M^2/day, Days 1-3
　　　Cytarabine 100 mg/M^2/day, Days 1-7
　　　6-Thioguanine 100 mg/M^2/day, Days 1-7
DHDA = Daunorubicin 45 mg/M^2, Day 1, and DHA as above
HDA = Cytarabine 3 gm/M^2 q 12 hrs × 6 doses
VP/AZ = Etoposide 250 mg/M^2, Days 1-3
　　　　5-AZ 350 mg/M^2, Days 4-5
[*]Treatment results published in Y. Ravindranath, et al. New Engl J Med 334:1478, 1996.

cluding the genes for deoxycytidine kinase and therefore up-regulation of the transcription of deoxycytidine kinase. Work by Jeffrey Taub in our institution clearly shows that this hypothesis of endogenous modulation of Ara-C metabolism is valid as, our data show, that deoxycytidine triphosphate pools are lower in DS cell lines and DS patients with AML compared to diploid cell lines in other AML patients.[8]

3. Is High-Dose Ara-C Necessary for the AML Treatment in DS Children?

The observations of Slørdahl and Lie from the Nordic countries,[9] and from Creutzig et al. from the BFM group[10] are of interest in this regard. Thirteen of seventeen DS children treated with high-dose Ara-C containing regimens in the NOPHO studies are alive, disease-free, 5–89+ months, while in contrast only 2 of 8 patients treated with other protocols are alive. There were no survivors in the untreated DS children with AML. Similar observations were made by Creutzig et al., from the BFM group. It is important, however, to recognize there is generalized increased toxicity with treatment in DS children (see Table 1). Counts recovery and the timing of the next course are generally delayed in DS children. Therefore, it is critical that DS children be given vigorous supportive care, and one should recognize that full counts recovery be permitted prior to initiation of the next chemotherapy course in order to prevent serious infectious complications.

4. Is the Increased Chemo-Sensitivity in DS Multifactorial?

Subsequent to our publication of the 1992 Blood manuscript, Kojima et al. from Japan[11] reported on the long survival of six of seven children with DS treated with multiple courses of conventional-dose 3+7 regimens of anthracycline and Ara-C, and Ara-C plus Etoposide. Subsequent studies by us have clearly shown that in in vitro cytotoxicity studies using the MTT assay (pioneered by the hosts of this conference), DS myeloblasts show enhanced sensitivity not only to cytarabine but also to daunorubicin.[12] Our studies have shown that in DS children, the mean IC50 value for Ara-C is 66 nmol compared to 550 nmol in non-DS children, and the IC50 values for daunorubicin are 8.2 nmol versus 187 nmol in non-DS children, with both differences being highly significant with p values less than 0.001. We have not done any studies with MTT cytotoxicity studies with VP-16.

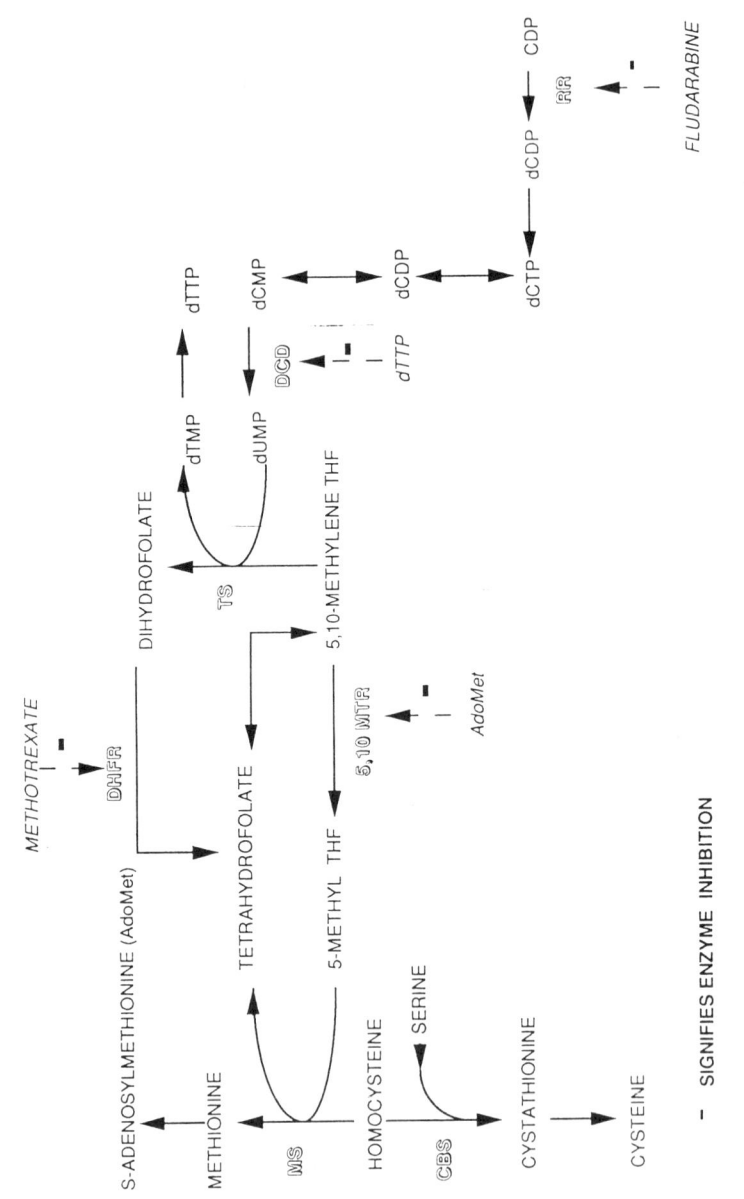

Figure 1. Inter-relationship of folate metabolism and deoxynucleotides.

5. What Is the Linkage of Sensitivity to Daunorubin and Ara-C; Is It Linked to Genes on Chromosome 21?

In addition to cystathionine b-synthase, the genes for superoxide dismutase (SOD) and carbonyl reductase (CBR) are both localized to 21q 22.1. CBR catalyzes the reduction of daunorubicin to daunorubicinol which is generally considered to be more potent in producing oxygen-free radicals than the primary drug. While SOD should normally result in detoxification of oxygen radicals, low levels of increased expression are associated with actually increased generation of hydroxyl radicals, the most toxic of the oxygen radicals species. Data exists in bacterial systems that transfection with superoxide dismutase may be associated with increased susceptibility to cytotoxicity.[13] Up to 9-fold increase in SOD in resealed ghosts of RBC did not protect against methenoglobin generation and membrane damage when superoxide generation was induced.[14] Thus, increased activity of SOD in the absence of a concomitant increase in enzymatic degradation of H_2O_2 (e.g. catalase) will result in increased production of free oxygen radicals and additional cellular damage. Suppression of membrane phospholipid synthesis a significant component of cytotoxicity for Ara-C.[15] Thus, it is possible that increased activity of both SOD and CBR might further enhance the cytotoxic effect of daunorubicin and Ara-C and enhance the synergy of the two drugs given in combination.[12,16]

6. What Are the Differences in Constitutional Trisomy 21 versus Acquired Trisomy 21?

Cortes et al.[17] from M.D. Anderson reported in 1995 about the lack of a superior outcome in adult AML patients with acquired Trisomy 21, observations later confirmed in pediatric patients by CCG[18] and POG data.[19] Preliminary studies[20] of relative transcript levels of chromosome 21 localized genes have shown that cystathionine B-synthase, superoxide dismutase, and carbonyl reductase were 9.4, 7.1, and 1.8 fold higher is DS myeloblasts compared to non-DS cases. This differential expression was unexpected, and mechanisms for the same remain to be elucidated. Similar studies need to be conducted in patients with acquired Trisomy 21 determine the mechanisms of lack of a superior clinical response given the same regimens.

SUMMARY

AML in DS children is uniquely sensitive to cytarabine and daunorubicin.

- This increased sensitivity is apparently linked to increased gene dosage effect of certain key enzymes localized to chr 21q22.1–22.3 — cystationine beta synthase, superoxide dismutase and carbonyl reductase.
- There appears to be a differential expression of these enzymes.
- The increased expression of superoxide dismutase several fold over that expected from gene dosage effect alone may lead to excess free oxygen radical generation and subsequent cellular damage.

Lessons from Down Syndrome Children

Experience with DS children has started a new way to look at chromosomal events and their impact on the metabolism of critical drugs. Thus, understanding the drug metabolism in good prognosis cytogenetic subgroups of leukemia, may lead to the development of improved therapeutic strategies. Some examples are:

1. Modulation of Ara-C and daunorubicin metabolism in constitutional Trisomy 21: is there a role for gene hypomethylation and if so, explore further the role of agents such as 5-azacytidine.
2. Why is there not improved response in acquired Trisomy 21 AML—what is the role of AML1 gene in constitutional versus acquired Trisomy 21,and what are the differences in the transcription of CBS, SOD, and CBR in acquired versus constitutional Trisomy 21.
3. What is the basis for the improved response to high-dose Ara-C in t(8;21)—is the translocation associated with *cis* activation of CBS, SOD and CBR, or is it transactivation of these genes by the hybrid AML1 - ETO fusion product.

These are but some of the possible avenues for research, which should further help us in designing new and better ways of therapy for childhood leukemias.

ACKNOWLEDGMENTS

This manuscript is based on an invited presentation (by Y. Ravindranath) at the 3rd International Symposium on Drug Resistance in Leukemia and Lymphoma, March 4–7, 1998, Amsterdam. The work is supported in part by grants to Y. Ravindranath from Leukemia, Research, Life, Inc. (Detroit); Pediatric Oncology Group (POG) Novel New Initiatives Program (NCI-CA-29691), and grants to J. Taub from Children's Cancer Research Fund, and Leukemia Society of America (6203-98). Ms. Julie Nucci prepared this manuscript.

REFERENCES

1. Robison L. Leukemia 6:5,1992.
2. Zipursky A, Thorner P, DeHarven E, Christensen H, Doyle J. Leuk Res 18:163, 1964.
3. Levitt GA, Stiller CA, Chessells JM. Arch Dis Child 65:212–216, 1990.
4. Ravindranath Y, Abella E, Krischer J, et al. Blood 76 (suppl. 1):311a, abstract # 1235, 1990.
5. Ravindranath Y, Abella E, Krischer JP, et al. Blood 80:2210–2214, 1992.
6. Lie SO. European J Paediatrics 148:382–388, 1989.
7. Lampkin B, Wells R, Woods W, et al. Proceed of ASCO 9:216, abstract # 834, 1990.
8. Taub JW, Matherly LH, Stout ML, Buck S, Gurvey J, Ravindranath Y. Blood 87:3395–3403, 1996.
9. Slordahl SH, Gustaffsson G, Janmundsson E, Mellander L, Siimes MA, Yssing M, Lie SO. Med Ped Oncol 20:373, abstract # P-10, 1992.
10. Creutzig CL, Ritter J, Vormorj WD, Niemeyer E, Reinsich I, Stohlmann-Gibbels B, Zimmerman M, Harlott J. Leukemia 10:1677, 1996.
11. Kojima S, Kato K, Matsuyama T, Yoshikawa T, Honibe K. Blood 81:3164, 1993.
12. Taub JW, Stout ML, Buck SA, Juang XI, Vega RA, Becton DL, Ravindranath Y. Leukemia 11:1594,1997.
13. Scott MD, Meshnick SR, Eaton JW. J Biol Chemi 262:3640–45, 1987.
14. Scott MD, Eaton JW, Kuypers FA, Chiu DT, Lubin BH. Blood 74:2542–49,1989.
15. Kucera GL, Capizzi EL. Cancer Res 52:3886, 1992.
16. Taub JW, Ravindranath Y. Bailliere's Clin Haematol 9:129, 1996.
17. Cortes JE, Kantarjian H, O'Brien S, Keating M, Pierce S, Freireich EJ, Estey E. Leukemia 9:115–1157, 1995.
18. Lange BJ, Kobrinsky N, Barnard DR, Arthur DC, Buckley JD, Howells WB, Gold S, Sanders J, Neudorf S, Smith FO, Woods WG. Blood 91:608–615, 1998.
19. Ravindranath Y, Chang M, Weinstein H. Unpublished data.
20. Taub JW, Huang XI, Stout ML, Buck S, Massey G, Becton D, Matherly LH, Ravindranath Y. Blood 90 (suppl. 1):496a, abstract # 2212, 1997.

44

CELLULAR DRUG RESISTANCE IN CHILDHOOD ACUTE MYELOID LEUKEMIA

A Mini-Review with Emphasis on Cell Culture Assays

G. J. L. Kaspers,[*] Ch. M. Zwaan, R. Pieters, and A. J. P. Veerman

Department of Pediatric Hematology/Oncology
University Hospital Vrije Universiteit
De Boelelaan 1117, 1081 HV Amsterdam, The Netherlands

Keywords: Acute myeloid leukemia, childhood, drug resistance, review, cytarabine, anthracyclines.

1. ABSTRACT

Cellular drug resistance is an important limiting factor in the success of chemotherapy in childhood acute myeloid leukemia (AML). We summarize the results of the studies published sofar that have focussed on drug resistance in childhood AML, using cell culture assays. We also briefly report our own results of an ongoing study. Finally, potential applications of cellular drug resistance testing are discussed. It appears that cellular drug resistance differs between AML and acute lymphoblastic leukemia and between subgroups of AML patients, that AML cells of relapsed patients are more resistant to cytarabine than those of untreated patients, and that in vitro resistance to cytarabine and daunorubicin is related to a worse prognosis. However, more and larger studies are required to determine the exact role of cellular drug resistance testing in the treatment of childhood AML.

---

[*] Phone: +31 - 20 444 2420; Fax: +31 - 20 444 2422; E-mail: gjl.kaspers@azvu.nl

Drug Resistance in Leukemia and Lymphoma III, edited by Kaspers *et al.*
Kluwer Academic / Plenum Publishers, New York, 1999.

2. INTRODUCTION

Despite major improvements, chemotherapy is not as successful in childhood acute myeloid leukemia (AML) as it is in childhood acute lymphoblastic leukemia (ALL). Overall survival for AML is about 50%, in contrast to up to 80% in case of ALL.[1–3] Considering the causes of unsuccessful chemotherapy, three factors emerge.[4,5] Firstly, the pharmacokinetics of the drugs administered, which determines the extent of drug exposure of the leukemic cells. Secondly, the cellular resistance of the leukemic cells: are leukemic cells eradicated upon the drug exposure. Finally, the capacity of (minimal) residual leukemic cells to give a relapse: regrowth resistance. There is a surprising lack of knowledge about cellular drug resistance in childhood AML. The studies that have been done focussed on cell culture drug resistance testing, mechanisms of resistance, and modulation or circumvention of resistance. In this review, we will summarize the data available with regard to cell culture drug resistance testing, including own preliminary observations. In addition, we will discuss its possible applications.

3. CELL CULTURE DRUG RESISTANCE ASSAYS

These assays can be divided into those that study inhibition of proliferation (e.g. clonogenic and thymidine incorporation assays) and those that study the total leukemic cell population.[6,7] The latter concern either apoptosis assays or total cell kill assays. Clonogenic assays have mainly been used in the past, because of the assumption that it is most important to study the inhibition of mitosis of clonogenic cells by anticancer agents. However, the results of clonogenic assays have never been shown to be superior to those of non-clonogenic assays. Therefore, and because clonogenic assays are labour-intensive, they are now used less often. Apoptosis is a new field of intensive research, and all sorts of assays have been adapted to determine the extent of drug-induced apoptosis. Examples are flowcytometry (Annexine V with propidium iodide staining, the TdT-mediated dUTP nick end labeling [TUNEL] assay, DNA histogram analysis), DNA fragmentation analysis, and morphology. Total cell kill assays have become quite popular.[6] The methyl-thiazol-tetrazolium (MTT) assay, the differential staining cytotoxicity (DiSC) assay and the fluorometric cytotoxicity assay (FMCA) are typical examples. The advantage of the total cell kill assays in general is that they are relatively simple, fast, and objective, and that they determine the end-point of drug cytotoxicity, cell kill.

4. RESULTS OF CELL CULTURE DRUG RESISTANCE TESTING IN CHILDHOOD AML

A total of 11 studies focussed on this subject. Different assays were used, and patients sometimes included adults. In general, the number of cases studied was small, and any conclusion should be drawn with caution. The results of the published studies will be briefly summarized. In addition, we will highlight some results of ongoing studies done at our laboratory in cooperation with the German AML-BFM group (Prof. J. Ritter, Prof. U. Creutzig).

4.1. In Vitro Drug Resistance in AML versus ALL Samples

Weisenthal et al.[8] compared samples of 41 AML patients (including adults), taken at either initial diagnosis or at relapse, with ALL samples. At arbitrary in vitro concentrations, AML samples were more often resistant than ALL samples to dexamethasone and vincristine, while differences for cytarabine and doxorubicin were not significant. These in vitro data are in good agreement with clinical experience. We also reported different drug resistance profiles in childhood ALL (n=125) and AML (n=28) samples, with AML cells being >75-fold more resistant to glucocorticoids, and 2-fold more resistant to vincristine.[9] Glucocorticoids even induced cell proliferation (or at least prevented spontaneous cell death) in more than 30% of the AML samples, compared to only 2% of ALL samples.[9] Results for 9 other drugs (cytarabine, anthracyclines, thiopurines, teniposide, asparaginase, vindesine) were not significantly different. These results suggest that the lack of sensitivity to one or more drugs in AML may at least partly explain its relatively poor prognosis. Exceptions may be cyclofosfamide and ifosfamide, because Miller et al. found that AML colony forming units were more sensitive to 4-OH-cyclofosfamide than ALL cells.[10] However, these drugs are not used intensively in the treatment of AML.

4.2. In Vitro Drug Resistance in Relation to Disease Status and Cell Biological Features

Hongo et al. found that FAB M4 and M5 samples taken at relapse were more resistant to etoposide and cytarabine than samples of similar FAB type taken at initial diagnosis.[11] We compared 29 untreated AML samples and 16 relapsed AML samples and showed that the latter were 3-fold more resistant to cytarabine.[12] For the other drugs (including anthracyclines, thioguanine and etoposide) no significant differences were found. This resistance to cytarabine may partly explain the worse prognosis of AML once it has relapsed. In a more recent analysis, relapsed AML samples were again more resistant (median 2.5-fold) to cytarabine than untreated samples, but such a difference was not seen for 2-chlorodeoxy-adenosine (2-CdA), despite a significant cross-resistance between the two drugs.[13] This suggests that at least in subgroups of relapsed AML patients resistant to cytarabine, 2-CdA may still have antileukemic activity.

At an analysis of 55 samples of newly diagnosed children with AML, FAB M5 samples were more sensitive to vincristine (8-fold) and l-asparaginase (3-fold) than the remaining samples.[14] The in vitro drug resistance profiles of AML FAB M5 samples thus resemble those of ALL samples, except that the former are more resistant to glucocorticoids. The relative sensitivity to vincristine may be explained by the low activity of myeloperoxydase in AML M5 samples, an enzyme that confers resistance to vincristine.[15,16] The relative sensitivity of AML M5 samples to l-asparaginase may be explained by the low asparagine synthetase activity in this particular type of AML samples.[17] Of particular interest, Hongo et al. found that only patients with AML FAB M1 or M2 type and the translocation (8;21) had AML cells relatively sensitive to prednisolone.[11] This is in agreement with the recent report that an AML cell line with the t(8;21) was relatively in vitro sensitive to prednisolone.[18]

AML cells of children with Down syndrome were 10-fold more sensitive to cytarabine compared to non-Down syndrome AML patients.[19] This correlated wih higher intracellular levels of the triphosphate-form of cytarabine, its active metabolite, and increased relative numbers of double DNA strand breaks. The same authors more recently reported their extended experience.[20] Children with both Down syndrome and AML (n=8) had AML cells that were 8-fold more sensitive to cytarabine and 23-fold more sensitive to daunorubicin than AML cells of children without Down syndrome. We could confirm these results, and found that AML cells of 4 Down syndrome patients were also more sensitive to all other drugs used in their treatment, including idarubicin and mitoxantrone, thioguanine, etoposide, vincristine, prednisolone and ifosfamide (Figure 1).[21] The superior

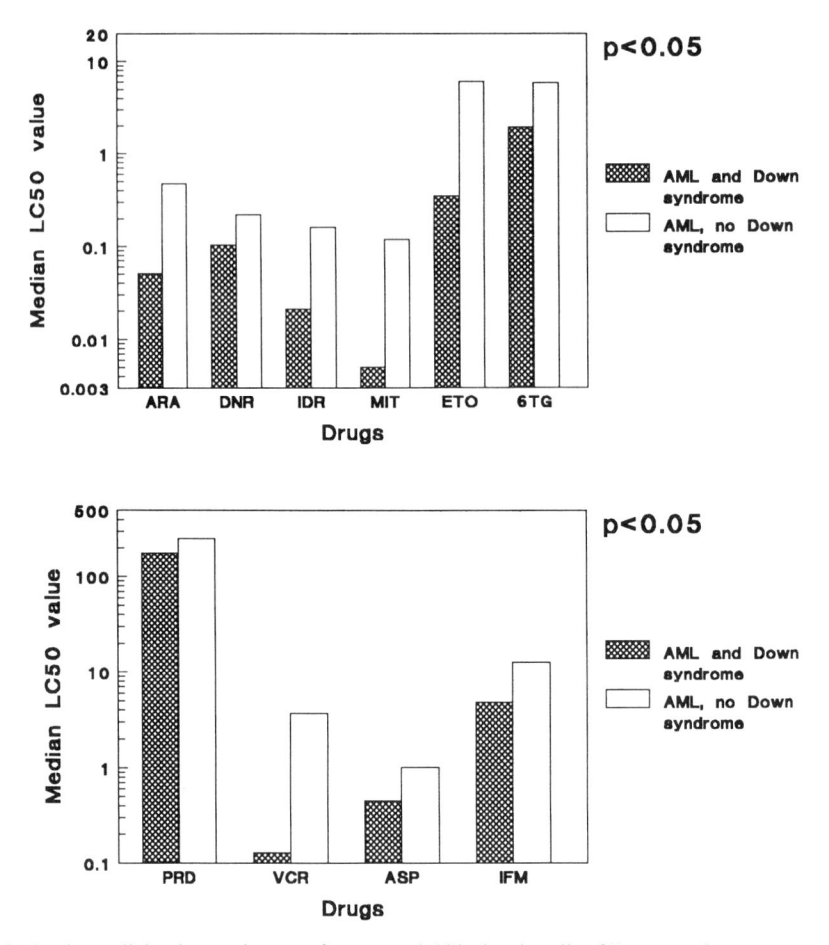

Figure 1. In vitro cellular drug resistance of acute myeloid leukemia cells of Down syndrome versus non-Down syndrome children. Abbreviations: ARA=cytarabine, DNR=daunorubicin, IDR=idarubicin, MIT=mitoxantrone, ETO=etoposide, 6TG=thioguanine, PRD=prednisolone, VCR=vincristine, ASP=l-asparaginase and IFM=4-hydroperoxy-ifosfamide.

outcome of AML in children with Down syndrome may be explained by this favorable drug resistance profile. Of interest, we also found that the leukemic cells of 6 children with Down syndrome and ALL were more sensitive to anthracyclines than those of up to 471 non-Down children with ALL.[21]

4.3. In Vitro Drug Resistance in Relation to Clinical Outcome

Several authors described the relation between in vitro drug resistance and clinical outcome after chemotherapy. In 41 AML children, in vitro resistance to daunorubicin, but not to cytarabine, was related to the response to remission induction chemotherapy.[22] In addition, the probability of continuous complete remission was significantly related to the extent of in vitro resistance to both daunorubicin and cytarabine. Smith and Lihou reported on 9 children, 6 achieving complete remission and 3 having clinically resistant disease.[23] In 8 out of 9 cases, the clinical response was predicted correctly based on the in vitro resistance to a combination of cytarabine and daunorubicin. In the remaining patient, resistant disease was predicted by the in vitro assay, but the patient achieved a complete remission. However, this child did suffer the earliest relapse of all patients that got into complete remission. Rosanda et al. described a total of 13 single agent vitro-vivo comparisons made in 11 AML children.[24] The true negative rate was 100% (11/11 relatively resistant), the true positive rate 100% (2/2 relatively sensitive), and thus the predictive accuracy was also 100%. In the study reported by Miller et al., in vitro drug resistance of occult leukemic colony-forming units was tested prior to stem cell transplantation in 35 patients (partly children).[10] Conditioning included cyclofosfamide. The 13 patients with in vitro 4-OH-cyclofosfamide (the active metabolite) resistant cells had a probability of relapse of 86% compared to 18% for the in vitro sensitive patients. Hongo et al. studied 63 children with AML.[11] Vitro-vivo correlations showed a true negative rate of 62%, a true positive rate of 70%, and a predictive accuracy of 68%. These authors also reported that assay-directed chemotherapy in relapsed cases resulted in a 50% (11/22) response rate, in contrast to 0% (0/8) in case of local hospital protocols.[11] In newly diagnosed AML patients, poor responders (n=14) to remission induction chemotherapy had AML cells that were 3-fold more resistant to cytarabine than the 15 good responders.[12] For the other drugs, no significant differences were found. We more recently showed that newly diagnosed patients with more than 5% blasts in the bone marrow at day 15 of remission induction chemotherapy had AML cells that were relatively resistant to daunorubicin, idarubicin, etoposide and cytarabine than the patients with less than 5% blasts.[14]

In summary, although a large study including multivariate analysis of potential prognostic factors is lacking, there seems to be a good correlation between in vitro drug resistance and clinical outcome after chemotherapy in childhood AML. This may not be surprising in view of our experiences in childhood ALL.[25–27]

5. POSSIBLE APPLICATIONS OF CELL CULTURE DRUG RESISTANCE TESTING (TABLE 1) AND CONCLUSIONS

In the first place, cellular drug resistance testing may provide a prognostic factor that can be used for risk-group stratification and subsequent risk-group adapted treatment. Good prognostic factors are scarce in AML. Certain chromosomal abnormalities have prognostic significance, but occur in a minority of the patients. A multivariate analysis of potential prognostic factors should be done before we may conclude that cellular drug resistance is an independent prognostic factor in childhood AML. Secondly, cellular drug resistance may be used to tailor chemotherapy for different subgroups. This concept is based on the fact that cellular drug resistance differs between subgroups of AML, such as among different FAB types.[11,14] This is in agreement with our experience in childhood ALL, in

Table 1. Possible applications of cellular drug resistance testing

- Prognostic factor to be used for risk-group stratification
- Tailored therapy for subgroups of patients
- Individualized tailored therapy
  curative
  palliative
- Selection of patients for phase II trials
- Drug screening
- Study of cross-resistance between both related and unrelated drugs

which we showed that e.g. age, immunophenotype and DNA ploidy subtypes have markedly different cellular drug resistance profiles.[28-30] Therefore, chemotherapy may be tailored for subgroups based on the in vitro data. Thirdly, such a tailored therapy may also be individualized. Hongo et al. reported that such individualized tailored therapy gave better treatment results than standard treatment in relapsed childhood AML.[11] To the best of our knowledge, other similar studies in childhood AML have not been performed. We have evaluated a similar approach in high risk relapsed ALL with a dismal prognosis, in cooperation with the German ALL-BFM Relapse group (Prof. G. Henze), but did not find an advantage of tailored therapy in these children compared to patients treated according to the standard protocol.[31] It also seems reasonable to use cellular drug resistance testing in the choice of one or more drugs for palliative chemotherapy. The fourth application is to select patients for phase II trials of new potential anticancer agents. Patients which have malignant cells that are markedly resistant in vitro to the agent to be tested should then be excluded from that particular phase II study. A fifth application is the use of cellular resistance testing in drug screening, for which purpose most often cell lines are being used. Finally, drug resistance testing can be used to study the cross-resistance patterns of known compounds and their new analogues, and non-related other anticancer agents.[32]

In conclusion, the data reported sofar demonstrate the clinical relevance of cellular drug resistance testing in childhood AML. However, more and larger studies are required to establish the role of this particular type of in vitro studies in the treatment of children with AML. The ultimate goal of this research is to further improve the success of chemotherapy, in terms of both efficacy and side-effects.

REFERENCES

1. Creutzig U, Rittter J, Schellong G. Identification of two risk groups in childhood acute myelogeneous leukemia after therapy intensification in study AML-BFM-83 as compared with study AML-BFM-78. Blood 1990, 75: 1932–1940
2. Pui Ch. Childhood leukemias. New Engl J Med 1995, 332: 1618–1630
3. Stevens RF, Hann IM, Wheatley K, Gray RG, on behalf of the MRC Childhood Leakemia Working Party. Marked improvements in outcome with chemotherapy alone in paediatric acute myeloid leukaemia: results of the United Kingdom Medical research Council's 10th AML trial. Br J Haematol 1998, 101: 130–140
4. Pieters R, Kaspers GJL, Veerman AJP. Drug sensitivity culture assays in childhood leukemia: A review of the results and applications. Int J Pediatr Hematol Oncol 1997, 4: 531–541
5. Preisler HD, Gopal V. Regrowth resistance in leukemia and lymphoma: the need for a new system to classify treatment failure and for new approaches to treatment. Leuk Res 1994, 18: 149–160
6. Bosanquet AG. Short-term in vitro drug sensitivity tests for cancer chemotherapy. A summary of correlations of test results with both patient response and survival. Trends in Experimental and Clinical Medicine 1994, 4: 179–195
7. Veerman AJP, Pieters R. Drug sensitivity assays in leukaemia and lymphoma. Br J Haematol 1990, 74: 381–384
8. Weisenthal LM, Dill PL, Finklestein JZ, Duarte TE, Baker JA, Moran EM. Laboratory detection of primary and acquired drug resistance in human lymphatic neoplasms. Cancer Treatm Rep 1986, 70: 1283–1295
9. Kaspers GJL, Kardos G, Pieters R, Van Zantwijk CH, Klumper E, Hählen K, De Waal FC, Van Wering ER, Veerman AJP. Different cellular drug resistance profiles in childhood lymphoblastic and non-lymphoblastic leukemia: A preliminary report. Leukemia 1994, 8: 1224–1229
10. Miller CB, Zehnbauer BA, Piantadosi S, Rowley SD, Jones RJ. Correlation of occult clonogenic leukemia drug sensitivity with relapse after autologous bone marrow transplantation. Blood 1991, 78: 1125–1131
11. Hongo T, Fujii Y, Yajima S. In vitro chemosensitivity of childhood leukemic cells and the clinical value of assay directed chemotherapy. In: Kaspers et al. (eds). Drug Resistance in Leukemia and Lymphoma I. Harwood, 1993: 313–319

12. Klumper E, Pieters R, Kaspers GJL, Huismans DR, Loonen AH, Rottier MMA, Van Wering ER, Van Der Does-Van Den Berg A, Hählen K, Creutzig U, Veerman AJP. In vitro chemosensitivity testing in childhood acute non-lymphoblastic leukemia using the MTT assay. Leukemia 1995, 9: 1864–1869
13. Zwaan CM, Kaspers GJL, Rottier MMA, Wünsche R, Hählen K, Creutzig U, Pieters R, Veerman AJP. Circumvention of ARA-C resistance in childhood acute non-lymphoblastic leukemia (ANLL) by the use of 2-chloro-deoxyadenosine: an in vitro study. Med Pediatr Oncol 1998, 31: 230 (abstract 0–144)
14. Kaspers GJL, Zwaan ChM, Creutzig U, Ritter J, Rottier MMA, Pieters R, Veerman AJP. In vitro drug resistance in childhood acute myeloid leukemia: A preliminary analysis. In: Hiddemann et al. (eds). Acute Leukemias VII. Springer-Verlag, 1998: 491–495
15. Schlaifer D, Cooper MR, Attal M, Sartor AO, Trepel JB, Laurent G, Myers CE. Myeloperoxydase: an enzyme involved in intrinsic vincristine resistance in human myeloblastic leukemia. Blood 1993, 81: 482–489
16. Schlaifer D, Meyer K, Muller C, Attal M, Smith MT, Tamaki S, Weimels J, Pris J, Jaffrezou JP, Laurent G, et al. Antisense inhibition of myeloperoxidase increases the sensitivity of the HL-60 cell line to vincristine. Leukemia 1994, 8: 289–291
17. Dübbers A, Schulze-Westhoff P, Kurzknabe E, Creutzig U, Ritter J, Boos J. Asparagine-synthetase in paediatric acute leukemias: AML-M5-subtype shows lowest activity. Ann Hematol 1997, 74 (suppl I): A37 (abstract #148)
18. Miyoshi H, Ohki M, Nakagawa T, Honma Y. Glucocorticoids induce apoptosis in acute myeloid leukemia cell lines with a t(8;21) chromosome translocation. Leuk Res 1997, 21: 45–50
19. Taub JW, Matherly LH, Stout ML, Buck SA, Gurney JG, Ravindranath Y. Enhanced metabolism of 1-beta-D-arabinofuranosylcytosine in Down syndrome cells - a contributing factor to the superior event free survival of Down syndrome children with acute myeloid leukemia. Blood 1996, 87: 3395–3403
20. Taub JW, Stout ML, Buck SA, Huang X, Vega RA, Becton DL, Ravindranath Y. Myeloblasts from Down syndrome children with acute myeloid leukemia have increased in vitro sensitivity to cytosine arabinoside and daunorubicin. Leukemia 1997, 11: 1594–1595 [letter]
21. Zwaan CM, Ramakers-Van Woerden NL, Kaspers GJL, Pieters R, Wünsche R, Rottier MMA, Hählen K, Janka-Schaub G, Creutzig U, Veerman AJP. Favourable drug resistance profiles in children with Down's syndrome (DS) and acute leukemia. Br J Haematol 1998, 102: 226 (poster 904)
22. Dow LW, Dahl GV, Kalwinsky DK, Mirro J, Nash MB, Roberson PK. Correlation of drug sensitivity in vitro with clinical responses in childhood acute myeloid leukemia. Blood 1986, 68: 400–405
23. Smith PJ, Lihou MG. Prediction of remission induction in childhood acute myeloid leukemia. Aust N Z J Med 1986, 16: 39–42
24. Rosanda C, Garaventa A, Pasino M, Strigini P, De Bernardi B. A short-term in vitro drug sensitivity assay in pediatric malignancies. Anticancer Res 1987, 7: 365–368
25. Pieters R, Huismans DR, Loonen AH, Hählen K, Van Der Does-Van Den Berg A, Van Wering ER, Veerman AJP. Relation of cellular drug resistance to long-term clinical outcome in childhood acute lymphoblastic leukaemia. Lancet 1991, 338: 399–403
26. Kaspers GJL, AJP Veerman, R Pieters, Van Zantwijk CH, LA Smets, ER Van Wering, A Van Der Does-Van Den Berg. In vitro cellular drug resistance and prognosis in childhood acute lymphoblastic leukemia. Blood 1997, 90: 2723–2729
27. Kaspers GJL, Pieters R, Van Zantwijk CH, Van Wering ER, Van Der Does-Van Den Berg A, Veerman AJP. Prednisolone in childhood acute lymphoblastic leukemia: vitro-vivo correlations and cross-resistance to other anticancer agents. Blood 1998, 92: 259–266
28. Pieters R, Den Boer ML, Durian M, Janka G, Schmiegelow K, Kaspers GJL, Van Wering ER, veerman AJP. In vitro drug resistance testing in infant acute lymphoblastic leukemia cells - implications for treatment. Leukemia 1998, 12: 1344–1348
29. Kaspers GJL, Pieters R, Van Zantwijk CH, Van Wering ER, Veerman AJP. Clinical and cell biological features related to cellular drug resistance of childhood acute lymphoblastic leukemia cells. Leukemia & Lymphoma 1995, 19: 407–417
30. Kaspers GJL, Smets LA, Pieters R, Van Zantwijk CH, Van Wering ER, Veerman AJP. Favorable prognosis of hyperdiploid common acute lymphoblastic leukemia may be explained by sensitivity to antimetabolites and other drugs: Results of an in vitro study. Blood 1995, 85: 751–756
31. Dörffel W, Hartmann R, Schober S, Veerman AJP, Pieters R, Klumper E, Henze G. Drug resistance testing as a basis for tailored therapy in children with refractory or relapsed acute lymphoblastic leukemia. In: Kaspers et al. (eds). Drug Resistance in Leukemia and Lymphoma I. Harwood, 1993: 353–357
32. Klumper E, Pieters R, Loonen AH, Huismans DR, Veerman AJP. In vitro anthracycline cross-resistance pattern in childhood acute lymphoblastic leukaemia. Br J Cancer 1995, 71: 1188–1193

45

IS *IN VITRO* SENSITIVITY OF BLAST CELLS CORRELATED TO THERAPEUTIC EFFECT IN CHILDHOOD ACUTE LYMPHOBLASTIC LEUKEMIA?

Britt-Marie Frost,[1] Rolf Larsson,[2] Peter Nygren,[3] and Gudmar Lönnerholm[1]

[1]Department of Pediatrics
[2]Department of Clinical Pharmacology
[3]Department of Oncology
University Hospital, Uppsala, Sweden

Keywords: Acute lymphoblastic leukemia, children, in vitro sensitivity, cytotoxic drugs.

ABSTRACT

Our aim is to study whether or not in vitro sensitivity of leukemic cells correlates with clinical effect; if so, in vitro testing might be used for stratification of treatment. During 1995–1997 bone marrow samples from 145 Swedish children with newly diagnosed acute lymphoblastic leukemia were analysed by the automated fluorometric microculture cytotoxicity assay. Therapeutic effect was evaluated by bone marrow morphology day 15 and 29. Preliminary results indicate that marrow samples from patients with poor response to induction therapy show a higher degree of in vitro resistance to several cytotoxic drugs at diagnosis than good responders.

INTRODUCTION

Modern combination chemotherapy can cure 70–80% of children suffering from acute lymphoblastic leukemia (ALL). A substantial number of relapses still occur in the so called "low risk" or "standard risk" groups, suggesting that there are patients who might benefit from a more intense therapy. On the other hand, there are most probably patients who are overtreated, thereby risking unnecessary side effects. These facts indicate a need for a more individualised therapy. Possibly, there is a role for in vitro sensitivity testing of leukemic cells in such efforts.

In a recent publication, Kaspers et al reported the relation between in vitro resistance, measured with the MTT method, and long-term clinical response in 152 children with newly diagnosed ALL (1). The drug resistance profile at diagnosis had prognostic independent significance superior to that of any other factor, and the authors concluded that treatment failure in newly diagnosed childhood ALL can be predicted from cellular drug resistance data. Since this is the only prospective study comprising a large number of patients, there is a need for other centre(s) to confirm these data. In the present study, we used the automated fluorometric microculture cytotoxicity assay (FMCA), which has been found suitable for drug sensitivity testing of leukemic cells (2,3). There are some technical differences between the FMCA and the MTT-assay, but in essence they are similar, and when run in parallel they have yielded almost identical results (4). The aim of the present study is to correlate in vitro sensitivity to drugs with treatment response. Plasma samples for determination of cytotoxic drug levels have also been collected, but these data are not included in the following presentation. Since this is an interim analysis of an ongoing study, no formal statistics have been performed.

PATIENTS AND METHODS

During 1995–1997 samples for in vitro sensitivity testing were collected from children <17 years old with newly diagnosed or relapsing ALL. All Swedish pediatric oncology centres participated. 164 samples were successfully analysed (79% technical success rate), 145 de novo ALL and 19 relapses. The patients were treated according to the Nordic ALL protocol (NOPHO ALL-92), where induction therapy for all risk groups includes prednisolone, vincristine, doxorubicin, asparaginase and intrathecal methotrexate. Clinical data for the patients, including bone marrow morphology day 15 and 29, were obtained from the NOPHO (Nordic Society of Pediatric Hematology and Oncology) registry.

In Vitro Sensitivity Testing

Bone marrow aspirates or peripheral blood were collected in heparinized glass tubes. The samples generally reached the analysing laboratory in Uppsala so that cell preparation could start within 24 hours. Mononuclear cells were obtained by 1.077 g/ml Ficoll-Isopaque (Pharmacia-Upjohn, Uppsala, Sweden) density gradient centrifugation. Viability was determined by trypan blue exclusion test and the density gradient centrifugation generally yielded cell suspensions of >85% leukemic cells. Mostly, fresh samples were used for the in vitro assay, but some samples were cryopreserved in culture medium containing 10% dimetylsulphoxide (dMso) and 50% fetal calf serum by initial freezing for 24 h in -70°C followed by storage in liquid nitrogen. Cryopreservation does not affect drug sensitivity (2,3).

The semi-automated fluorometric microculture cytotoxicity assay (FMCA) is based on the measurement of fluorescence generated from hydrolysis of fluorescein diacetate to fluorescein by living cells. The principal steps of the assay procedure have been described previously (2,3). Microtiter plates were prepared by addition of 20 µl/well of the drug solution at 10 times the desired final concentration.

The cytotoxic drug concentrations used were established from a pilot series of dose-response curves obtained in ALL samples (2,3). These empirically derived drug concentrations (generally 2–10 times the clinically achievable concentration time products) were chosen to give optimal conditions for separation of sensitive from resistant samples. On day one, 180 µl of the leukemic cell preparation at 5.6×10^5 cells/ml in culture medium were seeded into the wells of the microtiter plates, giving 100×10^3 cells per well. Six blank wells received only culture medium and six wells with cells but without drugs served as controls. After 72 h incubation the plates were centrifuged and the medium removed. After one wash with phosphate buffered saline, fluorescein diacetate was added. Subsequently the plates were incubated for 40 min before reading the fluorescence in a scanning fluorometer. Quality criteria for a successful assay included a signal in control cultures of >3 x mean blank values, mean coefficient of variation in control cultures of <30% and a proportion of leukemic cells of >70% prior to and at the end of incubation.

The results are presented as survival index (SI), denoting the proportion of surviving cells. SI is defined as fluorescence of experimental as a percentage of control cultures (fluorescence in test well/fluorescence in control well, with blank values subtracted).

The study was approved by the local ethics committee at each participating centre.

RESULTS

Figure 1 shows mean values for in vitro sensitivity at diagnosis correlated to bone marrow morphology after 29 days of induction therapy. Leukemic cells of good responders (<5% blasts cells) tended to be more sensitive than those of slow responders (>5% blasts cells) for all drugs tested. The slow responders were relatively few (n = 10) and this is not surprising, since modern treatment protocols for ALL are highly effective in inducing complete morphological remission.

Figure 2 gives more detailed data. The box plots demonstrate the differences in median values for good and slow responders, but they also show that there are a number of outliers in the "good responder" group, which appear quite resistant to some of the drugs, especially the corticosteroids. It will be of great interest to follow such patients and see whether this finding correlates to an increased risk for relapse. Furthermore, frozen samples of day 29 bone marrow will be analysed by PCR to see if minimal residual disease can be detected in some patients classified as good responders by morphological criteria.

As evident from Figures 1 and 2, data for prednisolone and dexamethasone are similar. This was true also when data for individual patients were compared.

Infants with ALL differ from children above 1 year of age in their response to therapy. In a separate analysis we compared the in vitro sensitivity of the infants (n = 9) with

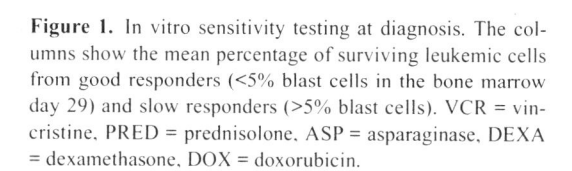

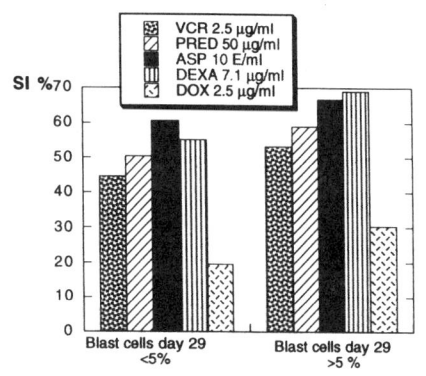

Figure 1. In vitro sensitivity testing at diagnosis. The columns show the mean percentage of surviving leukemic cells from good responders (<5% blast cells in the bone marrow day 29) and slow responders (>5% blast cells). VCR = vincristine, PRED = prednisolone, ASP = asparaginase, DEXA = dexamethasone, DOX = doxorubicin.

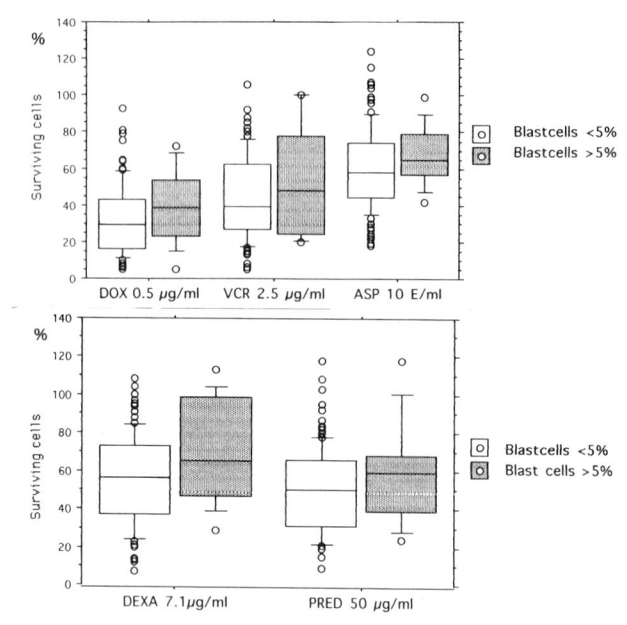

Figure 2. Box plot showing in vitro sensitivity data for "good" and "slow" responders (medium values together with 10th, 25th, 75th and 90th percentiles). Outliers are individually shown.

that of older children. Unexpectedly, blast cells of the infants tended to be more sensitive than those of older patients.

An important question is, whether in vitro sensitivity testing at diagnosis can be used to predict response to therapy. Kaspers et al reported that the combination of data for prednisolone, vincristine and asparaginase could provide a drug-resistance profile with prognostic independent significance superior to that of any single drug (1). In a similar way, we calculated a drug sensitivity profile score for these three drugs. For each drug the patients were divided into three groups and a sensitive result was counted as 1, an intermediate result as 2, and a resistant result as 3. The score was calculated by adding up these counts, and consequently the score ranged from 3 (sensitive to all three drugs) to 9 (resistant to all three drugs). Table 1 shows the sensitivity score for the ten patients classified as slow responders day 29 by morphological criteria. Five out of ten slow responders had a score of 8–9, i.e., they were highly resistant at diagnosis, and three had an intermediate score. The two slow responders who had a low score, indicating high in vitro sensitivity, were both infants.

In the presently used Nordic ALL protocol, bone marrow samples are collected also day 15, to allow an early evaluation of therapeutic effect. Patients with < 5% blast cells day 15 tended to have a more sensitive in vitro profile than those with > 5% blast cells, al-

Table 1. Drug sensitivity profile score for 10 slow responders (>5% blast cells on day 29)

Score	No. of patients with >5% blast cells day 29
3–4	2 (2 infants)
5–7	3
8–9	5

Data for prednisolone, vincristine and asparaginase were used.

In Vitro Sensitivity of Blast Cells

Table 2. Drug sensitivity profile score for 26 slow responders (>5% blast cells on day 15). Data for prednisolone, vincristine and asparaginase were used

Score	No of patients with >5% blast cells day 15
3–4	5 (3 infants)
5–7	10 (2 infants)
8–9	11

though the correlation was less obvious than day 29. Table 2 shows the sensitivity score for the 26 patients with >5% blast cells day 15. Evidently, high scores (= in vitro resistance) tended to be more frequent than low scores among "slow responders" day 15, at least for children above 1 year of age.

DISCUSSION

Follow-up time is still relatively short for most patients included in the present study, and the final clinical outcome is not known. We have therefore used bone marrow morphology after 15 and 29 days of treatment to evaluate the effect of induction therapy. Consequently, we have focused this report on in vitro sensitivity data for drugs used during the induction phase. We are aware of the limitations of this approach, and the final report will include both long-term clinical follow-up and in vitro data for all drugs used. The only exception will be methotrexate, because this drug is not cytotoxic to human leukemia samples in non-clonogenic assays.

Our main finding was that the effect of induction therapy appeared to correlate with in vitro sensitivity of leukemic cells at diagnosis. Good responders tended to be more sensitive than slow responders for prednisolone, vincristine, asparaginase, doxorubicin and dexamethasone. This agrees with recently published data by Kaspers et al. (1) who reported that in vitro resistance to prednisolone, asparaginase and vincristine were each significantly related to the probability of disease-free survival after combination chemotherapy for childhood ALL. The combination of data for these three drugs provided a drug-resistance profile with prognostic significance. We similarly calculated a drug resistance profile score and found that slow responders more often than expected had a high score, i.e. were more resistant than good responders.

An obvious exception were infants below 1 year of age. As a group they tended to be more sensitive in vitro than patients >1 year of age, and some infants with slow response had a highly sensitive profile. Due to the small number of infants these data must be considered preliminary, but they suggest that factors other than drug resistance at the cellular level might explain the well known fact, that infants with ALL have a lower cure rate than older children. Differences in pharmacokinetic parameters, with more rapid elimination of drugs in infants, as well as fast cellular re-growth between treatment courses, are possible mechanisms. As to variability in pharmacokinetics between different age groups, we hope that the present study will provide some useful data, since plasma samples have been collected at start of induction therapy to determine the levels of vincristine and doxorubicin. A number of samples have been analysed, but statistical analysis must await further data collection.

In conclusion, preliminary results from a large, prospective study agree with previously published data, that in vitro sensitivity testing at diagnosis correlates with response to therapy.

ACKNOWLEDGMENTS

This study was supported by the Children's Cancer Foundation in Sweden.

REFERENCES

1. Kaspers GJL, Veerman AJP, Pieters R, van Zantwijk CH, Smets LA, van Wering ER, van der Does-van den Berg A: In vitro cellular drug resistance and prognosis in newly diagnosed childhood acute lymphoblastic leukemia. Blood 1997;90:2723–2729.
2. Nygren P, Christensen J, Jansson B, Sundström C, Lönnerholm G, Kreuger A, Larsson R: Feasibility of the Fluorometric Microculture Cytotoxicity Assay (FMC) for Cytotoxic Drug Sensitivity Testing of Tumor Cells from Patients with Acute Lymphoblastic Leukemia. Leukemia 1992;11:1121–1128.
3. Larsson R, Kristensen J, Sandberg C, Nygren P: Laboratory determination of chemotherapeutic drug resistance in tumor cells from patients with leukemia using a fluorometric microculture cytotoxicity assay (FMCA). Int J Cancer 1992;50:177–185.
4. Larsson R, Nygren P, Ekberg M, Slater L: Chemotherapeutic drug sensitivity testing of human leukemia cells in vitro using a semi-automated fluorometric assay. Leukemia 1990; 4: 567–571.

46

IN VITRO CYTOTOXIC DRUG ACTIVITY AND IN VIVO PHARMACOKINETICS IN CHILDHOOD ACUTE MYELOID LEUKEMIA

Gudmar Lönnerholm,[1] Britt-Marie Frost,[1] Rolf Larsson,[2] E. Liliemark,[3] Peter Nygren,[4] and Curt Peterson[3]

[1]Department of Pediatrics
 University Children's Hospital, Uppsala, Sweden
[2]Department of Clinical Pharmacology
 University Hospital, Uppsala, Sweden
[3]Department of Clinical Pharmacology
 Karolinska Hospital, Stockholm, Sweden
[4]Department of Oncology
 University Hospital, Uppsala, Sweden

Keywords: acute myeloid leukemia, children, in vitro sensitivity, pharmacokinetics, cytotoxic drugs.

ABSTRACT

Since May 1996 all Nordic countries have been participating in a study of childhood acute myeloid leukemia (AML). The aim is to correlate the in vitro sensitivity of leukemic cells and individual plasma concentrations of cytotoxic drugs with clinical effect. Blast cells from bone marrow and/or peripheral blood are tested against a panel of cytotoxic agents using the fluorometric microculture cytotoxicity assay (FMCA). Plasma concentrations of cytotoxic drugs are analysed during induction therapy.

Bone marrow samples from the participating centres generally reached the analysing laboratory within 24 hours. 61 out of 71 (86%) samples were successfully analysed, 47 de novo AML and 14 relapses. Relapsing patients tended to have a more resistant test profile than newly diagnosed patients. Steady state plasma levels of doxorubicin, etoposide and 6-thioguanine nucleotide varied about 10-fold between patients. The intra-individual variation was much less, suggesting that dose adjustment based on pharmacokinetic data might be useful in the future.

INTRODUCTION

The cure rate for children with acute myeloid leukemia (AML) needs further improvement. With most current protocols about 50% of the children with AML will become long-time survivors (1). Therapeutic failure is mainly caused by resistant disease, toxic death or relapsing leukemia. All protocols use dosages of drugs based on body size only, in spite of the well known clinical experience that patients differ widely with respect to therapeutic effect and side effects. Possible explanations for differences in effect and toxicity include inter-individual differences in plasma concentrations (pharmacokinetic variability) and differences in sensitivity to cytotoxic drugs at the cellular level.

A few previous studies of in vitro chemosensitivity in AML have been published (2,3) but available data are far from conclusive. Pharmacokinetic studies in children with the cytotoxic agents used in current protocols are few, and only a small number of patients are included. These studies indicate, however, like similar studies in adults, that plasma concentrations in individuals receiving similar doses might differ considerably (4,5). In the present study, we used the semi-automated fluorometric microculture cytotoxicity assay (FMCA), which has been found suitable for drug sensitivity testing of leukemic cells. In a number of patients we also determined cytotoxic drug levels in plasma during induction therapy. The ultimate clinical endpoint, disease-free survival, has not been reached and therapeutic effect was therefore evaluated by studying bone marrow morphology after the first induction therapy. Since this is an interim analysis of an ongoing study, no formal statistics have been performed, and all results must be considered preliminary.

PATIENTS AND METHODS

Since 1996 all five Nordic countries (Denmark, Finland, Iceland, Norway, Sweden) participate in the study. The population of these countries is about 25 million people, with a yearly incidence of childhood AML of 30–40 cases.

Samples for in vitro sensitivity testing were obtained from 71 children and 61 (86%) were successfully analyzed, 47 de novo AML and 14 relapses. Clinical data, including bone marrow morphology after each course of induction therapy, were obtained from the NOPHO (Nordic Society of Pediatric Hematology and Oncology) registry. All children with de novo AML were treated according to the NOPHO 1993 AML protocol (1).

In Vitro Sensitivity Testing

Bone marrow aspirates (or sometimes peripheral blood) were collected in heparinized glass tubes. The samples generally reached the analysing laboratory in Uppsala so that cell preparation could start within 24 hours. Mononuclear cells were obtained by 1.077 g/ml Ficoll-Isopaque (Pharmacia-Upjohn, Uppsala, Sweden) density gradient centrifugation. Viability was determined by trypan blue exclusion test and the density gradient centrifugation generally yielded cell suspensions of >85% leukemic cells. Mostly, fresh samples were used for the in vitro assay, but some samples were cryopreserved in culture medium containing 10% dimethylsulphoxide (dMso) and 50% fetal calf serum by initial freezing for 24 h in -70°C followed by storage in liquid nitrogen. It has been shown that cryopreservation does not affect drug sensitivity (6).

The semi-automated fluorometric microculture cytotoxicity assay (FMCA) is based on the measurement of fluorescence generated from hydrolysis of fluorescein diacetate to fluorescein by living cells. The principal steps of the assay procedure have been described previously (6,7). Microtiter plates were prepared by addition of 20 µl/well of the drug solution at 10 times the desired final concentration.

The cytotoxic drug concentrations used were established from a pilot series of dose-response curves obtained in AML samples (7). These empirically derived drug concentrations (generally 2–10 times the clinically achievable concentration time products) were chosen to give optimal conditions for separation of sensitive from resistant samples. On day one, 180 µl of the leukemic cell preparation at 2.8×10^5 cells/ml in culture medium were seeded into the wells of the microtiter plates, giving 50×10^3 cells per well. Six blank wells received only culture medium and six wells with cells but without drugs served as controls. After 72 h incubation the plates were centrifuged and the medium removed. After one wash with phosphate buffered saline, fluorescein diacetate was added. Subsequently the plates were incubated for 40 min before reading the fluorescence in a scanning fluorometer. Quality criteria for a successful assay included a signal in control cultures of >3 x mean blank values, mean coefficient of variation in control cultures of <30% and a proportion of leukemic cells of >70% prior to and at the end of incubation.

The results are presented as survival index (SI), denoting the proportion of surviving cells. SI is defined as fluorescence of experimental as a percentage of control cultures (fluorescence in test well/fluorescence in control well, with blank values subtracted).

Pharmacokinetics

Blood samples were collected from 17 children during the first course of induction therapy. In eight children it was possible to repeat the sampling during an identical second course 3–4 weeks later. These courses included a 96-h continuous i.v. infusion of Ara-C, 200 mg/m² body surface area/day, day 1–4, and etoposide (VP 16), 100 mg/m²/day, day 1–4, plus 6-thioguanine 100 mg/m² orally twice daily, day 1–4 plus doxorubicin 75 mg/m² as an 8-h i.v. infusion day 5, plus methotrexate 12 mg intrathecally day 1. Blood samples were collected day 2,3 and 4 for determination of Ara-C, etoposide and 6-thioguanine nucleotide (6-TGN) steady state concentrations, and at the end of the doxorubicin infusion day 5. Blood from day 0 served as a blank. 3–4 ml of blood were collected in EDTA-tubes and immediately cooled by ice water. Within 60 min the samples were centrifuged to allow separate freezing of plasma and red blood cells.

High-pressure liquid chromatography (HPLC) was used for analysis of etoposide (total and free plasma concentrations), plasma doxorubicin and its main metabolite doxorubicinol, and 6-TGN in red blood cells (8). The concentrations of 6-TGN were calculated as µmol 6-TGN/mmol Hb. The analysis of Ara-C has not yet been performed.

The study has been approved by the Ethics committee at each participating center.

RESULTS AND DISCUSSION

Leukemic blast cells were tested in vitro against a panel of cytotoxic drugs. In this preliminary report we have concentrated on the drugs used during induction therapy in the NOPHO protocol, plus amsacrine, which is commonly used in relapse protocols. As shown in Figure 1, leukemic cells appeared more resistant at relapse than at diagnosis, especially against amsacrine and etoposide (VP 16). Interestingly, both these drugs are topoisomerase II inhibitors, and the decrease in sensitivity might suggest the induction of topoisomerase II mediated resistance mechanism(s) in relapse patients.

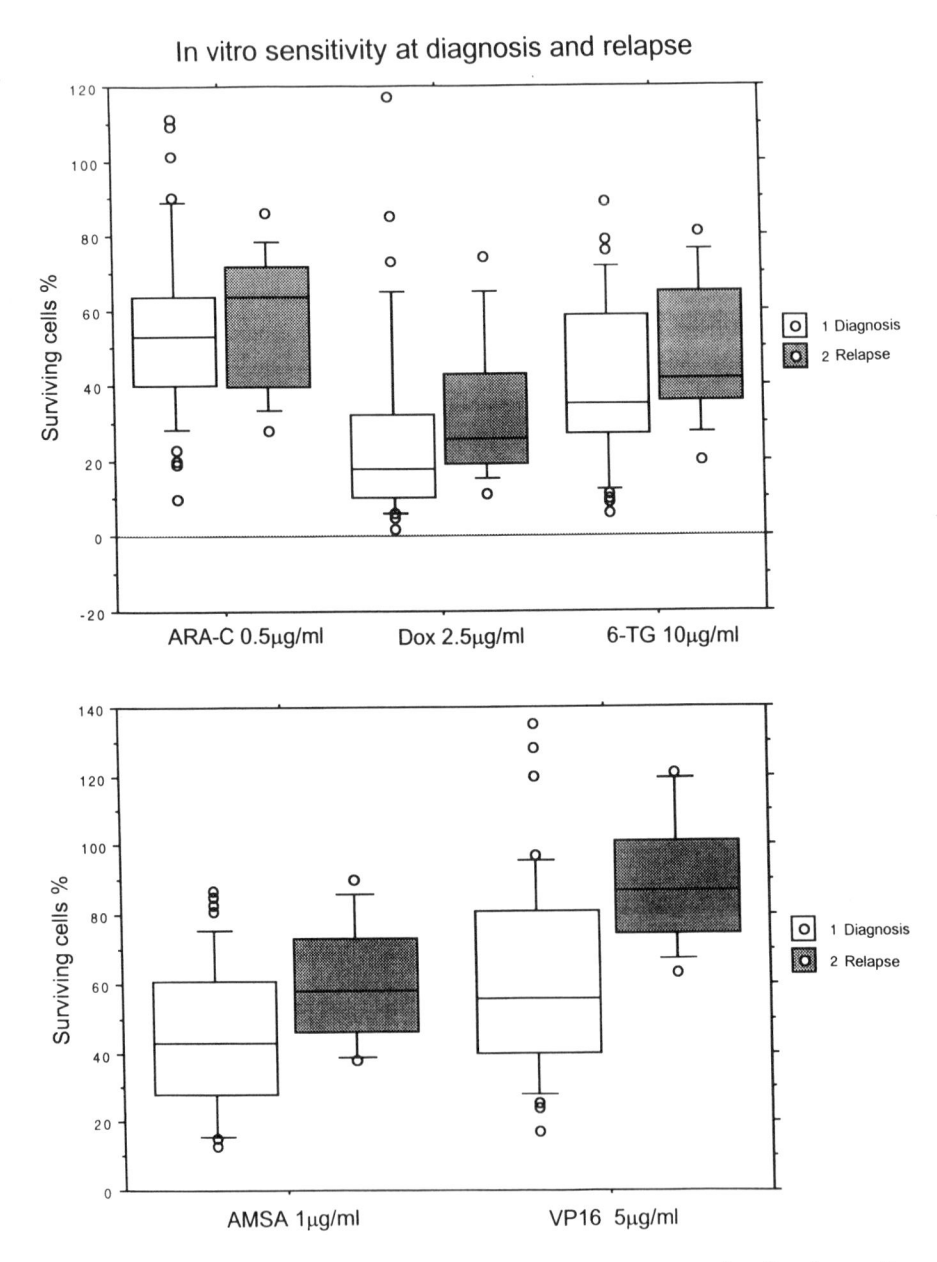

Figure 1. Box plot showing the distribution of data (median values together with 10th, 25th, 75th and 90th percentiles). Outliers are individually shown. AMSA = amsacrine, DOX = doxorubicin, 6-TG = 6-thioguanine and VP 16 = etoposide.

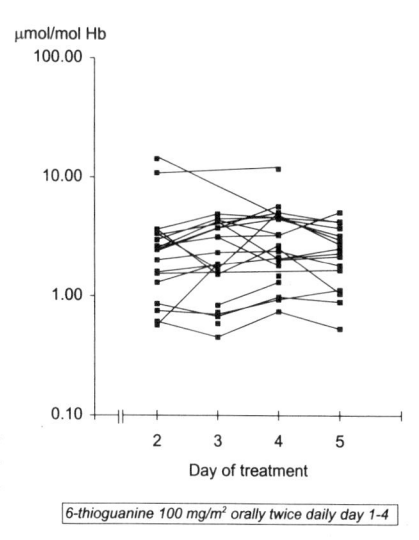

Figure 2. Etoposide plasma concentrations (total and free). Lines connect values of individual patients. In a few cases the concentration of free drug was determined after ultrafiltration of the plasma samples.

When in vitro sensitivity at diagnosis was correlated to bone marrow morphology after the first induction course (usually about 3 weeks after start of therapy), no difference was found between good responders (<5% blast cells in the marrow) and slow responders (>5% blast cells). Several explanations for this lack of correlation are possible: 1) More patients are needed (beta-error). 2) Bone marrow morphology at this point in time is not good enough to measure clinical effect, which instead must be judged by clinical long-term follow-up. 3) Factors not measured by the in vitro method are more important, e.g. differences in pharmacokinetics and/or cellular regrowth.

Figure 2 shows individual etoposide plasma concentrations. In most patients, steady state levels were reached on day 2 of the 4-d i.v. infusion, and concentrations remained essentially unchanged during day 2–4. There was an approximately 10-fold difference in steady state concentrations of total etoposide between individuals. The free concentration of etoposide was determined in 5 patients, and it was 1–3% of the total drug concentration. Repeated sampling at two consecutive courses was performed in eight patients. The results demonstrated only minor intra-individual course-to-course variability.

6-thioguanine was administered orally twice daily, which makes pharmacokinetic studies of the unchanged drug difficult, due to fluctuations in plasma concentration during the dose interval. Instead, the concentration of the major cytotoxic metabolite 6-TGN can be measured, since it is known to accumulate intra-cellularly, also in erythrocytes. Data displayed in Figure 3 show that "steady-state" concentrations of 6-TGN in erythrocytes were reached already the second day of treatment for most patients. The intra-patient variation between day 2–5 values was small (the day 5 sample was obtained 12 h after the last dose), but the inter-individual variability was at least 10-fold. Eight retested individuals had very similar mean erythrocyte 6-TGN concentrations at two consecutive treatment courses.

The plasma concentration of doxorubicin at the end of the 8-h infusion showed greater inter-individual than intra-individual variation (Figure 4).

To summarize, the findings for the three analysed drugs were similar, with an about 10-fold difference in steady-state concentrations between individuals, but a much smaller course-to-course variation in individual patients. Consequently, differences in steady-state concentrations might explain some of the differences in response to therapy. When the study is closed, statistical analysis of the correlation between concentration and clinical

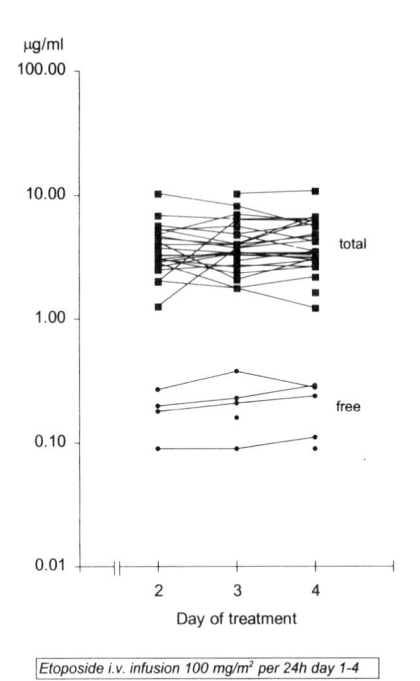

Figure 3. 6-thioguanine nucleotide (6-TGN) erythrocyte concentrations. Lines connect values of individual patients.

effect will be done. If such correlations are found, the next question is whether plasma concentrations can be used to monitor therapy and adjust dosage. In a recent publication Evans et al (9) reported that adjusting the dose of methotrexate to account for the patient´s ability to clear the drug improved the outcome in children with B-lineage acute lymphoblastic leukemia. Since all three drugs tested here showed relatively small intra-individual course-to-course variability, such manoeuvres appear quite feasible (sampling and analysis during one course, dose adjustment at next). For etoposide and 6-TG, even sampling during a course with rapid analysis and immediate dose adjustment might be possible. Such measures would be steps towards the ultimate goal of giving all patients appropriate doses of the chemotherapeutic agents used.

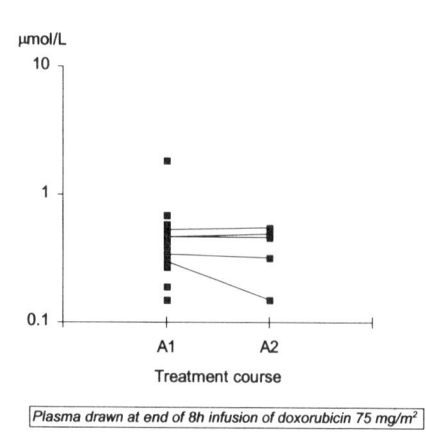

Figure 4. Doxorubicin plasma concentrations. Lines connect values in five patients, where samples were obtained during two identical treatment courses.

ACKNOWLEDGMENTS

This study was supported by the Children's Cancer Foundation in Sweden.

REFERENCES

1. Lie SO, Jonmundsson G, Mellander L, Siimes MA, Yssing M, Gustafsson G: A population based study of 272 children with acute myeloid leukaemia. Brit J Haematol 1996;94:82–88.
2. Klumper E, Pieters R, Kaspers GJL, Huismans DR, Loonen AH, Rottier MMA, van Wering ER, van der Does-van den Berg A, Hählen K, Creutzig U, Veerman AJP: In vitro chemosensitivity assessed with the MTT assay in childhood acute non-lymphoblastic leukemia. Leukemia 1995;9:1864–1869.
3. Sargent J, Elgie A, Williamson C, Bowen S, Taylor C: The use of the MTT assay to study drug resistance in AML, an update. Leukemia 1995;9:532.
4. Eksborg S, Strandler HS, Edsmyr F, Näslund I, Tahvanainen P: Pharmacokinetic Study of IV Infusions of Adriamycin. Eur J Clin Pharmacol 1985;28:205–212.
5. Liliemark E: Studies on podophyllotoxin derivatives; etoposide pharmacokinetics and liopsomal formulation of teniposide. Dissertation, Karolinska Hospital and Institute, Stockholm 1995.
6. Nygren P, Christensen J, Jansson B, Sundström C, Lönnerholm G, Kreuger A, Larsson R: Feasibility of the Fluorometric Microculture Cytotoxicity Assay (FMC) for Cytotoxic Drug Sensitivity Testing of Tumor Cells from Patients with Acute Lymphoblastic Leukemia. Leukemia 1992;11:1121–1128
7. Larsson R, Kristensen J, Sandberg C, Nygren P: Laboratory determination of chemotherapeutic drug resistance in tumor cells from patients with leukemia using a fluorometric microculture cytotoxicity assay (FMCA). Int J Cancer 1992;50:177–185.
8. Liliemark E, Pettersson B, Peterson C, Liliemark J: High Performance Liquid Chromatography with fluorometric detection for monitoring of etoposide and its cis-isomer in plasma and leukemic cells. J Chromatogr B; Biomed Appl 1995; 669(2):311–317.
9. Evans WE, Relling MV, Rodman JH, Crom WR, Boyett JM, Pui C-H: Conventional compared with individualized chemotherapy for childhood acute lymphoblastic leukemia. N Engl J Med 1998; 338:499–505.

PROGNOSIS IN ADULT AML IS PRECISELY PREDICTED BY THE DISC-ASSAY USING THE CHEMOSENSITIVITY-INDEX C_I

Peter Staib, Bernd Lathan, Timo Schinköthe, Sabine Wiedenmann, Bernhard Pantke, Thomas Dimski, Dimitris Voliotis, and Volker Diehl

Clinic I for Internal Medicine
University of Cologne
D-50924 Cologne, Germany

Keywords: acute myeloid leukemia, *in vitro* drug sensitivity, chemosensitivity index C_i, DISC-assay, prognosis.

1. ABSTRACT

We prospectively investigated the correlation between DISC-assay results and clinical response and also survival in patients with AML using a new method of evaluation.

1.1. Patients and Methods

Patients with de-novo AML were treated according to the TAD-HAM regimen (thioguanine, ara-C, daunorubicin—high dose ara-C, mitoxantrone) and patients with relapsed or secondary AML according to the Ida-FLAG regimen (idarubicin, fludarabine, ara-C, G-CSF). DISC assay was performed as described by Weisenthal and coworkers using minor modifications. All drugs used for treatment were tested at 5 concentrations in primary cell cultures in triplicate. Dose-response curves for each drug were obtained by logarithm and linear regression of assay results measured in percent tumor cell survival (TCS). The area under the curve (AUC) as a measure for the *in-vitro* dose-response relation was transformed into an index called chemosensitivity index C_i. If C_i was >0.5 probability of clinical response to that drug was defined to be high; if C_i was ≤0.5 to be low. Survival was estimated according to the Kaplan-Meier method.

1.2. Results

83 of 107 patients were eligible for evaluation; 66 received TAD-HAM and 17 Ida-FLAG for induction therapy. 55 pts. (66%) achieved CR and 19 (23%) BM-blast reduction below 10%, in both groups the maximum C_i (C_i-max) was >0,5 for at least one drug clinically used (TP=true positive correlation). 9 pts. (11%) were nonresponders and identified with C_i-max ≤0.5 of all drugs given for therapy (TN=true negative). TP=74, TN=9, correlations were highly significant (χ^2: p<0,001). Overall predictive accuracy was 100%. Median survival of the group with C_i-max >0.5 was significantly longer with 767 days as compared to 104 days in the group with C_i-max ≤0.5 (logrank, p<0,001).

1.3. Conclusions

The C_i may provide a more accurate evaluation of the DISC-assay, since clinical response was precisely predicted and assay results were also significantly correlated with patients' survival. Prospective clinical trials using the DISC-assay for treatment stratification and/or assay directed therapy strategies are justified.

2. INTRODUCTION

In-vitro drug sensitivity tests were developed for identifying the sensitivity of individual patients to anticancer chemotherapy. Stem cell or colony assays used to be the "gold-standard"[1], but since the early 1980s a variety of short-term tests, e.g. the colorimetric methyl-thiazol-tetrazolium (MTT) assay or the differential staining cytotoxicity (DISC) assay, have been devised to study *in-vitro* cellular drug resistance.[2–8] The DISC assay and the MTT assay were shown to be the short term *in-vitro* drug sensitivity tests of choice in acute leukemias.[4–7,9–12] We adapted the DISC assay which allows direct evaluation of the cells tested by light microscopy.

Since the individual prognosis in acute myeloid leukemia may still not be determined by known prognostic factors such as age or karyotype, the *in-vitro* chemosensitivtiy test result may help to predict individual treatment outcome more precisely.[5–6,11,13–16]

For *in-vitro* assays, defining a cut off point between sensitive and resistant is difficult as the results will usually make up a continuum from very sensitive through very resistant.[11,14] This may compromise the accuracy of an *in-vitro* assay, especially if preset cut off points such as a certain percentage of tumor cell survival (TCS) or various levels of inhibitory concentrations (IC_{50}, IC_{90}) are used for the evaluation of test results.[11,14] We, therefore, developed an evaluation system for the interpretation of DISC assay results that takes the complete dose-response relation into account.[16]

The accuracy of an *in-vitro* assay and its evaluation system should be assessed not only by correlation of assay results with response rates but also with survival.[11,14] We, therefore, conducted a prospective study to correlate response to therapy and overall survival with DISC-assay results in adult patients with AML applying this new evaluation methodology, that we called "chemosensitivity index C_i".

3. MATERIALS AND METHODS

3.1. Patients and Treatment

At our institution patients with de-novo AML were included into the German prospective randomized multicenter trial of the AML-Cooperative Group (AMLCG-'92 trial).[17] Induction therapy consisted of the TAD-HAM double induction regimen containing thioguanine, Ara-C, daunorubicin—high dose Ara-C, mitoxantrone. Patients suffering from relapsed AML or AML with a history of preexisting myelodysplastic syndrorme (MDS-AML) were treated with the Ida-FLAG regimen consisting of idarubicin, fludarabine, Ara-C and G-CSF.[18]

3.2. DISC Assay

The DISC-assay was performed according to the methods described by Weisenthal et al. with minor modifications.[1–2,9] Briefly, bone marrow or peripheral blood specimens from each patient with AML were collected into heparin prior to the administration of chemotherapy. Leukemic blast cells were isolated by Ficoll density gradient centrifugation, washed and suspended in RPMI 1640 culture medium supplemented with fetal calf serum (FCS). Drugs were tested at five concentrations in triplicate.[19] All drugs used for treatment in the TAD-HAM or the Ida-FLAG regimen were routinely tested: thioguanine, Ara-C, daunorubicin, mitoxantrone, idarubicin and fludarabine.[17–18] The middle test concentration of each drug was chosen within the range of clinically relevant steady state plasma levels.[19] Drug (20 µl) was added to 90,000 cells in 180 µl medium; phosphate-buffered saline (PBS) in medium served as a control. After 94 hours of incubation (37°C, humidified 5% CO_2), 50,000 fixed duck erythrocytes (DRBCs) were added to each tube in 10 µl PBS containing 2% fast-green and 1% nigrosin. The cells were transferred to collagen surfaced microscope slides by cytocentrifugation, air-dried and counterstained with May-Grünwald-Giemsa stain. Subsequent evaluation of slides by light microscopy facilitated the determination of drug efficacy at each concentration compared with controls. Assay results are expressed as percent tumor cell survival (% TCS).

3.3. New Evaluation System: Chemosensitivity Index C_i

TCS-data were transformed into the following mathematical equation by logarithm and linear regression for description of the dose response curve:

$$TCS(conc) = e^{-dist + rise * conc}$$

(conc = drug test concentration; e = Euler number; TCS = percent tumor cell survival; dist = y-intercept; rise = gradient)

The dose-response curve allowed the determination of the area under the curve (AUC), which is an exact measure of the complete dose-response relation. In order to compare the various drugs tested the AUC was transformed into an index ranging from 0 to 1. We called this index "chemosensitivity index C_i". The cut off point between resistance and sensitivity was adjusted at 0.5 for each drug by the AUC data of clinically resistant patients, since in these patients obviously all cytotoxic agents given for treatment are ineffective. If the C_i is ≤ 0.5 resistance to the particular drug is predicted, and if the C_i is > 0.5 sensitivity to the drug is postulated. The whole data processing is illustrated in Figure 1.

3.4. Clinical Correlation

The highest scoring C_i of those drugs clinically used was called C_i-max. The C_i-max was correlated with clinical outcome after induction chemotherapy in terms of complete remission (CR), reduction of bone marrow blasts less than 10%, refractory disease and also, most importantly, overall survival.

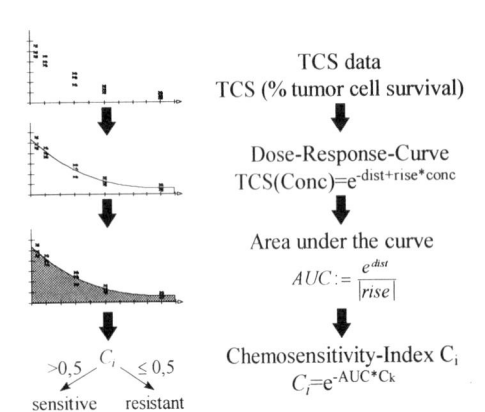

Figure 1. Flowsheet of data processing for the chemosensitivity index C_i; (conc = drug test concentration; e = Euler number; TCS = percent tumor cell survival; dist = y-intercept; rise = gradient; C_k = drug specific constant).

Steps shown in the flowsheet:
- TCS data: TCS (% tumor cell survival)
- Dose-Response-Curve: $TCS(Conc) = e^{-dist + rise \cdot conc}$
- Area under the curve: $AUC := \dfrac{e^{dist}}{|rise|}$
- Chemosensitivity-Index C_i: $C_i = e^{-AUC \cdot C_k}$
- $C_i > 0.5$ sensitive; $C_i \leq 0.5$ resistant

Overall survival curves were estimated according to the method described by Kaplan and Meier. Differences in survival between patients with C_i-max $\leq$ or $>$ 0.5 were assessed by the logrank test.

4. RESULTS

A total of 107 patients with AML were examined, in 85 patients the clinical outcome after chemotherapy was evaluable, whereas the DISC assay was successfully performed in 104 patients. Correlation between DISC assay results and clinical response was possible in 83 patients.

Of these 83 evaluable patients, 68 had de novo AML, the corresponding FAB subtypes are listed in Table 1. Four patients suffered from relapsed AML, 8 patients from secondary AML and 3 from biphenotypic acute leukemia. 66 patients received the TAD-HAM regimen and 17 patients the Ida-FLAG regimen for induction therapy. Ida-FLAG was used for high-risk AML such as relapse, secondary AML or AML with trilineage dysplasia.

After induction therapy 55 patients (66%) reached a complete remission and another 19 patients (23%) an effective reduction of bone marrow blasts below 10%, whereas 9 patients had refractory disease. The correlation between the C_i-max of only those drugs clinically used and the three response categories is shown in Figure 2. The non-responders were precisely identified from the total group of patients, and no difference of C_i-max values was found for the two responder-groups. The correlation of C_i-max with immediate treatment outcome is highly significant in the chi-square test. All the 74 patients in the responder group were found with a C_i-max value > 0.5 of at least one drug given for therapy, and all the 9 non-responders showed C_i-max values below 0.5 (see Table 2). Thus, the overall predictive accuracy was 100%.

Correlation of C_i-max with overall survival is shown in Figure 3. Median survival of patients with C_i-max > 0.5 was 767 days as compared to 104 days in patients with C_i-max

Table 1. FAB subtypes of patients with de-novo AML

FAB-subtype	M0	M1	M2	M3	M4	M5	M6	M7
n = 68		4	8	26	4	16	8	1	1

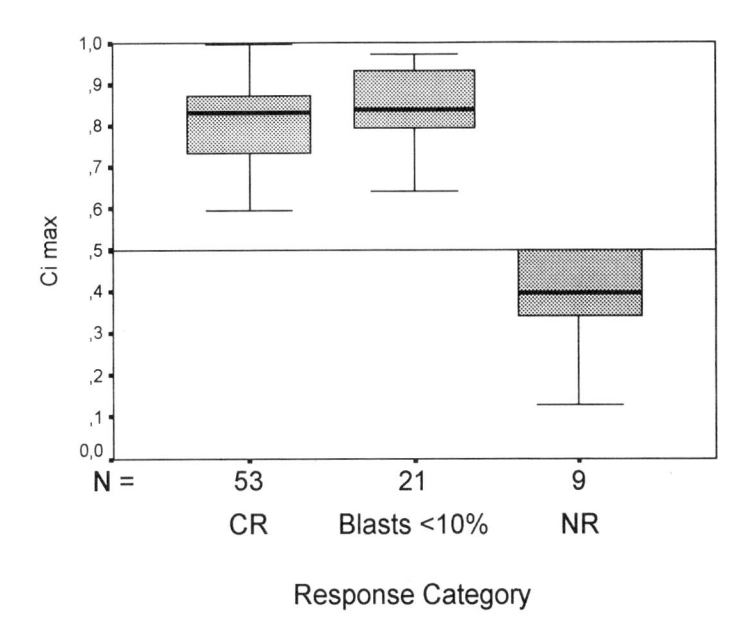

Figure 2. Median (=thick bar), interquartile range (=box), minimum and maximum (thin bars) of C_i-max in correlation with the three response categories.

≤ 0.5. The difference in survival between the two groups was statistically highly significant (p<0,001; logrank).

There were no favourable karyotypes found among the non-responders, and the rate of 56% unfavourable karyotypes in this group was twice as high as in the responder group with a rate of 28% (see Table 3).

5. DISCUSSION

In-vitro chemosensitivity assays have been developed with the ultimate aim of predicting clinical drug resistance and to tailor chemotherapy in individual patients with resistant disease or poor prognosis.[1–14,15–16,19–20] For the assessment of the accuracy of an *in-vitro* chemosensitivity assay it is necessary to compare the test results not only with short term outcome in terms of complete remission or persistent disease, but also with patient survival.[11,14] This clinical correlation is usually obtained by categorising into sensitive or resistant both test results and patient response and comparing the two. The definition of patient response is usually easy (response = CR or PR) whilst test results are not so easily categorized as the test results will usually make up a continuum from very sensitive through very resistant.[11,14] Defining a cut off point between sensitive and resis-

Table 2. Correlation between C_i-max and clinical outcome

Treatment outcome	C_i-max > 0.5	C_i-max $\leq$ 0.5	p-value
CR, BM-Blasts < 10%	74 (89%) (true positive, TP)	0	χ^2: p<0,001
Non-response	0	9 (11%) (true negative, TN)	

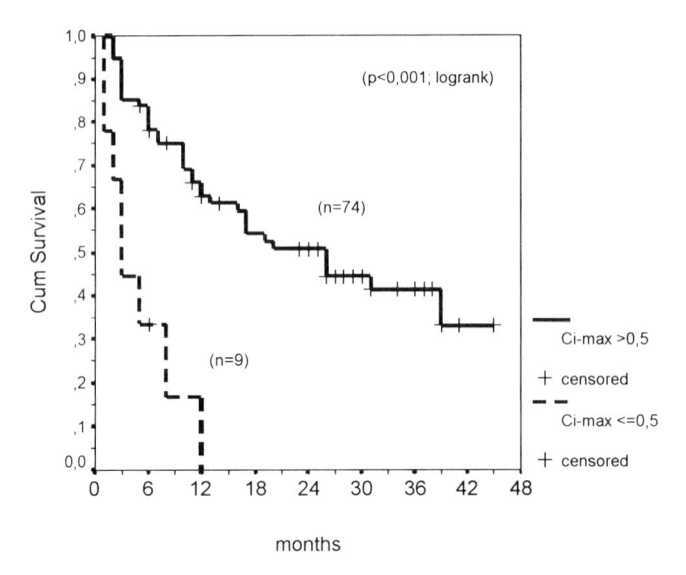

Figure 3. Overall survival of AML patients related to their C_i-max.

tant in vitro can in many cases only be done by comparison with the clinical data. In many studies the percentage of surviving tumor cells (e.g. 30%) at a particular drug concentration or the inhibitory drug concentration to achieve a certain percentage of killed tumor cells (e.g. IC_{90}) were used for cut off points.[2–7,10,12,15] In contrast to these conventional, rigid cut off point systems the newly developed chemosensitivity index C_i takes the total dose response relation into account by using the AUC.[16]

The application of the C_i methodology for analysing DISC-assay results in this series of AML patients demonstrated a correct prediction of clinical response to induction chemotherapy. Furthermore, we found that patients with a C_i-max over 0,5 lived significantly longer than patients with a C_i-max below 0.5. It is very important to notice that 9 patients with primary resistant disease were precisely identified within a few days. Thus, the predictive accuracy of 100% is promising, but this result is certainly due to the relatively small number of patients. No *in-vitro* test can hope to mimic the complexities of drug delivery, metabolism and excretion, that a perfect predictive accuracy results.

The majority (56%) of the non-responders had prognostic unfavourable cytogenetic abnormalities. Nevertheless, the rate of 28% of unfavourable karyotypes in the responder-group implies that the karyotype—although one of the strongest prognostic factors—is not the only determinant of the biology in AML.

Table 3. Frequencies of cytogenetic subgroups in relation to clinical outcome

Karyotype	Non-responders (n=6/9)		Responders (n=57/74)	
Favourable	0		5	(7%)
Intermediate	1	(11%)	31	(42%)
Unfavourable	5	(56%)	21	(28%)
N.D.	3	(33%)	17	(23%)

Favourable: t(15;17), t(8;21), inv16. Unfavourable: complex ($\geq$ 3) abnormalities, deletions of chromosome 5 or 7. Intermediate: other abnormalities, normal karyotype.

Our data confirm that the DISC-assay is one of the most suitable *in-vitro* drug sensitivity test for acute myeloid leukemias. By the application of the chemosensitivity index C_i evalutation methodology the DISC-assay provides a valuable tool for the prediction of individual treatment outcome in adult AML in terms of clinical response and also survival. Further studies are needed to find out whether the C_i is an independent prognostic factor and may serve for the stratification in prospective clinical trials where: 1) patients are randomised to receive best available therapy or assay directed therapy or 2) treatment is stratified according to risk groups identified by assay results.[13,20]

ACKNOWLEDGMENTS

This work was partly supported by the Deutsche Krebshilfe e.V. Bonn, Germany, and partly by the Frauke-Weiskam-Stiftung, Stifterverband für die deutsche Wissenschaft e.V., Essen, Germany.

REFERENCES

1. Delmer A, Marie JP, Thevenin D, Cadiou M, Viguie F and Zittoun R. Multivariate analysis of prognostic factors in acute myeloid leukemia: value of clonogenic leukemic cell properties. J Clin Onc 1989, 7, 738–746.
2. Weisenthal LM, Dill PL, Kurnick NB and Lippman ME. Comparison of dye exclusion assays with a clonogenic assay in the determination of drug-induced cytotoxicity. Cancer Res 1983, 43, 258–264.
3. Weisenthal LM, Marsden JA, Dill PL and Macaluso CK. A novel dye exclusion test for testing *in-vitro* chemosensitivity of human tumors. Cancer Res 1983, 43, 749–757.
4. Kirkpatrick DL, Duke M, Goh TS. Chemosensitivity testing of fresh human leukemia cells using both a dye exclusion assay and a tetrazolium dye (MTT) assay. Leukemia Res 1990, 14, 459–466.
5. Klumper E, Ossenkoppele GJ, Pieters R, Huismans DR, Loonen AH, Rottier A, Westra G and Veerman AJP. In vitro resistance to cytosine arabinoside, not to daunorubicin, is associated with the risk of relapse in de novo acute myeloid leukaemia. Br J Haematol 1996, 93, 903–910.
6. Pieters R, Huismans DR, Loonen AH, Hählen K, van der Does-van den Berg A, van Wering ER and Veerman AJP. Relation of cellular drug resistance to long-term clinical outcome in childhood acute lymphoblastic leukaemia. Lancet 1991, 338, 399–403.
7. Sargent JM, Taylor CG. Appraisal of the MTT assay as a rapid test of chemosensitivity in acute myeloid leukaemia. Br J Cancer 1989, 60, 206–210.
8. Bird MC, Godwin VAJ, Antrobus JH, Bosanquet AG. Comparison of *in-vitro* drug sensitivity by the differential staining cytotoxicity (DISC) assay and colony-forming assays. Br J Cancer 1987, 55, 429–431.
9. Bird MC, Bosanquet AG, Forskitt S, Gilby ED. Semi-micro adaption of a 4-day differential staining cytotoxicity (DISC) assay for determining the *in-vitro* chemosensitivity of haematological malignancies. Leuk Res 1986, 10, 445–449.
10. Bosanquet AG. The DISC assay—10 years and 2000 tests further on. In: Kaspers GJL, Pieters R, Twentyman PR, Weisenthal LM & Veerman AJP, Eds. Drug Resistance in Leukemia and Lymphoma. The Clinical Value of Laboratory Studies. Harwood, London. 1993, 373–384.
11. Bosanquet AG. Correlations between therapeutic response of leukaemias and *in-vitro* drug sensitivity assay. Lancet 1991, 337, 711–714.
12. Kaspers GJL, Pieters R, Van Zantwijk CH, De Laat PAJM, De Waal FC, Van Wering ER and Veerman AJP. *In-vitro* drug sensitivity of normal peripheral blood lymphocytes and childhood leukaemic cells from bone marrow and peripheral blood. Br J Cancer 1991, 64, 469–474.
13. Bosanquet AG. *In-vitro* drug sensitivity testing for the individual patient: an ideal adjunct to current methods of treatment choice. Clin Oncol 1993, 5, 195–197.
14. Bosanquet AG. Short-term *in-vitro* drug sensitivity tests for cancer chemotherapy. A summary of correlations ot test result with both patient response and survival. Forum Trends Exp. Clin. Med. 1994, 4, 179–189.

15. Lathan B, von Tettau M, Verpoort K, Diehl V. Pretherapeutic drug testing in acute leukemias for prediction of individual prognosis. In: Büchner T, Schellong G, Hiddemann W, Ritter J. eds. Haematology and Blood Transfusion. Vol. 33. Acute Leukemias II. Springer Verlag, Berlin, Heidelberg, 1990, 295–298.
16. Staib P., Lathan B., Michel K., Janz E., Schinköthe T. and Diehl V. Predictive value of pretherapeutic *in-vitro* chemosensitivity testing in adult AML. Haematology and Blood Transfusion 1998, 39, 509–519.
17. Büchner T, Hiddemann W, Wörmann B, Löffler H, Gassmann W et al. Intensive consolidation versus prolonged maintenance following intensive induction and conventional consolidation in primary AML: a study by AMLCG. Blood 1996, 88, No 10, Suppl. 1, 214a.
18. Wickramanayke PD, Steinmetz HT, Katay I, Glasmacher A, Staib P and Diehl V. Phase II trial of idarubicine, fludarabine, Ara-C and filgrastim (G-CSF) (Ida-FLAG) for the treatment of poor prognosis acut myeloid leukemia (AML). Blood 1995, 86, No 10, suppl. 1, 755a.
19. Tidefelt U, Sundman-Engberg B, Rhedin AS, Paul C. In vitro drug testing in patients with acute leukemia with incubations mimicking in vitro intracellular drug concentrations. Eur J Haematol 1989, 43, 374–384.
20. Veerman AJP and Pieters R. Drug sensitivity assays in leukemia and lymphoma. Br J Haematol 1990, 74, 381–384.

DRUG RESISTANCE TESTING OF ACUTE MYELOID LEUKEMIA IN ADULTS USING THE MTT ASSAY

N. Stute, T. Köhler, L. Lehmann, W. Wetzstein, and G. Ehninger

Medical Clinic I
Technical University Dresden
Fetscherstr. 74, 01307 Dresden, Germany

Keywords: acute myeloid leukemia, adult AML, MTT assay, drug resistance, topoisomerase II inhibitors, prognostic factors.

ABSTRACT

Objective: We want to evaluate the MTT in vitro assay for newly diagnosed AML in adults, in particular its prognostic significance. Methods: MTT tests were performed according to Pieters et al., Blood 76: 2327, 1990. Up to 18 cytostatic drugs were tested in a wide range of concentrations over 4 days and compared with controls. If necessary, blasts were enriched > 80 % by negative selection with dynabeads (Kaspers et al., Br. J. Cancer 70: 1047, 1994). Percent S-phase was measured at begin of assay and after 4 days. Results: Technical success rate was 80–85 % and the assay took about one day of work. IC_{50} values as a measure for drug resistance were highly reproducible with an interassay CV (range) of 28 % (13–47) between days. Median cell viability of controls after 4 days was 80 % (44–97); % S-phase at begin of assay was 3 % (0.1–15) and after 4 days 9 % (1–39). Leukemic blasts from 57 adult AML patients were prospectively tested in vitro at diagnosis. Large interindividual differences in drug resistance were observed (over 1000 fold on average). There was a trend for greater IC_{50} with higher cytogenetic risk and nonresponders to induction. Other clinical prognostic factors such as patient age, initial WBC, FAB subtype, prior MDS and % S-phase did not show a relationship with the in vitro data. There was a high correlation between the topoisomerase II related drugs regarding in vitro resistance. Conclusion: In vitro sensitivity tests like the MTT assay may provide a valuable tool for prediction of individual therapy outcome in combination with cytogenetics. However, longer follow-up is required.

Drug Resistance in Leukemia and Lymphoma III, edited by Kaspers et al.
Kluwer Academic / Plenum Publishers, New York, 1999.

INTRODUCTION

Drug resistance is a major cause of treatment failure. Drug sensitivity in vitro can serve as a valuable prognostic parameter in leukemias, as has been shown in prospective studies especially in children with ALL.[1] In adults there are relatively few data regarding short-term assays in AML,[2–8] but there is also emerging evidence of the prognostic relevance of in vitro testing in adult AML.[9,10] Short term assays like the MTT test could provide valuable information for better risk group stratification or aid in the rational and individualized selection of drugs, and thus perhaps improve therapy outcome. A major aim of our study is to evaluate the MTT in vitro test for newly diagnosed AML in adults within cooperative SHG (Süddeutsche Hämoblastosegruppe) study AML 96. In particular, we want to investigate its feasibility, reproducibility, interindividual variability and prognostic significance—like correlations with known prognostic factors, initial clinical response and ultimately disease free survival.

PATIENTS AND METHODS

Up to now, samples from 57 adult patients with AML at diagnosis have been prospectively tested in vitro, including 2 patients with secondary leukemia and 4 patients with prior MDS. Median age (range) was 55 years (17–77) and WBC $53 \times 10^9/l$ (7–359); there were five M0, eighteen M1, seventeen M2, three M3v, seven M4, five M5 and two M6 according to FAB classification. Patients were treated according to cooperative SHG study AML 91/96 or EORTC APL 93 protocol.

MTT tests were performed according to Pieters et al.:[11] MNC were obtained from peripheral blood or bone marrow after density centrifugation. Each drug and concentration was tested on microtiter plates in duplicate with $8-16 \times 10^4$ cells per well over 4 days and compared with controls without drug on day 4 (= 100 % cell survival). Up to 18 cytostatic drugs were tested over a wide range of concentrations: ara-C, mitoxantrone, busulfan, daunorubicin, amsacrine, etoposide, prednisolone, dexamethasone, L-asparaginase, 6-MP, 6-TG, teniposide, idarubicin, vincristine, cladribine, mafosfamide, treosulfan, and fludarabine. Drugs were stored in dilutions at -20 °C for < 3 months prior to testing. Less than 10^7 blasts are needed to test 3 cytostatic drugs. If necessary, RBC lysis was performed and blasts were enriched > 80 % by negative selection with dynabeads.[12] Blasts were then incubated for 4 days at 37 °C with 5 % CO_2 in RPMI-1640 DM with 15 % FCS and addition of ITS (insulin, transferrin, selenite).

MTT—a tetrazolium dye—was added after 4 days, and cells were incubated for another 6 hours. Living cells metabolize the dye and form coloured crystals, which were dissolved by the addition of acidic isopropanol. Absorption was measured by ELISA reader at 570 nm. Samples were considered evaluable if the drug-free control wells contain > 80 % leukemic cells before and > 70 % leukemic cells after 4 days of culture, and if control optical density (OD) on day 4 exceeds 0.15. Data was obtained by Mikrowin software (from Mikrotek), and concentration-survival data were analyzed by sigmoid regression using the 4-parameter function with Sigma-Plot (from Jandel Scientific). IC_{50} and IC_{80} values were calculated—the concentration at which 50 % or 80 % of cells are killed—and serve as a measure for the degree of cytostatic drug resistance. Using Sigma-Plot also AUC (area under the concentration-survival-curve) was calculated for each drug tested in vitro. Percent S-phase of leukemic blasts was determined by methods described elsewhere.[13]

RESULTS

Median cell viability of control (range) at start of assay was 97% (88–99) and after 4 days 80% (44–97); optical density of controls after 4 days was 0.40 (0.13–0.94). Technical success rate was 80–85% in fresh samples even if sent by overnight mail, so that the MTT assay could be successfully performed in most patients. A low control OD < 0.15 after 4 days was the most common reason for technical failure. Percent S-phase at begin of assay was 3 % (0.1–15) and after 4 days 9% (1–39). In vitro results were highly reproducible. Interday and interperson variability of measured IC_{50} values was small. Median CV in % (range) of the IC_{50} for n=9 experiments and several drugs tested was 28% (13–47) over a period of one year.

Leukemic blasts from 57 adults with newly diagnosed AML were tested in vitro up to now. Interindividual differences in cytostatic drug resistance were large (Figure 1), with individual resistance profiles for each patient. IC_{80} values could be generated for all drugs, except busulfan, prednisolone, dexamethasone, L-asparaginase and 6-MP, and highly correlated with IC_{50} values (data not shown).

Patients resistant to one drug are not necessarily so to another. However, in vitro resistance to mitoxantrone, unlike ara-C, correlated with resistance to daunorubicin, idarubicin, etoposide, teniposide and amsacrine (Figure 2).

48/57 of newly diagnosed patients with de novo AML were treated according to cooperative SHG study AML 96: induction therapy consisted of MAV (mitoxantrone, ara-C, etoposide) and MAMAC (amsacrine, ara-C), or DA (daunorubicin, ara-C) for patients > 65 years. For better comparison IC_{50} values of AML blasts from individuals were divided by the median IC_{50} values of patients with newly diagnosed AML. A large relative IC_{50} means that patient blasts are relatively resistant in vitro compared with other patients with AML and vice versa.

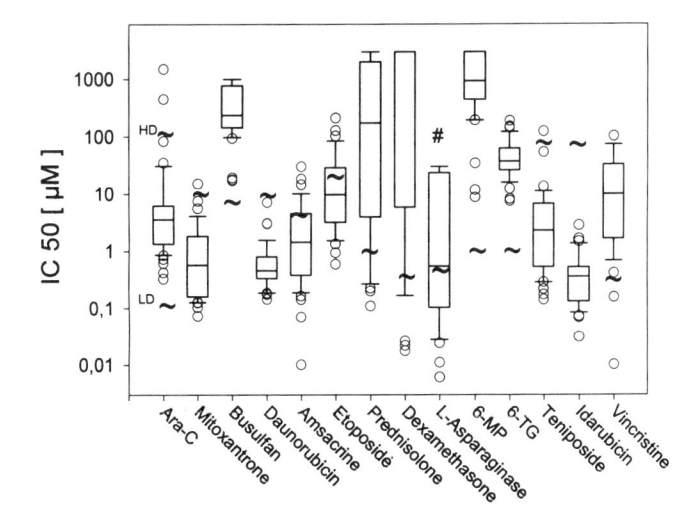

Figure 1. Distribution of IC_{50} values as measure of cytostatic drug resistance of adult AML in vitro (n=57). Shown are the 10, 25, 75 and 90 th percentiles and individual values outside this range. For orientation, population peak levels from the literature of cytostatic drugs at usual dosages are inserted (≈). HD = high dose, LD = low dose. However, in the clinical evaluation other factors also have to be taken into account: e.g. IC_{80}, pharmacokinetics and variability, infusion duration, drug stability, protein binding, metabolism and mechanism of action. # Concentration of L-asparaginase in IU/ml.

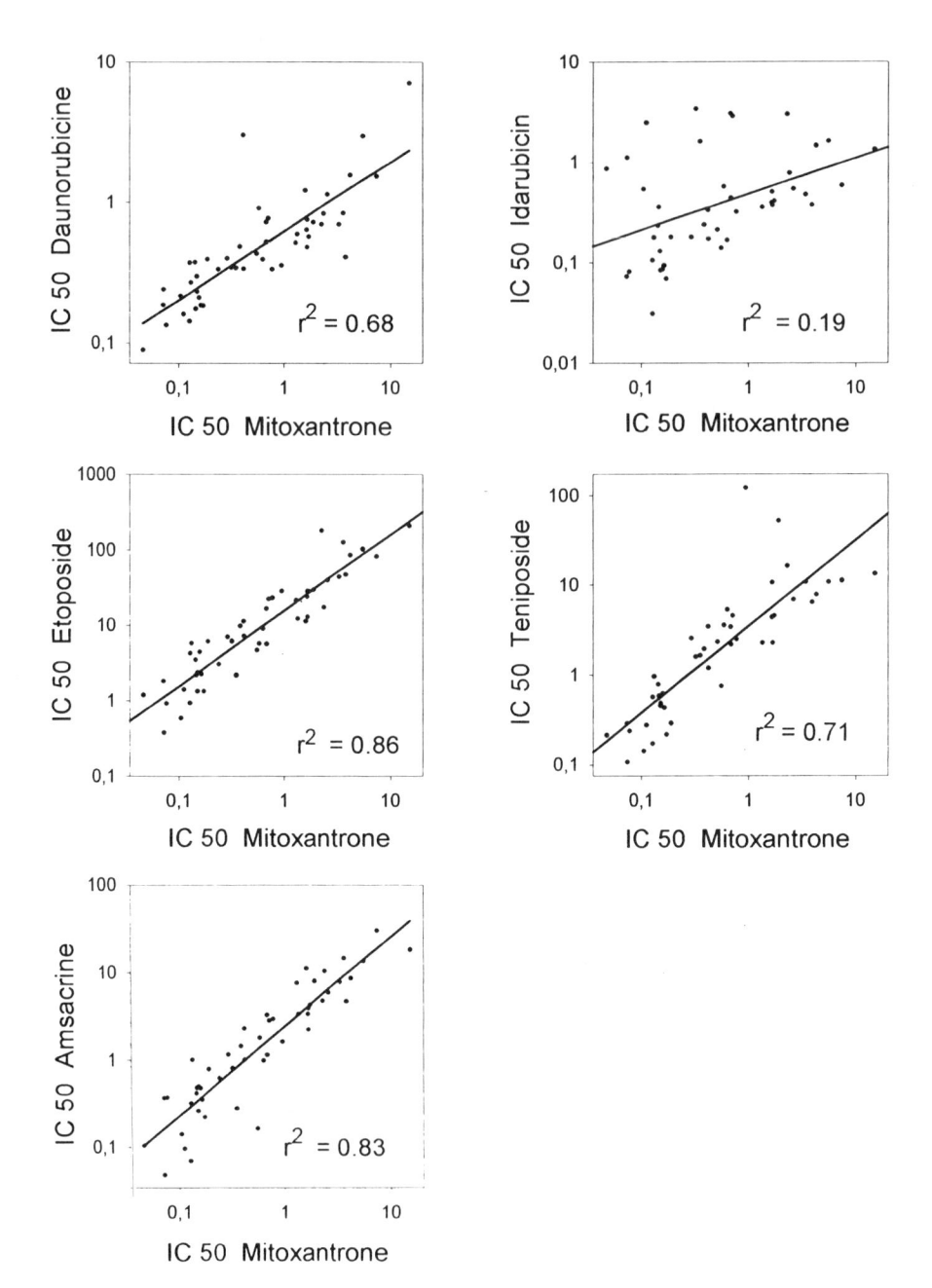

Figure 2. Comparison between in vitro sensitivity to mitoxantrone and other topoisomerase II related drugs: daunorubicin, idarubicin, etoposide, teniposide and amsacrine (n = 57).

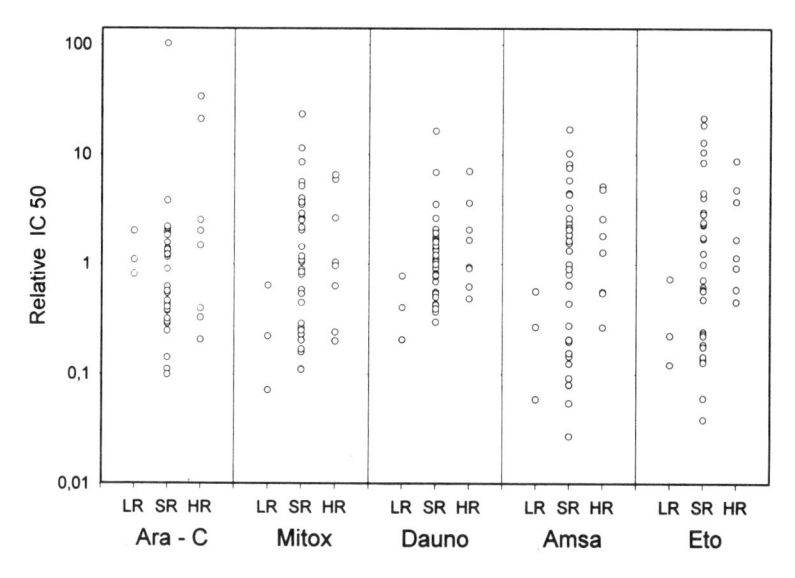

Figure 3. Relationship between AML in vitro drug resistance (relative IC_{50}) and cytogenetic risk (n = 57). In vitro data for cytostatic drugs commonly used in induction regimens for AML are shown. In order to enable comparisons between patients across several cytostatic drugs relative blast resistance for each drug was calculated by dividing IC_{50} values of individual adult patients by median IC_{50} values of all patients tested. Cytogenetic risk groups as defined by cooperative SHG study AML 96 : **LR** = low risk: t(8;21) without other abnormalities except -Y (M3 is being included here). **SR** = standard risk: all patients with no LR or HR abnormalities (including non-evaluable cases). **HR** = high risk: -5/del(5q), -7/del(7q), other monosomies, inv(3q), abnl 12p, abnl 11q, +11, +13, +21, +22, t(6;9), t(9;22), t(9;11), t(3;3), multiple aberrations or documented MDS.

So far no correlation could be found between in vitro drug sensitivity and clinical risk factors such as patient age, initial WBC, FAB classification, prior MDS and % S-phase (data not shown). There was a trend towards increasing drug resistance with increasing cytogenetic risk for several cytostatic drugs (Figure 3). However, AML blasts with high risk genetics were not more resistant in vitro than those with standard risk genetics.

Looking at initial clinical outcome, i.e. response after induction there was a trend for greater IC_{50} in nonresponders compared with patients in complete remission (Figure 4). The same holds true when looking at AUC (area under the concentration-survival-curve) as a measure of drug resistance and when looking at patients with standard risk cytogenetics only. Overall there was a good correlation between AUC and IC_{50} for the drugs shown, with a few exceptions. Looking across the cytostatic drugs used in induction for the lowest relative IC_{50} resulted in a better separation between patients regarding response, but did not change the picture completely (data not shown).

The relative IC_{50} (or AUC) were often either in the high, middle or low range for most drugs when comparing different patients with some variation and a few notable exceptions (data not shown).

DISCUSSION

Over eighty percent of AML samples can be assayed by the MTT test; this is a relatively high technical success rate compared to data published for ALL. Only 10–20 million leukemic cells are needed to test six cytostatic drugs, which equals on average 1 ml of bone marrow or a

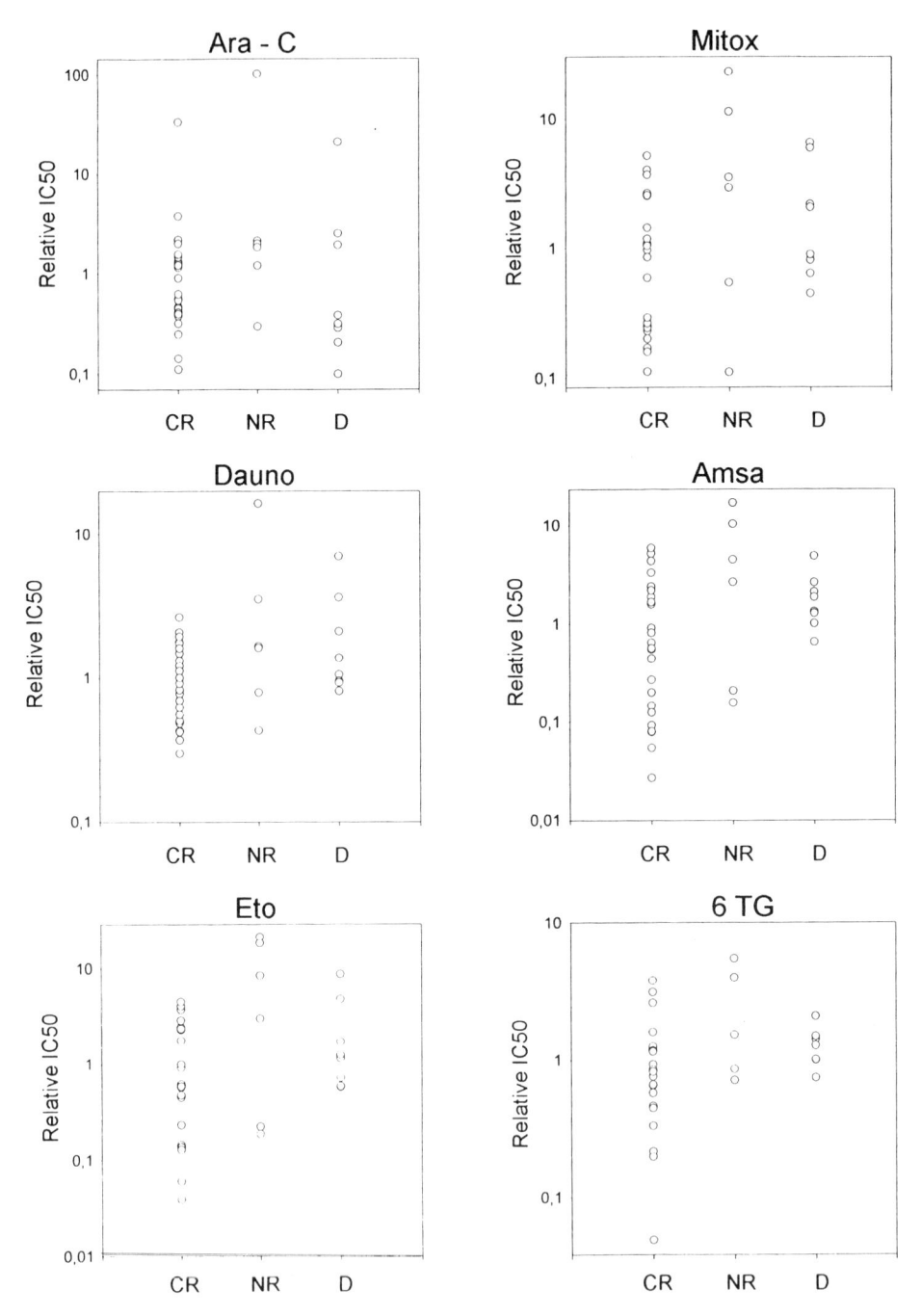

Figure 4. Relationship between AML in vitro drug resistance (relative IC$_{50}$) and initial clinical response (n<48). Results of induction therapy were evaluated after the second induction cycle as follows: **CR** = complete remission with normocellular bone marrow and < 5 % blasts, no blasts in the peripheral blood or extramedullary—including nominal CR with < 5 % blasts and persistent a- or hypoplasia. **NR** = nonresponse with > 5 % blasts in the bone marrow or blasts in the peripheral blood or extramedullary—induction failure, partial response or relapse during induction. **D** = death during induction. Of note, there was a trend towards higher IC$_{50}$ for some drugs with the group of patients who died during induction therapy (and nonresponders) when compared with patients who achieved a complete remission.

few mls of peripheral blood. Reproducibility of the in vitro data in our hands was remarkable for biological assays with an average CV of ≈ 25 % between days and technicians.

Large interindividual differences exist in drug sensitivity between AML patient samples; IC_{50} values varied by a factor of over 1000 (25–300.000) depending on the drug. It is likely that these differences somehow translate into different clinical response and therapy outcome. In vitro results in part reflect clinical experience in AML and pharmacological knowledge. The poor response to steroids in adult AML, for instance, is mirrored in vitro; also the better response of AML to 6-TG than 6-MP. Interestingly, resistance to mitoxantrone in vitro highly correlated with resistance to daunorubicin, idarubicin, etoposide, teniposide and amsacrine—all drugs which inhibit topoisomerase II—whereas there was no correlation between mitoxantrone and the antimetabolites ara-C and 6-TG. A similar observation was made by Klumper et al.[9]

In vitro drug resistance did not correlate with clinical prognostic factors such as patient age, initial WBC, FAB classification, prior MDS and % S-phase. Cytogenetics of leukemic blasts are a well known prognostic factor in AML. The differences in prognosis between cytogenetic risk groups might be explained, at least in part, by the differences of in vitro sensitivity to cytostatic drugs. However longer follow-up is required. Other risk factors like immunophenotype and mdr-1 expression will also be evaluated.

Comparing in vitro drug resistance with initial clinical response after induction therapy some, but no major differences in the IC_{50} between the patients with complete remission and the nonresponders were observed, which makes it difficult to predict initial response from our data. The same holds true for IC_{80} and AUC (data not shown). Since there was a high correlation between AUC and IC_{50} for the drugs shown this is not surprising. Unlike Staib et al.[10] with the DiSC assay in adult AML we can not, therefore, readily predict initial clinical outcome based on our in vitro data. Basically because one or two nonresponders had sensitive blasts in vitro, which in our opinion can not be attributed to differences between MTT and DiSC assay.

Correlations between in vitro results and disease-free survival (DFS) are still too early to allow conclusions regarding the prognostic value of MTT in vitro testing in adults with de novo AML from our data; further patient accrual and longer follow-up are required. Whether the patients with standard risk cytogenetics can be divided into a low and high risk group by in vitro data remains to be seen. Another open question is whether in vitro data may help to distinguish, with regards to DFS, between a low and high risk group within those patients who achieve a complete remission. If in vitro data contain prognostically relevant information in addition to cytogenetic risk, this could then be used for better risk group stratification in the future.

ACKNOWLEDGMENTS

This work is supported by the 'Deutsche Krebshilfe'. The authors wish to thank Verona Schwarze for her technical assistance with the MTT assay and people from the clinic and laboratory (morphology, flow cytometry and cytogenetics) who are involved. We also thank Gertjan Kaspers, Rob Pieters and Lokie Huismans from the group of Prof. Veerman in Amsterdam for helpful advice regarding technical details of MTT testing.

REFERENCES

1. Kaspers GJL, Veerman AJP, Pieters R, van Zantwijk CH, Smets LA, van Wering ER, van der Does-van den Berg A. In vitro cellular drug resistance and prognosis in newly diagnosed childhood acute lymphoblastic leukemia. Blood 1997; 90: 2723–29

2. Sargent JM, Taylor CG. Appraisal of the MTT assay as a rapid test of chemosensitivity in acute myeloid leukaemia. Br J Cancer 1989; 60: 206–10
3. Tidefelt U, Sundman-Engberg B, Rhedin AS, Paul C. In vitro drug testing in patients with acute leukemia with incubations mimicking in vivo intracellular drug concentrations. Eur J Haematol 1989; 43: 374–84
4. Santini V, Bernabei PA, Silvestro L, Dal-Pozzo O, Bezzini R, Viano I, Gattei V, Saccardi R, Ferrini PR. In vitro chemosensitivity testing of leukemic cells: prediction of response to chemotherapy in patients with acute non-lymphocytic leukemia. Hematol-Oncol 1989; 7: 287–93
5. Bosanquet AG. Correlations between therapeutic response of leukaemias and in-vitro drug-sensitivity assay. Lancet 1991; 337: 711–4
6. Larsson R, Fridborg H, Kristensen J, Sundstrom C, Nygren-P. In vitro testing of chemotherapeutic drug combinations in acute myelocytic leukaemia using the fluorometric microculture cytotoxicity assay (FMCA). Br J Cancer, 1993; 67: 969–74
7. Hwang W-S, Chen L-M, Huang S-H, Wang C-C, Tseng MT. Prediction of chemotherapy response in human leukemia using in vitro chemosensitivity test. Leuk Res 1993; 17: 685–8
8. Norgaard JM, Langkjer ST, Palshof T, Clausen N, Pedersen B, Hokland P. Relation of blast cell survival and proliferation to chemotherapy resistance in AML. Br J Haematol 1996; 93: 888–97
9. Klumper E, Ossenkoppele GJ, Pieters R, Huismans DR, Loonen AH, Rottier A, Westra G, Veerman AJ. In vitro resistance to cytosine arabinoside, not to daunorubicin, is associated with the risk of relapse in de novo acute myeloid leukaemia. Br J Haematol 1996; 93: 903–10
10. Staib P, Lathan B, Michel K, Janz E, Schinköthe T, Diehl V. Prognostic relevance of pretherapeutic in vitro chemosensitivity testing in adult AML. Blood 1996; 88(10), suppl 1: #1447
11. Pieters R, Loonen AH, Huismans DR, Broekema GJ, Dirven MWJ, Heyenbrok MW, Hählen K, Veerman AJP. In vitro sensitivity of cells from children with leukemia using the MTT assay with improved culture conditions. Blood 1990; 11:2327–36
12. Kaspers GJL, Veerman AJP, Pieters R, Broekema GJ, Huismans DR, Kazemier KM, Loonen AH, Rottier MAA, van Zantwijk CH, Hählen K, van Wering ER. Mononuclear cells contaminating acute lymphoblastic leukaemic samples tested for cellular drug resistance using the methyl-thiazol-tetrazolium assay. Br J Cancer 1994; 70: 1047–52
13. Nowak R, Oelschlaegel U, Hofmann R, Zengler H, Huhn R. Detection of aneuploid cells in acute lymphoblastic leukemia with flow cytometry before and after therapy. Leuk Res 1994; 18: 897–901

MTT ASSAY FOR DRUG RESISTANCE IN CHILDHOOD ACUTE LEUKEMIA AND EFFECT OF CYCLOSPORIN AND INTERFERON

A Preliminary Report

Zeynep Karakaş,[1,*] Leyla Ağaoğlu,[1] Serap Erdem,[2] Sema Anak,[1] Ayşegül Hacıbektaşoğlu,[2] and Gündüz Gedikoğlu[3]

I.U. School of Medicine
[1]Department of Pediatric Hematology/Oncology
[2]Department of Physiology
[3]Our Children Leukemia Foundation
Capa 34390 Istanbul, Turkey

INTRODUCTION

Cellular drug resistance is thought to be an important cause of the poor prognosis in childhood leukemia.[4] Drug resistance in leukemic cells may occur primary or may be acquired. To develop more effective treatment regimens for resistance patients is necessary, but it is difficult to use many drugs at same time in patients.[2,3] Therefore, it is more easy to use in vitro systems for various drug treatment of cells so that individual chemotherapy may be designed.[3] A rapid colorimetric assay based on the ability of viable cells to reduce a tetrazolium-based compound (MTT) to a blue formazan product is an increasingly used assay for testing in vitro chemosensitivity of leukemic samples.[2,3,4,5,7,8] MTT assay provides a good correlation between in vitro resistance to cytotoxic drugs and prognosis in childhood leukemia.[1]

In this preliminary report we describe in vitro resistance of fresh cells from patients with leukemia with MTT assay and its correlation with clinical resistance.

---

[*] Corresponding Author: Dr. Zeynep Karakas, Istanbul University School of Medicine, Department of Hematology/Oncology; Our Children Leukemia Foundation; Capa 34390 Istanbul, Turkey; fax: 0212 631312

MATERIALS AND METHODS

Samples

Bone marrow of leukemic cells was obtained from 15 children with acute leukemia: 6 ALL, 3 AML, 2 relapse, 4 remission of ALL. The bone marrow samples were isolated by density gradient centrifugation (200 rpm/20 min.) with Histopaque (Sigma). Then the cells were washed three times in medium RPMI-1640.

Drugs

All drugs were obtained from commercial sources which is used in clinic and aliquatus were stored at -20°C. The dilutions used in assay are 1, 0.1, 0.01, 0,001. Maximum concentrations of drugs[2] were as are followed:

DNR	(Daunorubicin)	1 µg/ml
IDA	(Idarubicin)	1 µg/ml
ADR	(Adriamycin)	1 µg/ml
L-ASP	(L-asparaginase)	20 µg/ml
PRD	(Prednisolone)	100 µg/ml
VCR	(Vincristine)	1 µg/ml
ETO	(Etoposide)	20 µg/ml
CPM	(Cyclophosphamide)	40 µg/ml
FN	(Interferon-(2b)	1000 U/ml
CSA	(Cyclosporin)	3 µMol/ml

Short Term Culture

Leukemic cells were suspended at 2×10^6 cells/ml RPMI-1640 (Sigma) that contained 10% fetal bovine serum (Sigma), penicillin, streptomycin and 2 mmol/L L-glutamine. One of microculture plates included 50 µl cell suspension and 10 µl of drugs and 40 µl of only medium. In addition control wells were prepared without drugs. After 4 day of incubation period at 5% CO_2, 37°C, MTT (Sigma) was added to microwells. The plates were incubated 4 hours. Then 100 µl DMSO (Sigma) was added to each wells. Overnight, optical density was measured using a ELISA (Pasteur) reader with a 550 nm test wavelength and a 620 nm reference wavelength. The mean values triplate prepared control wells and treated wells were calculated and the leukemic cell survival was evaluated with below formula:

$$LCS \% = OD \text{ treated wells} / OD \text{ control wells} \times 100$$

RESULTS

Leukemic cells survival was dose dependent with drugs. There are individual differences for the number of viable cells for ALL and AML patients although the cells were treated with same doses. The ratio of resistant cells that were treated with DNR in vitro were higher in patients with relapse and remission than initial ALL and AML (Figure 1). We obtained similar results in some cases when we use IDA. In addition, IDA doses were not low when compared to DNR but IDA increased cytotoxic effect in 1 ALL and 2 AML

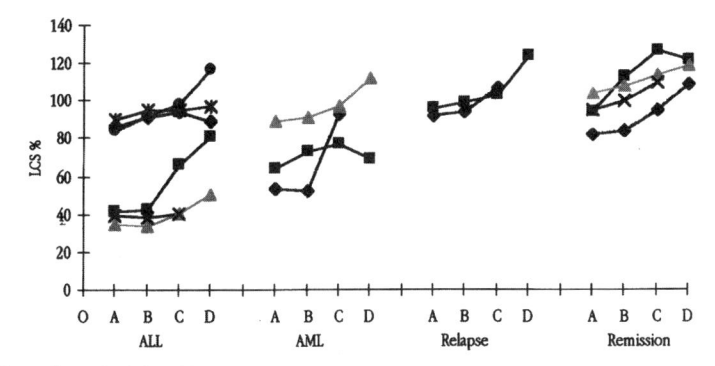

Figure 1. The cell survival for all patients treated with DNR. A= 1 µg; B=0,1 µg; C= 0,01 µg; D= 0,001 µg.

patients (Figure 2). At the initial cases with ALL and AML, individual differences were observed especially in ALL samples with PRD (Figure 3). We treated VCR and ADR in only ALL and remission cases, because cells obtained from other patients were limited (Figure 4, 5). The cell viability decrease to 80% in some patients cells when treated with ETO (Figure 6). Therefore, ETO is thought to be more effective. It is noticed that CSA and IFN had an increasing cytotoxic effect since cell viability decrease from 90% to 60% in DNR resistant cells. (Figure 7). As given in Table 1, in vitro drug sensitivity compared with clinical findings for all patients. Figure 8 gives an impression of cross-resistance to 4 drugs in 6 ALL patients.

DISCUSSION

Childhood leukemia can show varying degrees of sensitivity to a specific cytostatic agent.[4] This variation is an important consideration in attempts to develop individualized chemotherapy protocols.[3] Sensitivity testing is assumed to be an important aid in planning chemotherapy and in vitro drug resistance assays might be useful for predicting the responsiveness to standard chemotherapy.[3] Relapsed or refractory acute leukemia requires the development of a method for the rapid and accurate prediction of clinical response to specific chemotherapuetic agents for assessing drug sensitivity in leukemic patients.[7]

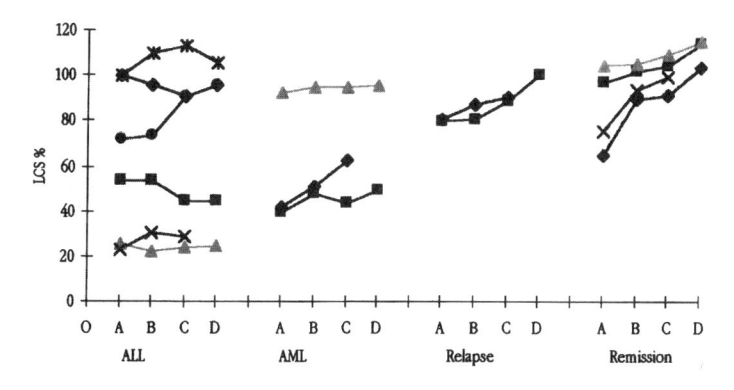

Figure 2. The cell survival for all patients treated with IDA. A= 1 µg; B=0,1 µg; C= 0,01 µg; D= 0,001 µg.

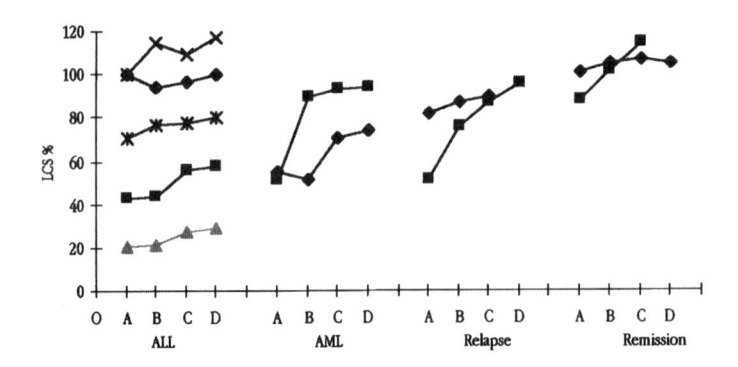

Figure 3. The cell survival for all patients treated with PRD. A= 1 µg; B=0,1 µg; C= 0,01 µg; D= 0,001 µg.

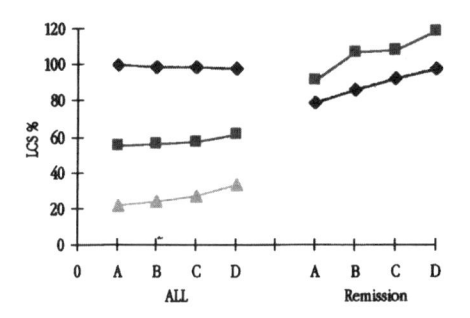

Figure 4. The cell survival of ALL and remission patients treated with VCR. A= 1 µg; B=0,1 µg; C= 0,01 µg; D= 0,001 µg.

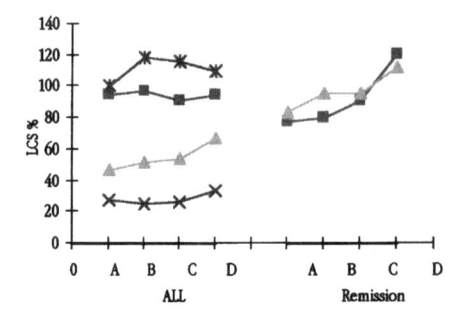

Figure 5. The cell survival of ALL and remission patients treated with ADR. A= 1 µg; B=0,1 µg; C= 0,01 µg; D= 0,001 µg.

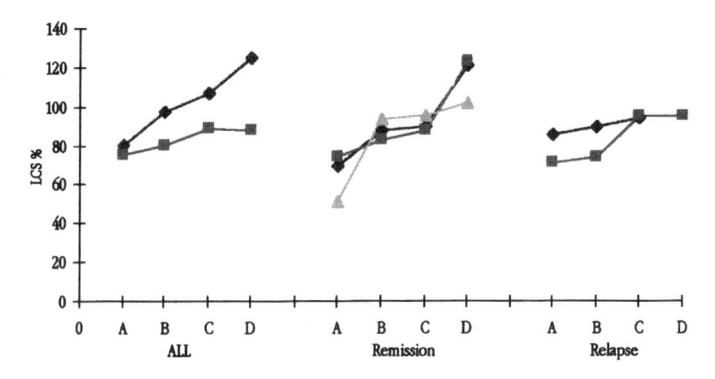

Figure 6. The cell survival of ALL, remission and relapse patients treated with ETO. A= 1 µg; B=0,1 µg; C= 0,01 µg; D= 0,001 µg.

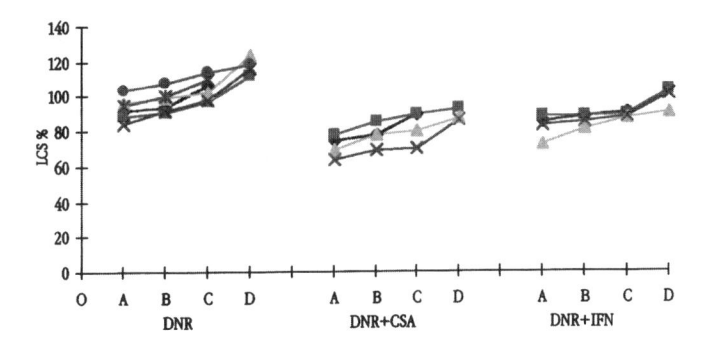

Figure 7. The cell survival of ALL and AML patients treated with DNR, DNR+CSA, DNR+IFN. A= 1 µg; B=0,1 µg; C= 0,01 µg; D= 0,001 µg.

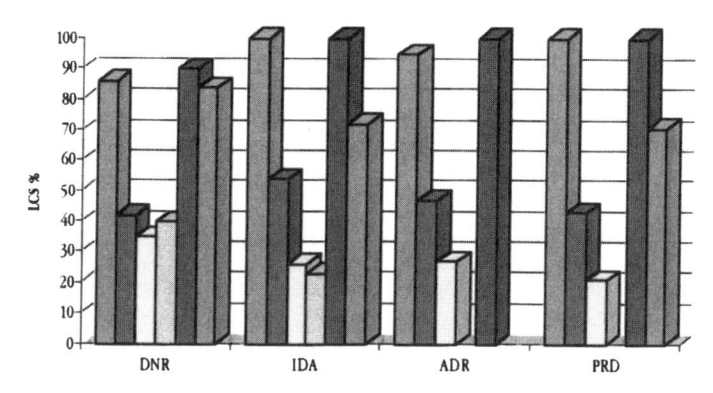

Figure 8. The cell survival of patients with ALL treated with maximum drug doses.

Table 1. In vitro drug sensitivity and clinical results

n	Disease	DNR	IDA	ADR	VCR	PRED	L-ASP	CPM	ETO	DNR + CSA	DNR + INF	Immuno-phenotype	Risk group	P-gp	Clinical sensitivity
1	ALL	R	R	R	R	R	R	R	—	—	—	Pre B, MM	G2	—	S
2	ALL	S	S	S*	S*	S	S	R	—	—	—	T, MM	G3	+	S
3*	ALL	S	S	S	S	S	S	R	—	—	—	Pre B Calla +	G2	—	S**
4	ALL	S	S	—	—	—	—	—	—	—	—	Pre Pre B	G3	+	S**
5	ALL	R	R	R	R	R	R	R	—	—	—	T, MDS	G3	+	S
6	ALL	R	R	—	—	R	R	—	R	R	R	Pre B Calla +	G3	Nonsps. binding	S
7	AML	S*	S*	—	—	—	—	—	—	—	—	CD 34 +	M5	+	S
8	AML	S*	S	—	—	S*	—	—	S	—	—	CD 34 —	M5	—	S
9	AML	R	R	—	—	S*	S*	—	R	R	R	CD 34 —	Transmission from CML	+	R
10	Rel ALL	R	R	—	—	R	R	—	R	R	R	Pre Pre B	G3	+	S
11	Rel AML	R	R	—	—	S*	R	—	R	R	R	CD 7 + CD 34 +	M4	+	R
12	Rem. ALL	R	R	R	R	—	R	—	R	—	—	—	G3	—	S
13	Rem. ALL	R	R	R	R	—	R	—	R	—	—	—	G2	—	S
14	Rem. ALL	R	R	—	—	R	—	R	S*	R	R	—	G2	+	S
15	Rem. ALL	R	R	—	—	R	R	—	—	R	R	—	G2	—	S

S*: Sensitive in high doses; S: Sensitive; R: Resistance; 3*: This patient had relapsed; S**: No response at day of 14, but remission achieved by the end of the induction therapy.

We performed the MTT assay for a total of 15 patients; 6 ALL, 3 AML, 2 relapse and 4 remission cases. Leukemic cells were cultured with nine anticancer-drugs for four days. In addition, we treated the cells with cyclosporin and interferon as MDR modulating agents which have potentiate DNR effect in 1 ALL, 1 AML, and 2 relapse cases. There are individual differences in chemosensitivities of leukemic cells in ALL and AML patients with all tested drugs. This was observed clearly in leukemic cells exposed to DNR, IDA, ADR and PRD. We have used in vitro doses which calculated from the maximal serum concentration reported by Hongo et al.[2] We did not want to use over doses provoked LC_{50} to stand by clinical convenient doses. The cell survival ratio with different concentrations of drugs are presented in Figure 1–6. Therefore, in this preliminary study we tried to establish a standardized MTT assay in childhood leukemia.

ACKNOWLEDGMENTS

This study is supported by Istanbul University Research Fund and Our Children Leukemia Foundation.

REFERENCES

1. Dow LW, Dahl GV, Kalwinsky DK, Mirro J, Nash MB, Robenson PK. Correlation of drug sensitivity in vitro with clinical responses in childhood acute myeloid leukemia. Blood 1986; 68: 400–405.
2. Hongo T, Fujii Y, Igarashi Y. An in vitro chemosensitivity test for the screening of anti-cancer drugs in childhood leukemia. Cancer 1996; 65:1263–1272.
3. Pieters R, Kaspers GJL, Klumper E, Veerman AJP. Clinical relevance of in vitro drug resistance testing in childhood acute lymphoblastic leukemia (ALL): The state of the art. SIOP Seventh schwe›sguth prize winning paper 1992; Hannover. Med Pediatr Oncol 1994; 22:299–308.
4. Klumper E, Pieters R, Kaspers GLJ, Huismans DR, Loonen AH, Rottier MA, Van Wering ER, Van der does-van den Berg A, H(hlen K, Creutzig U, Veerman A J P. In vitro chemosensitivity assessed with the MTT assay in childhood acute non-lymphoblastic leukemia. Leukemia 1995; 9:1864–1869.
5. Twentyman PR, Fox NE, Rees JKH. Chemosensitivity testing of fresh Leukemia cells using the MTT colorimetric assay. British Journal of Hematology 1989; 71; 19–24.
6. Pieters R, Kaspers GJL, Van Wering ER, Huismans DR, Loonen A H, Hählen K, Veerman A P J. Cellular drug resistance profiles that might explain the prognostic value of immunophenotype and age in childhood acute lmphoblastic leukemia, Leukemia 1993; 7:392–397
7. Klumper E, Pieters R, Veerman APJ, Huismans DR, Loonen AH, Hählen K, Kaspers GJL, Van Wering ER, Hartmann R, Henze G. In vitro cellular drug resistance in children with relapsed/refactory acute lymphoblastic leukemia. Blood 1995; 86:3861–3868
8. Klumper E, Pieters R, Den Boer ML, Huismans DR, Loonen AH, Veerman AJP. In vitro anthracycline cross-resistance pattern in childhood acute lymphoblastic leukemia. British Journal of Cancer 1995; 71:1188–1193

50

DIFFERENTIAL ANTILEUKEMIC ACTIVITY OF PREDNISOLONE AND DEXAMETHASONE IN FRESHLY ISOLATED LEUKEMIC CELLS

Vladimír Mihál,[1] Marián Hajdúch,[1,*] Věra Nosková,[1] Gabriela Feketová,[1] Kassmine Jess,[1] Libuše Gojová,[1] Ivo Kašpárek,[1] Jan Starý,[2] Bohumír Blažek,[3] Dagmar Pospíšilová,[1] and Zbynik Novák[1]

[1]Laboratory of Experimental Medicine
Department of Pediatrics, Palacký University
775 20 Olomouc, Czech Republic
[2]Faculty of Medicine
Department of Pediatrics, Charles University
Prague, Czech Republic
[3]Faculty Hospital
Department of Pediatrics
Ostrava, Czech Republic

Keywords: glucocorticoid, ALL, MTT assay, drug resistance, prednisolone, dexamethasone.

1. ABSTRACT

This study was designed to compare the antileukemic activity of prednisolone and dexamethasone in childhood acute lymphoblastic leukemia (ALL) under *in vitro* conditions. The chemoresistance of leukemic cells was ascertained by means of a MTT assay in 69 ALL children at diagnosis and the concentration killing 50% of leukemic cells (LCS$_{50}$) was determined. The children were treated using the protocol ALL-BFM 90/95. Statistical correlations were made among prednisolone (PRED) and/or dexamethasone (DEX) LCS$_{50}$

---

[*] Corresponding author: Laboratory of Experimental Medicine, Department of Pediatrics, Faculty of Medicine, Palacký University and Faculty Hospital Olomouc, Puškinova 6, 775 20 Olomouc, Czech Republic; Tel.: +420-68-585 4473; Fax: +420-68-585 2505; e-mail: marian@risc.upol.cz

Drug Resistance in Leukemia and Lymphoma III, edited by Kaspers *et al.*
Kluwer Academic / Plenum Publishers, New York, 1999.

and absolute number of blast cells (ANB) on day 0/8 and a new parameter named blast cells clearance (BCC, BCC8 [%] = ANB8 : ANB0 x 100) on day 8. Despite the previously published results of Ito et al. (J.Clin.Oncol. 14:2370–2376,1996) and Kaspers et al. (MPO 27:114–121,1996) on a positive correlation of DEX versus PRED LCS_{50} ($p<0.002$), in our study, we identified 30% of children (21/69) with differential *in vitro* responsiveness to PRED and DEX. 16% of patients (11/69) were highly sensitive to DEX and resistant to PRED, while 14% of them (10/69) were resistant to DEX and highly sensitive to PRED. The major difference found in our and the other studies was in the processing of leukemic cells. These results were confirmed in a model experiment using the CCRF-CEM line, where we showed that sensitivity to PRED and DEX, but not to other anti-cancer drugs critically depends on manipulation with tumor cells (cryopreservation). Correlation of PRED/DEX *in vitro* sensitivity values with parameters of *in vivo* patient's response to PRED monotherapy identified significant association of PRED LCS_{50} with BCC8 ($p<0.02$). It indicates strong linkage of *in vitro* sensitivity to PRED with percentage of blast cells eliminated from patient blood within the first 8 days of PRED monotherapy.

2. INTRODUCTION

Glucocorticoids (GCs) are highly efficient drugs in the treatment of childhood acute lymphoblastic leukemia, although they are not curative when used in single agent therapy. These drugs were introduced into hemato-oncological practice in the late 1940's and early 1950's.[1] Since that time GCs have been one of the most important components of ALL treatment protocols. The mechanism of the action relies upon diffusion of GCs through cytoplasmatic membrane and binding of the drugs to cytoplasmatic GC receptors (GCRs).[2] The GC-GCR complex is translocated into the nucleus, where it binds to DNA and transactivates a number of GC inducible genes.[2] In GCs sensitive leukemias, the drug induced apoptosis is the major cellular response,[2,3,4] although GCs do not always induce cell death and may exert biological activity via induction/repression of expression of other genes or proteins. For instance, DEX can down regulate expression of mdr genes in drug resistant cells and thus can sensitize tumor tissue to chemotherapy.[4,5,6,7,8] Nonetheless, a significant portion of patients exhibit primary or secondary resistance to corticoids. For instance, at diagnosis, 80% of patients respond to steroids as a single agent therapy, while only 35% of responses were observed in ALL relapsed children.[2] A range of mechanisms of resistance to GCs were described, which include *mdr1* mediated efflux of GCs with both 11- and 17-hydroxyl groups,[4] aberrant GCRs,[2] altered expression of hsp90 and hsp70 proteins,[9] etc. From clinical point of view, there is an emerging importance of prediction of patient's response to GCs. There are two basic questions, which are important to address: 1) whether the individual patient is responding to GCs therapy; and 2) whether there is an individual variability in patient's response to various corticoids, for instance PRED versus DEX.

To predict and further separate responders and non-responders to PRED under *in vivo* conditions, the Berlin-Frankfurt-Munster (BFM-) group and Dutch Childhood Leukemia Study Group have introduced "PRED window". It is one week PRED monotherapy, where the cut-off value defining clinical response is decrease of ANB in patient blood under $1000/mm^3$ on day 8.[10] The overall response rates were 92%, and the majority of non-responders were males, children with high white blood cell count (WBC) and patients with T-ALL.[10] Non-responders are treated with high-risk protocols. However, some of the ALL children were not eligible for PRED response analysis, because their initial ANB is under $1000/mm^3$.

Other efforts were performed to avoid the complications of *in vivo* GC response assessment, and *in vitro* assays were developed. These include quantification of GCRs in the cytoplasm of tumor cells,[2,11] activation and translocation of GC-GCR complexes[2] and induction of DNA fragmentation following steroid treatment.[2,3] However, the prediction of patient's response based upon *in vitro* examinations was only variably successful and/or the *in vitro* analyses were inappropriate for clinical routine due to high cost and labor demands. Nonetheless, a few years ago semi-automated *in vitro* MTT assay for analysis of drug resistance in primary tumor cells was introduced.[3,12,13,14,15,16] This is an cytotoxicity based cost-effective method which determines drug concentrations lethal to 50% of leukemic cells under *in vitro* conditions.[16] Despite, the fact that the assay possess only cellular mechanisms of GC resistance, it showed significant association between *in vitro* drug sensitivity to PRED and long term survival of ALL children.[14] This assay also demonstrated that there is a strong correlation between *in vitro* anti-leukemic activity of PRED and DEX, and provided indirect evidence that substitution of PRED with DEX would not increase the percentage of GC responses *in vivo*.[3,13]

Although the positive correlation between PRED and DEX LCS$_{50}$ was also found in our study, the level of significance was much lower that that in the papers of Kaspers et al.[13] and Ito et al.[3] Moreover, we have identified a substantial portion of patients with different *in vitro* responses to PRED and DEX. The reasons and clinical significance of our observations are described and discussed in this report.

3. MATERIALS AND METHODS

3.1. Samples and Patients

The bone marrow and peripheral blood samples were collected from children newly diagnosed with ALL in the Departments of Pediatrics in Olomouc, Prague and Ostrava and were transported within 6 hours to the Laboratory for Drug Resistance, Faculty of Medicine, Palacký University in Olomouc. The diagnosis of ALL was based on cytomorphology, cytochemistry, CD classification and cytogenetics. The clinical prognostic factors included risk factor calculated according to ALL-BFM 90 protocol guidelines [6], age, sex, the total number of white blood cells at diagnosis (WBC), absolute number of blast cells at diagnosis (ANB0) and on the 8th day of the treatment (ANB8), the percentage of blast cells in patient's bone marrow 15 (BM15) and 33 days (BM33) after initiation of the therapy. To better characterize the percentage of reduction of tumor mass, a new parameter named blast cell clearance on day 8 (BCC8) was introduced. BCC8 was calculated from ANB0 and ANB8 using the following equitation: BCC8[%] = ANB8 : ANB0 × 100. The following CD markers were examined in leukemic cells of patients included in this study: CD79a, cytoplasmatic IgM, cytoplasmatic CD22, CD19, CD10, CD20, TdT, CD24, CD3 (cytoplasmatic and membrane), anti-TCR, CD2, CD4, CD5, CD7, CD8, CD1a, anti-MPO, CD13, CD33, CDw65, CD14, CD15, CD64, CD117.

3.2. Cell Line

Human T-lymphoblastic cell line CCRF-CEM was kindly provided by Dr. W.T. Beck (St. Jude Children Research Hospital). Cells were cultured in their log phase in Dulbeco's modified essential medium with 5 g/l glucose, 2mM glutamine, sodium bicarbonate, 100 U/ml penicillin, 100 µg/ml streptomycin (Sigma, Czech Republic), 15% fetal calf serum (Biocom, Czech Republic).

3.3. MTT Assay

The 3-day MTT assay was used to determine the *in vitro* drug sensitivity of leukemic cells to anti-cancer drugs as described elsewhere.[16] Briefly, mononuclear cells were separated by density centrifugation on Ficoll Paque (density 1.077 g/ml; Pharmacia Sweeden) and washed twice in RPMI 1640 with 2mM glutamine, sodium bicarbonate, penicillin (100 U/ml), and streptomycin (100 µg/ml) (Sigma, USA). After the second wash, the cell pellet was suspended in a culture medium (RPMI 1640 with 2mM glutamine, sodium bicarbonate, 100 U/ml penicillin, 100 µg/ml streptomycin (Sigma, USA), 15% fetal calf serum (Biocom, Czech Republic), 5 µg/ml insulin, and 5 µg/ml transferrin) at the final concentration 1–2.10^6/ml (patient's cells) or 5.10^{-4}/ml (CCRF-CEM line). Aliquots (80 µl) of cell suspension were added to 96-well microculture plates containing 20 µl aliquots of drug solutions. Leukemic cells were exposed to six concentrations of each drug in duplicate for three days. Control tumor cells were cultured in the absence of drugs. At the end of culture, 10 µl of MTT (5 mg/ml) were pipetted into each well, and incubated another 6 hours. The yellow tetrazolium salt MTT was reduced to dark blue formazan by viable cells only. Formazan crystals were dissolved by 100 µl 10% sodium dodecylsulphate/water (pH=5.0) overnight at 37°C. The optical density (OD) was measured at 540 nm with the Labsystem iEMS Reader MF (UK). The leukemic cell survival (LCS) was calculated using the following equation: $LCS = (OD_{drug\ exposed\ well} / mean\ OD_{control\ wells}) \times 100\%$. The LCS_{50} value, the drug concentration lethal to 50% of the tumor cells, was calculated from the obtained dose response curves.

3.4. Statistics

To analyze positive or negative associations among individual parameters examined, we applied multivariate correlation analysis (Pearson product-moment correlation; STATGRAPHICS, version 5.0). The program has calculated the correlation coefficient (r) and its statistical significance (p). In cases when the LCS_{50} values were higher/lower than the maximum/minimum concentration tested, maximum/minimum values were entered as LCS_{50} for statistical analysis.

4. RESULTS

4.1. Patient Characteristics

The study included a group of 53 children, newly diagnosed as having ALL. All of them were completely examined for the analyzed parameters. This group was further processed to exclude patients with ANB0=0 (4; 8.7%) and children whose death was not due to leukemia, e.g. treatment induced sepsis (3; 5.7%). The remaining group of patients (46; Table 1) consisted of 22 boys (47.8%) and 24 girls (52.2%). Twenty children (43.5%) were older than six years of age. Only two children failed to accomplish hematological remission (4.3%). 36 children (78.3%) had a good clinical response to glucocorticoids (BC8<10^9/l). 5 patients (12.2%) had a BM15 over 16% of nucleated cells and 26 (63.4%) of them reached hematological remission on day 15 (blast cells in bone marrow < 5%). Three children were found to bear chromosomal translocation t(4;11), two t(9;22) and two children were diagnosed as having complex chromosomal changes. Five patients (10.9%) were suffering from proB-ALL, 6 (13.0%) had preB-ALL, 25 children had c-ALL (54.4%), 2 (4.3%) B-ALL and 8 patients (17.4%) were diagnosed with T-ALL.

Table 1. Clinical and laboratory characteristics of patients included in the study

Patient no.	PRED [µg/ml]	DEX [µg/ml]	PRED/DEX	WBC0 [x10⁹/l]	ANB0 [/µl]	ANB8 [/µl]	BCC8 [%]	CD classification	Cytogenetics	Age [years]	Sex	RG	Clinical outcome*	BM0 [%]	BM15 [%]	BM33 [%]
1	1,0878	0,1861	8,183	143	126840	43990	65,32	T-ALL	46XY	14	M	HRG	>24,1CR	100	62	3,2
2	0,0189	0,0035	7,560	23,3	1631	0	100,00	B-ALL	46XY,t(8;14)	6	M	SRG	<24,1CR	100	<5	<5
3	0,0073	0,1	0,102	7,7	2310	96	95,84	c-ALL	47XX,+der19,del13,t(1;19)	11	F	HRG	3,dead	94,8	1	0,5
4	0,0145	0,001	20,300	32,9	2277	13	99,43	c-ALL	47XY,+M	5	M	MRG	>24,1CR	96	1,1	0,4
5	241,25	6	56,292	6,4	256	112	56,25	preB-ALL,My+	46XX,t(12;21)	4	F	SRG	<24,1CR	90	<5	<5
6	50,11	6	11,692	57,8	4624	0	100,00	proB-ALL	46XY,t(4;11)	18	M	MRG	>24,1CR	98	6,8	1,2
7	16,2368	0,0429	529,872	8,1	329	0	100,00	c-ALL	54XX	6	F	SRG	>24,1CR	84	5,6	0,8
8	241,25	6	56,292	191,6	180104	4080	97,73	proB-ALL,My+	46XY,t(4;11)	1	M	HRG	<24,1CR	100	<5	<5
9	0,0077	0,0006	17,967	300	2700000	0	100,00	T-ALL	46XY	14	M	HRG	>24,1CR	95	<5	<5
10	0,1713	0,0076	31,555	27,2	2180	288	86,79	c-ALL	46XX,CCC	12	F	SRG	14,dead	84,8	7,2	<5
11	0,4496	0,0121	52,020	182	87000	950	98,91	preB-ALL	46XX,t(9;22)	11	F	HRG	<24,1CR	98	9	<5
12	0,0516	0,0189	3,822	53,5	49312	4758	90,35	preB-ALL	46XX,CCC	13	F	HRG	<24,1CR	97	52	11
13	0,001	0,0002	7,000	6,8	2652	186	92,99	c-ALL	46XY	11	M	SRG	>24,1CR	95	ND	4,4
14	0,0073	6	0,002	25,2	2520	0	100,00	c-ALL	46XX,t(1;19)	2	F	MRG	<24,1CR	92	<5	<5
15	241,25	0,143	2361,888	7	41	0	100,00	c-ALL	56XY	8	M	SRG	>24,1CR	94,4	0,8	1,2
16	10	6	2,333	188,6	1546652	0	100,00	T-ALL	46XY	15	M	HRG	>24,1CR	94	<5	<5
17	241,25	6	56,292	4,8	2112	1584	25,00	c-ALL	ND	2	F	HRG	>24,1CR	91,6	9,2	0,4
18	0,0073	6	0,002	66,1	59490	378	99,36	preB-ALL	46XY,19+der19,t(1;19)	9	M	MRG	<24,1CR	98	1,2	2
19	1,0613	0,0041	362,395	114,6	77928	870	98,88	c-ALL	46XY,t(9;22)	10	M	HRG	>24,1CR	99	30	<5
20	0,8918	0,0003	4161,733	64,5	52890	48	99,91	c-ALL	ND	2	F	MRG	<24,1CR	97	<5	<5
21	0,11	0,0016	96,250	75,4	62831	9796	84,41	c-ALL	46XX,X+M	10	F	HRG	<24,1CR	75	21	4,4
22	241,25	0,0149	22667,785	2,3	92	0	100,00	preB-ALL	ND	17	M	MRG	<24,1CR	100	ND	<5
23	0,0073	0,0327	0,313	35,1	26300	1140	95,67	c-ALL	46XX	3	F	HRG	0,5;dead	76,8	-	-
24	0,8728	0,0335	36,475	29,9	23920	198	99,17	c-ALL	46XX	16	F	MRG	>24,1CR	98	<5	<5
25	0,0344	0,1987	0,242	219,8	149464	120	99,92	T-ALL	46XY,t(12;21)	14	M	MRG	<24,1CR	95	<5	<5
26	241,25	6	56,292	5	2100	280	86,67	c-ALL	46XX	4	F	MRG	>24,1CR	97	16	<5
27	241,25	0,0002	1688750	67	60970	1940	96,82	c-ALL	ND	6	M	HRG	>24,1CR	92	<5	<5
28	0,558	6	0,130	6,9	1770	1	99,94	preB-ALL,My+	46XY,t(12;21)	10	M	MRG	>24,1CR	98	14	<5
29	0,0357	0,0004	124,950	2,1	42	0	100,00	c-ALL	46XX,t(12;21)	3	F	SRG	<24,1CR	100	<5	<5
30	241,25	0,4789	705,262	1,2	12	0	100,00	c-ALL	48XY,+21+22	5	M	SRG	>24,1CR	75	4,4	3,6
31	0,0779	0,0022	49,573	2,7	432	25	94,21	c-ALL	46XY,t(12;21)	5	M	SRG	<24,1CR	89	<5	<5
32	0,0073	0,0002	51,100	37,1	33292	0	100,00	c-ALL	47XY,+M	2	F	MRG	<24,1CR	98	2	0,4
33	11,22	0,044	357,000	246	24600	4940	79,92	T-ALL	46XX	4	F	MRG	>24,1CR	79	<5	<5
34	0,25	0,0032	109,375	20,5	17425	288	98,35	c-ALL	56-58XX	6	F	MRG	>24,1CR	84	18,8	1,6
35	0,0073	0,0039	2,621	11,8	236	0	100,00	B-ALL	46XY,t(8;14)	4	M	SRG	<24,1CR	92,8	2,4	<5
36	0,794	0,0079	140,709	1,6	576	0	100,00	c-ALL	46XY	7	M	MRG	>24,1CR	91	<5	<5
37	241,25	6	56,292	7,8	2340	40	98,29	c-ALL	46XY,t(12;21)	3	M	SRG	>24,1CR	98	<5	<5
38	2,8	3,548	1,105	5,6	1120	0	100,00	T-ALL	46XX,dub1q	7	F	MRG	19,dead	79	<5	<5
39	1,77	0,0398	62,261	10,1	8282	300	96,38	c-ALL	47XY,+21	4	F	MRG	>24,1CR	97,6	17,6	0,4
40	241,25	6	56,292	47,5	39425	5278	86,61	proB-ALL,My+	ND	<1	F	HRG	1;dead	100	-	-
41	0,0088	1,0305	0,012	1,4	448	0	100,00	T-ALL,My+	46XY	16	M	MRG	<24,1CR	95	12	<5
42	0,0074	0,0002	51,800	323,6	268588	638	99,76	T-ALL	46XY	7	M	MRG	<24,1CR	99	<5	<5
43	5,0624	0,0457	155,084	20,2	10032	714	92,88	proB-ALL	46XX	3	F	MRG	<24,1CR	94	13	<5
44	2,27	0,11	28,891	15,4	7238	1095	84,87	c-ALL	56-63XY	3	M	HRG	<24,1CR	92,8	<5	<5
45	0,0217	0,0002	151,900	146,2	130118	0	100,00	c-ALL	46XX,t(4;11)	1	F	HRG	6;dead	94	ND	<5
46	0,1618	0,0023	98,487	9,2	7636	0	100,00	c-ALL	46XX,t(12;21)	8	F	MRG	<24,1CR	92	<5	<5
Median	0,676	0,03665	51,9099	24,25	7437	104	99,27			6				95	5	5
Average	54,754	1,5678	37425,16	62,23	42574,72	1829,26	93,49			7,46				93,06	9,81	4,12
Minimum	0,001	0,0002	0,0017	1,2	12	0	25			1				75	0,8	0,4
Maximum	241,25	6	1688750	323,6	270000	43990	100			18				100	62	11

Legend: BM 0/15/33 - percentage of blast cells in bone marrow 0/15/33 days after diagnosis, RG - risk group, CCC - complex chromosomal changes
PRED/DEX - molar ratio of in vitro LC50, My+ - myeloid marker(s), F - female, M - male, ND - not done
SRG - standard risk group, MRG - medium risk group, HRG - high risk group, CR - complete remission

* Clinical outcome is reported in months of survival after diagnosis of ALL, and it indicates patients death or number of CRs

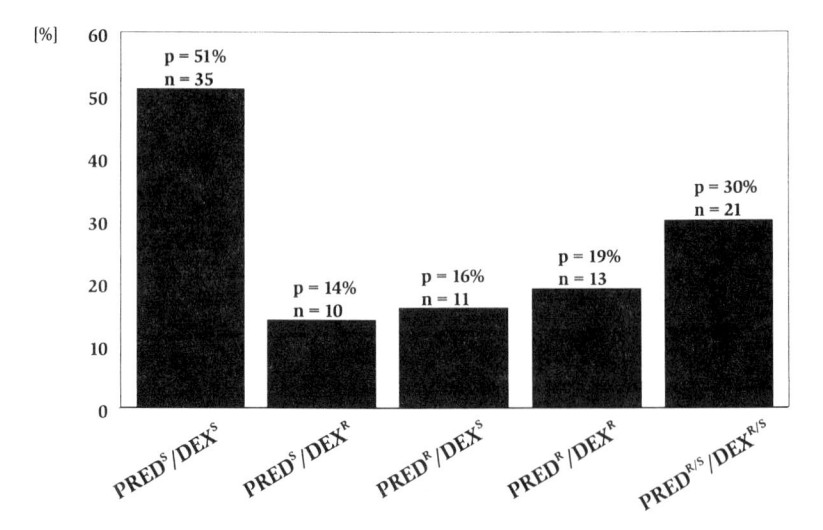

Figure 1. Proportion of PRED and DEX *in vitro* sensitive patients (PRED^s/DEX^s); PRED sensitive, but DEX resistant (PRED^s/DEX^r); PRED resistant, but DEX sensitive(PRED^r/DEX^s); PRED resistant, and DEX resistant (PRED^r/DEX^r); and total percentage/number of patients showing opposite *in vitro* response to GCs (PRED$^{r/s}$/DEX$^{r/s}$) included in the study.

4.2. Glucocorticoid Resistance *in Vitro*

The cut-off values for *in vitro* resistance/sensitivity to PRED/DEX were determined by classification of patients into two groups as sensitive (66% lowest LCS$_{50}$ values) and resistant (33% highest LCS$_{50}$ values), and they were calculated as 12.0/0.15 µg/ml respectively. The range of GC resistance values (Table 1) showed generally good *in vitro* responsiveness of children with ALL at diagnosis to GCs compared to AML and adult ALL[16]. However, an important portion of children showed differential *in vitro* response to PRED/DEX (21; 30%). Ten patients (14%) were sensitive to PRED and resistant to DEX, and 11 (16%) children were resistant to PRED while good response to DEX was observed (Table 1, Figure 1).

4.3. Correlation of PRED and DEX *in Vitro* Drug Resistance Values with Patient Characteristics

Multivariate correlation analysis (Pearson product-moment correlation) was applied to investigate positive or negative correlations among PRED and/or DEX LCS$_{50}$, ANB0, ANB8, and a new parameter named blast cells clearance on day 8. Figure 2 demonstrates positive correlation between DEX and PRED LCS$_{50}$ values (r=0.4497; p<0.002), however, the level of significance is much lower than in the papers of Ito et al.[3] and Kaspers et al.[13] Although there was no significant linkage between PRED/DEX *in vitro* response and ANB8, the PRED LCS$_{50}$ significantly correlated with the blast cell clearance (r=-0.3340; p<0.02). Nonetheless, the correlation of BCC8 with DEX LCS$_{50}$ was not significant.

4.4. The Effect of Cryopreservation on Sensitivity of CCRF-CEM Cells to Anti-Cancer drugs

Although we confirmed a significant correlation of PRED and DEX LCS$_{50}$ in patient leukemia cells (r=0.4497; p<0.002), there was a portion of patients with differential sensi-

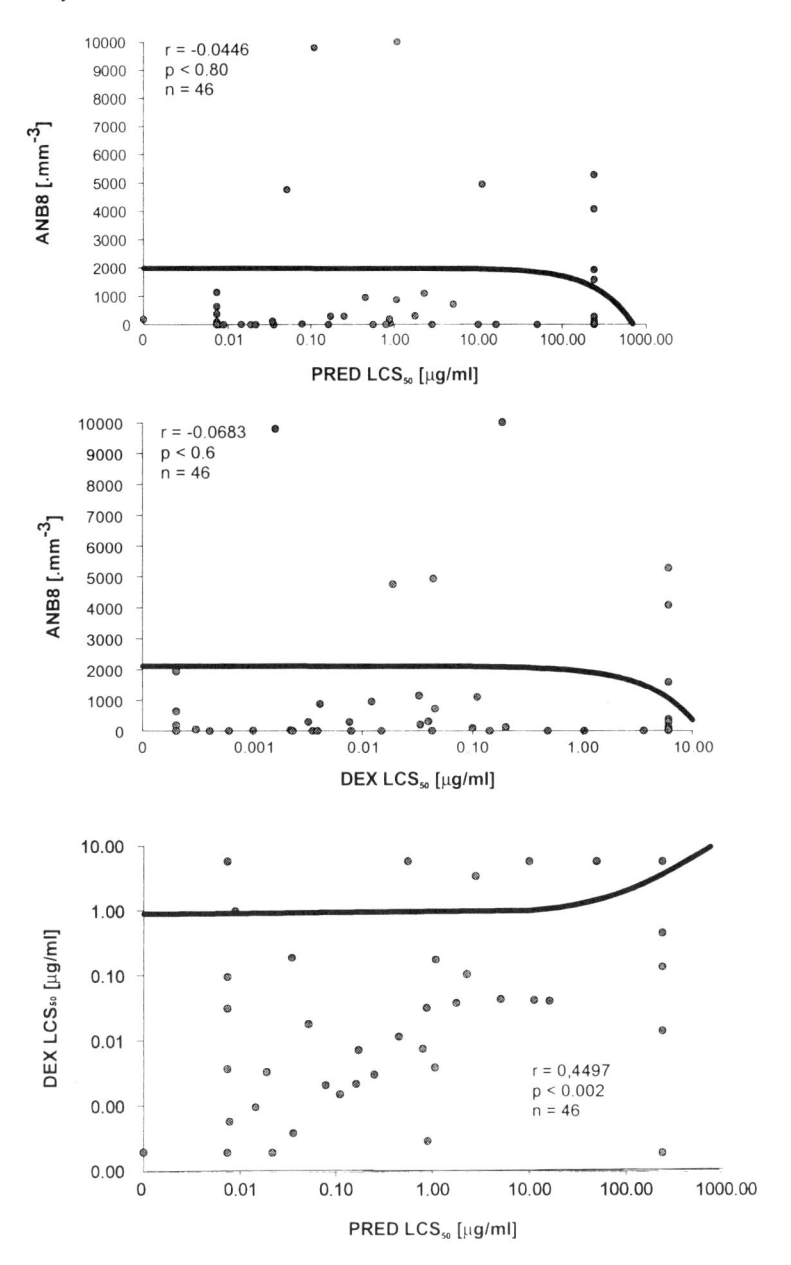

Figure 2. Correlation of clinical patient response characteristics with PRED/DEX LCS$_{50}$ values.

tivity to PRED versus DEX. This opposes previously published data of Ito et al.[3] and Kaspers et al.[13] When analyzing both these papers, we realized that the experiments were performed on cryopreserved and long-term transported patient cells, while only freshly isolated cells were used in our study. We show here on the model of T-lymphoblastic leukemia cell line CCRF-CEM that cryopreservation significantly decreased ($p<0.01$) PRED resistance compared with the drug resistance in freshly processed cells (Figure3). To our surprise, the differences in LCS$_{50}$ in fresh versus cryopreserved cells were not significant in the cases of other anti-cancer drugs (Figure3).

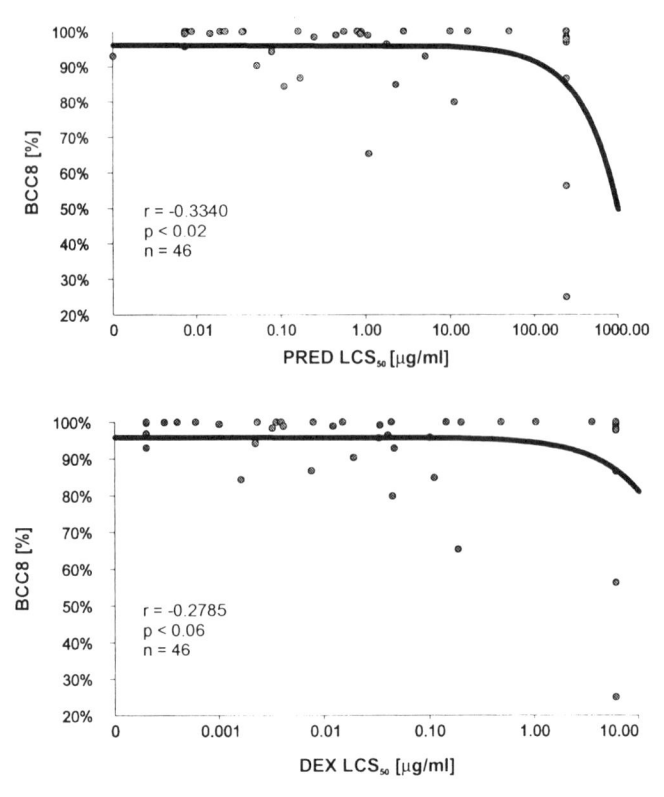

Figure 2. (*Continued*)

5. DISCUSSION

Biological activities of GCs differ considerably in their estimated glucocorticoid and mineralocorticoid potencies[2]. Moreover, there are substantial differences among individual GCs in their ability to reduce inflammation,[17] thymolysis,[17] glycogenesis[18] etc. In the example of PRED and DEX, the generally accepted ratio is that 1 mg of DEX is equivalent to 5–10 mg of PRED.[2] More specifically, DEX was 5.5 to 16 times more cytotoxic to leukemic cells than PRED (on a molar basis) under *in vitro* conditions.[1,13] In our study, the DEX/PRED molar ratio in patient cells was 51.9. In the case of fresh versus cryopreserved CCRF-CEM cells it was 44.0 and 15.3 respectively. Previously published papers of Ito at al.[3] and Kaspers et al.[13] reported median ratio of DEX to PRED LCS_{50} tested on primary leukemic cells 5.5 and 16.2 respectively, however, DEX/PRED molar ratio reported for CCRF-CEM cells was 15.9[3] and it is similar to ours data. We suppose that much higher antileukemic activity of DEX described in this study is on account of fresh processing of tumor cells as discussed later.

By contrast, others have reported a strong correlation between PRED and DEX LCS_{50},[3,13] but a much lower level of significance was found in our study. This was due to a large number of patients with differential sensitivity/resistance do PRED and DEX. The reason for these differences seems to be distinct processing of leukemic cells in ours (fresh samples) and the other studies (cryopreserved[3] or long-term transported[13]), which resulted in increased sensitivity of cryopreserved tumor cells to PRED (Figure 3). We suppose that

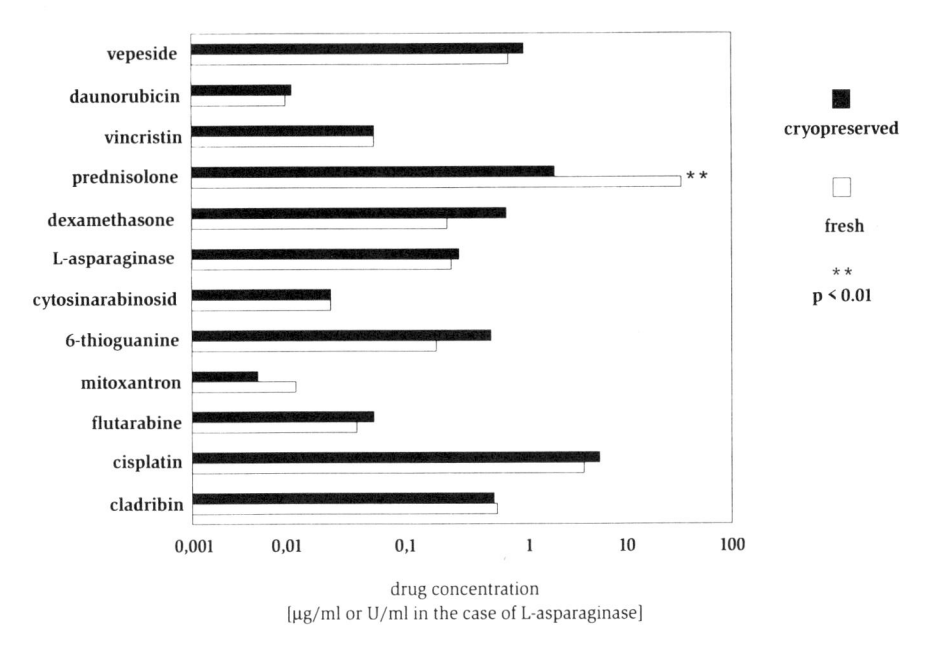

Figure 3. Effect of cryopreservation on LCS$_{50}$ concentrations of various anti-cancer drugs analyzed on CCRF-CEM cells.

a possible explanation of this event is an impairment of energetic metabolism of cryopreserved or long-term transported cells followed by a decrease in intracellular levels of ATP, a well known source of energy for cellular drug transporters, for instance Pgp and MRP.[19] Another possibility is that the cell manipulation can increase susceptibility to PRED induced apoptosis. Nonetheless, we realize that more detailed experiments are needed to elucidate specific reasons of increased PRED sensitivity in cryopreserved or long-term storage cells.

To better characterize patient's response to PRED *in vivo*, we introduced a new parameter—the percentage of blast cell clearance on day 8. This parameter indicates the portion of tumor mass eliminated by PRED monotherapy within the first 8 days of treatment. We assume that the BCC8 describes patient's response to therapy much better than the identification of non-responders according to an arbitrary cut-off point of more than 1000 leukemic cells/mm^3 in the peripheral blood, since the parameter is more quantitative, and it enables to evaluate PRED response in patients which already have ANB0<1000/mm^3 (22% in our study) and would be recorded as a good responders by definition.[10] Nonetheless, BCC8 is not applicable to patients with zero ANB0 at diagnosis (4 children, 8.7% in our study), and blast cell clearance in these patients can be evaluated by a bone marrow biopsy at day 8 or 7. The significance of this parameter for long-term survival has already been reported.[20] Importantly, PRED LCS$_{50}$ values significantly correlated with the percentage of BCC8, although no association with ANB8 was observed (Figure 2). Furthermore, no significant correlation was found for DEX LCS$_{50}$ and BCC8, since PRED but not DEX was applied within the first 8 days of treatment and a large number of PRED *in vitro* sensitive patients was DEX resistant (Table 1, Figure 1). However, it should be noted, that it is not dealt with true monotherapy since at day zero, an intrathecal injection of methorexate is given, and children are medicated with allopurinol, both the drugs have also systemic antileukemic activity.[21,22] In agreement with this is the higher percentage of PRED non-responders (close to 20%) in the EORTC trial, where methotrexate is given after PRED monotherapy, compared to the BFM trials.[21]

We expect that the most significant impact of our study is in the identification of a subset of patients with differential *in vitro* sensitivity to PRED compared to DEX. Despite the long-term clinical outcome information are not yet available, based on this data we conclude that individual patient's *in vitro* glucocorticoid resistance profile should be respected in the treatment of ALL.

ACKNOWLEDGMENTS

This study was supported in parts by the Grant Agency of Ministry of Health, the Czech Republic and the Cancer Research Foundation in Olomouc. We are grateful to Mária Šafářová and Anna Janošťáková for excellent technical assistance and to Richard Kořínek for editorial help.

REFERENCES

1. Bell, P.A.: Glucocorticoids in the therapy of leukemia and lymphoma. Clin. Oncol., 1, 131–148
2. Kaspers, G.J.L., Pieters, R., Klumper, E., De Waal, F.C., Veerman, A.J.P.: Glucocorticoid resistance in childhood leukemia. Leuk. Lymph., 1994, 13, 187–201
3. Ito, C., Evans, W.E., McNinch, L., Coustat-Smith, E., Mahmoud, H., Pui, C.-H., Campana, D.: Comparative cytotoxicity of dexamethasone and prednisolone in childhood acute lymphoblastic leukemia. J Clin Oncol, 1996, 14, 2370–2376
4. Bourgeois, S., Gruol, D.J., Newby, R.F., Rajah, F.M.: Expression of a mdr gene is associated with a new form of resistance to dexamethasone-induced apoptosis. Mol Endocrinol 1993, 7, 840–851
5. Fardel, O., Lecureur, V., Guillouzo, A.: Regulation by dexamethasone of P-glycoprotein expression in cultured rat hepatocytes. FEBS Lett, 1993, 327, 1898–193
6. Barancik, M., Docolomansky, P., Slezak, J., Breier, A.: Overcoming of vincristine resistance in L1210/VCR cells by several corticosteroids. Collateral sensitivity of resistant cells. Neoplasma, 1993, 40, 21–25
7. Zhao, J.Y., Ikeguchi, M., Eckersberg, T., Kuo, M.T.: Modulation of multidrug resistance gene expression by dexamethasone in cultured hepatoma cells. Endocrinol, 1993, 133, 521–528
8. Danel-Moore, L., Bronnegard, M., Gustafsson, J.A.: Dexamethasone reverses glucocorticoid receptor RNA depression in multi-drug resistant (MDR) myeloma cell lines. Med Oncol Tumor Pharmacother, 1992, 9, 199–204
9. Kojika, S., Sugita, K., Inukai, T., Saito, M., Iijima, K., Tezuka, T., Goi, K., Shiraishi, K., Mori, T., Okazaki, T., Kagami, K., Ohyama, K., Nakazawa, S.: Mechanisms of glucocorticoid resistance in human leukemic cells: implication of abnormal 90 and 70 kDa heat shock proteins. Leukemia, 1996, 10, 994–999
10. Riehm, H., Reiter, A., Schrappe, M., Berthold, F., Dopfer, R., Gerein, V., Ludwig, R., Ritter, J., Stollmann, B., Henze, G.: Die corticosteroid-abhangige dezimierung der leukamiezellzahl im blut als prognosefaktor bei der akuten lymphoblastischen leukamie im kindesalter. (Therapiestudie ALL-BFM 83). Klin. Pad., 1986, 199, 151–160
11. Mastrangelo, R., Malandrino, R., Riccardi, R., Longo, P., Ranelletti, F.O., Iacobelli, S.: Clinical implications of glucocorticoid receptor studies in childhood acute lymphoblastic leukemia. Blood, 1980, 56, 1036–1040
12. Kaspers, G.J.L., Veerman, A.J.P., Pieters, R., Van Zantwijk, C.H., Smets, L.A., Van Wering, E.R., Van Der Does-Van Den Berg, A.: *In vitro* cellular drug resistance and prognosis in newly diagnosed childhood acute lymphoblastic leukemia. Blood, 1997, 90, 2723–2729
13. Kaspers, G.J.L., Veerman, A.J.P., Popp-Snijders, C., Lomecky, M., Van Zantwijk, C.H., Swinkels, L.M.J.W., Van Wering, E.R., Pieters R.: Comparison of the antileukemic activity *in vitro* of dexamethasone and prednisolone in childhood acute lymphoblastic leukemia. Med Pediatr Oncol, 1996, 27, 114–121

14. Pieters, R., Huismans, D.R., Loonen, A.H., Hahlen, K., Van Der Does-Van Den Berg, A., Van Wering, E.R., Veerman, A.J.P.: Relation of cellular drug resistance to long-term clinical outcome in childhood acute lymphoblastic leukemia. Lancet, 1991, 338, 399–403.
15. Pieters, R., Huismans, D.R., Loonen, A.H., Hählen, K., van der Does-van den Berg, A., van Wering, E.R., Veerman, A.J.P.: Relation of cellular drug resistance to long-term clinical outcome in childhood acute lymphoblastic leukaemia. Lancet, 1991, 338, 399–403
16. Hajdúch, M., Mihál, V., Minaøík, J., Fáber, E., Šafåøová, M., Weigl, E., Antálek, P.: Decreased *in vitro* chemosensitivity of tumor cells in patients suffering from malignant diseases with a poor prognosis. Cytotechnology, 1996, 19, 243–245
17. Ichii, S., Satoh, Y., Izawa, M., Iwasaki, K.: Stability of receptor complexes in the rat liver bound to glucocorticoids of different biopotencies. Endocrinol. Jpn., 1984, 5, 583–594
18. Ortega, E.: Effects of clopenrednol and other corticosteroids on hypothalamic-pituitary-adrenal axis function. J. Int. Med. Res., 1976, 4, 326–337
19. Hall, A., Cattan, A.R., Proctor, S.J.: Mechanisms of drug resistance in acute leukemia. Leuk. Res., 1989, 13, 351–356
20. Schultz, K.R., Massing, B., Spinelli, J.J., Gaynon, P.S., Wadsworth, L.: Importance of the day 7 bone marrow biopsy as a prognostic measure of the outcome in children with acute lymphoblastic leukemia. Med. Ped. Oncol., 1997, 29, 16–22
21. Thyss, A., Suciu, S., Bertrand, Y., Mazingue, F., Robert, A., Vilmer, E., Mechinaud, F., Benoit, Y., Brock, P., Ferster, A., Lutz, P., Boutard, P., Marguerite, G., Plouvier, E., Michel, G., Plantaz, D., Munzer, M., Rialland, X., Chantraine, J.- M., Norton, L., Solbu, G., Philippe, N., Otten, J.: J. Clin. Oncol., 1997, 15, 1824–1830
22. Masson, E., Synold, T. W., Relling, M. V., Schuetz, J. D., Sandlund, J. T., Pui, C.-H., Evans, W. E.: Leukemia, 1996, 10, 56–60

51

ACTIVITY OF VINORELBINE ON B-CHRONIC LYMPHOCYTIC LEUKEMIA CELLS *IN VITRO*

P. A. Bernabei, I. Landini, B. Bartolozzi, I. Banchelli,
A. Degli Innocenti o Nocentini, and V. Santini

U.O. Ematologia
Università degli Studi-Azienda Ospedaliera di Careggi
Firenze, Italy

Keywords: Vinorelbine, *In vitro* sensitivity testing, INT assay, Chronic Lymphocytic Leukemia.

SUMMARY

Vinorelbine (VNR) is a new semi-synthetic *Vinca rosea* alkaloid that has been employed both in combination and as a single agent, showing a significant antitumour activity. Since little is known about VNR in human leukemia, we studied the *in vitro* cytotoxic effect of VNR on peripheral blood lymphocytes from 18 patients affected by B-chronic lymphocytic leukemia (CLL), employing the INT assay. VNR inhibited fresh B-CLL cells from 15/18 patients in primary cultures, the ID50 doses ranging from 4 ng/ml to 83 µg/ml. These data strongly suggest that VNR could be effective in the treatment of B-CLL.

INTRODUCTION

Vinorelbine (VNR), a semi-synthetic *Vinca rosea* alkaloid-derived drug, has been recently introduced in clinics as antitumour agent. Like other *V. rosea* alkaloids, VNR exerts its activity by binding to α and β tubulin, thus inhibiting microtubule assembly, impairing metaphasic tumour cell division (1) and showing, at the same time, greater lipophility and *in vitro* wider spectrum (2). Moreover, VNR shows lower blocking activity against axonal microtubules, and thus it has less neurotoxicity compared with other members of its class (3, 4).

VNR is currently used in clinics for treatment of Non-Small Cell Lung Cancer, in breast and ovarian cancer and in relapsed or refractory Hodgkin lymphoma (2). As natural

V. rosea alkaloids are widely employed for treatment of lymphoid malignancies, in this *in vitro* preclinical study we tested the effects of VNR on cells collected from patients affected by chronic lymphocytic leukemia (CLL), with the aim of prospecting a new indication for this drug.

MATERIALS AND METHODS

Peripheral blood cells were collected, after informed consent, from 18 patients suffering from CLL. Diagnosis of CLL was performed according to the following criteria (5):

1. An absolute lymphocytosis in the blood, with a count of $\geq 5 \times 10^9/L$, and cells morphologically mature in appearance, sustained over at least 4-week period.
2. Normocellular or hypercellular bone marrow with lymphocytes $\geq 30\%$.
3. A monoclonal B-cell phenotype expressed by the preponderant population of blood lymphocytes with low levels of surface immunoglobulins, simultaneously showing CD5 positivity.

In Table 1 age, sex and clinical stage according to Rai classification (6) of patient are presented.

Mononuclear cells were isolated by discontinous density gradient, 1.077 g/ml., from peripheral blood collected in heparin containing tubes. Cells were washed twice and resuspended in RPMI 1640 without phenol red, with 10% foetal calf serum (FCS). Viability determined by trypan blue exclusion test, was in all the experiments greater than 95%.

VNR bitartrate was diluted with RPMI without phenol red with 10% FCS to the concentration required.

The colorimetric assay, based on the cleavage of the tetrazolium salt (2–4-iodophenil)-3-(4-nitrophenil)-5-pheniltetrazolium violet (INT) (7), was used to evaluate the *in vitro* citotoxicity of VNR. Cells were plated in a total volume of 200 µl, at the density of 2×10^5 /well, in 96-flat-bottom microwell plates. The following drug concentrations were employed: 10 ng/ml, 100 ng/ml, 1 µg/ml, 10 µg/ml, 100µg/ml. After 24 hours of incubation at 37 °C, 100 % humidity and 5 % CO_2, 50 µl of 1 mg/ml INT solution were added to each well, and the colour developed by INT reduction was measured, after 18 hours incubation, by an automated microplates spectrophotometer.

The ID50 (the drug dose able to reduce the cells viability of 50 %) was calculated for each case from the equation of correlation line obtained by semilogarithimic computation and assumed as the VNR cytotoxicity index. The lack of INT reduction, sign of a non interference of VNR with the viability of the cells, was assumed as resistance to the drug.

RESULTS AND DISCUSSION

Table 1 summarizes the INT *in vitro* sensitivity testing of VNR on cells obtained from 18 CLL cases.

We observed that only three cases showed resistance to the exposition to VNR, i.e absence of a significant reduction of cellular viability in comparison with controls.

In all the other cases an increasing cytotoxicity was demonstrated by INT assay, semilogarithmically correlated with the drug concentrations. The ID50s obtained ranged from 4 ng/ml to 83 µg/ml. VNR pharmacodinamics studies have previously indicated that the C_{max} after i.v. infusion of 30 mg/m² range from 0.78 to 1.13 mg/l (2). In 9 out of 15 sen-

Table 1. Effects of VNR on cells obtained from patients suffering from B-CLL

Case	Age	Sex	RAI*	N°Cells** (x 10^9/l)	VNR ID50***
1	58	m	II	135	100 ng/ml
2	63	m	0	42	21 ng/ml
3	68	f	II	13	15 ng/ml
4	73	m	II	28	17 µg/ml
5	51	f	II	37	83 µg/ml
6	66	m	I	345	18 ng/ml
7	71	f	II	64	R****
8	62	f	III	37	82 ng/ml
9	49	m	I	22	66 µg/ml
10	55	m	0	84	1 µg/ml
11	74	m	II	34	6 µg/ml
12	55	f	IV	47	R
13	63	m	0	18	R
14	62	f	II	39	88 ng/ml
15	56	m	0	12	4 ng/ml
16	78	m	I	33	18 µg/ml
17	59	m	II	71	26 µg/ml
18	65	m	III	48	50 µg/ml

*Clinical staging according to Rai classification (6).
** Leukemic cells in peripheral blood.
*** The ID50 is the drug dose able to reduce the cells viability of 50%.
**** Resistance.

sitive CLL cell samples the *in vitro* ID 50 obtained was lower than 10 µg/ml, i.e. in the order of magnitude of the plasma C_{max}.

A drug may find an indication in clinics for a particular type of tumour, if laboratory studies have indicated its effectiveness in inhibiting first the growth of cell lines belonging to the same tumour type, and secondly of tumoural cells freshly obtained from patients and mantained in primary cultures (8). The possible effectiveness is also related to the *in vitro* cytotoxic concentrations, that have to be comparable to drug plasma levels obtainable in patients. A sharp correlation between *in vitro* sensitivity and *in vivo* results in treatment of many malignancies, included those of the lympho-hematopoietic system, as been previously well assessed (9,10). It has been finally reported that VNR is active in some lymphoid neoplasms. Indeed, 90% of refractory Hodgkin's disease, resistant to natural *Vinca* alkaloids, show a significant response to VNR (11).

We demonstrated an *in vitro* sensitivity of CLL cells to VNR, which in many cases was present for doses comparable to the therapeutic plasma levels. This may be the starting point for further clinical studies.

REFERENCES

1. Potier P. The synthesis of Navelbine-prototype of a new series of vinblastine derivates. Semin. Oncol. 16 Supp. 4:2–4, 1989.
2. Goa K.L. and Foulds D. Vinorelbine. A review of its pharmacological properties and clinical use in cancer therapy. Drug and Aging 5 (3):200–234, 1994.
3. Meininger V., Binet S., Chaineau E., et al. In situ response to vinca alkaloids by microtubules in coltured post-implanted mouse embryos. Biol. Cell 60:21–9, 1990.
4. Binet S., Chaineau E., Fellus A., et al. Immunofluorescence study of the action of navelbine, vincristine and vinblastine on mitotic and axonal microtubules. Int. J. Cancer 46:262–6, 1990.

5. Cheson B.D:, Bennet J.M:, Rai K.R., et al. Guidelines for clinical protocols for chronic lymphocytic leukemia (CLL). Recommandation of the NCI-Sponsored Working Group. Am. J. Hematol. 29:152, 1988.
6. Rai K.R., Sawitsky A., Cronkite E.P., et al. Clinical staging of chronic lymphocytic leukemia. Blood 46:219, 1975.
7. Bernabei P.A., Santini V., Silvestro L., Dal Pozzo O., Bezzini R:, Gattei V., Saccardi R., Rossi Ferrini P. *In vitro* chemosensivity testing of leukemic cells. Development of a semiautomated colorimetric assay. Hematol. Onc. 7:243–253, 1989.
8. Salomon S.E: Application of the human tumour stem cell assay to new drug evaluation and screening. In Salomon S.E. (ed), Cloning of human stem cell. New York: Alan R. Liss Inc. 223, 1980.
9. Santini V., Bernabei P.A., Silvestri L., Dal Pozzo O., Bezzini R., Viano I., Gattei V., Saccardi R., Rossi Ferrini P. *In Vitro* Chemosensivity testing of leukemic cells: prediction of response to chemotherapy in patients whit acute non-lymphoblastic leukemia. Hematological Oncology vol. 7 287–293, 1989.
10. Kaspers G.J.L., Veerman A.P.J., Van Zantwijk C.H., Smets L.A., Van Wering E.K., Van Der-Does-Van Den Berg. *In vitro* cellular drug resistance and prognosis in newly diagnosed childhood Acute Lymphoblastic Leukemia. Blood 2723–2729, 1997.
11. Bruno S., Savignano R., Corrado C., et al. Vinorelbine (VNR): a new vinka alkaloid active in refractary/relapsed Lymphomas. A phase II study (Abstract n° 1300) Proceeding of ASCO 13:383, 1995.

STUDIES OF SOME MECHANISMS OF DRUG RESISTANCE IN CHRONIC MYELOID LEUKEMIA (CML)

Anna G. Turkina,[1] Natalia P. Logacheva,[2] Tatjana P. Stromskaya,[2] Tatjana N. Zabotina,[1] Sergei V. Kuznetzov,[1] Kuralay K. Sachibzadaeva,[1] Akshin Tagiev,[1] Vacheslav S. Juravlev,[1] Nina D. Khoroshko,[1] Anatoly Y. Baryshnikov,[2] and Alla A. Stavrovskaya[2]

[1]Haematological Research Centre of Russian Academy of Medical Sciences
[2]Cancer Research Centre of Russian Academy of Medical Sciences
Moscow, Russia

Keywords: CML, BCR-ABL translocation variants, apoptosis, drug resistance, P-glycoprotein.

1. ABSTRACT

CML is the myeloproliferative disorder connected with the specific chromosome translocation (9;22) and occurrence of the fusion gene/protein BCR-ABL. BCR-ABL protein is believed to inhibit apoptosis and to cause drug resistance. We investigated the correlation of two different forms of BCR-ABL mRNA in 94 pts with their overall survival. It was found that b2a2 (but not b2a3) mRNA expression correlates with longer survival of patients treated with chemotherapy. We did not find an influence of different types of BCR/ABL mRNA on the survival of pts treated with interferon-α. FAS/APO-1 antigen was expressed by the cells of 34% of the pts in CML blast crisis (BC) and directly correlated with the expression of CD34, CD13 and CD14 differentiation antigens. FAS/APO-1 non-expression correlated with higher rate of remissions in BC. We investigated P-glycoprotein (Pgp) expression and functional activity in 40 BC CML pts. 2-fold shorter survival was found in the pts with Pgp expression. Pgp expression strongly correlated with CD13 antigen. Consecutive studies of pts in BC CML show that Pgp expressing cells often do not multiply in the course of BC CML. We postulate that Pgp may be regarded as differentiation marker of the cells and the unfavorable prognostic factor in BC CML.

2. INTRODUCTION

Chronic myeloid leukemia (CML) is a stem cell disorder which progresses from the monoclonal chronic phase (CP) to highly malignant polyclonal terminal stage - blast crisis (BC), one of the worth kinds of acute leukemia. CML is clinically heterogeneous disease, characterised by very different prognosis for different patients: some patients live for 10–15 years while 5–8% die in 12 months. The causes of this heterogeneity are unclear. CML is a good example of refractoriness to chemotherapy developing in the course of disease progression, especially during the terminal stages of CML. It is well established that the treatment of BC CML patients is extremely difficult, thus it is crucial to understand the mechanisms underlying chemotherapy resistance in CML patients.

CML is probably the best characterised form of human leukemia. It is well known that more than in 90% of cases it occurs due to the specific reciprocal chromosome translocations, mainly - translocation 9;22 (q34;q11), involving two genes *BCR* and *ABL*. Cytogenetically this translocation usually is demonstrated by the occurrence in of the Philadelphia chromosome (Ph'-chromosome) - the well known hallmark of CML. Ph' chromosome contains *BCR-ABL* fusion gene which is translated into BCR-ABL 210 kD fusion protein with elevated tyrosine kinase activity.[1,2] This protein is regarded as central mechanism which underlies CML. *BCR-ABL* fusion gene is found also in 10 to 20% of acute lymphoblastic leukemia and in some cases of acute myeloid leukemia, lymphoma and myeloma.[3] Some data suggest that the precise location of the breakpoint in *BCR* and thus the composition of the fusion BCR-ABL protein may determine the disease phenotype—the immunophenotype of the cells with this chromosome translocation and treatment outcome. However, these data are debatable and this problem needs further investigation.[3]

For years, the mechanism by which BCR-ABL fusion protein deregulates cell growth in CML was unknown. In the last years the data were obtained showing that this protein primarily produces clonal expansion not by stimulating proliferation but by inhibiting apoptosis.[4,5] It was shown that transfected *BCR-ABL* will protect growth-factor dependent cells from the apoptosis in growth factor depleted medium.[3,6] The transfection of this gene increased cell resistance to ionising radiation, and to some cytostatic drugs.[7] However, evidently, some kinds of apoptosis are not inhibited: in CML cells, for example, apoptosis induced by immunocytes is not blocked by BCR-ABL.[8] Biological effects of BCR-ABL fusion protein on apoptosis can not be the only explanations of refractoriness of CML patients (especially BC CML patients) to different kinds of the therapy, different mechanisms of drug resistance have to be investigated.

The aim of this study was to investigate some probable causes of drug resistance and differences in CML patient's surwival. Here we present the results of the following studies: 1) Investigation of the influence of two different locations of breakpoint *BCR/ABL* translocation on patients' overall survival and therapy outcome. 2) Studies of the correlation of Fas/APO-1 antigen expression by patients' peripheral blood (PB) cells in BC CML with their survival and response to the therapy. 3) Studies of the expression and functional activity of P-glycoprotein (multidrug resistance protein, Pgp) in connection with patients' survival and sensitivity to the treatment.

3. MATERIALS AND METHODS

3.1. Patients

94 patients in various stages of CML (40 males and 54 females) were examined for the variants of BCR-ABL mRNA; 37 patients (17 males and 20 females) in BC CML were

studied for the expression of Fas/APO-1 (CD95) antigen; 40 patients (19 males and 21 females) in BC CML were examined for Pgp expression. The age of the patients was between 16 and 71 years. The diagnosis of CML was based on the history, physical examination results, and studies of bone marrow aspirate or biopsy samples, peripheral blood smears, and chromosome analysis or molecular verification of the presence of BCR-ABL fusion transcript. We examined only Ph'-positive or BCR-ABL positive patients)

3.2. Reverse Transcriptase-Polymerase Chain Reaction

(RT-PCR) amplification of the hybrid gene. The method used to detect the various BCR-ABL hybrid mRNAs was based on the RT-PCR. Total RNA was extracted from cells by the guanidinium thiocyonate and phenol/chloroform method. cDNAs were transcribed with random hexamer primers. To detect the b2a2 and b3a2 type of BCR/ABL transcripts encoding the p210 chimeric protein, an additional amplification step with the nested primers of the first-step amplified products was used. The PCR was perfomed in standart buffer with 30 cycles , with each cycle consisting of 94^0 for 1min, 56^0 for 1 min, 72^0 for 2 min for external primers pair and 94^0 for 1min, 63^0 for 1 min, 72^0 for 2 min for internal primers pair. Final size of fragments was 303bp for b2a2 type and 378 for b3a2 type of BCR/ABL mRNA

Oligonucleotides: The following primers were used for RT-PCR amplification of BCR/ABL hybrid transcripts: (external) 10bcr1: exon 10 (BCR) sense primer 5'TGGAT-GAACTGGAGGCAG3'; 3abl1: exon 3 (ABL) antisense primer 5'TGACTGGCG-TGATGTAGTTG3'; (internal) D1: exon b2 (BCR) sense primer 5'GGAGCTGCAGATG-CTGACCAAC3'; 3abl2: exon 3 antisense primer 5'GCTTCACACCATTCCCCATT3'.

3.3. Monoclonal Antibodies

For evaluation of Fas/APO-1, Pgp expression and immunophenotyping of blast cells monoclonal antibodies (Mabs) against cell surface antigens (Table 1) were used. Anti-CD95 mouse Mabs IPO-4 were characterized at Fifth International Workshop and Conference on Human Leukocyte Differentiation Antigens. Anti-Pgp mouse Mab UIC2 recognises an extracellular epitope of human Pgp[9] and is specific for MDR1 gene product.[10] Mabs against human leukocyte differentiation antigens gave the possibility to characterise various differentiation stages of blast cells (from hematopoietic precursors to the mature cells.[11] Each marker was regarded as diagnostic valuable if it was detected on 20% (or more) of the cells. The following immunophenotypic variants of BC CML were evaluated: 1/. Primitive ("P" in Table 3): CD34+ , CD33-, CD13-, CD14-, CD15-, CD19-, CD10-. 2/. Myeloid : CD34+-, CD33+, CD13+, CD14+-, CD15+-, CD19-, CD10-.3/. Lymphoid : CD34+-, CD33-, CD13-, CD14-, CD15-, CD19+, CD10+..4/. Mixed: CD34+-, CD33+-, CD13+, CD14+-, CD15+, CD19+, CD10+. 5/. Undifferentiated all above markers were not expressed on the surface of blast cells.

3.4. Immunofluorescence Assays

Antigens expression was studied by indirect immunofluorescence technique and FACScan analysis. The blood samples (10 ml) were separated by gelatine sedimentation for 45 min at 37 C, plasma with leukocytes was collected, centrifuged, and leukocytes were resuspended in 0.5 ml of lysing solution (for total lysis of erythrocytes), incubated for 4 min, washed in and resuspended in PBS. Cells were used either for the analysis of the antigens expression or for studies of Fas/APO-1 or Pgp activity. Indirect immunofluorescence technique: 500000 cells were incubated with 20 ml of Mab for 30 min at 4 C and washed twice

Table 1. Monoclonal antibodies used in the study

Antibody	Antigen	Main distribution
IPO-4[a], ICO-160[b]	CD95	Broad expression
UIC2[d]	Pgp	MDR cells, early progenitors, some lymphocytes
ICO-115[b]	CD34	Progenitor cells
Anti-CD33[c]	CD33	Myelomonocytic progenitors
My32	CD13	Myelomonocytic progenitors
My1[c]	CD15	Myeloid cells
Anti-CD14[c]	CD14	Monocytes
ICO-124[b]	CD10	Lymphoblastic cells
ICO-1[b]	HLA-DR	HLA-DR
ICO-150[b]	CD24	B cells, granulocytes

a Mabs kindly provided by Dr D.Gluzman
b Mabs kindly provided by "MedBioSpectr", Moscow, Russia
c Mabs kindly provided by Dr T.Trishman, Johns Hopkins Oncology Center, Baltimore, USA
d Mabs kindly provided by Dr. E. Mechetner, INGENEX inc. Menlo Park, Ca. USA

in PBS. Then cells were incubated for 30 min at 4 C with 20 ml F(ab')2 fragments rabbit-anti-mouse serum conjugated with FITC (fluorescein isothiocyanate) or isotype specific antiserum conjugated with FITC or phycoerythrin (PE). At the next stage cells were washed twice in PBS and resuspended in PBS solution of formaldehyde (1 %). An expression of antigens on the cells surface was detected by flow cytometry (FACScan, Beckton Dickinson) using two flow cytometric parameters as light scatter and size of cells.

3.5. Two-Color Immunofluorescence Analysis

Two-color flow cytometry analysis was performed using a combination of Mabs IPO-4 (anti Fas/Apo-1) and isotype-specific anti-mouse IgM FITC-conjugate (Sigma) and then the second Mabs directly conjugated with phycoerythrin(PE) (CD34PE).We used a combination of anti-CD34 Mab My10 (IgG1) conjugated with PE and the second Mab, anti-Pgp UIC2 (IgG2a), and isotype-specific antiserum conjugated with FITC. Mouse immunoglobulins of the same isotype as Mab and directly conjugated with FITC or PE were used as controls. Sorting windows were established for four separate parameters: forward and light scatter, FITC and PE fluorescence.

3.6. Pgp Function Evaluation

For evaluation of Pgp activity the fluorescent dye Rhodamine 123 (Sigma) (Rh123) and the technique described[12,13] was used. Cells were stained with Rh123 (5 mg/ml) for 15

Table 2. Median duration of various CML stages in patients with different types of *BCR/ABL mRNA*

mRNA type	Total number of pts studied	Chronic	Accelaration	Blast crisis	Median survival
b2a2	46	45	6	4	61
b3a2	48	38	8	6	52
Statistical significance[*]		p = 0.5	p = 0.5	p = 0.5	p > 0.2

*Student's criterium.

Table 3. CD95 (Fas\APO-1) expression by the cells of patients in CML blast crisis and immunophenotypic variants of blast crisis

Variant of blast crisis	Number of patients studied	
	Total	CD95 + (%)
Lymphoid	5	1 (20%)
Mixed	10	6 (60%)
Non-lymphoid	22	13 (59%)

min, then washed twice with PBS and put into dye-free medium for 30–60 min. Pgp inhibitor verapamil (20 mg/ml) was added into dye-free medium in one of the experimental groups. The fluorescence intensity of Rh123 in the cells was measured in FACScan (FACScan, Beckton Dickinson).

4. RESULTS

4.1. Different Locations of Breakpoints in BCR-ABL Translocation (Different Forms of BCR-ABL mRNA) and Patients' Overall Survival and Response to the Treatment

The breakpoints in the major breakpoint cluster region (M-bcr) were studied in 94 patients with Ph' positive CML by means of RT-PCR. According to breakpoint position several types of mRNA's are usually found, most often transcript with b2a2 junction (120 bp) and with b3a2 junction (200 bp) types.[14] Table 2 shows that the duration of chronic phase and blast crisis as well as median survival did not statistically differ in patients with b2a2 and b3a2 types of mRNA. However when we analysed this material according to the different types of treatment of patients, the significant differences between two groups of patients were found (Figure 1). It was found that the overall survival of patients with b2a2 translocation treated with bysulfan was greater than the overall survival of the patients with b3a2 type of mRNA. However, we did not found the influence of different types of BCR-ABL mRNAs on the survival of patients treated with interferon-α. We did not revealed any correlations between mRNA variants and immunological and cytochemical types of CML blast transformation.

4.2. Studies of the Correlation of FAS/APO-1 Antigen Expression by Patients' PB Cells with Their Survival and Response to the Therapy

CD95 Fas/APO-1) antigen was absent in CML chronic stage; its expression was found in 34 % (12 of 35) of our patients with CML BC on peripheral blood blasts. This antigen expressed on the CML BC blast cells was functionally active, that was proved by results of apoptosis induction by Mabs ICO-160 and IPO-4 against CD95(Fas/APO-1) antigen using flow cytometric method of measurement of hypodiploid DNA, labeled by propidium iodide. The percentage of apoptosis, induced by Mabs in CD95(Fas/APO-1)-positive, cultivated with Mabs (10 µg/ml) for 24 hrs, cells of 6 of 7 CML BC patients was 17–60%.

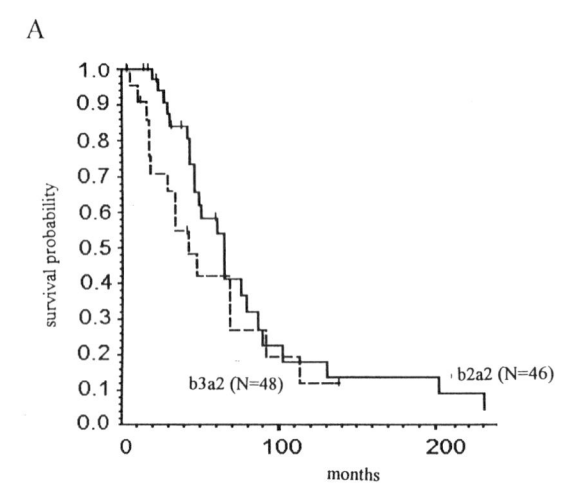

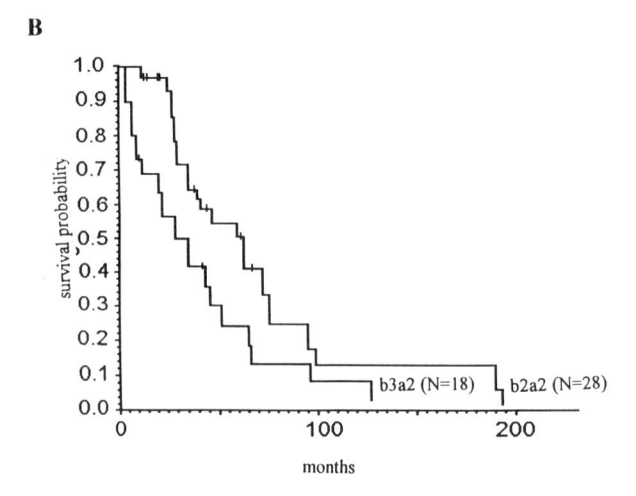

Figure 1. Overall survival of CML patients with different types of BCR-ABL mRNA. a. Overall survival of all patients studied (comparison of patients with b2a2 and b3a2 types of mRNA). b. Overall survival of patients treated with busulfan (comparison of patients with b2a2 and b3a2 types of mRNA).

We studied the associations of CD95(Fas/APO-1) antigen and other differentiation antigens and found a direct correlation between the percentage of CD34+ and CD95(Fas/APO-1)+ cells in PB (r = 0.44, p = 0.05) of newly diagnosed CML BC patients. With the use of the two-color immunofluorescence we have shown that these antigens are coexpressed on the same cells (data not shown). We also revealed a significant correlation of CD95(Fas/APO-1) (r = 0.7, p<0.05) in PB with CD10– phenotype in untreated patients. Besides CD34, CD95(Fas/APO-1)-antigen also correlated with CD13 and CD14 (r = 0.48 and r = 0.47, p<0.05), but not CD15 and CD11b. (r = 0.82, p<0.05).

Different immunological variants of CML BC - lymphoid (positive for 1 or more of lymphoid antigens (CD10, CD19, CD20, CD22) and negative for all of myeloid (CD33, CD13, CD14, CD15, CD11b)), myeloid (positive for 1 or more of myeloid antigens and negative for all of the lymphoid), mixed (positive for 1 or more of both lymphoid and myeloid antigens), primitive (expressing only CD34) and undifferentiated (expressing no differentiation antigens) were described.[11] According to clinical significance of CD10 antigen here we analyzed patients in accord of this antigen expression. Into non-lymphoid

Table 4. Median duration of various CML stages and number of therapeutic remissions in patients with different FAS/APO-1 phenotype of PB cells

Phenotype	Number of patients	Remissions complete	Remissions partial	Median duration of phases (months) chronic	accelereted	blast
CD95+	11	1	0	39	3,6	3,6
CD95-	18	3	2	38	3,1	5,4

(CD10-) group myeloid, primitive and undifferentiated variants are included. The analysis of lymphocytic antigens and CD95(Fas/APO-1) expression according to this classification is shown in Table 3. It is evident that high frequency of CD95(Fas/APO-1) antigen expression was found in mixed and non-lymphoid variants, while in lympoid it is comparatively rare (20% of cases).

Remissions in CML BC are infrequent. We have obtained only 5 (3 complete and 2 partial) remissions in our patients. All of them were achieved in the lymphoid and mixed variants (Table 4). The phenotype of these patients was CD10+CD13– CD95(Fas/APO-1)– No remissions were obtained in CD13+ and CD95(Fas/APO-1) + groups regardless of CD10 expression; CD34 expression had no influence on survival (4 vs. 3 months, p>0.05). In the mixed variant (i.e. positive for both CD10 or CD22 and one or more of the myeloid antigens), where 6 of 9 patients were CD95(Fas/APO-1)-positive, the remissions were obtained only in CD95(Fas/APO-1) -negative subgroup. Surprisingly, the median survival in the CD95(Fas/APO-1)+ and CD95(Fas/APO-1)– patients was nearly equal: 3.5 vs. 3 months in the whole group, and 8 vs. 9 months in the CD10+ patients (all differences not significant). Only CD10-positivity had prognostic significance for the survival in CML BC (8 vs. 3 months, p<0.05). Interestingly, the CD10+ group had also significantly shorter acceleration phase (0 vs. 3.5 months, p<0.01).

4.3. Studies of the Correlation of P-Glycoprotein Expression by Patients' PB Cells with Their Survival and Response to the Therapy

We investigated P-glycoprotein (Pgp) expression in 40 BC CML patients. The number of Pgp positive (Pgp+) cases in BC at 20% threshold of positivity was 13 (approximately 1/3). Addition of the Pgp+/- cases (> 10% and < 19 % of Pgp-expressing cells in the studied cell population) gives around 50% of Pgp positivity in BC and makes our data comparable with the results of Weide et al.[15] and Michelutti et al.[16] who also studied comparatively large groups of CML patients. Rhodamine 123 (Rh123) test revealed functional Pgp in all Pgp+ cases studied.

The question is: does Pgp positivity occurs due to the treatment of CML patients or Pgp+ cells appear spontaneously, independently of therapy? Our data show that although in some cases the treatment of the patients might explain the presence of Pgp+ cells in their PB, significant numbers of Pgp expressing cells might emerge spontaneously: in 2 untreated patients in BC CML we have found Pgp+ phenotype of PB blasts. The next question is: does the number of Pgp+ cells increase during the course of the treatment of BC CML patients? We investigated 14 patients sequentially during the course of BC. All these patients received polychemotherapy including drugs known to select for MDR. Table 5 shows that at the first examination 5 cases were Pgp positive and that 4 of them demonstrated Pgp-negative phenotype at the second analysis. Of 9 Pgp- samples 7 remained

Table 5. Sequential studies of Pgp expression in blast crisis of CML

Examination	Number of patients		
	Total	Pgp+	Pgp-
I	14	5	9
II	14	3	11

Pgp-negative at the second analysis and only 2 became Pgp-positive. These data suggest that the Pgp+ phenotype in most cases does not confer a selective advantage to the blasts in BC CML when polychemotherapy is given. Although the number of the patients studied is not large, the tendency seems evident: only in a small number of sequentially studied cases did Pgp+ cells become dominant during the course of BC progression and treatment.

Examination of the correlations of Pgp expression with the expression of lymphocytes differentiation markers revealed that In BC 20% of patients demonstrated a Pgp+CD34+ phenotype. Among these were 4 of 5 cases with a large fraction of Pgp expressing blasts (more than 50% of PB cells expressing Pgp). Using double staining of the cells with anti-Pgp and anti-CD34 Mabs we have shown that Pgp and CD34 antigens are expressed on the same cells (data not shown).

We had not found a the correlation between the expression of the majority of other antigens of hematopoietic cell differentiation (CD10, CD19, CD22, CD11b, CD14, HLA-DR were studied). However the antigen of early myeloblasts CD13 did give a significant correlation with Pgp expression (n = 40; correlation coefficient 0.31).

Among 40 patients with BC 8 Pgp+ and 17 Pgp- samples were studied at the time of diagnosis of BC. Figure 2a shows the overall survival of these two groups of patients according to the Pgp phenotype illustrating that survival is statistically lower in the Pgp+ group ($p<0.02$). Although the median survival of patients in both groups was not too long (1.9 and 4.3 months), it is evident that Pgp positivity found at diagnosis of BC may reflect negative prognostic influence. CD13 expression shown above to correlate with Pgp positivity was also found to influence the overall survival of BC patients (Figure 2b; $p<0.03$). Statistical significance of the differences between antigen-positive and -negative cases increased when Pgp+CD13+ cases were compared with Pgp-CD13- cases ($p<0.01$). It is known that the myeloid type of BC is most unfavourable in terms of treatment outcome[17] and from this point of view the negative prognostic value of early myeloid antigen CD13 is understandable. The probable explanation of our data is that the negative prognostic value of CD13 may often be explained by the presence of Pgp-mediated drug resistance in CD13+ cells.

5. DISCUSSION

We have examined three factors which could influence the survival and sensitivity of CML patients to therapy: variants of BCR-ABL translocation, FAS/APO-1 and Pgp expression. We have found that all three factors are connected in some way or the other with patient's survival or peculiarities of their response to the treatment. First, if the patients were treated with cytostatic, than the overall survival of the persons with BCR-ABL transcript with b2a2 junction was greater than the overall survival of the patients with b3a2 type of mRNA. These differences were not revealed in patients treated with interferon-α. Thus our data suggest that the variants of BCR-ABL translocation can influence CML pa-

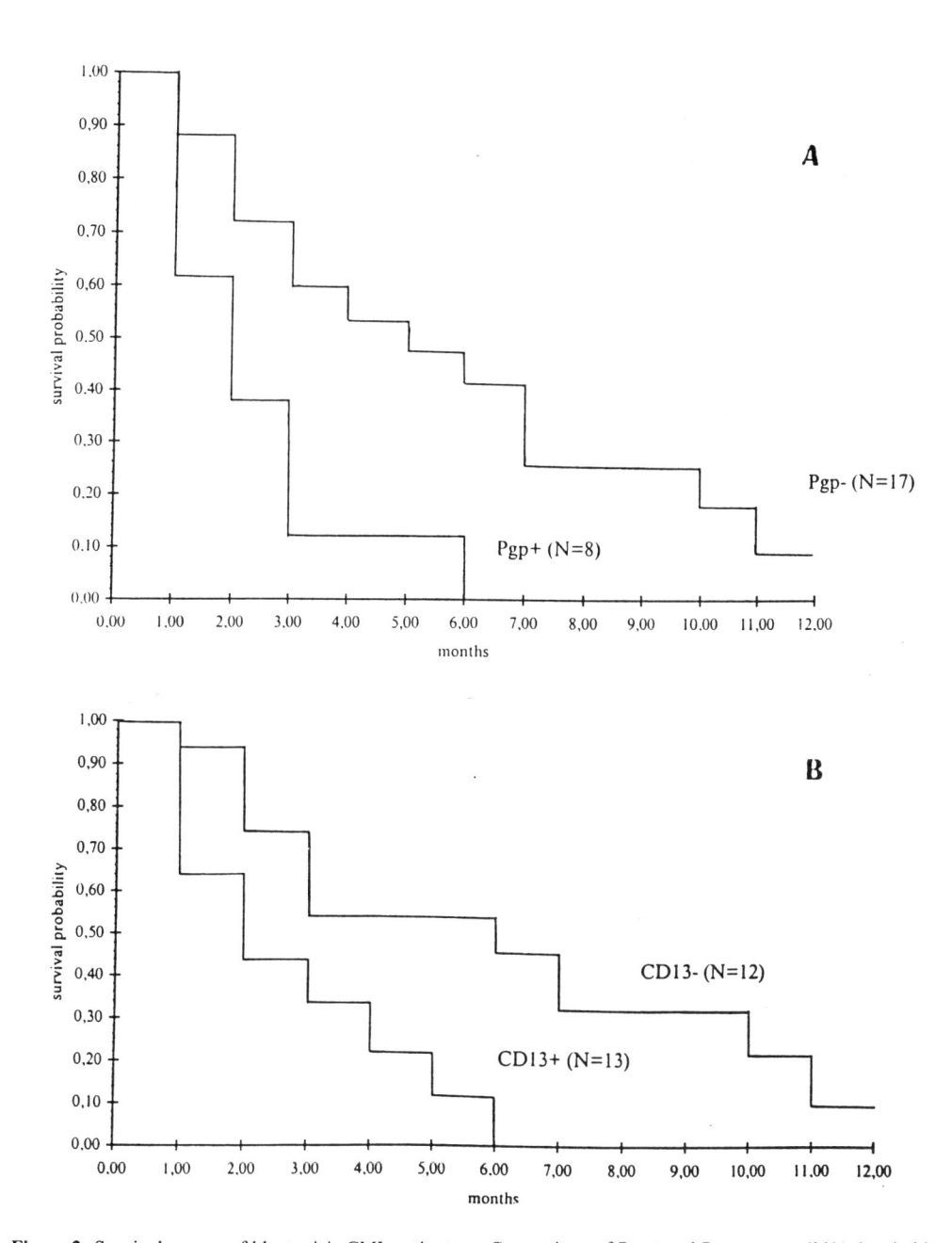

Figure 2. Survival curves of blast crisis CML patients. a. Comparison of Pgp+ and Pgp- groups (20% threshold level of Pgp expression found at diagnosis of blast crisis). b. Comparison of CD13+ and CD13- groups (20% threshold level of CD13 expression).

tients' response on some kinds of the treatment. The available data suggest that one can distinguish at least three clinico-hamatological entities among the chronic and two among the acute Ph+ myeloid leukemias depending on the type of BCR-ABL fusion protein produced by different BCR breakpoints.[14] However we have not found any clinico-hematological differences in our two groups of patients besides the differences in overall survival.[18]

Second, the studies of Fas/APO-1 expression by the cells of PB have revealed the differences in the remissions frequency and the immunophenotype of the patients between CD95 (Fas/APO-1)+ and CD95(Fas/APO-1)- groups. Surprisingly, in Fas/APO-1 negative group of patients the remission frequency was higher than among Fas/APO-1 positive. Abrogation of apoptosis due to non-expression of Fas ligand receptor must give cells the possibility to proliferate and survive. We obtained the opposite results. The number of remissions was higher in Fas/APO-1 negative patients. The duration of BC did not significantly differ between two groups of patients, although some tendency to the longer terminal stage was registered in Fas/APO negative persons. The explanation of this discrepancy can be the following: Fas-mediated apoptosis is suppressed in the cells of CML patients due to another mechanism (expressed below of the Fas ligand receptor). Indeed, it was shown that cell mediated apoptosis of cells expressing BCR-ABL is independent of Fas and that BCR-ABL blocks Fas-induced death.[3,19] We suppose that Fas/APO-1 expression by the PB cells of CML patients may be regarded as some differentiation marker and not as mechanism of the programmed cell death. Indeed, we have found that Fas/APO-1 was expressed more often in myeloid or mixed, but not in lymphoid variants of BC CML. The peculiarities of patient's response on the therapy (the chance to have a remission) is dependent on cell immuniphenotype and one of the markers of this phenotype is, probably, Fas/APO-1 antigen.

Pgp+ cases may occur both spontaneously and as a result of the therapy. Pgp-positive cases constitute about 20% of all BC cases studied showing that the Pgp-mediated MDR is not the main cause of therapy failure of BC CML. The results of sequential studies in the same patients suggest that Pgp+ cells have no selective advantage and their number do not often increase when BC patients receive polychemotherapy. Meanwhile Pgp expression in BC correlated with the expression of the stem cell antigen CD34 and the marker of early myeloid cells CD13. This suggests that Pgp is expressed by an immature cell population. Pgp and CD13 positivity at the time of BC diagnosis was shown to have prognostic value for BC duration: 2-fold shorter BC was found in the patients with Pgp expression. We propose that Pgp may be regarded as differentiation marker of the cells and the prognostic factor in BC CML. Several explanations of our data may be offered. It is probable that either polychemotherapy kills Pgp+ cells, or that Pgp- cells have some benefit in comparison with their Pgp-positive variants. Perhaps Pgp+ cells proliferate more slowly, and it is probable that they have collateral sensitivity to some non-MDR drugs. It is also possible that the therapy leads to the occurrence of more differentiated cell populations with down regulated Pgp. Moreover it is known that the populations of blasts in BC CML patients is extremely heterogeneous and highly variable.[11,17] In our sequential studies most of the cases were examined twice. Accordingly it can not be excluded that the later examinations might have revealed an increase of the Pgp+ cell portion. It is also probable that in some cases the smaller number of Pgp+ cells with a higher rate of Pgp expression or an higher functional activity of Pgp might survive and eventually can determine their resistance to the therapy. Nevertheless our data show that in BC CML chemotherapy using MDR drugs is not the main selective factor and does not invariably lead to the accumulation of Pgp expressing cells.

Thus although all three factors examined in this study seems to have some influence on patients' survival and/or sensitivity to treatment, this influence was not strong. It seems that all these factors can be regarded as modifiers of CML evolution. It is evident that some other cause (main cause) underlay CML, and especially BC CML refractoriness to the therapy. It is doubtful that this factor is only the activity of BCR-ABL fusion protein and its anti-apoptotic effects. CP CML is characterised by the presence of BCR-ABL translocation, but it can be treated by different drugs. In BC CML there is the same translocation. There are cases of BC CML without elevation or even with decrease in the levels of BCR-ABL transcripts.[6] It seems that factor(s) other than only BCR-ABL may be responsible for the evolution of the terminal stage of CML. This factor is not known. Nevertheless it is important to understand the mechanisms modifying its (their) effects.

ACKNOWLEDGMENTS

This work in part was supported by grants of Russian Foundation for Basic Research.

REFERENCES

1. Konopka, J.B., Watanabe, S.M., Witte, O.N. An alteration of the human ABL protein in K562 leukemia cells unmasks associated tyrosine kinase activity. Cell, 1984, 37, 1035–1043.
2. Kloetzer,W., Kurzrock, R., Smith, I., Talpaz, M., Spiller, M., Gutterman, I., Arlinghaus, R. The human cellular ABL gene product in chronic myelogeneous leukemia cell line K562 has an associated tyrosine protein kinase activity.Virology, 1985, 140, 230–238.
3. Jones, R.J. Biology and treatment of chronic myeloid leukemia. Current Opinion in Oncology, 1997, 9, 3–7.
4. Bedi, A., Zehnbauer, B.A., Barber, J.P., Sharkis, S.J., Jones, R.J. Inhibition of apoptosis by BCR-ABL in chronic myeloid leukemia. Blood, 1994, 83, 2038- 2044.
5. Mc Gahon, A., Bissonnette, R., Schmitt, M., Cotter, K.M., Green, D.R., Cotter, T.G. BCR-ABL maintains resistance of chronic myeloid leukemia cells to apoptotic death. Blood, 1994, 83, 1179–1187.
6. Gordon, M.Y., Goldman, J.M. Cellular and molecular mechanisms in chronic myeloid leukemia: biology and treatment. Br. J. Haemat.1996, 95, 10–20.
7. Bedi, A., Barber, J.P., Bedi, G.C., El-Deiry, W.S., Sidransky, D., Vala, M.S., Akhtar, A.J., Hilton, J., Jones, R.J. BCR-ABL-mediated inhibition of apoptosis with delay of G2/M transition following DNA damage: a mechanism of resistance to multiple anticancer agents. Blood, 1995, 86, 1148–1158.
8. Roger, R., Issaad, C., Pallardy, M., Turhan, A.Gg, Beroglio, J., Breard, J. BCR-ABL does not prevent apoptotic death induced by human natural killer or lymphokine-activated killer cells. Blood, 1996, 87, 1113–1122.
9. Mechetner, E.B., Roninson, I.B. Efficient inhibition of P-glycoprotein -mediated multidrug resistance with a monoclonal antibody. Proc. Natl. Acad. Sci. USA, 1992, 89, 5824–5828.
10. Schinkel, A.H., Arceci, R.J., Smith, J.J.M., Wagenaar, E., Baas, F., Doll, M., Tsuruo, T., Mechetner, E.B., Roninson, I.B., Borst, P. Binding properties of monoclonal antibodies recognazing external epitopes of the human MDR1 P-glycoprotein. Int.J.Cancer, 1993, 55, 478–484.
11. Frolova, E. A., Baryshnikov, A.Yu., Moiseenkova, I.N., Tupitsin, N.N., Turkina A.G. Heterogeneity in immunological types of chronic myeloid blast crisis. Haematologia i Transfusiologia, 1992, 5, 6–11 (in Russian).
12. Neyfakh, A.A. Use of fluorescent dyes as molecular probes for the study of multidrug resistance. Exp. Cell Res., 1988, 174, 168–176.
13. Egudina S.V., Stromskaya, T.P., Frolova E.A., Stavrovskaya, A.A. Early steps of P-glycoprotein expression in cell cultures studied with vital fluorochrome. FEBS Letters, 1993, 329, 63–66.
14. Melo, J.V. The diversity of BCR-ABL fusion proteins and their relationship to leukemia phenotype. Blood, 1996, 88, 2375–2784.

15. Weide, R., Dowding, C., Paulsen, W., Goldman, J. The role of MDR-1/P-170 mechanism in development of multidrug resistance in chronic myeloid leukemia. Leukemia, 1990, 4, 695–699.
16. Michelutti, A., Michieli, M., Damiani., D., Melli, C., Geromin, A., Russo, D., Fanin, R., Baccarani, M. Overexpression of MDR-related P-170 glycoprotein in chronic myeloid leukemia. Haematologica, 1994, 79, 200–204.
17. Baryshnikov, A.Ju., Turkina A.G., Michailova, I.N., Sedyakhina, N.P., Shishkin, Ju.V., Korolyova, A.M., Palkina, T.N., Ivanov, P.K., Frolova, E.A., Mokeyeva, R.A., Khoroshko, N.D. In: Gene Technology. Stem Cell and Leukemia Research, 1996, Edited by A.R.Zander, W.Ostertag, B.V.Afanasiev, F.Grosveld, NATO ASI Series, Series H: Cell biology, vol. 94, 475–484. Springer-Verlag Berlin Heidelberg.
18. Turkina, A.G., Domninsky, D.A., Pokrovskaya, E.S., Babushkina, E.A., Moiseenkova, I.N., Zacharova, A.V., Archipova, N.V., Grineva, N.I., Khorochko, N.D. Prognostic value of the structure of the variants of chromosome translocation t(9;22) in chronic myeloid leukemia. Gematologia, 199 , 3, 8–11 (in Russian).
19. McGahon, A.J., Nishioka, W.K., Martin, S.J., Mahboubi, A., Cotter, T.G., Green, D.R. Regulation of the Fas apoptotic cell death patway by Abl. J.Biol.Chem., 1995, 270, 22625–22631.

53

CLINICAL SENSITIVITY TO ANTHRACYCLINES IN PH/BCR+ ACUTE LYMPHOBLASTIC LEUKEMIA

Renato Bassan,[1] Ama Z. S. Rohatiner,[2] Alessandro Rambaldi,[1] Teresa Lerede,[1] Eros Di Bona,[3] Maxine Carter,[2] Giuseppe Rossi,[4] Enrico Pogliani,[5] Giorgio Lambertenghi-Deliliers,[6] Piero Fabris,[7] Adolfo Porcellini,[8] T. Andrew Lister,[2] and Tiziano Barbui[1]

[1]Division of Hematology
Ospedali Riuniti, Bergamo, Italy
[2]ICRF Department of Medical Oncology, St. Bartholomew's Hospital
London, United Kingdom
[3]Division/Unit of Hematology/Bone Marrow Transplant
Ospedale Civile, Vicenza
[4]Spedali Civili, Brescia
[5]Nuovo Ospedale San Gerardo, Monza
[6]Clinica Medica Università di Milano, Milan
[7]Ospedale Civile, Bolzano
[8]Ospedale Civile, Cremona, Italy

Keywords: Ph+/BCR+ ALL, anthracyclines, prognostic factors, survival.

1. ABSTRACT

Translocation t(9;22) or Philadelphia chromosome (Ph)/BCR-ABL rearrangement positive acute lymphoblastic leukemia (Ph/BCR+ ALL) is associated with a very short survival of about one year in most patients. We analyzed long-term outcome of 76 adults with Ph/BCR+ ALL, in order to detect which factors were associated with longer survival. Modifiable prognostic factors included type of treatment, allogeneic marrow transplant (allo-BMT), and early anthracycline dose intensity (high=H/A, low=L/A); unmodifiable factors were age, gender, FAB morphology, phenotype, blast count, P190/210 transcript, hepato-spleno-lymphadenopathy, LDH level. Median patient age was 43 years (range 15–71). Four favorable prognostic factors (FPF) were found associated with greater likelihood of complete remission (blast count $<50 \times 10^9$/l, p= 0.08), longer remission duration (age <50 years, p<0.001; H/A, p<0.05), and lower relapse rate (allo-BMT, p=0.017). Age and anthracycline dose intensity exerted a synergistic prognostic effect. According to the cumulative incidence of FPF in each patient (FPF 0–1=29, 2–3=42, 4=5), the probability of survival increased from nil to 0.22 to 0.60 at 5 years (p<0.005). Adult Ph/BCR+ ALL is relatively sensitive to anthracyclines, which therefore should be prescribed at full dosage to patients not eligible to allo-BMT or in the waiting list for unrelated donor transplantation.

2. INTRODUCTION

Many adult acute lymphoblastic leukemia (ALL) cases express the Philadelphia (Ph+) chromosome translocation between chromosomes 9 and 22 (q34; q11), in which ABL and BCR proto-oncogenes give typically rise to the new activated BCR-ABL fusion gene. The BCR-ABL (BCR+) gene product has a variable molecular weight of 190 kD (P190) or 210 kD (P210). The rearrangement, for diagnostic purposes, is detectable by the polymerase chain reaction (PCR) technique.

In adult Ph/BCR+ ALL, complete remission (CR) rates range from 56%-96%, the median duration of first CR is 5–11 months, and less than 20% of patients survive >2 years (1–8). The prognostic profile, however, may be more heterogeneous than initially reported. A relatively better outcome was in fact associated with a hyperdiploid karyotype (9), the achievement of an early PCR- status (10,11), the lack of a myeloid cell component (12) or, on the contrary, with stem-cell features as shown by concurrent Ph/BCR positivity of nonlymphoid cells (13). In a recent childhood series, a white cell count <25 × 10^9/l conferred a very good outlook to some patients treated with intensive postremission consolidation (14). In general, survival rates are improved by allogeneic bone marrow transplantation (allo-BMT), but the high post-transplant relapse rate, the advanced age of many patients and the paucity of donors prevent this procedure from having a determinant prognostic impact, although the reported long-term disease-free survival rates are 40–50% (15,16). The interest towards very high-dose treatments supported by autologous bone marrow/peripheral blood cell transplants (ABMT/ABCT) is therefore increasing, but data insofar produced are scanty and inconclusive as concerns a real prolongation of survival by this treatment method (17–21).

Here we analyze the long-term results obtained in an unselected series of 76 adults with Ph/BCR+ patients, who were treated over a 25 year period with the ALL-directed regimens developed by the L-B-V Group (London, UK, St. Bartholomew's Hospital; Bergamo, Italy, Ospedali Riuniti; Vicenza, Italy, Ospedale Civile). Our aim was to investigate further the clinical and prognostic heterogeneity of Ph/BCR+ ALL of adults, and particularly to assess which treatments and drugs could be specifically associated with an improved therapeutic outcome and could therefore suggest a hitherto unrecognized chemosensitivity pattern.

3. MATERIALS AND METHODS

3.1. Ph/BCR+ ALL Diagnosis

ALL was defined by French-American-British (FAB) criteria (22). Blast cell immunophenotype was evaluated to confirm ALL diagnosis. No Ph/BCR+ case had T-cell ALL or B-ALL with FAB-L3 morphology and clonal surface immunoglobulin/SIg expression). Accordingly, cases were subdivided in pre-B CD10+ ALL (TdT, nuclear terminal-deoxynucleotidyl-transferase+, SIg-, HLA-DR+, CD19+, CD20+, CD10+), and pre-B CD10- ALL. Most cases were examined for the co-expression of CD13, CD33, and CD34 myeloid and stem cell associated antigens. The cytogenetic analysis was performed by means of standard banding techniques. BCR-ABL rearrangements were identified by means of reverse-transcriptase PCR (RT-PCR), as previously detailed (23). Ph/BCR+ positivity was defined by cytogenetic analysis, RT-PCR, or both.

3.2. Patient Selection

Three hundred forty nine adult patients with ALL were enroled into five subsequent prospective chemotherapy trials between 1979 and 1996 at Bergamo Hospital and collaborating centers. One hundred ninety-three cases were examined by RT-PCR and/or cytogenetics for Ph/BCR expression, and 57 were found positive. Nineteen additional Ph/BCR+ patients identified by cytogenetic analysis were from St. Bartholomew's Hospital. Seventy six total Ph/BCR+ ALL cases formed the study group.

3.3. Treatment Programs

All patients were treated with one of seven OPAL-derived, ALL-directed regimens adopted between 1972–1996 (24–26). The general outline of these programs is reported in Table 1. HEAV'D and R-HEAV'D regimens were characterized by an early dose-intensive anthracycline administration (total adriamycin 360–405 mg/m^2) (24,28). The OPAL-Hi-DAC regimen included high-dose cytarabine (HiDAC) 2 g/m^2/bd on days 1–6 as early consolidation course (28). The IVAP protocol consisted of a dose-intensive idarubicin-containing induction and early consolidation phase (total idarubicin 132 mg/m^2, IVAP-1; and 116 mg/m^2, IVAP-2), followed by high-dose BCNU-etoposide-melphalan with ABMT (only patients <50 year-old), continuation weekly therapy for three months, and standard low-dose maintenance (29); the bone marrow harvest was performed after the four early consolidation cycles and was unpurged; a low intensity idarubicin schedule (IVAP-3) was adopted for patients older than 60 years (30). The STT (short term therapy) regimen consisted of 6 total intensive cycles with vincristine-adriamycin-prednisone alternating with HiDAC-etoposide pulses, without maintenance therapy (31); total adriamycin dosage was 360 mg/m^2. The 07/93 regimen consisted of IVAP-type induction followed by 6 total idarubicin-vincristine-cyclophosphamide and intermediate-dose cytarabine-etoposide

Table 1. Summary of treatment regimens, 1972–1993

Denomination, year introduced	Induction drugs	Consolidation drugs (no. of cycles)	CNS phase	ABMT/ABST	Maintenance drugs (mos.)
OPAL*, 1972	D,A,V,P	D,V (2)	RT+LP	–	MP,M,C (36)
HEAVD, 1978	D,A,V,P	D,V,C (4)	RT+LP	–	MP,M,C (36)
OPAL-HD-ara-C, 1984	D,A,V,P	D,V, HD-ara-C (3)	LP	–	MP,M,C (36)
R-HEAV'D, 1987	D,A,V,P	D,V,C,ara-C,T (4+12w)	RT+LP	–	MP,M (36)
IVAP*, 1991	I,A,V,P,G	I,A,V,C,ara-C,T (4+12w)	RT+LP	B,E,ML (BM)	MP,M (ABMT y/n: 6/18)
STT*, 1991	D,A,V,P,GM	D,V,HD-ara-C,E (5)	LP	–	–
07/93, 1993	I,A,V,P,G	I,V,Dx,C,ara-C,E (6)	RT+LP	C,E,ML (PB)	MP,M (18)

pulses, followed by high-dose cyclophosphamide-etoposide-melphalan with unpurged ABCT support and mid-term low-dose maintenance (32). Allo-BMT was offered in first CR to patients with a histocompatible sibling donor.

3.4. Definitions and Statistics

The definition of CR required an untransfused hemoglobin >10 g/dl, neutrophils >1 × 10^9/l, platelets >100 × 10^9/L, a normocellular or slightly hypocellular regenerating bone marrow with trilineage normal hemopoiesis without ALL cells (marrow blasts <5%), and a clear cerebrospinal fluid (CSF) in patients with CNS involvement. An early pancytopenic death was due to infection, hemorrhage or other lethal complication developed before the assessment of antileukemic response. A recurrence was defined by the presence of >5% ALL blasts in the bone marrow, blasts in the CSF, or elsewhere (biopsy proven). Survival was taken from date of diagnosis to death, by any cause, and relapse-free survival (RFS) from date of CR to first relapse in any site or death in CR by any cause.

Results were analyzed by the treatment intention principle. The probabilities of achieving a CR were compared using the chi-squared test with Yate's correction. RFS and survival curves were plotted by the standard Kaplan and Meier method and compared by the log-rank method. Statistical significance was expressed by p values <0.05, and trends by a p value <0.1. Nonsignificant (ns) p values were not reported.

4. RESULTS

4.1. Diagnosis and Patients

Fifty seven Ph/BCR+ ALL patients were found to be registered in the Bergamo Hospital file. Eighteen were identified by the cytogenetic study only and a further 18 by RT-PCR only. Cytogenetic and PCR study were concurrently performed in 21 patients: 7 were positive by PCR only but no case was Ph+ and BCR-. Twenty seven of 39 patients examined by RT-PCR expressed the P190 type of molecular transcript (69.2%). Diagnostic study results are summarized in Table 2.

The clinical features of 76 evaluable patients with pre-B Ph/BCR+ ALL are reported in Table 3. By comparison with 92 pre-B Ph/BCR- adult patients registered at Bergamo Hospital (data not shown), higher age and CD10 plus CD34 positivity were strongly associated with the Ph/BCR+ status (p<0.05). Patient characteristics did not differ significantly by P190 or P210 molecular BCR-ABL transcript (data not shown).

4.2. Induction of CR

The number of patients treated with each of 7 regimens was OPAL 7, HEAV'D 4, OPAL-HiDAC 7, R-HEAV'D 7, IVAP 22, STT 4, and 07/93 25. The overall CR rate was 78.9% (60 patients), with a median time to CR of 31 days. Six patients aged 40–67 years (p=0.093) died early of complications (7.8%) and 10 had refractory disease (13.1%). Induction resistance was apparently associated with a blast cell count at presentation >50 × 10^9/l: 4/48 (8.3%) with blasts 0–49, 3/14 (21.4%) with blasts 50–100, and 3/8 (37.5%) with a blast cell count >100 (p=0.08). Response to adriamycin and idarubicin-based programs was similar. None of refractory patients achieved a CR with second line chemotherapy. Limitedly to patients from Bergamo Hospital, the comparative analysis

Table 2. Diagnostic results according to cytogenetic and RT-PCR analyses

Diagnostic tests	All cases N=76	London cases N=19	Bergamo cases N=56
Cytogenetics only:	37	19	18
RT-PCR only:	18	–	18
RT-PCR+/cytogenetics-:	7	–	7
RT-PCR+/cytogenetics+:	14	–	14

with pre-B Ph/BCR- cases confirmed the greater incidence of refractory ALL in the Ph/BCR+ subset (p<0.05, data not shown).

4.3. Postremission Therapy Results and RFS by Prognostic Factors

Two patients were lost to follow-up during early treatment. Eleven patients were submitted to allo-BMT after a short consolidation phase according to current treatment protocol. With a median observational time to relapse, death or last follow-up of 9.4 months (range 1 month-9.54 years), the median and 5-year RFS probability of 60 CR patients was 10.5 months and 0.15, respectively. Because 27% per cent of CR patients were noticed to be alive and disease-free at 4 years from CR and some remissions lasted up to 9.54+ years, we sought for the factors associated with an increased RFS probability. Among those considered for this analysis (age, gender, blast count, FAB type, immunophenotype, type of molecular transcript, hepatosplenomegaly and lymphadenopathy, CNS involvement, serum LDH concentration, treatment protocol, HiDAC, anthracycline dose intensity, anthracycline type, ABMT/ABCT, allo-BMT), only age <50 years and dose-intensive anthracycline therapy (see Table 4 for details) conferred a net prognostic benefit in the univariate analysis.

The significance of these findings is shown in Figure 1, also reporting the combined effect of age and high anthracycline dose intensity after censoring of patients undergoing allo-BMT or lost to follow-up. In the combined analysis, 4/17 patients (23.5%) with both these favorable prognostic factors (FPF) remained disease-free after 4–9.54+ years vs none in the other groups.

The median and long-term 6–8 years probability of RFS for the different prognostic groups were: age <50 years 1.37 years and 0.19; age >50 years 0.66 years and 0 (Figure

Table 3. Clinical features of 76 patients
(no. of evaluable cases indicated when necessary)

Diagnostic features	Values
Age, median and range (yr)	43 (15–71)
Male gender, no	42
FAB L2, no	64
Blasts x10^9/l, median (range)	13.3 (0–330)
Immunophenotype, no	
CD10+	68/74
CD34+	34/52
CD13+	16/59
CD33+	16/59
Hepatosplenomegaly, no.	36/75
Lymphadenopathy, no.	20/75
CNS involvement, no.	3/69

Table 4. Regimen-related anthracycline intensity (postremission consolidation phase)

Intesity	Regimens	Drug[1]	Cumulative mg/m^2	No. early consolidation cycles(mg/m^2/cycle)
High				
	HEAV'D	Dox	350	4 (87.5)
	R-HEAV'D	Dox	300	4 (75)
	STT	Dox	300	4 (75)
	IVAP-1/2	Ida	96	4 (24)
Low				
	OPAL	Dox	90	4 (22.5)
	OPAL-HiDAC	Dox	90	4 (22.5)
	IVAP-3	Ida	48	4 (12)
	07/93	Ida	72	6 (12)

[1]Dox, doxorubicin (adriamycin); Ida, idarubicin

1a); intensive anthracycline consolidation 1.45 years and 0.24; nonintensive anthracycline consolidation 0.75 years and 0 (Figure 1b); age <50 years and intensive anthracycline consolidation 2.22 years and 0.23; age <50 years or intensive anthracycline consolidation 0.97 years and 0; age >50 years and nonintensive anthracycline consolidation 0.67 years and 0 (Figure 1c, with censoring of allo-BMT patients); allo-BMT patients 0.93 years and 0.36; other treatments excluding allo-BMT 0.78 years and 0.08 (Figure 1d).

Performing an allo-BMT in first CR improved RFS, but the impact was statistically nonsignificant in view of the small patient number and the two toxic deaths. However, the analysis of relapse by postremission treatment and type of transplant was clearly favorable to allo-BMT (Table 5).

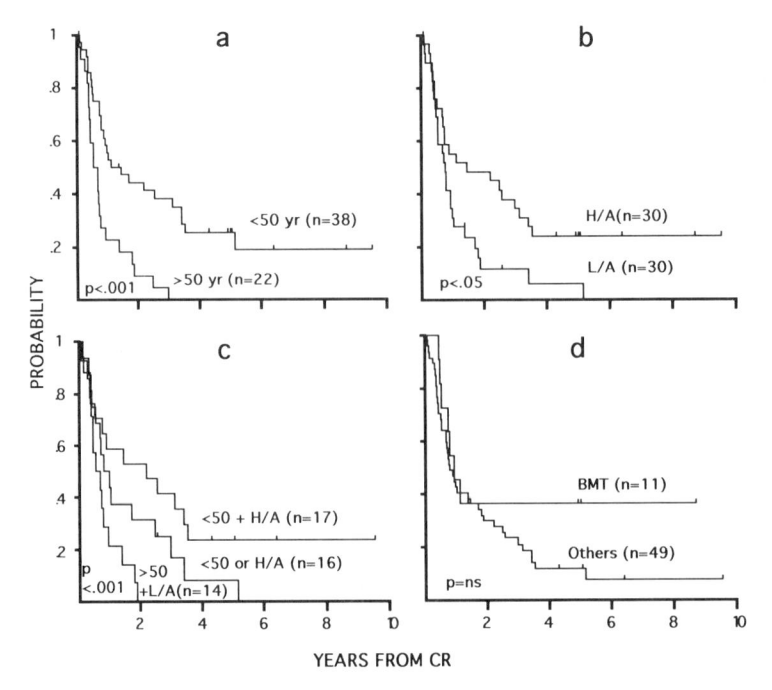

Figure 1. RFS probability according to patient age < or >50 years (a), high (H/A) or low (L/A) anthracycline dose intensity (b), age and anthracycline dose intensity (c), allo-BMT patients and those lost to follow-up censored), and allo-BMT in first CR (d).

Table 5. CR outcome by postremission treatment

	Chemotherapy N=41	ABMT/ABCT N=6	Allo-BMT N=11	p value
Relapse, no. (%)	35 (85.3)	5 (83.3)	5 (45.4)	0.017[1]
CR death, no. (%)	2 (4.8)	–	2 (18.1)	ns
Continued CR, no. (%)	4 (9.7)	1 (16.7)	4 (36.3)	0.08

[1] allo-BMT vs chemotherapy.

Nearly 35% of all CR cases relapsed within the first 6 months from CR. This was, for protocol 07/93 with a low anthracycline dose intensity, the reason why only one out of 17 CR patients underwent ABCT. Altogether, 7 CR patients are alive without recurrence, 4 after a chemotherapy consolidation program including anthracyclines at high cumulative dosage and 3 after allo-BMT.

4.4. Survival and Prognostic Profile by FPF

Median overall survival was 1.15 years and the projected 5-year probability 0.16. Median survival was 1.37 years for CR patients and 68 days for nonresponders (p<0.0001). The four factors exerting a favorable prognostic effect on CR achievement and RFS duration or relapse rate (FPF: blast count <50 × 10^9/l, age <50 years, intensive anthracycline consolidation, allo-BMT) were considered for a cumulative analysis of survival. The results are detailed in Table 6, which includes the analysis of the distribution of these variables in the whole patient population.

Because of the superimposable long-term survival rates of groups with 0–1 FPF and with 2–3 FPF, respectively, 3 different patterns of survival could be eventually identified by this model (Figure 2). The median and long-term survival probability were: 0–1 FPF 0.89 years and 0; 2–3 FPF 1.37 years and 0.08; 4 FPF not reached and 0.60. The prognostic difference between the 3 groups was highly significant (p<0.005).

5. DISCUSSION

In this retrospective survey on long-term treatment results of a relatively large series of adult patients with Ph/BCR+ ALL, we collected evidence for a response to anthracyclines when these drugs were intensively used in the early remission consolidation phase. In

Table 6. Cumulative distribution and prognostic effect of FPF on survival

FPF	No. of patients	FPF Bl <50	Age <50	H/A	BMT	Survival (yr) Median (5-yr probability)
4	5	5	5	5	5	NR (0.60)
3	15	15	15	14	1	1.78 (0.14)
2	27	21	18	11	4	1.37 (0.14)
1	27	7	17	2	1	0.9 (0)
0	2	0	0	0	0	0.7 (0)

[1] Bl, blast cells × 10^9/l; age in years; H/A, high anthracycline dose intensity; BMT, allo BMT. NR denotes not reached.

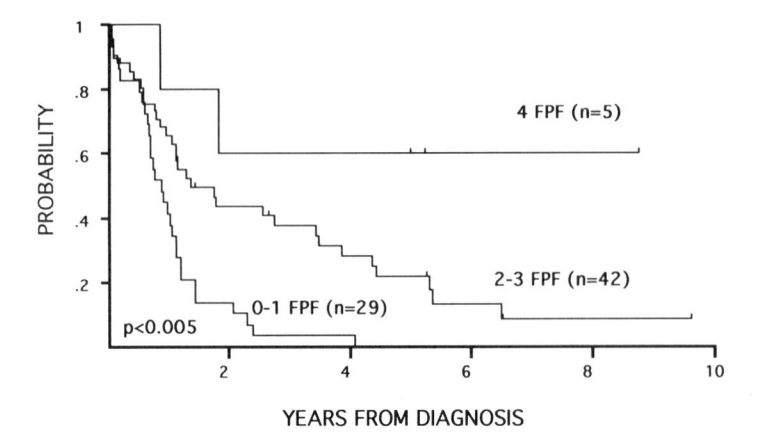

Figure 2. Overall patient survival by cumulative incidence of FPF.

Drug Resistance in Leukemia and Lymphoma II, we presented data in favor of anthracyclines in ALL of the pre-B type expressing the CD10 antigen and lacking t(9;22)/BCR rearrangement (33). Even in that preliminary report we noticed that a small group of Ph/BCR+ patients benefitted from intensive anthracycline consolidation, an observation that, with greater patient accrual and longer follow-up, is now extended and confirmed. A possible comment is that, regardless Ph/BCR expression, CD10+ pre-B ALL is more sensitive to dose-intensive anthracycline therapy than other ALL subtypes. By extrapolation, our attention should focus on other topoisomerase II inhibitors and, within the anthracycline subclass, on different members of this seemingly active drug family.

The role of single-drugs in Ph/BCR+ ALL is scarcely understood. Like the closely related entity lymphoid blast crisis of Ph/BCR+ chronic myelogenous leukemia (CML), Ph/BCR+ ALL is initially sensitive to ALL-directed chemotherapy. In the lymphoid blast crisis of CML, with a regimen similar to HEAV'D that contained a high cumulative dose of adriamycin, we obtained a high CR rate (9/10 patients) with a median CR duration of 12 months (range 2–17 months) and a median overall survival of 17 months (34). The data from the literature are scanty. Experience in 23 children with Ph/BCR+ ALL indicated that the majority of those with a low blast cell count could achieved "cure" following programs employing, as topoisomerase II inhibitors, etoposide and teniposide, but not anthracyclines (14). In view of the limited patient number in that study and the lack of prognostic significance of blast cell count in ours, these conclusions cannot be presently extended to the adult setting, but never the less they suggest that Ph/BCR+ ALL, under the best of circumstances, may be approached with curative intent even with chemotherapy only. A second, recent pediatric study indicated a heterogeneous response to pre-phase corticosteroids, that eventually predicted for a longer duration of response (35). In adult patients, data relative to single drugs were previously produced in favor of HiDAC, though this conclusion was based on the temporary efficacy of this treatment at time of recurrence (5). We underline that 3 of 4 long responders in our series were treated with the STT regimen, which included an intensive anthracycline consolidation plus both HiDAC and etoposide.

Hence, there is reason to believe that topoisomerase II inhibitors other than anthracyclines and HiDAC may be useful in the initial management of adult Ph/BCR+ ALL, particularly in patients with high blast count ($>50 \times 10^9$/l) that, in our experience, are more likely to manifest resistance to conventional ALL induction regimens. Primary induction failure and recurrence are obvious expressions of clinical drug resistance, that in acute leukemias is often associated with an overexpression of the MDR1 multidrug resistance mechanism or other. MDR1 substrates are all topoisomerase II inhibitors including anthracyclines and several other drugs, but not HiDAC. MDR1 positivity is frequently described in Ph/BCR+ ALL (36,37). Interestingly, we found a strict correlation between Ph/BCR+ ALL and cellular positivity for the stem cell antigen CD34. In healthy subjects, CD34+ bone marrow stem cells are normally protected by environmental toxic damage by the MDR1 mechanism (38). Therefore, it is not surprising that, in patients with acute myelogenous leukemia, the expression of CD34 antigen correlates well with MDR1 expression and clinical drug resistance (39). By analogy, Ph/BCR+ ALL could be intrinsically characterized by the expression of the MDR1 resistance mechanism. In the light of the direct blast cell count-clinical drug resistance relationship, like that we have observed, a higher blast cell count might confer an increased risk for the occurrence of clonal evolution phenomena with cells overexpressing MDR1, eventually responsible for both overt primary drug resistance or very short, transient response to chemotherapy.

In this retrospective analysis of 60 CR patients and 76 overall patients, a dose-intensive anthracycline treatment prolonged significantly both RFS and survival duration, even if the vast majority of the cases had a recurence and died of the disease. This is probably the first demonstration of a specific drug sensitivity pattern in Ph/BCR+ ALL of adults, and as such it may represent a valuable clinical information since a prolongation of early response can be crucial for many patients, for instance while unrelated bone marrow donors are being sought for (40).

Moreover a prognostic model for survival was proposed for the first time by combining the four identified FPF: blast count at diagnosis, patient age, anthracycline dose intensity, and allo-BMT. The prognostic pattern correlated explicitly with both unmodifiable (age, blast-count) and modifiable (anthracycline dose intensity, allo-BMT) factors. These findings push towards a more rational exploitation of the latter. In this respect, more active and less MDR1 vulnerable anthracyclines (idarubicin, annamycin) (41,42), higher drug dosages, and/or the concurrent therapeutic use of MDR1 functional down regulators (cyclosporin A, SDZ PSC 833) (43) could all be advantageous therapeutic steps. Our experience with idarubicin is still insufficient to provide conclusive data, and the exact place of etoposide and HiDAC is not known.

The management of Ph/BCR+ ALL in adult patients remains an outstanding clinical task. While we and others (44) are presently investigating in patients not eligible to allo-BMT the role of very high dose regimens supported by highly purified autologous stem cell rescue (45), the historical experience herein reviewed indicates that survival can be improved in many patients by the appropriate choice and scheduling of the drugs to which the disease appears to be at least partially sensitive. While the curability of this otherwise rapidly fatal condition rests exclusively on different and hopefully newer therapeutic applications, the achievement of a more durable palliation represents, for the time being an for aged patients, a sensible clinical goal.

REFERENCES

1. Jain, K., Arlin, Z., Mertelsmann, R., et al. (1983) Philadelphia chromosome and terminal transferase-positive acute leukemia: similarity of terminal phase of chronic myelogenous leukemia and de novo acute presentation. J Clin Oncol, 1, 669–676.

2. Raza, A., Minowada, J., Barcos, M., Rakowsky, I., Preisler, H.D. (1984) Ph-positive acute leukemia. Eur J Cancer Clin Oncol, 12, 1509–1516.
3. Gotz, G., Weh, H.J., Walter, T.A., et al. (1992) Clinical and prognostic significance of the Philadelphia chromosome in adult patients with acute lymphoblastic leukemia. Ann Hematol, 64, 97–100.
4. Annino, L., Ferrari, A., Cedrone M., et al. (1994) Adult Philadelphia-chromosome-positive acute lymphoblastic leukemia: experience of treatment during a ten-year period. Leukemia, 8, 664–667.
5. Preti, H.A., O'Brien, S., Giralt, S., et al. (1994) Philadelphia-chromosome-positive adult acute lymphoblastic leukemia: characteristics, treatement results, and prognosis in 41 patients. Am J Med, 97, 60–65.
6. Larson, R.A., Dodge, R.K., Burns, C.P., et al. (1995) A five-drug remission induction regimen with intensive consolidation for adults with acute lymphoblastic leukemia: Cancer and Leukemia Group B study 8811. Blood, 85, 2025–2037.
7. The Groupe Francais de Cytogénétique Hématologique. (1996) Cytogenetic abnormalities in adult acute lymphoblastic leukemia: correlations with hematologic findings and outcome. A collaborative study of the Groupe Francais de Cytogénétique Hématologique. Blood, 87, 3135–3142.
8. Secker-Walker, L.M., Prentice, H.G., Durrant, J., Richards, S., Hall, E., Harrison, G. (1997) Cytogenetics adds independent prognostic information in adults with acute lymphoblastic leukaemia on MRC trial UKALL XA. Br J Haematol, 96, 601–610.
9. Rieder, H., Ludwig, W-D., Gassmann, W., et al. (1996) Prognostic significance of additional chromosome abnormalities in adult Philadelphia chromosome positive acute lymphoblastic leukaemia. Br J Haematol, 95, 678–691.
10. Westbrook, C.A., Dodge, R., Szatrowski, T.P., et al. (1996) Acute lymphoblastic leukemia- detection of minimal residual disease (Abstract). Blood, 88 (suppl.1), 477a.
11. Preudhomme, C., Henic, N., Cazin, B., et al. (1997) Good correlation beteween RT-PCR analysis and relapse in Philadelphia (Ph1)-positive acute lymphoblastic leukemia (ALL). Leukemia, 11, 294–298.
12. Cuneo, A., Demuynck, H., Ferrant, A., et al. (1994) Minor myeloid component in Ph chromosome-positive acute lymphoblastic leukaemia: correlation with cytogenetic pattern and implication for poor response to therapy. Br J Haematol, 97, 515–522.
13. Secker-Walker, L.M., Craig, J.M. (1993) Prognostic implication of breakpoint and lineage heterogeneity in Philadelphia positive adult acute lymphoblastic leukemia: a review. Leukemia, 7, 147–151.
14. Ribeiro, R.C., Broniscer, A., Rivera, G.K., et al. (1997) Philadelphia chromosome-positive acute lymphoblastic leukemia in children: durable responses to chemotherapy associated with low initial white blood cell counts. Leukemia, 11, 1493–1496.
15. Barrett, A.J., Horowitz M.M., Ash, R.C., et al. (1992) Bone marrow transplantation for Philadelphia chromosome-positive acute lymphoblastic leukemia. Blood, 79, 3067–3070.
16. Dunlop, L.C., Powles, R., Singhal, S., et al. (1996) Bone marrow transplantation for Philadelphia chromosome-positive acute lymphoblastic leukemia. Bone Marrow Transplant, 17, 365–369.
17. Grigg, A.P. Approaches to treatment of Philadelphia-positive acute lymphoblastic leukemia. Bone Marrow Transplant, 12, 431–435.
18. Martin, H., Hoelzer, D., Atta, J., Elsner, S., Claudé, R., Bruecher, J. Autologous bone marrow trasplantation for Ph-positive/BCR-ABL positive acute lymphoblastic leukemia. Blood, 81 (suppl.1), 167a.
19. Carella, A.M., Frassoni, F., Pollicardo, N., et al. (1995) Philadelphia-chromosome-negative peripheral blood stem cells can be mobilized in the early phase of recovery after a myelosuppressive chemotherapy in Philadelphia-chromosome-positive acute lymphoblastic leukaemia. Br J Haematol, 89, 535–538.
20. Stockschadlader, M., Hegewisch-Becker, S., Kruger, W., et al. (1995) Bone marrow transplantation for Philadelphia-chromosome-positive acute lymphoblastic leukemia. Bone Marrow Transplant, 16, 663–667.
21. Baruchel, A., Auclerc, M.F., Bordigoni, P., et al. (1996) Potential value of autologous bone marrow transplantation for Philadelphia chromosome positive acute lymphoblastic leukemia (Ph+ ALL) in childhood (Abstract). Blood, (Suppl.1), 125a.
22. Bennett J.M., Catovsky, D., Daniel, M.T., et al (1981) The morphologic classification of acute lymphoblastic leukaemia: concordance among observers and clinical correlations. Br J Haematol, 47, 553–558.
23. Rambaldi, A., Attuati, V., Bassan, R., et al. (1996) Molecular diagnosis and clinical relevance of t(9;22), t(4;11) and t(1;19) chromosome abnormalities in a consecutive group of 141 adult patients with acute lymphoblastic leukemia. Leuk Lymphoma, 21, 457–466.
24. Lister, T.A., Whitehouse, J.M.A, Beard, M.E.J., et al. (1978) Combination chemotherapy for acute lymphoblastic leukaemia in adults. Br Med J, 1, 199–203.
25. Barnett, M.J., Greaves, M.F., Amess, J.A.L., et al (1986) Treatment of acute lymphoblastic leukaemia in adults. Br J Haematol, 33, 451–458.
26. Bassan, R., Battista, R., Rohatiner, A.Z.S., et al. (1992) Treatment of adult acute lymphoblastic leukaemia (ALL) over a 16 year period. Leukemia, 6 (suppl. 2), 186–190.

27. Bassan, R., Battista, R., Montaldi, A., et al. (1993) Reinforced HEAV'D therapy for adult acute lymphoblastic leukemia: improved results and revised prognostic criteria. Hematol Oncol, 11, 169–177.
28. Rohatiner, A.Z.S., Bassan, R., Battista, R., et al. (1990) High dose cytosine arabinoside in the initial treatment of adults with acute lymphoblastic leukaemia. Br J Cancer, 62, 454–458.
29. Bassan, R., Battista, R., Viero, P. et al. (1993) Intensive therapy for adult acute lymphoblastic leukemia: preliminary results of the idarubicin/vincristine/L-asparaginase/prednisolone regimen. Semin Oncol, 20 (suppl. 8), 39–46.
30. Bassan, R., Di Bona, E., Lerede, T., et al. (1996) Age-adapted moderate-dose induction and flexible outpatient postremission therapy for elderly patients with acute lymphoblastic leukemia. Leuk Lymphoma, 22, 295–301.
31. Papamichael, D., Andrews, T., Owen, D., et al. (1993) Intensive chemotherapy for adult acute lymphoblastic leukaemia (ALL) given with or without granulocyte/macrophage colony stimulating factor (GM-CSF). Br J Haematol, (Suppl.3), 60.
32. Lerede, T., Bassan, R., Rossi, A., et al. (1996) Therapeutic impact of adult-type acute lymphoblastic leukemia regimens in B-cell/L3 acute leukemia and advanced-stage Burkitt's lymphoma. Haematologica, 81, 442–449.
33. Bassan, R., Rambaldi, A., Lerede, T., et al. (1997) Correlation between early anthracycline dose intensity and clinical outcome identifies specific chemo-resistance patterns in adult acute lymphoblastic leukemia. In: Pieters, R., Kaspers, G.J.L., Veerman, A.J.P. (Eds.) Drug resistance in Leukemia and lymphoma II. Harwood Academic Publishers, Amsterdam, pp. 395–402.
34. Bassan, R., Battista, R., Comotti, B., et al. (1987) Treatment of the lymphoid blast crisis of chronic myeloid leukemia. Eur J Cancer Clin Oncol, 23, 513–515.
35. Aricò, M., Schrappe, M., Harbott, J., et al. (1997) Prednisone good response (PGR) identifies a subset of t(9;22) childhood acute lymphoblastic leukemia (ALL) at lower risk for early leukemia relapse. Blood, 90 (suppl. 1), 560a.
36. Goasguen, J.E., Dossot, J.M., Fardel, O., et al. (1993) Expression of the multidrug resistance-associated P-glycoprotein (P-170) in 59 cases of de novo acute lymphoblastic leukemia: prognostic implications. Blood, 81, 2394–2398.
37. Savignano, C., Geromin, A., Michieli, M., et al. (1993) The expression of the multidrug resistance related glycoprotein in adult acute lymphoblastic leukemia. Haematologica, 78, 261–263.
38. Marks, D.C., Su, G.M.I., Davey, R.A., Davey, M.W. Extended multidrug resistance in haemopoietic cells. Br J Haematol, 95, 587–595.
39. te Boekhorst, P.A.W., Lowenberg, B., van Kapel, J., Nooter, K., Sonneveld, P. (1995) Multidrug resistant cells with high proliferative capacity determine response to therapy in acute myeloid leukemia. Leukemia, 9, 1025–1031.
40. Sierra, J., Radich, J., Hansen, J., et al. (1997) Marrow transplant from unrelated donors for treatment of Philadelphia chromosome-positive acute lymphoblastic leukemia. Blood, 90, 1410–1414.
41. Ross, D., Tong, Y., Cornblatt, B. (1993) Idarubicin (IDA) is less vulnerable to transport-mediated multidrug resistance (MDR) than its metabolite idarubicinol (IDAol) or daunorubicin (DNR). Blood, 82 (suppl. 1), 257a.
42. Consoli, U., Priebe, W., Ling, Y.H., et al. (1996) The novel anthracyclin annamycin is not affected by P-glycoprotein-related multidrug reistance: comparison with idarubicin and doxorubicin in HL-60 leukemia cell lines. Blood, 88, 633–644.
43. Chiodini, B., Bassan, R., Borleri, G., Lerede, T., Barbui, T. (1998) Idarubicin activity against multidrug-resistant (mdr-1+) cells is increased by cyclosporin A. In: Hiddemann, W., et al. (Eds.) Acute Leukemias VII. Springer, Berlin, pp. 475–482.
44. Martin, H., Goekburget, N., Atta, J., Ludwig, W.D., Hoelzer, D. (1998) Treatment of Ph+ and t(4;11)+ acute lymphoblastic leukemia in adults. In: Hiddemann, W., et al. (Eds.) Acute Leukemias VII. Springer, Berlin, pp. 771–778.
45. Rambaldi, A., Borleri, G., Dotti, G. et al. (1998) Innovative two-step negative selection of G-CSF mobilized circulating progenitor cells: adequacy for autologous and allogeneic transplantation. Blood, 91, 2189–2196.

54

DIFFERENTIAL KINETICS OF DRUG RESISTANCE IN HUMAN LEUKAEMIC CELLS MEASURED BY SCGE/CLSM

Lynne M. Ball, Christopher L. Lannon, G. Ross Langley, Allen F. Pyesmany, Margaret Yhap, and Dick van Velzen

Department of Clinical Haemato-Oncology
Dalhousie University, IWK Grace Health Centre
5850 University Avenue
B3J 3G9, Halifax, Nova Scotia, Canada

Keywords: single cell gel electrophoresis, confocal laser scanning microscopy, human leukaemia, drug resistance, DNA excision repair.

1. ABSTRACT

1.1. Background

New analogues of DNA directed chemotherapy moieties are available for comparative efficacy testing in human neoplastic disease. In addition to MTT testing direct assessment of DNA excision repair activity after direct exposure of marrow cells may provide information on relative DNA effects in vitro.

1.2. Aims

To assess the ability of SCGE/high resolution CLSM to detect differences in drug resistance between human neoplastic cell lines in the DNA excision repair response to chemotherapy.

1.3. Methods

Eight human leukaemia samples (4 childhood, 4 adult) were exposed to 1 hour of single concentrations of daunorubicin, DaunoXome (courtesy NeXstar Pharmaceuticals

Inc, USA), cyclophosphamide and 4-hydroperoxycyclophosphamide (4-HC, courtesy Dr. M. Colvin, Duke University, USA), followed by SCGE/high resolution CLSM with quantitation of total excised DNA. Differences between cases/drug moieties/exposures were analysed.

1.4. Results

Although generally equal effect dose levels for DaunoXome were lower than for standard daunorubicin, patients/individual neoplastic cells differed considerably in optimal dose levels. Conventional cyclophosphamide in comparison to 4-HC showed inconsistent results indicating considerable differences in the level of drug resistance to the conventional product.

1.5. Conclusions

Direct testing for drug resistance patterns in DNA directed drug moieties by SCGE/CLSM reveals individual variability of human malignant cell lines warranting comparison with results of MTT testing and in-vivo patient response.

2. INTRODUCTION

An important phase in the development of any new (chemotherapeutic) agent is drug activity screening. At this stage large numbers of drug candidates are screened for comparative efficacy using a battery of neoplastic and normal cells usually in immortalized forms of cell culture. In addition to comparing dose-response curves to established standard reference drugs with similar properties as well those with an entirely different mechanism of action, no observed effect levels (NOEL) and necrosis levels are usually independently established.

Studies for the relative ability of new or established drugs to affect, in-vitro, neoplastic cells obtained from an actual patient, were first carried out by Von Limburgh in 1963 using fluid suspension cultures of mainly ovarian tumour cells.

In clinical practice these experimental approaches, with the advent of a wide range of new and highly effective drugs, were replaced by a drive towards polychemotherapy in which the number of agents used and the dosing schedules gradually became more complex.

It is only recently, that sensitivity testing of neoplasms on an individual patient base has been re-addressed, implicitly recognizing the often unique biological nature and thus therapeutic response to treatment of an individual patient's tumour.

Many lesions are multi clonal and may demonstrate great variability in proliferation rates and DNA abnormalities between the clones. In addition, individual cells may vary greatly in the ability to carry out effective DNA excision repair. Some lesions have abnormal quantities of cell surface receptors for binding of specific drug. Alternatively, as in multi drug resistant gene mutations, cells may develop the ability to survive relatively high levels of specific drug exposure by an effective up regulation of drug expulsion. Some cell lines vary in their ability to survive excessive amounts of DNA damage by regulation of DNA excision repair.

In this light, a recently developed approach emphasises (in analogy to developments in medical microbiology almost a century earlier) the need for reduction of the highly toxic side effects of polychemotherapy. The obvious alternative strategy is then to reduce the total number of chemotherapeutic agents in an individual patient by eliminating those agents that show no evidence of in-vitro effectivity.[1,2]

As a result MTT testing has been studied and developed to considerable levels of sophistication.[3] The choice of leukaemia for this development may not necessarily have been a random one as these lesions are considered to be relatively homogenous. In addition, they often are uniclonal at least on karyotype assessment or flow cytometry. Finally, any sample taken of the lesions by marrow aspiration or trephine biopsy, due to the suspended nature of tumour cells, will be highly homogenous and representative of the original tumour or its relapses. It is also easier to culture leukaemic cells in-vitro as these cells do not necessarily require a long initial establishment phase to achieve monolayer status or the development of a complex organoid architectural integration either with each other or with a second cell culture layer or substrate of artificial type. Short term drug toxicity or drug resistance testing with overall cell growth/cell death as the test parameter, has the advantage of being able to test virtually any presently used drug. The only limitations are that in some agents the an initially inactive agent requires extensive metabolization into active compounds before these can act on a drug. Some of these metabolites are extremely short lived especially in a watery environment and as such in-vitro testing is complicated.

DNA excision repair, following exposure of malignant cells to DNA directed drug moieties, until recently, could not be quantitated effectively. This was changed with the development of single cell gel electrophoresis (SCGE).[4–6] SCGE is carried out after causing a standardized DNA trauma to a living cell, for example by UV radiation[7–9] or drug exposure.[10,11] This is then followed by a standardize period of short term culture with activation of DNA excision repair. The intranuclear DNA fragments which result from DNA excision as part of the repair mechanisms can then be demonstrated. In SCGE these cells are embedded in a single cell gel layer, subsequently permeabilised and then submitted to electrophoretic conditions similar to those of normal DNA analysis. The small DNA fragments, in contrast to the bound large intact DNA belonging to the genome, will electrophorese out of the nuclear membrane confines and can be visualized adjacent to the nucleus.[4,12,13] This "stream" of nuclear fragments also named "comet tail" can then be visualized. Using modern optimised visualisation techniques (Lannon et all, this volume) these may then be assessed for fragment size distribution, total quantity of excised DNA and for maximum fragment size which is easily equated to total tail length.

With the advent of confocal laser scanning microscopy (CLSM) it becomes possible to objectively quantitate, through the use of fluorescent and stochastic DNA stains, the total content of the comet tail adjacent to the nucleus.[14] This opens the way for comparative assessment of the effect of different drugs on the same lesion.[11] In other circumstances the effects of a new candidate drug on different lesions may be investigated.[15] The techniques is sensitive enough to develop precise drug dose response curves by the combined methodological improvements we have developed (SCGE / High Resolution CLSM).[16–18]

Previously very labourious and time consuming, we have adapted this approach to a more practical form and presently have arrived at a stage where it becomes feasible to compare the ability of this technique to discriminate between different drug actions on a single lesion. If this were able to show in an efficient manner differences between patients and differences between the reaction of a tumour in individual patients to different drugs then SCGE/HR-CLSM might provide a rapid complementary method to the study of drug resistance in MTT. If applied immediately to a freshly acquired sample the whole procedure of SCGE/CLSM would take less than 8–12 hours to perform and in a number of clinical conditions such rapid testing may be of use. However, the limitation of this approach is that it only provides relevant information in those patients and lesions where the use of DNA directed drug moieties is beneficial.

We therefore chose to assess the ability of SCGE/High Resolution CLSM to detect differences in drug resistance in the form of measuring differences between the DNA excision repair activity of de-novo human leukaemic cells in response to exposure to chemotherapeutic agents.

3. METHODS AND MATERIALS

3.1. Study Populations

Eight pretreatment diagnostic bone marrow samples from patients with leukaemia (4 children, 4 adults) were included in the study.

3.2. Drug Exposure

Leukaemic cells were separate from the original aspirate samples through routine Ficoll separation. After initial dose range finding studies in a limited number of cases, patients and lesions were compared by exposure of the cell samples as obtained to a single dose / exposure variations / concentrations of daunorubicin, DaunoXome (courtesy NeXstar Pharmaceuticals Inc, USA) cyclophosphamide and 4-hydroperoxycyclophosphamide (4HC courtesy Dr. M. Colvin, Duke University, USA). See also Table 1.

3.3. Single Cell Gel Electrophoresis

Cell suspensions after two hours recovery culture in RPMI (Dutch modification) were suspended in 1% standard agar (1 part suspension, 3 parts agar) and poured into one of six punched out wells (diameter 6mm) in a normal 1 mm thick gel electrophoresis medium suspended on microscopy slides. After permeabilisation and under alkaline conditions, routine single cell gel electrophoresis (SCGE) was carried out at 150V with resulting amperages between 25–30 mA.

3.4. Confocal Laser Scanning Microscopy

The punched out wells were frozen to -30°C under cryoprotection to allow for the preparation of 30μm frozen sections. These were individually suspended on normal routine microscopy slides and embedded in a watery medium and stained with ethidium bromide. Using standard cover slips, they were immediately observed in a Zeiss Axioinvert

Table 1. Results SCGE/HR-CLSM assessment after multiple drug exposure of individual leukaemic cells in 8 patients

Agent	Tail length	Comment
Daunorubicin 0.20 μg/ml	++	consistent result
DaunoXome® 0.02 μg/ml	+ to +++	variable results
4-HC 4.00 μg/ml	++	limited number of cases
Cyclophosphamide 5.00 μg/ml	0	negative control
Cisplatin 3.30 μg/ml	+	limited number of cases

microscope integral to a LSM 410 Zeiss Confocal Laser Scanning Microscope (CLSM) with associated hard and software.

Using the 63X, N.A. 1.40 oil immersion objective, individual comet tails were analysed as a stacked series of 10–15, 1μm optical sections which were summated into single data sets and subjected to image analysis for quantitation purposes. 20 systematically random selected cells were analysed per sample for comparison between agents patients and drug levels.

4. RESULTS

The results of comet tail length measurement, reflecting maximal fragment size and total integrated tail signal, reflecting total DNA content of tail, are summarised in Table 1. and representative images are presented in Figure 1 and 2.

As is evident, patient responses vary considerably. In addition to variations in the response to identical drug exposure, there are differences between the response to the panel of 4 agents used. The use of cyclophosphamide, consistently associated with absence of any detectable DNA excision repair effectively functions as a negative control, showing the culture circumstance not to result in spurious DNA excision repair activity. The requirement for cyclophosphamide to be metabolised to an active compound is demonstrated by the results of exposure of the leukaemic cells to the 4-HC metabolite with which we were provided.

5. DISCUSSION

In this study we aimed to assess the ability of SCGE/HR-CLSM as we had optimised, to discriminate differences in the reaction of individual lesions to a standardised quantity and quality of DNA damage by candidate drugs or agents in use in clinical treatment of leukaemic disease. In this we feel we have succeeded. To establish SCGE/HR-CLSM to a level of clinical usefulness equivalent to that of MTT further experimentation is however required. Most importantly, before any clinical studies were to be considered it would seem to be of importance to carry out comparative studies in which the results of investigations of drug resistance in individual neoplastic lesions in the current MTT procedure are compared with the results of SCGE/HR-CLSM even if the latter can only carried out with those agents which have an effect on the genome of the malignant cell. However, anthracyline sensitivity testing as carried out within prognosis assessment of relapsed breast cancer, has been shown to be highly predictive of successful response to high dose ablative chemotherapy regimens. The current practice of using in-vivo response may be augmented by the study of the cells obtained from a confirmatory biopsy or fine needle aspirate, by comparison with the results of SCGE/HRCLSM.

ACKNOWLEDGMENTS

We would like to thank Mr. Alan Cooke, NeXstar, Cambridge, UK, for facilitating the release of DaunoXome®, Dr. M Colvin, Duke University, USA, for the provision of the 4-Hydro-peroxy-cyclophosphamide. We also are grateful for the support of the staff of the Department of Pharmacy of the IWK Grace Health Centre for the provision and prepara-

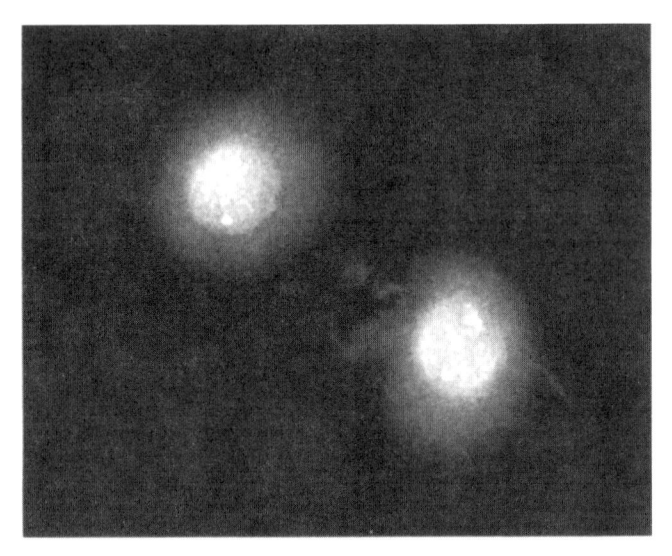

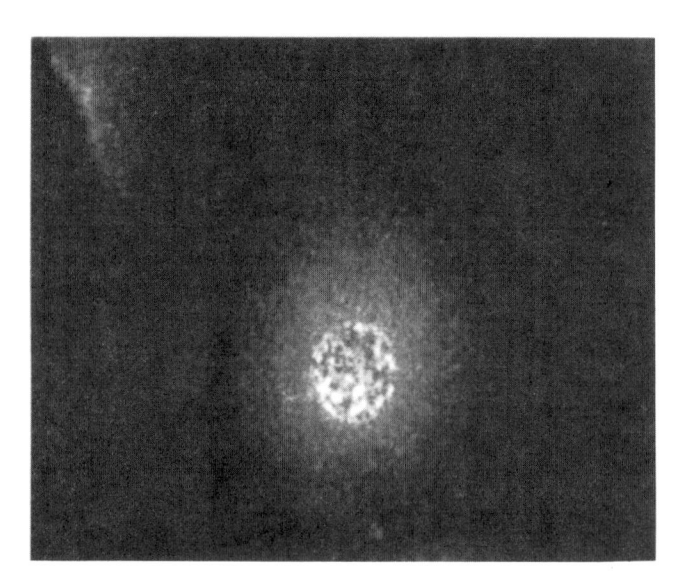

Figure 1. A and B. Results of SCGE/HR-CLSM analysis comparing of exposure to daunorubicin in 2 different patients. Note differences in tail length and position of fragments of maximal size. However, comet tail results within each patient are highly consistent. Different positions of fragments with equal signal strength, probably reflect differences in electrophoretic properties.

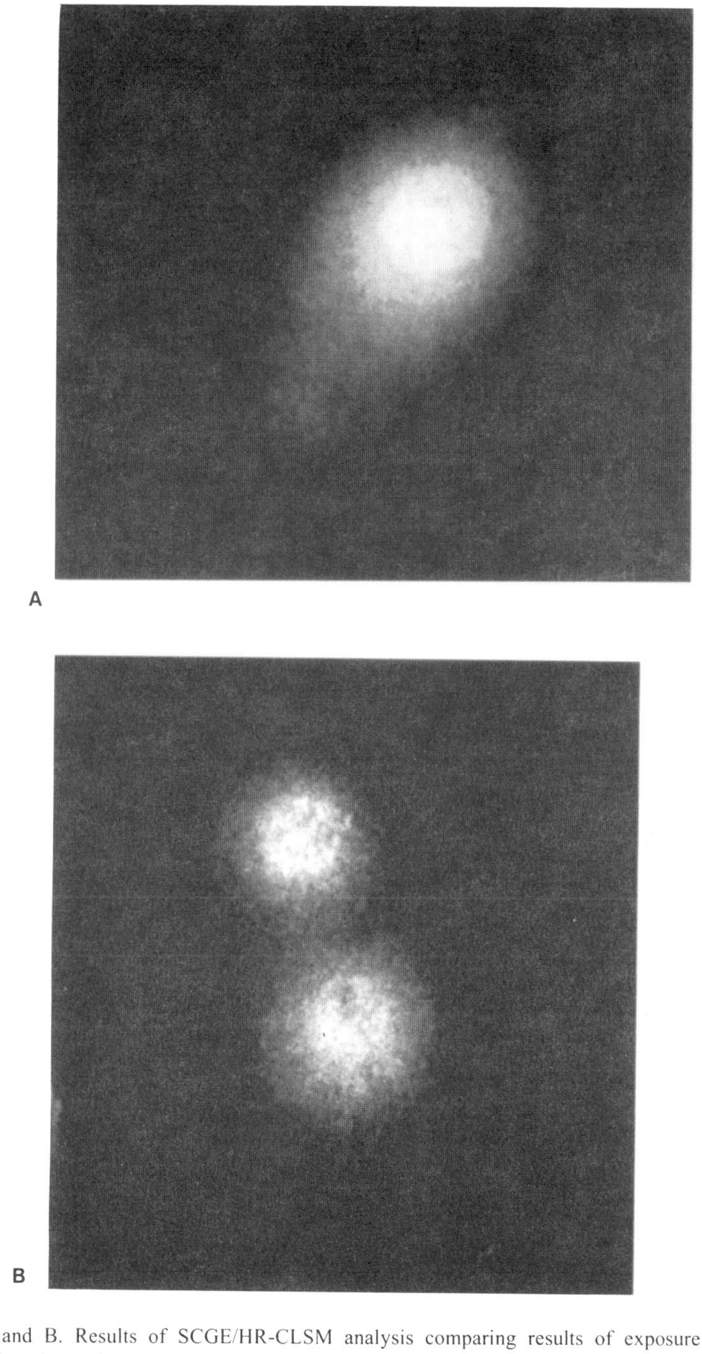

Differential Kinetics of Drug Resistance in Human Leukaemic Cells 507

Figure 2. A and B. Results of SCGE/HR-CLSM analysis comparing results of exposure to 0.02 μg / ml DaunoXome® to those of 4.0 μg/ml 4-HC in a single patient (adult CML transformed to ALL). Note differences in tail length and tail content which in addition to being visually noticeable can be objectified by the Fourier transformation analysis. 63 x, N.A. 1.40 Zeiss Oil immersion objective, Zeiss Axiovert, LSM 410 confocal laser scanning microscope, stacked set of 10, 1μm focal plane height, optical sections, 10 second scanning time per section.

tion of daunorubicin and cyclophosphamide. We acknowledge the assistance of the haematology medical staff of the QEII Health Sciences in obtaining samples. We are grateful to Mrs. Linda Lee Maughan for typing and preparation of the manuscript. Finally we acknowledge the financial assistance of this work by the IWK Grace Health Centre Research Foundation.

REFERENCES

1. Kaspers GJ, Veerman AJ, Pieters R, van Zantwijk CH, Smets LA, Van Wering ER, Van Der Does-Van Den Berg A. In vitro cellular drug resistance and prognosis in newly diagnosed childhood acute lymphoblastic leukemia. Blood, 1997, 90(7): 2723–2729.
2. Klumper E, Pieters R, Kaspers GJ, Huismans DR, Loonen AH, Rottier MM, van Wering ER, van der Does-van den Berg A, Hahlen K, Creutzig U et al. In vitro chemosensitivity assessed with the MTT assay in childhood acute non-lymphoblastic leukemia. Leukemia, 1995, 9(11): 1864–1869.
3. Hongo T, Yajima S, Sakurai M, Horikoshi Y, Hanada R. In vitro drug sensitivity testing can predict induction failure and early relapse of childhood acute lymphoblastic leukemia. Blood, 1997, 89(8):2959–2965.
4. Ostling O, Johanson KJ. Microelectrophoretic study of radiation-induced DNA damages in individual mammalian cells. Biochem Biophys Res Comm, 1984, 123(1):291–298.
5. Hara A, Zhang W, Kobayashi H, Niikawa S, Sakai N, Yamada H. A single cell gel electrophoresis technique for the detection of DNA damage induced by ACNU, an alkylating agent or irradiation in murine glioma cell lines. Neurological Res, 1994, 16:234–40.
6. Fairbairn DW, Olive PL, O'Neill KL. The comet assay: a comprehensive review. Mutat Res, 1995, 339:37–59.
7. Olive PL, Banath JP, Durand RE. Heterogeneity in radiation-induced DNA damage and repair in tumour and normal cells measured using the "comet" assay. Radiat Res, 1990, 122:86–94.
8. Olive PL, Frazer G, Banath JP. Radiation induced apoptosis measured in TK6 human B lymphoblast cells using the comet assay. Radiat Res, 1993, 136:130–136.
9. Olive PL, Banath JP, Durand RE. Development of apoptosis and polyploidy in human lymphoblast cells as a function of position in the cell cycle at the time of irradiation. Radiat Res, 1996, 146:595–602.
10. Olive PL, Banath JP, Durand RE. Detection of etoposide resistance by measuring DNA damage in individual Chinese Hamster cells. J Natl Cancer Inst, 1990, 82(9):779–783.
11. Tice RR, Strauss GHS, Peters WP. High dose combination alkylating agents with autologous bone marrow support in patients with breast cancer: preliminary assessment of DNA damage in individual peripheral lymphocytes using the single cell gel electrophoresis. Mutat Res, 1992, 271:101–113.
12. Singh NP, McCoy MT, Tice RR, Schneider EL. A simple technique for quantitation of low levels of DNA damage in individual cells. Exp Cell Res, 1988, 175:184–191.
13. Collins AR, Dobson VL, Dusinska M, Kennedy G, Stetina R. The comet assay: what can it really tell us? Mutat Res, 1997, 375:183–193.
14. O'Neill K, Fairbairn W, Standing MD. Analysis of single-cell gel electrophoresis using laser-scanning microscopy, Mutation Res, 1993, 319:129–134.
15. Vaghef H, Hellman B. Demonstration of chlorobenzene induced DNA damage in mouse lymphocytes using the single cell gel electrophoresis assay. Toxicology, 1995, 96:19–28.
16. Zheng H, Olive PL. Reduction of tumour hypoxia and inhibition of DNA repair by nicotinamide after irradiation of SCCVII murine tumours and normal tissues. Cancer Res, 1996, 56:2801–2808.
17. Hellman B, Vaghef H, Friis L, Edling C. Alkaline single cell electrophoresis of DNA fragments in biomonitoring for genotoxicity: an introductory study on healthy human volunteers. Int Arch Occup Environ Health, 1997, 69(3):185–92.
18. Muller WU, Bauch T, Streffer C, Niedereichholz F, Bocker W. Comet assay studies of radiation-induced DNA damage and repair in various tumor cell lines. Intl J Radiat Biol, 1994, 65(3):315–319.

55

DEMONSTRATION OF DIFFERENCES IN DRUG RESISTANCE BY DIRECT TESTING OF DNA EXCISION REPAIR ACTIVITY FOLLOWING STANDARD AND LIPOSOMAL DAUNORUBICIN EXPOSURE IN NORMAL PAEDIATRIC MARROW USING HIGH RESOLUTION CLSM

Christopher L. Lannon, Lynne M. Ball, Allen F. Pyesmany, Margaret Yhap, G. Ross Langley, and Dick van Velzen

Department of Pathology
Dalhousie University, IWK Grace Health Centre
5850 University Avenue
B3J 3G9, Halifax, Nova Scotia, Canada

Keywords: DNA excision repair, liposomal Daunorubicin, drug resistance, confocal laser scanning microscopy, single cell gel electrophoresis.

1. ABSTRACT

1.1. Background

High resolution Confocal Laser Scanning Microscopy (CLSM) may be applied to testing of drug resistance in vitro in clinical setting. Rapid analysis of DNA damage by precise quantitation of excised DNA in bone marrow samples exposed to potential treatment moieties directly after isolation but the relative sensitivity of the integrated method is as yet untested.

1.2. Aims

To test the clinical applicability of SCGE/high resolution CLSM for differences in drug resistance in marrow cells.

Drug Resistance in Leukemia and Lymphoma III, edited by Kaspers *et al.*
Kluwer Academic / Plenum Publishers, New York, 1999.

1.3. Methods

Cells from normal bone marrow samples were exposed for identical periods and at 4 concentrations to either 1 hour of standard Daunorubicin (.5, 1, 1.5, 2 µg/ml) or 8 hours DaunoXome® (courtesy of NeXstar Inc, USA) (.05, .1, .15, .2 µg/ml). After 2 and 6 hours recovery, cells were harvested for SCGE, randomization, analysis of tail length, total excised DNA and fragment size distribution using high resolution CLSM.

1.4. Results

Tail length and fragment size distribution was not, but total excised DNA was significantly increased after 0.1 µg/ml Liposomal Daunorubicin (DaunoXome®) compared to 1.0 µg/ml Daunorubicin.

1.5. Conclusion

SCGE/high resolution CLSM effectively demonstrated differences in Daunorubicin resistance of human marrow cells to alternative formulations. The method has potential for use in clinical testing of neoplastic cell drug resistance.

2. INTRODUCTION

Short or long term in vitro tumour tissue culture and exposure to various chemotherapeutic drug moieties was first experimented with in the study of ovarian tumour drug resistance as early as the 1960's. However, it was not until the early 1990's that practical applications for this technique were developed. This development was facilitated by choosing leukaemoid neoplasm and neoplastic disease as the field of application of nature a homogeneous self proliferation in which inter-lesion variability of differentiation and viability/proliferation rates are unknown. These malignancies are more suited to testing a sub sample without any question as to the representativeness of the findings for the sensitivities or resistance to various drug moieties of the lesion as a whole.

Technically the current methods generally depend on long term in vitro culture of tumour cells exposed to variable concentrations of the full range of drug moieties considered suitable for applications to this particular form of neoplastic disease (e.g., MTT assay[1,2,3]). The outcome parameter of the test is generally total or absolute cell numbers and vitality thereof following a standardized exposure time of four days or more. The number of clinical conditions would benefit from the ability to assess more rapidly sensitivity or resistance to at least a segment of the range of drug moieties, especially in those rapidly progressing conditions where high haematocrit values or rapid solid tumour growth of critically positioned lesions do not allow for a delay of more than 24 hours in initial treatment.

A simple method for the detection and quantitation of an individual cell's response to genomic damage, based on the technique of micro-electrophoresis was described by Ostling an Johanson in 1984.[4] Coined by Singh et al.,[5] "single cell gel electrophoresis" (SCGE) is a technique for the detection of excised, free intranuclear DNA in a single eukaryotic cell. Viewed under the fluorescent microscope, DNA strand breakage (following electrophoresis) results in a "comet" with a brightly fluorescent head and tail; consequently, it has been labelled the "comet assay".

SCGE is a highly sensitive test for the detection of DNA damage.[6,7,8,9] It has been a promising tool for the study of genomic damage induced by chemicals and radiation in culture[10,11,12] as well as in freshly isolated cells from experimental animals and humans.[13,14,15,16,17] SCGE is also a quick, simple and relatively inexpensive assay with a wide range of applications, ranging from mutagenesis and toxicology studies to disease monitoring for molecular epidemiology.[6] In the case of exposure to DNA directed drug moieties, preliminary research show that it is possible to compare different drugs and a major application for this technique has been in the rapid screening of new and novel candidate drug variants.

The application of confocal laser scanning microscopy, especially with recently developed adaptations to allow for high resolution scanning and quantitative analysis, raises the possibility of precise analysis of dose response curves and as such the comparison of relative drug sensitivity and/or resistance in a single cell lesion or the establishment of systematic drug sensitivities/resistance differences between drugs of various types within a single clinical condition. The advantage of this approach would in essence be that for drugs with a DNA damaging effect, such results could be available within 10 hours after bone marrow sampling. This would provide considerable clinical benefit in the occasion of very rapid lesional growth.

The ability to discriminate between alternate formulations of the same drug, either by differences in the total amount of damaged and repairing DNA, or through the analysis of the fragment size distribution of such nuclear content has not been demonstrated. We therefore chose to test the clinical applicability of the combination of single cell gel electrophoresis with high resolution confocal laser scanning microscope for accurately establishing differences in normal bone marrow cell drug resistance to different formulations of an established chemotherapeutic modality.

3. MATERIALS AND METHODS

3.1. Study Population

Cells from normal bone marrow samples obtained at orthopaedic surgery and collection of iliac crest bone marrow graft samples were used for isolation of normal human bone marrow of paediatric age donors. Mononuclear cells were isolated using Ficoll-Hypaque (Sigma) sedimentation, as outlined by the manufacturer. The final pellet of cells was suspended in RPMI 1640 (Gibco, Dutch modification[1,2]) containing 2mM L-glutamine, 100 UI ml^{-1} penicillin, 100 μg ml^{-1} streptomycin, 10 μg ml^{-1} insulin, 5.5 μg ml^{-1} transferrin, 6.7 ng ml^{-1} selenium (all obtained from Gibco) and 15% fetal bovine serum (Sigma). Viability was assessed at > 96% using the trypan blue exclusion test. Cells were incubated in 5% CO_2 at 37°C for less than 24h before drug exposure.

Normal bone marrow cells were exposed to either standard Daunorubicin or liposomal preparations of DaunoXome® (courtesy of NeXstar Inc. USA). Exposure concentrations where 0.5,1,1.5,2 µg/ml of standard Daunorubicin for 1 hour or .05, .1, .15, .2 µg/ml of DaunoXome for 8 hours (to allow sufficient time for liposomal pharmacokinetics). Cells were kept after exposure and one washing of cells for recovery.

3.2. Chemotherapeutic Exposure

Normal bone marrow cells (400 μl) were exposed to either standard Daunorubicin (obtained from pharmacy) preparations of DaunoXome® (courtesy of NeXstar Inc, USA) using 48-well microtitre plates (Falcon). Exposure concentrations were 0, 0.5, 1.0, 1.5, 2.0 µg/ml of standard Daunorubicin for 1 hour or 0.05, 0.1, 0.15, 0.2 µg/ml of DaunoXome for 8 hours. After exposure, cells were pelletized (centrifugation at 250 g, 5 min), resuspended in 100 μl fresh medium and incubated for two and six hours recovery before being harvested. This recovery period, based on our own laboratory experience, allows for the maximal accumulation of SCGE-associated intranuclear fragments.

3.3. Single Cell Gel Electrophoresis

Cells were fixed after harvesting and poured at high concentration into punched out wells of SCGE bedding gel, submitted to permeabilization under alkaline conditions and submitted to standardized single gel electrophoresis. 2.0 ml of 1% low melting point agarose (Sigma, prepared with distilled water and held at 40°C) was pipetted onto a half-frosted microscope slide and allowed to gel. Agar "wells" (5 per slide) were created in the agarose layer using a 6 mm cork borer. Following the two hours of post-exposure incubation, 0.5 ml of cell suspension was mixed with 1.5 ml agarose and 75 μl of this mixture was quickly pipetted into the agarose wells and allowed to gel (approximately 1 min). Slides were washed for 1 hour in three rinses of alkaline lysis solution, and electrophoresed in fresh alkaline buffer for 25 min.[16,17] Slides were rinsed twice in distilled H_2O, and stained for 20 min with ethidium bromide (20 μg/ml in 0.1 M NaCl).

3.4. Visualization

Following staining, contents of agar wells were removed from the slide with a scalpel, and 30 μm frozen sections prepared. Sections were wet mounted with 70 μl of PBS before coverslipping. Slides were examined using the Zeiss LSM-410 with a krypton/argon laser, mounted on a Zeiss Axiovert 100 microscope (excitation at 488 nm). Images were collected as the summation of 10–12 serial "optical" sections (4 sec scans) using a focal plane height ("section thickness") of 1 μm as defined by choice of beam diameter and pinhole setting.

4. RESULTS

For both agents, a clearly defined dose-response relationship was defined. Inhibition of DNA excision repair processes was observed (for both agents) at the maximum exposure levels. Further, maximal tail length and moment was achieved at concentrations of 1.0 μg/ml and 0.1 μg/ml, standard daunorubicin and DaunoXome®, respectively.

Comet tail length, on a dose by dose compariosn, did not differ between conventional daunorubicin and DaunoXome®. However, tail lengths in both series were maximal at a relatively low dose and were reduced before tails became absent with crossing of the apoptotic threshold (Table 1).

5. DISCUSSION

Clearly developed dose response relationships exist for both drug moieties in which effective levels of exposure for DaunoXome compares favourably to that of Daunorubicin. Further, it appears that the liposomal formulation (DaunoXome®) is effective, in vitro, at one-tenth the dosage of standard daunorubicin, reflecting in vivo experiences during clinical trials.

Table 1. Summary results of dose-response analysis in pediatric normal marrow by SCGE/HR-CLSM

Daunorubicin	Tail length	DaunoXome®	Tail length
2.0 µg/ml.	0	0.20 µg/ml.	0
1.5 µg/ml.	+	0.15 µg/ml.	+
1.0 µg/ml.	+++	0.10 µg/ml.	+++
0.5 µg/ml.	+	0.05 µg/ml.	+

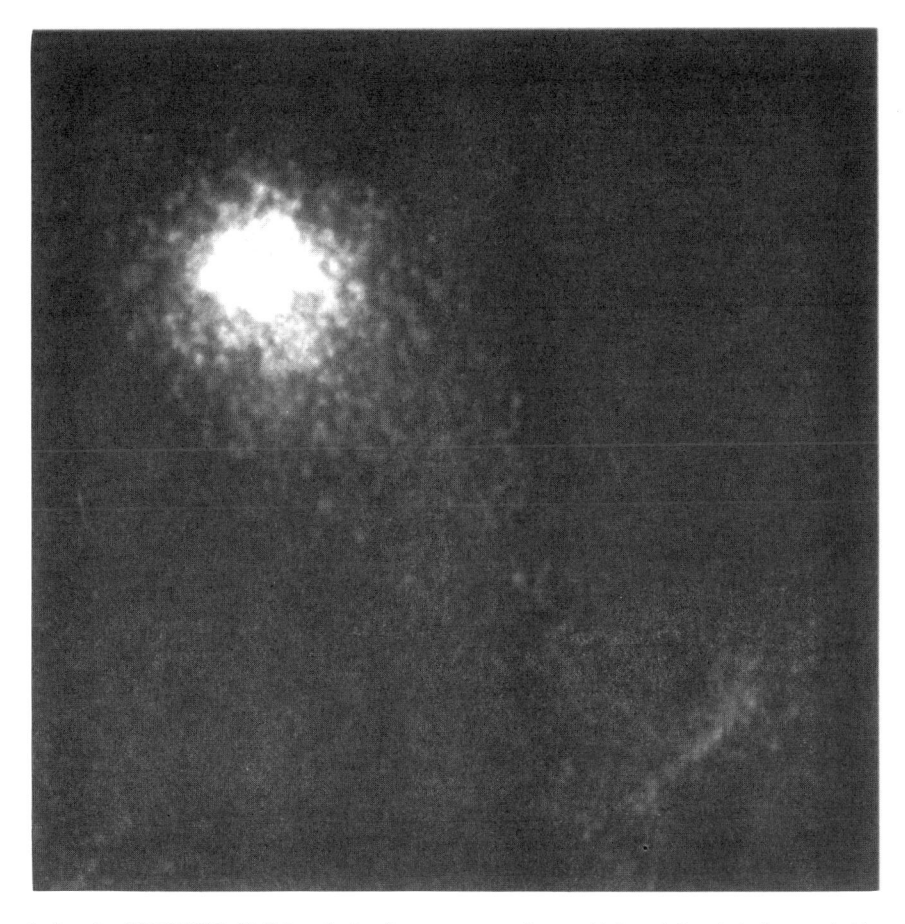

Figure 1. Result of SCGE/HR-CLSM analysis after exposure to daunorubicin at 1.0 µg/ml. Grey scaled image of results of summation of 15, 1 µm high focal plane section of a single nucleus and "comet tail" after 10 second scan assessments of each section. Note relatively long tail, indicating relatively large size of largest fragment and granular appearance of signal in tail, indicating variable electrophoretic movement of fragments of relatively large size, possibly reflecting configurational differences. 63 x, N.A. 1.4 Zeiss Objective, Axiovert / LSM410 Zeiss Confocal Laser Scanning Microscope.

Figure 2. Result of SCGE/HR-CLSM analysis after exposure to DaunoXome® at 0.10 µg/ml. Grey scaled image of results of summation of 15, 1 µm high focal plane section of a single nucleus and "comet tail" after 10 second scan assessments of each section. Note very comparable tail to that of Figure 1 indicating comparable size of the largest fragments and comparable granular appearance of signal in tail, indicating comparable size distribution and electrophoretic movement of larger DNA fragments. 63 x, N.A. 1.4 Zeiss Objective, Axiovert / LSM410 Zeiss Confocal Laser Scanning Microscope.

At this stage, it is evident that both curves have been taken to a exposure level where excision repair is not effectively obtained. These findings can only be interpreted at this stage as the result of supra critical DNA damage forcing all exposed cells that were exposed in vulnerable stages of cell cycle to enter apoptotic cell disassembly. It is of interest to note that the results of both drug variants are similar with respect to DNA fragment size as evidenced by tail length.

However, the finding of variable tail length with drug dose or exposure requires discussion. One of the potential explanations may be that with increasing dose, 2 separate processes contribute to the tail content. These may be the production of DNA excision repair derived fragments as compared to the induction of DNA strand breakage derived fragments. If these two processes have a different dose-response relationship and in addition result in DNA fragments which differ in the range of fragment size, the observed variation in tail length may be explained. This phenomenon may be studied in future through the use of fluorescent probes which are selective for either double stranded or single stranded DNA.

The findings of this study indicate that the technique of single cell gel electrophoresis with high resolution confocal laser scanning microscopy is an effective technique for the demonstration of differences in drug resistance. Further, this assay is sufficiently sensitive to detect differences between alternate formulations of the same chemotherapeutic drug. As such, this technique has potential for use in the rapid clinical testing of neoplastic cell drug resistance to DNA-directed modalities and warrants further investigation.

Single cell electrophoresis combined with high resolution of confocal laser scanning microscopy is able to effectively demonstrate differences in the dose response curve between different formulations of Daunorubicin in which differences if affectivity are based on differences in cell delivery. With the ability to have good intersample reproducibility and well defined drug dose response curves the method has potential for use in clinical testing of neoplastic cell drug resistance where urgency is required and where the limitation of to DNA-directed chemotherapeutic agents can be accepted.

ACKNOWLEDGMENTS

The project was supported in part by NeXstar Pharmaceuticals Inc. (USA) and the IWK Grace Research Committee. The authors are grateful to Mrs. Linda-Lee Maughan for her assistance in the typing of this manuscript. We would also like to express our gratitude for the help of Dr. Lorne Leahey, Department of Orthopaedic Surgery, who counselled patients and obtained their informed consent or parental permission for the procurement of normal bone marrow tissue obtained as part of routine corrective surgery.

The study was carried out with agreement of the Ethical Committee of the IWK Grace Health Centre.

REFERENCES

1. Kaspers GJ, Veerman AJ, Pieters R, van Zantwijk CH, Smets LA, van Wering ER, van der Does-van den Berg A. In vitro cellular drug resistance and prognosis in newly diagnosed childhood acute lymphoblastic leukemia. Blood, 1997, 90(7):2723–2729.
2. Klumper E, Pieters R, Kaspers GJ, Huismans DR, Loonen AH, Rottier MM, van Wering ER, van der Does-van den Berg A, Hahlen K, Creutzig U et al. In vitro chemosensitivity assessed with the MTT assay in childhood acute non-lymphoblastic leukemia. Leukemia, 1995, 9(11): 1864–1869.
3. Hongo T, Yajima S, Sakurai M, Horikoshi Y, Hanada R. In vitro drug sensitivity testing can predict induction failure and early relapse of childhood acute lymphoblastic leukemia. Blood, 1997, 89(8):2959–2965.
4. Ostling O, Johanson KJ. Microelectrophoretic study of radiation-induced DNA damages in individual mammalian cells. Biochem Biophys Res Comm, 1984, 123(1):291–298.
5. Singh NP, McCoy MT, Tice RR, Schneider EL. A simple technique for quantitation of low levels of DNA damage in individual cells. Exp Cell Res, 1988, 175:184–191.
6. Collins AR, Dobson VL, Dusinska M, Kennedy G, Stetina R. The comet assay: what can it really tell us? Mutat Res, 1997, 375:183–193.
7. Fairbairn DW, Olive PL, O'Neill KL. The comet assay: a comprehensive review. Mutat Res, 1995, 339:37–59.
8. Olive PL, Banath JP, Durand RE. Detection of etoposide resistance by measuring DNA damage in individual Chinese hamster cells. J Natl Cancer Inst, 1990, 82(9):779–783.

9. Olive PL, Frazer G, Banath JP. Radiation induced apoptosis measured in TK6 human B lymphoblast cells using the comet assay. Radiat Res, 1993, 136:130–136.
10. Hara A, Zhang W, Kobayashi H, Niikawa S, Sakai N, Yamada H. A single cell gel electrophoresis technique for the detection of DNA damage induced by ACNU, an alkylating agent or irradiation in murine glioma cell lines. Neurological Res, 1994, 16:234–40.
11. Muller WU, Bauch T, Streffer C, Niedereichholz F, Bocker W. Comet assay studies of radiation-induced DNA damage and repair in various tumor cell lines. Intl J Radiat Biol, 1994, 65(3):315–319.
12. Vaghef H, Hellman B. Demonstration of chlorobenzene induced DNA damage in mouse lymphocytes using the single cell gel electrophoresis assay. Toxicology, 1995, 96:19–28.
13. Tice RR, Strauss GHS, Peters WP. High dose combination alkylating agents with autologous bone marrow support in patients with breast cancer: preliminary assessment of DNA damage in individual peripheral lymphocytes using the single cell gel electrophoresis. Mutat Res, 1992, 271:101–113.
14. Olive PL, Banath JP, Durand RE. Development of apoptosis and polyploidy in human lymphoblast cells as a function of position in the cell cycle at the time of irradiation. Radiat Res, 1996, 146:595–602.
15. Olive PL, Banath JP, Durand RE. Heterogeneity in radiation-induced DNA damage and repair in tumor and normal cells measured using the "comet" assay. Radiat Res, 1990, 122:86–94.
16. Olive PL, Durand RE, le Riche J, Olivotto IA, Jackson SM. Gel electrophoresis of individual cells to quantify hypoxic fraction in human breast cancers. Cancer Res, 1993, 53:733–736.
17. Zheng H, Olive PL. Reduction of tumour hypoxia and inhibition of DNA repair by nicotinamide after irradiation of SCCVII murine tumours and normal tissues. Cancer Res, 1996, 56:2801–2808.

56

MICROSATELLITE INSTABILITY ASSESSMENT IN PREDICTION OF DRUG RESISTANCE IN CHILDHOOD BURKITT'S AND LARGE CELL DIFFUSE MALIGNANT NON-HODGKIN LYMPHOMA (MNHL)

Margaret Yhap, Allen F. Pyesmany, Lynne M. Ball, D. Christie Riddle, Jiang Mu, and Dick van Velzen

Department of Clinical Haemato-Oncology
Dalhousie University, IWK Grace Health Centre

Keywords: microsatellite, Burkitt's Lymphoma, large cell malignant non Hodgkin lymphoma, drug resistance, childhood.

1. ABSTRACT

1.1. Background

Genomic instability may, especially with DNA directed treatment, be associated with increased therapeutic response; absence may be associated with drug resistance. In childhood MNHL, drug response is variable. At present the degree of presence of microsatellite variation, i.e., intrinsic DNA instability is not known.

1.2. Aims

To determine presence and range of microsatellite variability in common childhood MNHL.

1.3. Methods

1.3.1. Study Populations. Consecutive, unselected (1976–96) cases of childhood Large Cell diffuse, N=16; (9T,7B), age range 1y5m-16y8m; Burkitt's Lymphoma, n=13, age range 4y2m-14y. Non-malignant/pre-treatment tissue of 20 cases, 13 LC, 7 Burkitt's MNHL.

1.3.2. Molecular Pathology. Routine DNA extraction, amplifications at loci D3S 1304 and D3S1537 (both closely distal to VHL, tumour suppressor gene); ELN gene D7S1870; IFNA D1S243 (1p36) which show microsatellite variation. Isotopic labelling in amplification, non-denaturing gel electrophoresis, autoradiography.

1.4. Results

Microsatellite variability was found 3/16 LC and 2/13 Burkitt's MNHL. LC MNHL, 4 abnormal areas: n=1, 3 abnormal areas: n=1, 2 abnormal areas n=1; Burkitt's MNHL, 3 abnormal areas: n=1, 1 abnormal area n=1. No variability was found in the normal (constitutional) DNA of any of the 20 patients studied.

1.5. Conclusions

Microsatellite variability occurred in 5/29 patients with common types of childhood MNHL, indicating a limited contribution to reduced drug resistance through this mechanism.

2. INTRODUCTION

Neoplastic disease arises from an accumulation of multiple genetic changes each of which may be mediated through rearrangements that result in mutations of either oncogenes, numerous suppressor genes or other cellular control genes. Some of these changes may result in changes of the stability of the genome in cancer cells which may accelerate the accumulation of mutations in critical target genes.

One form of genome instability in human tumours is characterised by defective DNA mismatch repair. This mechanism normally corrects errors in replication of DNA as part of cell division. The results of instability are highly polymorphic mono and di nucleotide micro satellites. The observed alterations in the length of such micro satellites result from accumulated frame shift mutations which are not corrected after replication. Defects of such post replication mismatch repair may be associated with the familial occurrence of neoplastic disease. When present, it usually occurs in an early stage of tumour development and alters the phenotype to be that of a general mutator. The absence of such post replication mismatch repair may then accelerate the accumulation of critical mutations in target genes in progression to malignant neoplastic disease. The human genome contains several hundred thousand non-informative sequences of up to six base pairs length.[1] These so-called micro satellites may accumulate neutral mutations as they are generally non coding and as such are highly polymorphic between humans.[2] Although relatively frequent subject of mutation it has become apparent that DNA repair limits the rate of micro-satellite variability.

The genomic instability that results from hereditary repair defective status, even if limited to tumours, results in a substantial destabilization of micro satellites. For example, in hereditary non polyposis colorectal cancer, although usually associated with diploid status and a fairly normal karyotype, the tumours show extremely polymorphic DNA micro satellites present in multiple loci on different chromosomes.[3,4] At least 90% of such colorectal tumours exhibit microsatellite instability[4] with error accumulation beginning early in tumour development as a persistent trait.[7] In non hereditary sporadic colon cancers, microsatellite instability occurs in approximately 15% and is observed in higher frequency in, for example, endometrial or gastric carcinoma if and when associated with the hereditary form of colon cancer.[8,9]

Subsequent research has shown that there are four DNA repair genes[10-13] which may be mutated in the germ lines of families affected by hereditary cancer forms.[5,6] The genes encode for protein structures that are involved in DNA mismatch repair. Such proteins are conserved from organisms such as Escherichia coli to man.[14,15] It has been shown that in hereditary colon cancer it is deficiencies in the correction of replication mistakes rather than an increased commission of polymerization errors that accounts for the variability of micro satellites. Micro satellite instability in affected genome or tumour cells, reflects a tendency to accumulate frame shifts in regions of reiterated sequences.

While this generalization is a useful guide to the underlying mechanism of micro satellites instability, recent research suggests that each family of micro satellites, be they mono, di or tri nucleotide repeats, are affected differently by different defects in the mismatch repair pathways.[16] While the relationship between DNA and mismatch correction defects and human cancer was only recently established,[17] it is clear that mismatch repair defects destabilize the genome in a highly selective fashion which does not result in the general derangement of genomic organization. However, the effects are profound.

While it is of interest to study mismatch repair defects in relation to understanding both the protection against malignant derailment and its causation, the potential of defective mismatch repair to confer a greater sensitivity to DNA drug moieties has as yet not been studied.

Very little literature exists with respect to the frequency of evident micro satellites-variability in non hereditary lesions. Especially in childhood, no significant studies have been undertaken or have been reported.

Childhood Burkitt's lymphoma and large cell diffuse Malignant Non-Hodgkin Lymphoma (MNHL) are two of the more common variants of neoplastic conditions in childhood. The sensitivity or resistance to chemotherapeutic treatment varies considerably between the two. As such we considered it of interest to study the relative frequency of microsatellite variability in a number of relevant genomic loci in a pilot study.

3. MATERIALS AND METHODS

3.1. Study Populations

All cases of childhood large cell diffuse or Burkitt's lymphoma diagnosed in a single centre between 1976 and 1996 where included in the study.

There were 16 patients with large cell diffuse large cell MNHL confirmed on review by two pathologists not involved in the original study. On immunophenotyping 9 were typed as T-cell and 7 of B-cell lineage. The age range of the patients varied from 1 year, 5 months to 16 years, 8 months of age at the time of diagnosis and biopsy. There were 13 cases of Burkitt's lymphoma in the same period with patients ranging in age from 4 years 2 months to 14 years of age. In 13 cases of large cell lymphoma and 7 cases of Burkitt's malignant non Hodgkin lymphoma sufficient non malignant tissue was available in the same or synchronous biopsies from the same patients and obtained prior to treatment with any form of therapy.

3.2. Molecular Pathology

Of all blocks representative sections were taken with strict measures to avoid cross contamination of samples from contact of paraffin blocks with instruments or the storage container. After de-paraffinization, 18 DNA extractions were carried out followed by amplifications of loci D3S1304 and A3S1537 (both closely distal to the VHL tumour suppression gene). Similarly, amplifications were carried out at the D7S1870 locus (for the ELM gene) and at the B1S243 (1B36) locus (for the IFNA gene). All of these loci are known to show microsatellite variation. With isotopic labelling in the amplification stage, non-denaturing gel electrophoresis of amplified and digested DNA was carried out. The gels were subsequently analysed by autoradiography.

4. RESULTS

No microsatellite variability was found in analysis of the normal constitutional DNA of any of the normal tissues of 20 patients for which such tissue was available. Microsatellite variability was found in 3/16 cases of large cell lymphoma and 2/13 cases of Burkitt's MNHL. The results are further illustrated in Figures 1 to 4.

In one case of large cell MNHL, variability was found in four areas. In one patient, three abnormal areas were detected and one patient two abnormal areas. In the case of Burkitt's MNHL, one patient was found to have three abnormal areas and in one patient abnormality was limited to one area.

5. DISCUSSION

Although the number of patients with affected microsatellite areas form a considerable minority of all patients, it is of interest to note that in 4/5 patients more than one locus is affected. Still the normal constitutional DNA showed no variability and as such these abnormalities must be limited to the neoplastic cell lines only. In view of the presence of multi-locular variability, a defect in the mismatch repair gene system, in analogy of that for hereditary colon carcinoma, is the most likely acquired underlying lesion in these cases with an associated likelihood of this abnormality being limited to the neoplastic cell line.

However, if the presence of such mismatch repair defects were to result in greater sensitivity to DNA directed moieties, this effect will then also only exist in a small fraction of the patients as in our study this phenomenon was limited to 5/29 cases under study.

However, at this stage this inference is not substantiated by results of fundamental research or long term follow up studies. However, with the ability to carry out analysis of microsatellite variability in a retrospective manner, long term follow up of results may already exist, a situation which would allow for rapid validation of this hypothesis or for its conclusive refutal.

ACKNOWLEDGMENTS

This study would not have been possible without the active support of Mrs. Constance Isenor and Mrs. Karen Sampson. We are grateful to Mrs. Linda-Lee Maughan for

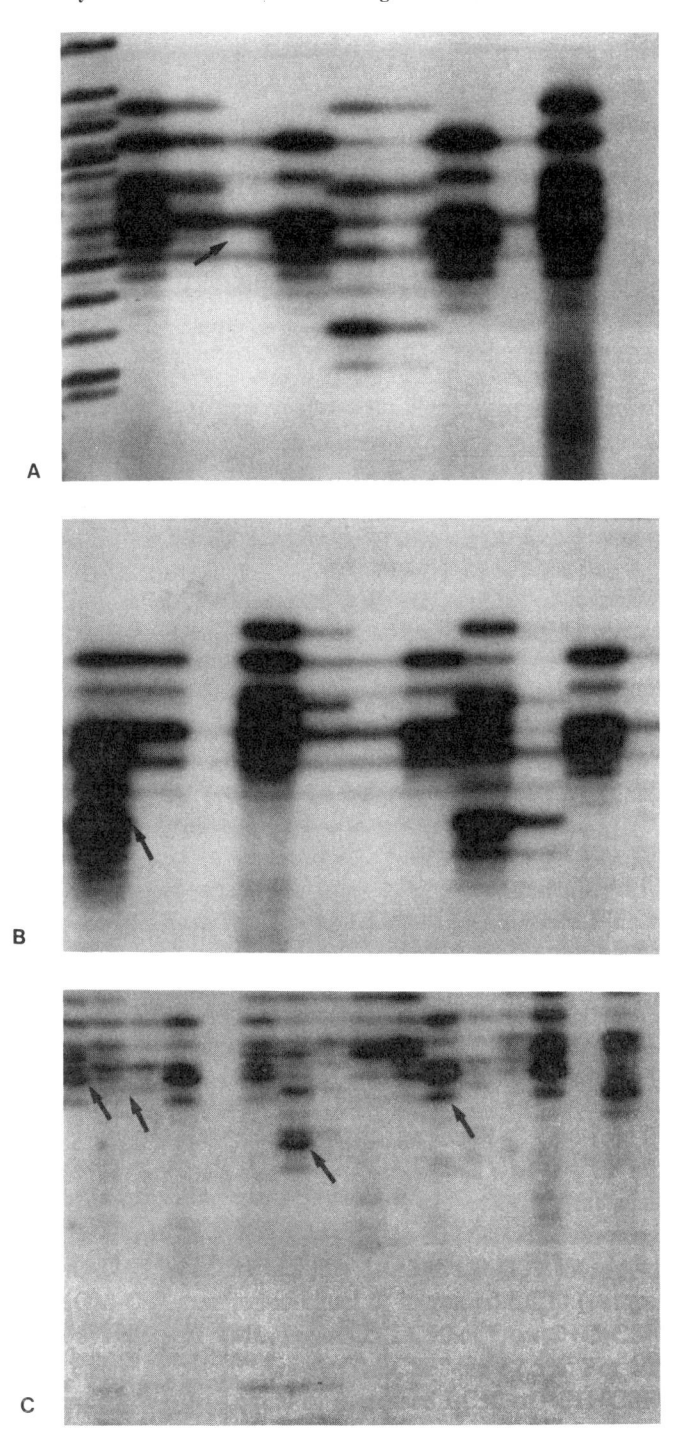

Microsatellite Instability Assessment in Prediction of Drug Resistance

Figure 1. A: Primer INFA; note missing band in tumour of lane 2 (arrow). B: Primer INFA; note band shift between tumour and control of lane 1 (arrow), loss of band by tumour of lane 2 (arrow), additional bands in tumours of lane 4 (arrow) and 6 (arrow). C: Primer INFA; note additional band in tumour in lane 1 (arrow).

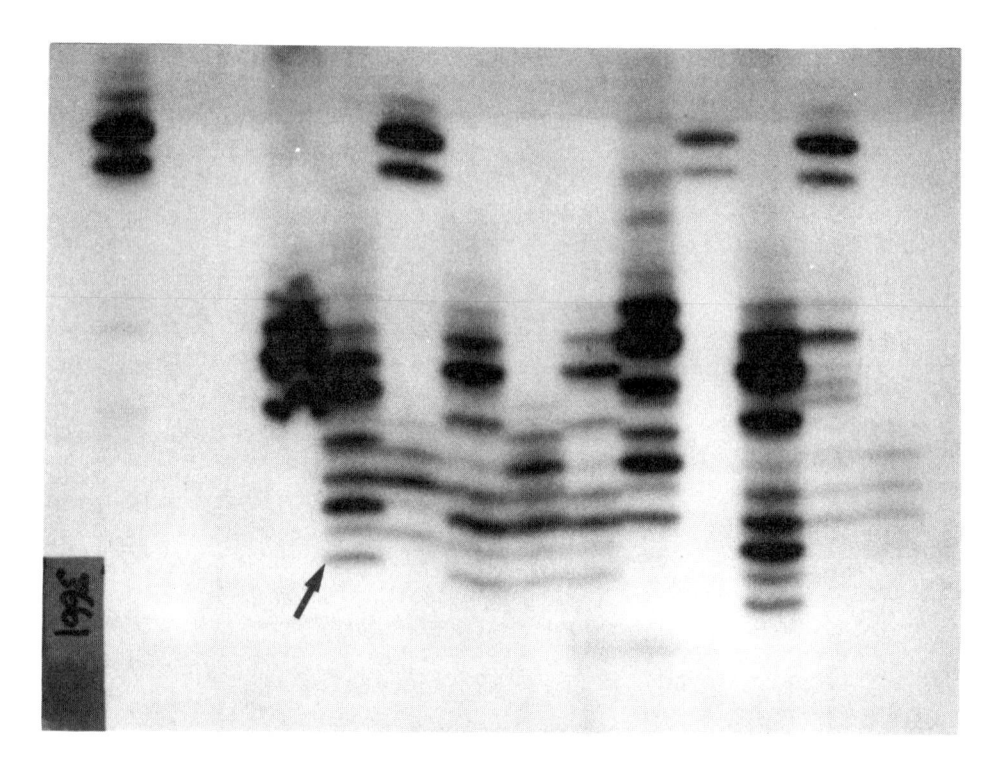

Figure 2. ELN gene, primers D7S1870; note additional bands in tumour of lane 3 (arrow).

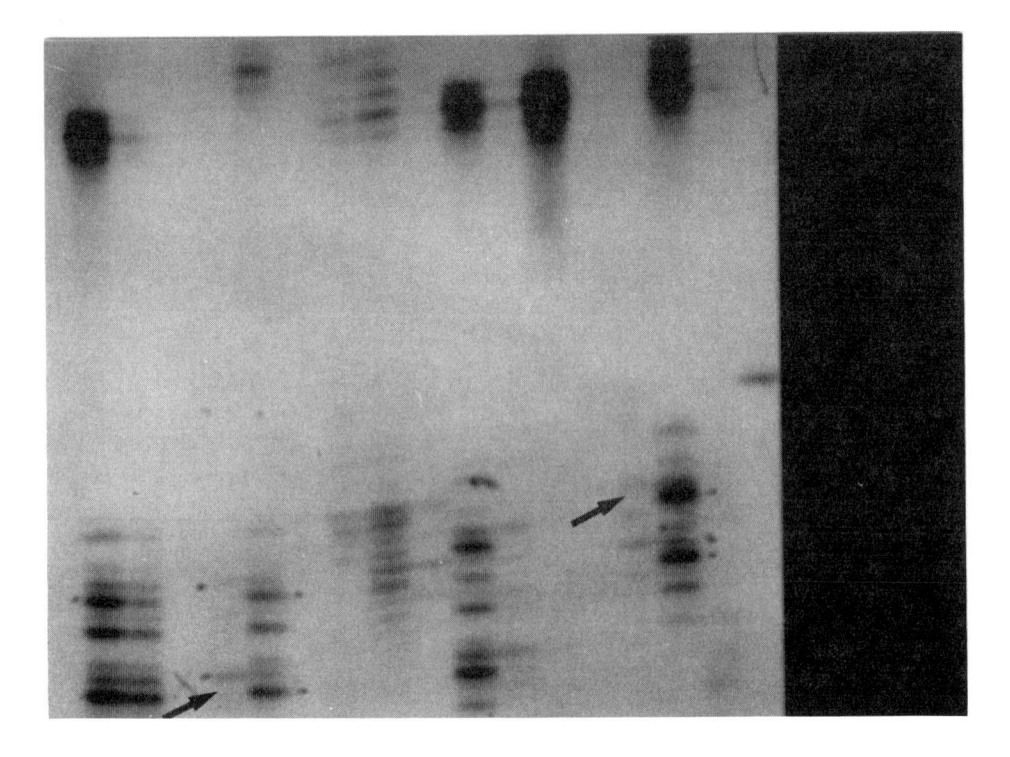

Figure 3. Primer Wms, Mpx; note repeated loss of bands in tumours of lane 3 and 8 (arrow).

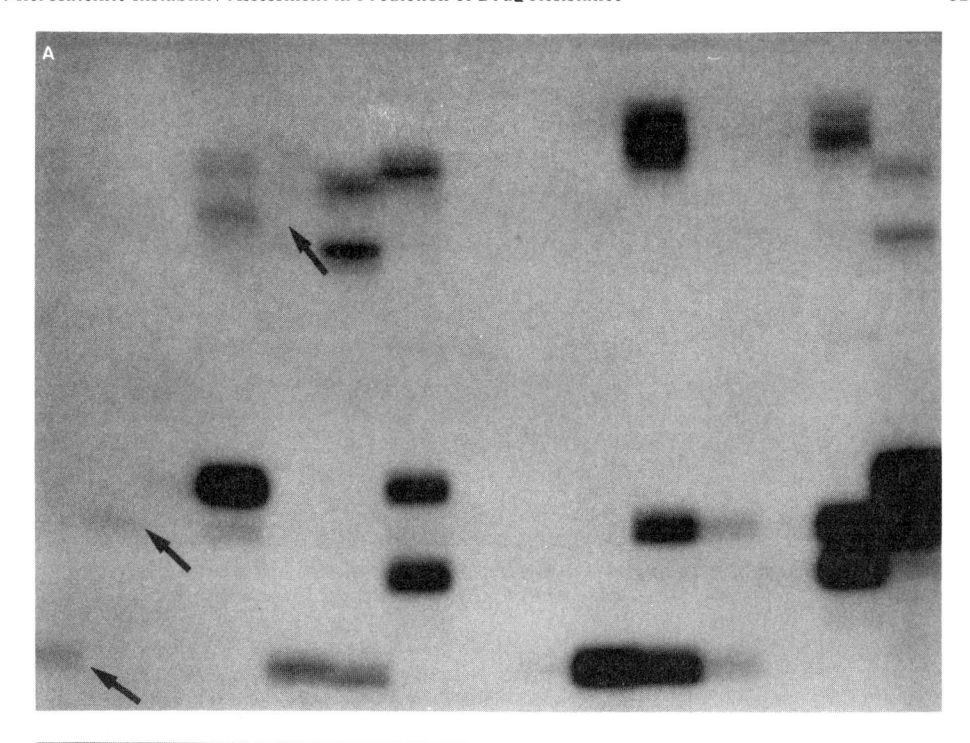

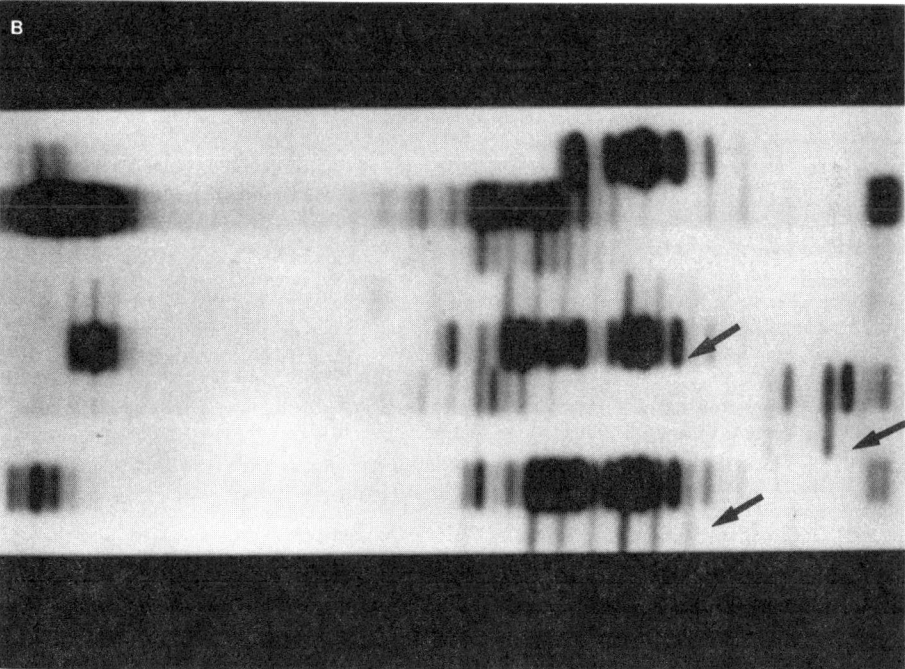

Microsatellite Instability Assessment in Prediction of Drug Resistance

Figure 4A, B. A (top): Primer VHL Mpx; Lane 1, note band switch between band in tumour (arrow left) and band in control (arrow right). Lane 3, note absence of two bands (arrow) in tumour (left). B (bottom): Primer VHL Mpx; Lane 1 and 2, note missing bands in tumours (arrows). Lane 3 extra band in tumour (arrow).

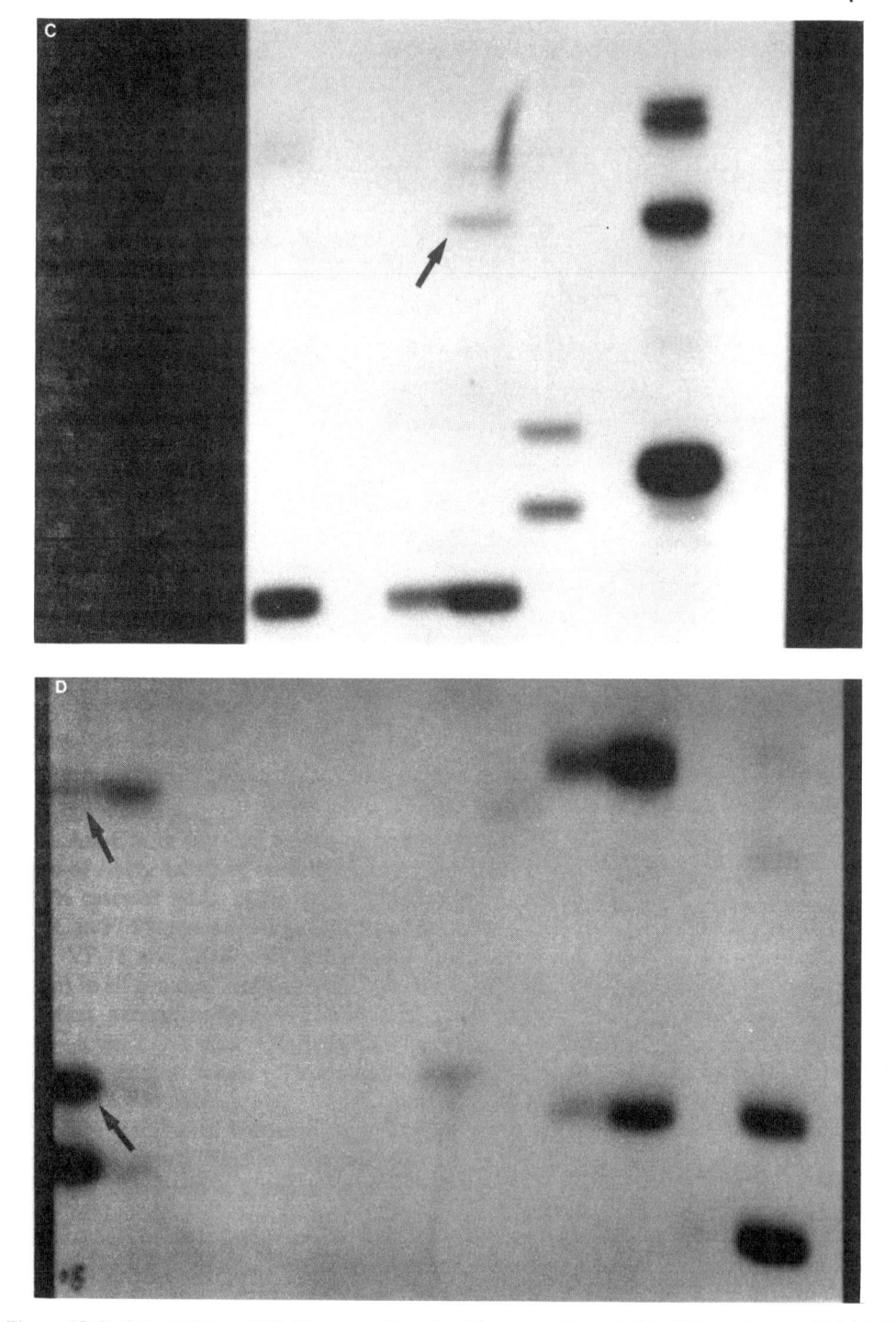

Figure 4C, D. C (top): Primer VHL Mpx; note absent band in tumour (arrow left) with band in control (right). D (bottom): Primer VHL Mpx; Lane 1, note band strength switch between band in tumour (arrow left) and band in control (arrow right).

typing this manuscript. The study was supported by the IWK Grace Research Foundation who funded part of the instrumentation required for the study.

REFERENCES

1. Hearne CM, Ghosh S, Todd JA. Microsatellites for linkage analysis of genetic traits. Trends Genet, 1992, 8:288–294.
2. Bowcock A, Osborne-Lawrence S, Barnes R, Chakravarti A, Washington S, et al. Microsatellite polymorphism linkage map of human chromosome 13q. Genomics, 1993, 15:376–386.
3. Lynch HT, Smyrk TC, Watson P, Lanspa SJ, Lynch JF, et al. Genetics, natural history, tumour spectrum and pathology of hereditary nonpolyposis colorectal cancer: an updated review. Gastroenterology, 1993, 104:1535–1549.
4. Bishop DT, Hall NR. The genetics of colorectal cancer. Eur J Cancer 1994, 30A:1946–1956.
5. Aaltaonen LA, Peltomaki P, Leach FS, Sistonen P, Pylkkanen L, et al. Clues to the pathogenesis of familial colorectal cancer. Science, 1993, 260:812–816.
6. Ionov Y, Peinado MA, Malkhosyan S, Shibata D, Perucho M. Ubiquitous somatic mutations in simple repeated sequences reveal a new mechanism for colonic carcinogenesis. Nature, 1993, 363:558–561.
7. Shibata D, Peinado MA, Ionov Y, Malkhosyan S, Perucho M. Genomic instability in repeated sequences is an early somatic event in colorectal tumourigenesis that persists after transformation. Nature Genetics, 1994, 6:273–281.
8. Burks RT, Kessis TD, Cho KR, Hedrick L. Microsatellite instability in endometrial carcinoma. Oncogene, 1994, 9:1163–1166.
9. Peltomaki P, Lothe RA, Altonen LA, Pylkkanen L, Nystrom-Lahti M, et al. Microsatellite instability is associated with tumours that characterise the hereditary non-polyposis colorectal carcinoma syndrome. Cancer Res, 1993, 53:5853–5855.
10. Peltomaki P, Aaltonen LA, Sistonen P, Pylkkanen L, Mecklin JP, et al. Genetic mapping of a locus predisposing to human colorectal cancer. Science, 1993, 260:810–812.
11. Lindblom A, Tannergard P, Werelius B, Nordenskjold M. Genetic mapping of a second locus predisposing to hereditary non-polyposis colon cancer. Nature Genet, 1993, 5:279–282.
12. Papadopoulos N, Nicolaides NC, Wei Y-F, Ruben SM, Carter KC, et al. Mutation in a *mutL* homolog in hereditary colon cancer. Science, 1994, 263:1625–1628.
13. Bronner CE, Baker SM, Morrison PT, Warren G, Smith LG., et al. Mutation in the DNA mismatch repair gene homolog hMLH1 is associated with hereditary non-polyposis colon cancer. Nature, 1994, 368:258–261.
14. Leach FS, Nicolaides NC, Papdopolulos N, Liu B, Jen J, et al. Mutations of mutS homolog in hereditary non-polyposis colorectal cancer. Cell, 1993, 75:1215–1225.
15. Fishel R, Lescoe MK, Rao MSR, Copeland NG, Jenkins NA, et al. The human mutator homolog MSH2 and its association with hereditary nonpolyposis colon cancer. Cell, 1993, 75:1027–1038.
16. Boon T, Pel Av, Plaen Ed, Chromez P, Lurquin C, et al. Genes encoding for T-cell defined Tum transplantation antigens: Point mutations, antigenic peptides and subgenic expression. Cold Spring Harbor Symp Quant Biol, 1989, LIV:587–596.
17. Wooster R, Cleton-Jansen AM, Collins N, Mangion J, Cornelis RS, et al. Instability of short tandem repeats (microsatellites) in human cancers. Nature Genet, 1994, 6:152–156.

HIGH RESOLUTION CONFOCAL LASER SCANNING MICROSCOPY ANALYSIS OF DNA EXCISION REPAIR CAPABILITY IN SMALL VOLUME MARROW SAMPLES EXPOSED TO DNA DIRECTED TREATMENT MOIETIES

Christopher L. Lannon, Lynne M. Ball, Allen F. Pyesmany, Margaret Yhap, Ross Langley, and Dick van Velzen

Department of Pathology
Dalhousie University, IWK Grace Health Centre
5850 University Avenue
B3J 3G9, Halifax, Nova Scotia, Canada

Keywords: DNA excision repair, drug treatment, leukaemia, confocal laser scanning microscopy, single cell gel electrophoresis, comet tail analysis.

1. ABSTRACT

1.1. Background

Assessment of resistance to drug moieties in tissue culture is complicated by limited sample, clonal selection and alteration of cycling fraction and cycle duration in clonally mixed lesions. DNA damage assessment by single cell gel electrophoresis (SCGE) of excised DNA is limited by non-linear analysis in fluorescent light microscopy. Confocal Laser Scanning Microscopy (CLSM) with high N.A. magnification allows for quantitation of total excised DNA fragment size distribution but is still limited by the large volume required for labour intensive SCGE, precluding multi-exposure clinical testing.

1.2. Aims

To optimise sample requirement for SCGE and CLS.

Drug Resistance in Leukemia and Lymphoma III, edited by Kaspers *et al.*
Kluwer Academic / Plenum Publishers, New York, 1999.

1.3. Methods

Standard slide mounted bed gels were punched with multiple coded 6 mm wells and filled with suspensions of cells subjected to drug/concentration variations. After SCGE, 30μm frozen sections were prepared of each well and mounted in ethidium bromide solution on multi-well hydrophilic slides to allow for short working distance of high resolution CLSM in a Zeiss Axiovert L410 SM. Testing for feasibility, reproducibility and consistency used both cultured standard leukaemic cell lines, normal human control marrow and clinical samples.

1.4. Results and Conclusion

Multiple well SCGE followed by frozen section, high resolution CLSM allows for rapid analysis of high numbers of multiple drug exposure permutations clinically required.

2. INTRODUCTION

Based on the technique of microelectrophoresis,[1] a simple method for the quantitation of cellular response to genomic damage in individual cells was developed and called single cell gel electrophoresis (SCGE).[2] This became the standardized technique for detection of the excised free nuclear DNA that may be separated by electrophoresis from the nuclear confines of eukaryotic cells. When viewed under the fluorescent microscope this results in a brightly fluorescent head (which contains the remainder of the genomic DNA) and a "tail" (electrophoresed nuclear fragments), and has consequently been named the comet tail assay (Figure 1).[3,4,5]

A highly sensitive test, the comet assay has been extensively explored for the study of genomic damage resulting from chemical and radiation exposure both in culture[6,7] as well as in cells isolated from exposed experimental animals and humans.[8,9,10] As it is relatively quick and inexpensive, it has been used for large scale studies on mutagenesis and disease monitoring.[11,12]

Fundamentally, two methodologies for SCGE exist: the agarose sandwich layer technique[2,8] and the dilute, single suspension technique.[5,6,7,10] However, both protocols ultimately produce a thick agarose suspension, in which the majority of cells for analysis are located beyond the working plane of routine microscopical objective lenses. Consequently, imaging thus requires the use of long working distance (low Numerical Aperture, N.A.) objectives which precludes the resolution of small nuclear fragments.

The application of confocal laser scanning microscopy to SCGE has been reported,[13] albeit without in-depth analysis of tail contents.

The practical application of SCGE to large sample numbers is presently restricted to the number of slides that can be placed in the electrophoresis chamber. Consequentially, there is a considerable degree of inter-specimen and inter-series variability in the electrophoretic condition. The establishment of precise dose response curves in drug affectivity screening and especially in comparative drug efficacy testing may be compromised under these circumstances. Further, the application of this method to the assessment of chemotherapeutic resistance of clinical samples (requiring dose response curves for variations in drug exposure time and concentration) is complicated.

As a result, the application of single cell gel electrophoresis and subsequent comet tail analysis to clinical practice has as yet not been effectively considered. The application

High Resolution Confocal Laser Scanning Microscopy Analysis of DNA Excision Repair

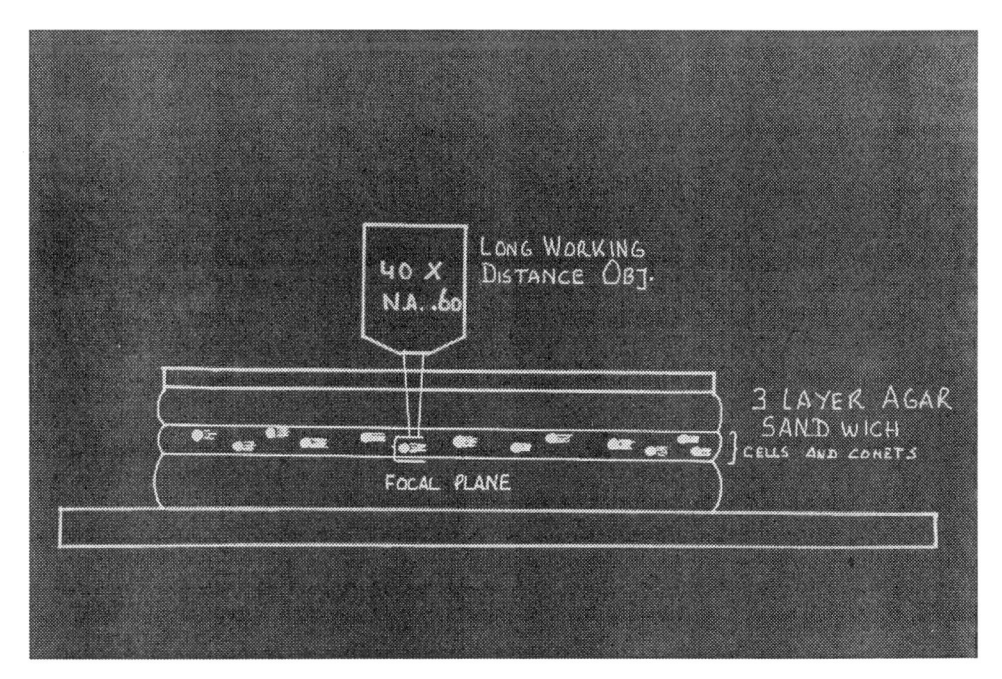

Figure 1. Schematic drawing of imaging problem encountered during imaging of comet tails from single, thick (2 mm high) suspension layer of electrophoresis agarose. Note that most nuclei/tails will be out of reach of high Numerical Aperture (N.A.), high resolution objectives with associated short working distances. As a result, long working distance objectives must be used, which will inevitably result in low N.A.

of single cell gel electrophoresis and confocal laser scanning microscopy based quantisation of the results is finally limited to those agents which directly cause genomic damage.

We therefore aimed to develop an approach to:

a) reduce the bottle neck in electrophoresis by increasing the capacity by altering the procedure of gel suspension of individual cell samples,
b) alter the imaging conditions of cells after single cell gel electrophoresis to allow for the use of the highest numerical aperture possible high resolution high magnification objectives in imaging procedures.

3. METHODS, MATERIALS AND EXPERIMENTATION

3.1. Single Cell Gel Electrophoresis Conditions

The essential problem within single cell electrophoresis of specimens suspended on routine microscopy slides is the size of the individual gel electrophoresis bath. Although enlargement of the electrophoresis chamber or the use of a number of instruments in parallel is technically feasible, both may introduce variability into the experimentation. The subsequent running of gels in the same bath will be associated with an increased variability.

Essentially, the number of cells that are to be tested and/or analysed is relatively limited and is defined by that number of cells that can be successfully retrieved from any in-vitro culture circumstance. The use of microtiter plates with small wells has allowed for standardization of culture conditions but also for the concentration of sufficiently large cell numbers in a relatively small sample. As such it is possible to suspend this sample after exposure and after allowance for DNA excision repair process to occur, in a relatively small volume of agar.

In order to maintain comparability with the existing SCGE, while increasing the sample capacity as well as decreasing the resultant specimen thickness (to allow for the use of high resolution objective lenses), we have developed the following protocol:

2.0 ml of 1% low melting point agarose (Sigma, prepared with distilled water and held at 40°C) was pipetted onto a half-frosted microscope slide and allowed to gel. Agar "wells" were created in the agarose using a 6 mm cork borer (VWR, Mississauga, Canada). 250 μl of cell suspension was mixed with 0.75 ml agarose, 75 μl of this mixture was quickly pipetted into the agarose wells, and the slide allowed to gel (approximately 1 min). Slides were carefully submersed in an alkaline lysis solution containing 1.2 M NaCl, 0.03 M NaOH, and 0.5% sarkosyl and kept for 1 hour in the dark, followed by a 1 hour wash in three rinses of 0.03 M NaOH and 2mM EDTA. Electrophoresis (0.6 V/cm, 40–50 mA) for 25 minutes was carried out in a fresh solution of 0.03 M NaOH and 2mM EDTA. Slides were rinsed twice in distilled H_2O and stained for 20 minutes with ethidium bromide (20 μg/ml in 0.1 M NaCl).

Following staining, agar wells were removed from the slide with a scalpel, and mounted on a prepared mount of frozen embedding medium, and sectioned with an Anglia Scientific (AS 620, Fisher, Ottawa, ON) cryotome (30 μm sections). Sections were thawed out by mounting on a warm microscope slide, and wet mounted with 70 μl of PBS before coverslipping.

Slides were examined using the Zeiss LSM-410 with a krypton/argon laser, mounted on a Zeiss Axiovert 100 microscope (excitation at 488 nm). Summary comet tail images were collected as the summation of 10–12 serial sections (individual focal plane height / optical section thickness of 1 μm).

We tested the reproducibility of well to well single cell gel electrophoresis conditions by pouring subsamples of a large cell culture exposed to a single dose of daunorubicin and provided with a two hour period for post exposure (1 hour) of recovery to allow for sufficient DNA excision to occur to result in significant comet tail development. This experiment was repeated a number of times with different times and concentrations to daunorubicin and different post exposure times for DNA excision repair and recovery. The test parameters for assessment of inter-sample SCGE variability were maximum comet tail length, totally integrated florescence or DNA content of the comet tail, and a distribution of these two parameters between individual cells within a single well. Differences between wells were compared using calculated means for population of at least 20 cells and t-test.

3.2. High Resolution Confocal Laser Scanning Microscopy

The intrinsic problem in achieving high resolution confocal laser scanning microscopy is to reduce the distance between cells under observation and the front surface of the objective in use. With the ability to punch out the wells which had been filled with individual cell suspensions, arose the possibility to punch the same samples out of the support medium after the conclusion of gel electrophoresis.

With the ability for cryotomy we chose to assess the feasibility of producing frozen sections of the agar plugs of sufficient thickness to include a suitable number of completely intact and completely included nuclei with their comet tails. As the comet tails are within the plane of the agar strictly parallel to the surface due to the direction of the electrophoretic voltage and current, tails will be completely contained within such sections as long as the original vertical diameters of the nucleus are completely contained.

As sections can be taken as deep within the plug as required the central part of the plugs, in which electrophoretic conditions are most optimal and standardized can be used for the preparation of subsections. The thickness of standard cover slips and the working distance of even the most high resolution objectives will then allow for the full thickness of the 30μm frozen section to be explored and visualized under optimum conditions.

We chose to assess the applicability of this procedure to three modern high resolution objectives in the current high end usage of confocal laser scanning microscope systems. A 40x (NA 1.3, oil immersion objective), 63x (NA 1.4 oil immersion objective) and 100x (NA 1.4 oil immersion objective) series of objectives was tested. Objectives were manufactured by Zeiss and applied to the Zeiss Axiovert microscope combined with a LSM 410 confocal laser scanning microscope. Variable pinhole settings to result in variable optical section thickness and various scanning and exposure modes as well as filter block and wave length settings were explored.

In order to avoid problems with ethidium bromide leaching into the agarose this stochastic DNA stain was applied to the sections only at the time of section mounting. The slides were then visualized immediately.

3.3. Results of Gel Electrophoresis Adaptations

Hardening of the gel and homogenous suspension of cells throughout the well was reproducibly achieved without difficulty.

On examination of the excised plugs and sections electrophoretic conditions were found to be homogenous throughout the plugs based on mean lengths of standard deviations of maximum comet tail length and integrated florescence that were within 5% of each other providing inter-sample reproducibility for the two important parameters are greater than 95%.

3.4. Results of Imaging Modifications

The placement of 30μm frozen sections results in a sample in which at least 50% of all nuclei are non-capped and are contained completely within the 30 μm sections. The presence of capping or the absence thereof can easily be ascertained by starting a z-series of optical sections beginning at the surface of the 30 μm section. Any nuclear profile present at that level is discarded and only nuclear profiles that start within optical sections of 1μm high that are at least 2–3 μm away from the surface of the gel section are included in the samples.

We found stacks of 12–15 optical sections to be required for complete inclusion of childhood as well as adult ALL cells, and with this approach, even using systematic random sampling as defined by XY coordinate altercations, protocols samples of 20–40 cells could be rapidly sampled from any frozen section without a problem.

The use of high viscosity mounting medium (e.g., D.P.X.) was attempted but resulted in extensive fragmentation of the gel sections. This is in contrast to frozen sections of organoid tissue and results from the complete absence within electrophoresis gel of any long collagen fibres which presumably provide support for the use of such media for solid tissue samples.

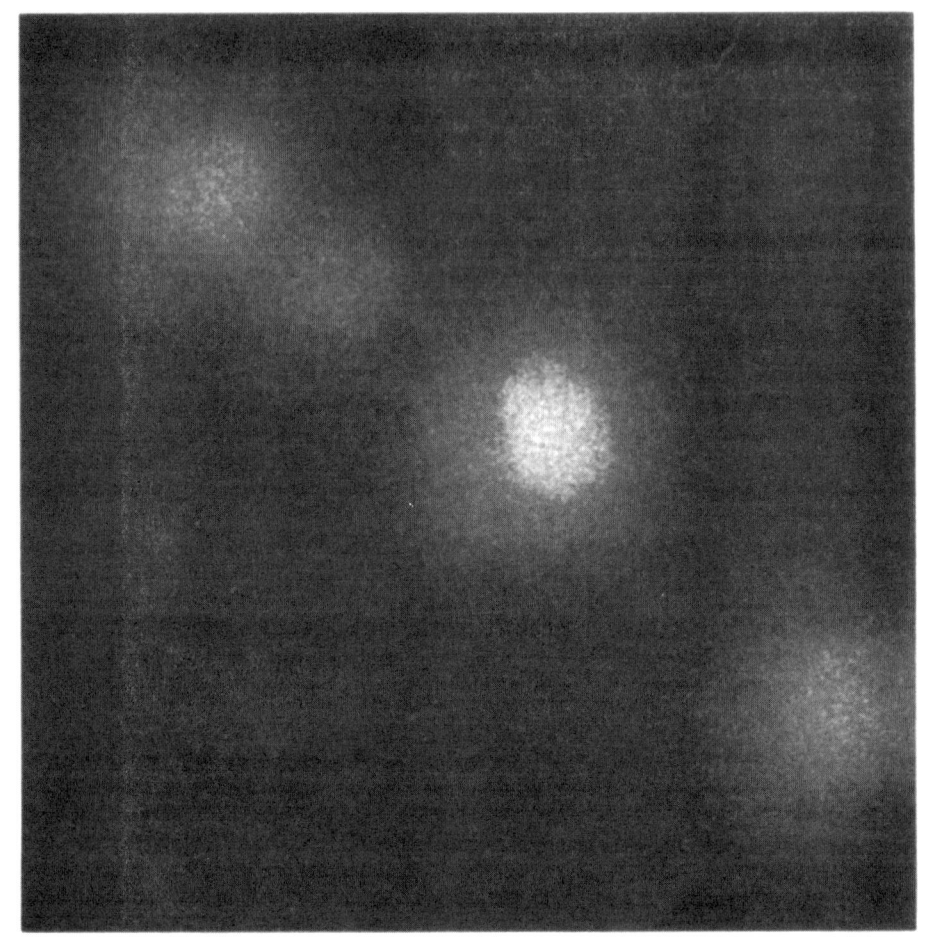

Figure 2. Microphotograph of results of assessment of thick agar section using low N.A. objective. Due to the high focal plane there is a risk of overlapping of images and, as a result of low N.A., no details of DNA fragments within the tails can be visualized.

As such, after initial experimentation, frozen sections were all mounted in a water medium. This does result in some limitations to the storage of such individual sections. However, individual samples of the agarose plug embedded in cryotomy support media, may be stored frozen for repeated sampling and future analysis.

Using this method, and as illustrated in Figures 4 and 5, there is a profound improvement in the now acieved high resolution of the comet tails. Further, nuclear membrane remnants and associated heterochromatin can easily be visualized. The resolution of the comet tail structure is now sufficient to recognize individual smaller and larger florescent signals and facilitate a true measurement of integrated florescence.

With individual images collected at 1 μm optical section height the total integrated florescence can now be easily calculated and reproducibility studies on this same stack of images result in values for the maximum length of comet tail and the integrated total florescence that are again within 95% of each other.

High Resolution Confocal Laser Scanning Microscopy Analysis of DNA Excision Repair 533

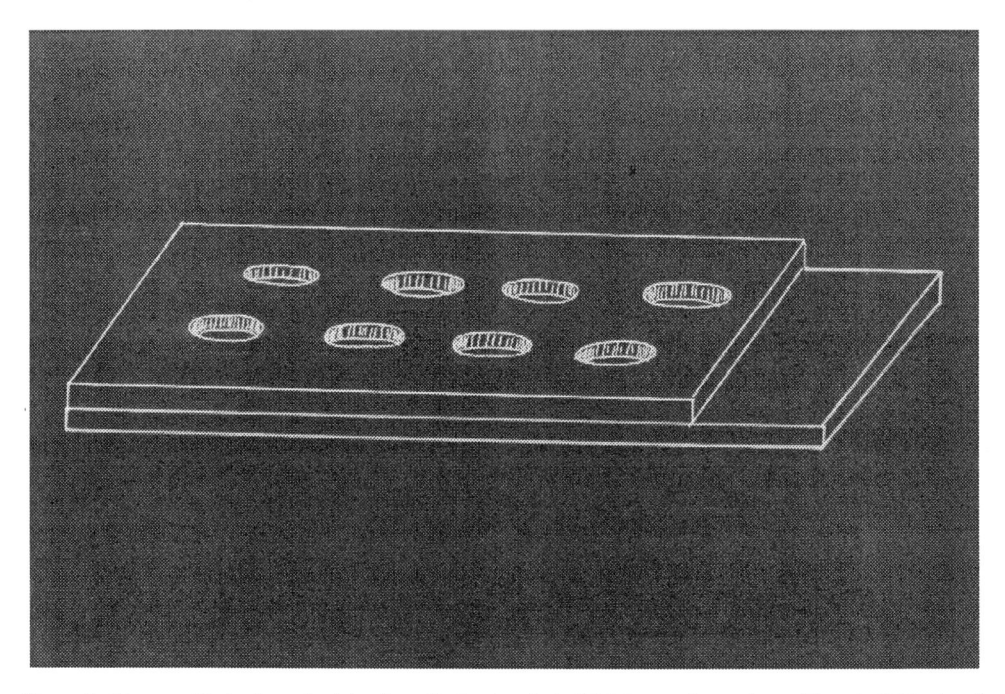

Figure 3. Diagram illustrating principle of punched out wells in thick (support) agar layer. These individual wells can then be filled with the SCGE cell-agarose suspension. The entire slide can then be placed within the standard electrophoresis chamber. As a result, the capacity of the assay is immediately increased by a factor of 6–8, depending on the number of wells punched.

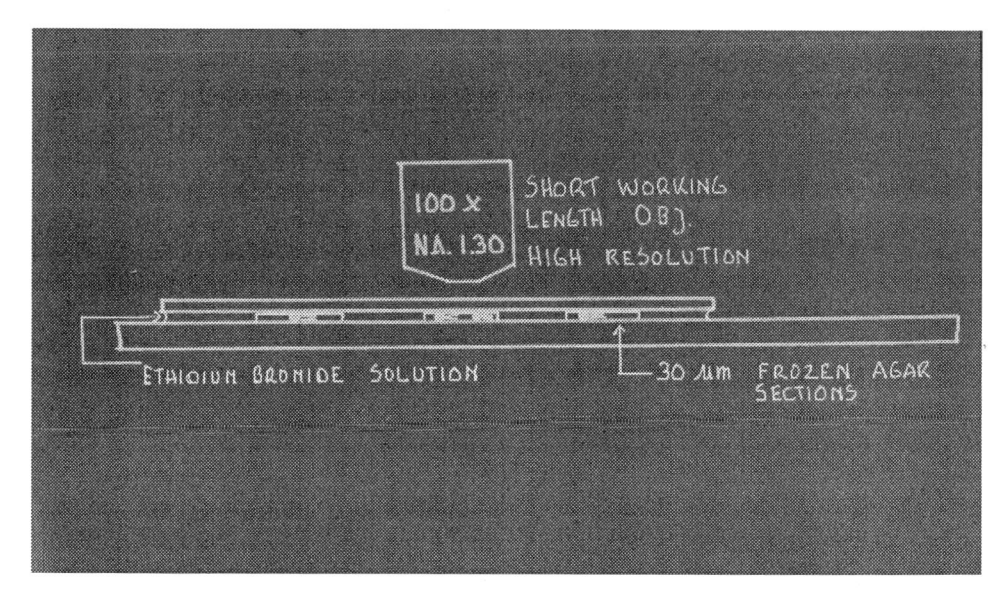

Figure 4. Diagram illustrating results of assessment of 30 μm frozen section of the agarose "plugs." Water-mounted and covered with a conventional coverslip, the nuclei / tails within the section are easily within the optical capacity of modern high N.A., high magnification objective lenses.

Figure 5. Printed results of digitized image of nuclei and comet tail obtained using 30 μm frozen section and high resolution confocal laser scanning microscopy (Zeiss Axiovert, LSM 410). Image is the result of 12 "stacked" sequential "optical sections" of 1 μm thickness. Note the well defined granularity within the tail, showing the variability of DNA fragment size and evidencing the benefit of the applicability of high N.A. objectives (compare to Figure 2).

4. CONCLUSIONS

The combination of punched out wells for single cell gel electrophoresis with high concentration cell samples, combined with high resolution confocal laser scanning microscopy based on 30 μm frozen sections placed in watery medium for direct visualization, augmented further by the usew of the most modern high resolution and high N.A. microscope objectives results in a considerable improvement of the combined procedure: single cell electrophoresis / high resolution confocal laser scanning microscopy.

ACKNOWLEDGMENTS

We would like to acknowledge Dr. Lorne Leahey, Department of Orthopaedic Surgery for his assistance in the procurement of normal bone marrow samples and the patients who with his counselling agreed to donate a sample of their marrow obtained as part of corrective surgery.

We are grateful for the help of Mrs. Linda Lee Maughan in the preparation of this manuscript.

This study was supported by the IWK Grace Health Centre Research Foundation under agreement of the Ethical Committee of the same institution.

REFERENCES

1. Ostling O, Johanson KJ. Microelectrophoretic study of radiation-induced DNA damages in individual mammalian cells. Biochem Biophys Res Comm, 1984, 123(1):291–298.
2. Singh NP, McCoy MT, Tice RR, Schneider EL. A simple technique for quantitation of low levels of DNA damage in individual cells. Exp Cell Res, 1988, 175:184–191.
3. Collins AR, Dobson VL, Dusinska M, Kennedy G, Stetina R. The comet assay: what can it really tell us? Mutat Res, 1997, 375:183–193.
4. Fairbairn DW, Olive PL, O'Neill KL. The comet assay: a comprehensive review. Mutat Res, 1995, 339:37–59.
5. Olive PL, Banath JP, Durand RE. Heterogeneity in radiation-induced DNA damage and repair in tumour and normal cells measured using the "comet" assay. Radiat Res, 1990, 122:86–94.
6. Olive PL, Banath JP, Durand RE. Detection of etoposide resistance by measuring DNA damage in individual Chinese Hamster cells. J Natl Cancer Inst, 1990, 82(9):779–783.
7. Olive PL, Frazer G, Banath JP. Radiation induced apoptosis measured in TK6 human B lymphoblast cells using the comet assay. Radiat Res, 1993, 136:130–136.
8. Singh NP, Banner DB, Tice RR, Brant L, Schneider EL. DNA damage and repair with age in individual human lymphocytes. Mutat Res, 1990, 237:123–130.
9. Tice RR, Strauss GHS, Peters WP. High dose combination alkylating agents with autologous bone marrow support in patients with breast cancer: preliminary assessment of DNA damage in individual peripheral lymphocytes using the single cell gel electrophoresis. Mutat Res, 1992, 271:101–113.
10. Zheng H, Olive PL. Reduction of tumour hypoxia and inhibition of DNA repair by nicotinamide after irradiation of SCCVII murine tumours and normal tissues. Cancer Res, 1996, 56:2801–2808.
11. Vaghef H, Hellman B. Demonstration of chlorobenzene induced DNA damage in mouse lymphocytes using the single cell gel electrophoresis assay. Toxicology, 1995, 96:19–28.
12. Hellman B, Vaghef H, Friis L, Edling C. Alkaline single cell electrophoresis of DNA fragments in biomonitoring for genotoxicity: an introductory study on healthy human volunteers. Int Arch Occup Environ Health, 1997, 69(3):185–92.
13. O'Neill K, Fairbairn W, Standing MD. Analysis of single-cell gel electrophoresis using laser-scanning microscopy, Mutation Res, 1993, 319:129–134.

58

DEFINING THE OPTIMAL DOSAGE OF METHOTREXATE FOR CHILDHOOD ACUTE LYMPHOBLASTIC LEUKEMIA*

New Insights from the Lab and Clinic

William E. Evans, Ching-Hon Pui, and Mary V. Relling

Departments of Pharmaceutical Sciences and Hematology-Oncology
The Hematological Malignancies Program
St. Jude Children's Research Hospital
University of Tennessee
Colleges of Pharmacy and Medicine
Memphis, Tennessee, 38105

1. INTRODUCTION

Until recently, relatively little was known about the intracellular disposition of methotrexate (MTX) in leukemic lymphoblasts in patients. One reason for the paucity of such data is the unavailability of blast cells after the initial 2–4 weeks of chemotherapy, at which time >95% of patients have achieved a complete remission. In the absence of cellular pharmacokinetic and pharmaco-dynamic studies in patients, selection of the optimal dosage, route, and schedule of antileukemic drugs must be based largely on imprecise clinical results and less than optimal preclinical models. For the past forty years, the dosage of MTX for children with acute lymphoblastic leukemia (ALL) has evolved largely on an empirical basis, such that today there is more than a 100-fold range in MTX dosages being used in different ALL treatment protocols worldwide (Table 1). Furthermore, childhood ALL comprises specific lineage and genetic subtypes that differ in their response to modern treatment protocols, yet little or no distinction is made for these differences in determining the dosage of MTX. This brief overview summarizes a series of clinical studies conducted at St. Jude Children's Research Hospital, focused on the intracellular disposition and effects of methotrexate in leukemic lymphoblasts of children with newly diagnosed ALL.

---

* Abbreviations as defined in text, except THF = tetrahydrofolate, DHF = dihydrofolate, GARtf = glycinamide ribonucleotide transformylase, AICARtf = aminoimidazole carboxamide ribonucleotide transformylase.

Table 1. Dosages of high-dose MTX currently used to treat childhood ALL

Group	Protocol	MTX Dosage
CCG	1882 (high risk)*	no HDMTX (0.04 gm/m^2)
CCG	1901 (high risk)	0.2 gm/m^2
CCG	1922 (low risk)	1.0 gm/m^2
CCG	1941 (relapsed)	1.0 gm/m^2
Germany	CoALL-05-92	1.0 gm/m^2
POG	9317 (B-cell ALL)	1.0 gm/m^2
POG	9605 (standard risk)	1.0 gm/m^2
Taiwan	TPOG-ALL-93	1.0 gm/m^2
St. Jude	Total XIII (window)	1.0 gm/m^2
France	FRALLE 93 (low risk)	1.5 gm/m^2
Italy	AIEOP95 (B-lineage)	2.0 gm/m^2
Dutch	DCLSG ALL9	2.0 gm/m^2
Brazil	GBTLI LLA-93	2.0 gm/m^2
St. Jude	Total XIII (continuation)	2.0 gm/m^2
POG	9405/9406 (high risk)	2.5 gm/m^2
Spain	ALL27/89	3.0 gm/m^2
Dana Farber 91-001	91-001	4.0 gm/m^2
POG	9404 (T-cell)	5.0 gm/m^2
Germany	BFM95	5.0 gm/m^2
Austria/Swiss BFM95	BFM95	5.0 gm/m^2
Italy	AIEOP95 (T-lineage)	5.0 gm/m^2
Argentina 1-LLA96-BT-M/HPG	1-LLA96-BT-M/HPG	5.0 gm/m^2
UK	UKALL-XI (age 4-15 y)	6.0 gm/m^2
UK	UKALL-XI (age 1-4 y)	8.0 gm/m^2
France	FRALLE (intermediate risk)	8.0 gm/m^2
Nordic	NOPHO92	8.0 gm/m^2

*example of ALL protocol without HDMTX

2. IS THE DOSAGE OF MTX IMPORTANT?

There are several lines of evidence indicating that it is important to establish the optimal dosage of MTX for children with different phenotypic and genotypic subtypes of ALL. Results of the St. Jude TOTAL-XS protocol indicated that the level of systemic exposure to high-dose MTX (HDMTX) can significantly influence the event-free survival (EFS) of children with B-lineage ALL, with a better outcome in children with MTX plasma concentrations (Cp$_{ss}$) > 16μM during their 24 hour MTX infusions (1). Our subsequent prospective trial (TOTAL-XII), in which patients were randomized to receive HDMTX at fixed doses (1.5 gm/m^2) or at doses individualized to ensure a MTX Cp$_{ss}$ >20 μM, revealed significantly better EFS in children with B-lineage ALL who received individualized doses of HDMTX, yet this difference was not evident in children with T-lineage ALL. Up-front "window" studies in the current St. Jude TOTAL XIII protocol provided new insights to explain this finding, as they revealed significant lineage differences in accumulation of methotrexate polyglutamates (MTXPG), active metabolites of MTX, in ALL blasts of children (2) (as reviewed below). Subsequent studies demonstrated that higher levels of MTXPG in ALL blasts translated into greater antileukemic effects, such as the inhibition of *de novo* purine synthesis and the decrease in circulating blasts (3). Based on these data, our working hypothesis is that the MTX plasma concentration necessary to achieve maximum MTXPG accumulation in ALL blasts differs by ALL lineage, such that the optimal dosage of HDMTX will be different in these subtypes of childhood ALL. Ongoing studies are designed to define the MTX plasma concentration (and hence dosage) required to maximize MTXPG accumulation in lymphoblasts of children with these major subtypes of ALL, and to elucidate the mechanism(s) underlying these differences in MTX intracellular disposition and effects.

3. WHAT FACTORS REGULATE MTX DISPOSITION IN LEUKEMIA CELLS?

MTX is a prodrug, requiring metabolism (anabolism) to MTX-polyglutamates for maximum cytotoxic effects (4). A simplified overview of the intracellular metabolism and effects of MTX is depicted in Figure 1. In brief, MTX entry into cells is mediated by three principal mechanisms: (1) the reduced folate carrier (RFC) with a micromolar Km, (2) the high-affinity low-capacity folate receptor (FR) with a nanomolar Km, and (3) passive diffusion (PD). Influx via the FR and PD are relatively minor at typical MTX plasma concentrations (1–30 μM) achieved clinically. Once inside cells, MTX either binds to target enzymes (e.g. dihydrofolate reductase) or is metabolized by cytosolic folylpolyglutamate synthetase (FPGS) to polyglutamylated MTX (MTXPG), with up to 5 additional glutamates (glu) sequentially added to the molecule in ALL blasts (2). These longer chain MTXPGs are retained longer in cells and inhibit additional target enzymes when compared to MTX; thus their formation is considered highly advantageous. MTXPGs are eventually hydrolyzed by gamma glutamyl hydrolase (GGH), a lysosomal enzyme that cleaves glutamic acid residues from MTXPG. The relative sensitivity or resistance of cancer cells to MTX is influenced by a number of mechanisms, including decreased entry into cells due to impaired RFC function, decreased formation of MTXPG via FPGS or increased hydrolysis of MTXPG via GGH. The extent to which these mechanisms contribute to differences in the intracellular disposition and effects of MTX in different subtypes of childhood ALL has not been fully elucidated, but is the focus of ongoing studies.

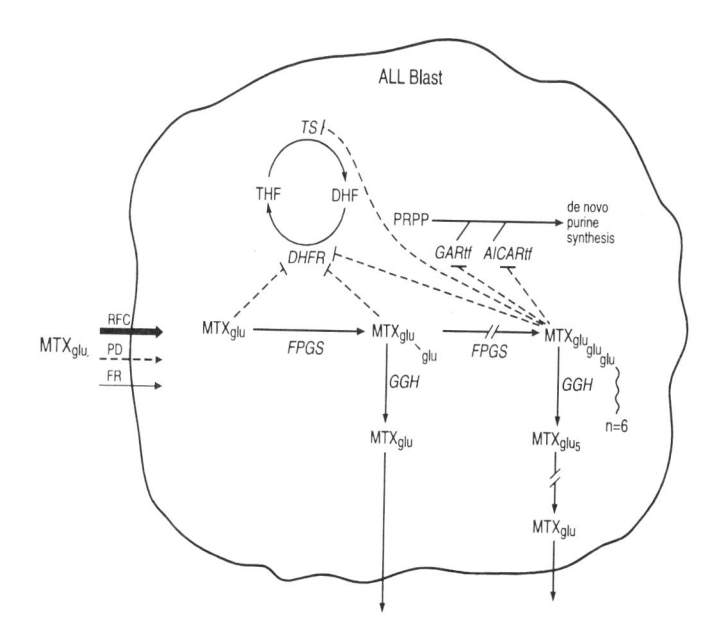

Figure 1. Overview of MTX disposition and effects in ALL blasts.

4. WHY NOT GIVE VERY HIGH DOSE MTX TO ALL CHILDREN WITH ALL?

Administering very high doses of MTX to all patients is not an acceptable strategy to avoid suboptimal MTX exposure, because of the increased risk of toxicity and the increased cost of therapy. HDMTX can produce a number of toxicities, including hepatic and renal dysfunction, myelosuppression and stomatitis, which is related to MTX concentrations and leucovorin dosage, among other factors. The most devastating adverse effect is the development of encephalopathy. Transient cerebral dysfunction following administration of 8–12.5 gm/m^2 of MTX has been reported in 5–15% of patients with osteosarcoma, a complication rarely observed with lower doses of HDMTX given to children with ALL. However, even 1.0 gm/m^2 HDMTX can produce unacceptable neurotoxicity if administered too frequently and if insufficient leucovorin rescue is administered. For these reasons, we feel it is wise to establish the optimal dosage of HDMTX by leukemic subtypes, to ensure appropriate levels of MTXPG in the target tissue (lymphoblasts) and yet avoid unnecessarily high dosages that are associated with greater toxicity.

5. INTRACELLULAR DISPOSITION OF MTX DIFFERS BY DOSAGE AND BY LYMPHOBLAST LINEAGE AND PLOIDY

In a randomized up-front "window" study (TOTAL-XIIIA), we found that 1.0 gm/m^2 HDMTX (IV over 24H) achieves significantly higher MTXPG concentrations in ALL blasts of children with newly diagnosed ALL, *in vivo*, when compared to lower-dose MTX (30 mg/m^2 Q6H x 6) (2). While these studies have resolved a long-standing debate as to whether HDMTX achieves higher MTXPG concentrations in ALL blasts compared to prolonged exposure to lower-dose MTX, several important questions remain unanswered. For example, these studies revealed significant lineage differences in MTXPG accumulation with either LDMTX or HDMTX, with B-lineage lymphoblasts accumulating significantly higher MTXPG than T-lineage blasts (2), but the highest dose evaluated in our previous studies was 1.0 gm/m^2 and we do not know whether higher doses might overcome some of these lineage differences. Furthermore, within B-lineage ALL, we found significantly higher MTXPG accumulation in hyperdiploid (> 50 chromosomes) ALL blasts, compared to non-hyperdiploid lymphoblasts, but we do not yet know the mechanisms for these ploidy differences. Our initial studies in a subset of these patients revealed higher activity of FPGS in B-lineage vs T-lineage lymphoblasts (5), but this difference in FPGS activity was not statistically significant at diagnosis and could not completely explain the lineage difference in MTXPG accumulation.

6. FUTURE STUDIES

Our ongoing studies are designed to establish the dosage of MTX required to maximize MTXPG accumulation in blasts of children with ALL of differing lineage and genetic characteristics. In our next protocol, we will systematically administer substantially higher doses of HDMTX (e.g., up to ~ 8.0 gm/m^2) to define the MTX plasma concentration (Cp_{ss}) required for maximum MTXPG accumulation in each of these major subtypes of childhood ALL, and investigate the biochemical mechanisms for differences in

MTXPG accumulation in patients. The goal is to further improve the cure rate of childhood ALL by more precisely defining the optimal dosage of HDMTX for the major subtypes of this heterogenous disease.

ACKNOWLEDGMENTS

This work was supported in part by the following NIH, NCI grants: R37 CA36401, Leukemia Program Project grant CA20180, Cancer Center CORE grant CA21765, by a State of Tennessee Center of Excellence grant, and by the American Lebanese Syrian Associated Charities (ALSAC). This work is adapted from a report for the ECC Newsletter, volume 7, number 1, 1998, pp. 8–10 (with permission).

REFERENCES

1. Evans WE, Crom WR, Abromowitch M, Dodge R, Look T, Bowman P, George SL, Clinical pharmacodynamics of high-dose methotrexate in acute lymphocytic leukemia: Identification of a concentration-effect relationship. N Engl J Med 314:471–477, 1986.
2. Synold TW, Relling MV, Boyett JM, Rivera GK, Sandlund J, Mahmoud H, Crist WM, Pui C-H and Evans WE. Blast cell methotrexate-polyglutamate accumulation *in vivo* differs by lineage, ploidy and methotrexate dose in acute lymphoblastic leukemia. J. Clin. Invest. 94:1996–2001, 1994.
3. Masson E, Relling MV, Synold TW, Liu Q, Schuetz JD, Sandlund JT, Pui C-H, Evans WE. Accumulation of methotrexate polyglutamates in lymphoblasts is a determinant of antileukemic effects in vivo: A rationale for high-dose methotrexate. J. Clin Invest 97(1):73–80, 1996.
4. Gorlick R, Goker E, Trippett T, Waltham M, Banerjee D, Bertino JR: Intrinsic and acquired resistance to methotrexate in acute leukemia. N. Engl. J. Med. 335: 1041–1048, 1996.
5. Barredo JC, Synold TW, Laver J, Relling MV, Pui C-H, Priest DG, Evans WE. Differences in constitutive and post-methotrexate folylpolyglutamate synthetase activity in B-lineage and T-lineage leukemia. Blood 84:564–569, 1994.

59

MECHANISMS OF METHOTREXATE RESISTANCE IN ACUTE LEUKEMIA

Decreased Transport and Polyglutamylation

Richard Gorlick,[1,*] Peter Cole,[1] Debabrata Banerjee,[2] Giuseppe Longo,[2] Wei Wei Li,[2] Daniel Hochhauser,[2] and Joseph R. Bertino[2]

[1]Department of Pediatrics
[2]Program of Molecular Pharmacology and Therapeutics
Memorial Sloan-Kettering Cancer Center
1275 York Avenue
New York, New York 10021

Keywords: Folylpolyglutamate synthetase, gamma-glutamyl hydrolase, methotrexate, reduced folate carrier, acute lymphocytic leukemia, acute myelocytic leukemia.

Abbreviations used: DHFR, dihydrofolate reductase; RFC, reduced folate carrier; FPGS, folylpolyglutamate synthetase; GGH, gamma-glutamyl hydrolase; MTX, methotrexate; ALL, acute lymphocytic leukemia; AML, acute myelocytic leukemia; TMTX, trimetrexate; GAR, glycinamide ribonucleotide; AICAR, aminoimidazole carboxamide; LV, leucovorin.

1. ABSTRACT

Drug resistance limits the effectiveness of methotrexate (MTX) for the treatment of acute leukemia. An increased understanding of the pathways involved in folate metabolism has allowed investigations of the mechanisms of resistance observed in leukemic blasts obtained from patients. Acute lymphocytic leukemia (ALL) was studied for mechanisms of acquired MTX resistance. MTX transport in 27 patients with untreated ALL and

---

[*] Corresponding Author: Richard Gorlick, M.D., Department of Pediatrics, Memorial Sloan-Kettering Cancer Center, 1275 York Avenue Box #376, New York, NY 10021. Phone # 212-639-8392. Fax # 212-639-2767. E-mail: gorlickr@mskcc.org.

31 patients with relapsed ALL was measured using a previously described competitive displacement assay. Only 13% of the untreated patients were considered to have impaired MTX transport whereas over 70% of the relapsed patients had evidence of impaired MTX transport. Northern analyses and quantitative RT-PCR for the reduced folate carrier (RFC) were performed on the RNA available from the leukemic blasts of 24 patients in whom MTX transport had been measured. Six of 9 samples with impaired MTX transport had decreased RFC expression (one had no detectable RFC expression), while three had no decrease in RFC expression. Acute myelocytic leukemia (AML) was studied to determine the basis of the decreased MTX polyglutamylation. Enzyme kinetics of the enzyme folylpolyglutamate synthetase (FPGS) were studied, demonstrating FPGS in the myeloid cell lines and patient samples had a higher K_m for MTX as a substrate than lymphoid cells. Measuring gamma-glutamyl hydrolase enzyme activity allowed a more accurate prediction of steady state levels of MTX polyglutamates. A knowledge of the mechanisms of MTX resistance that occur in leukemic blasts obtained from patients may allow the development of therapeutic strategies to circumvent resistance.

2. INTRODUCTION

Methotrexate (MTX), an antifolate drug that replaced aminopterin in the clinic in 1956, continues to be an essential drug in the curative regimen used to treat acute lymphocytic leukemia (ALL).[1] It is used during the continuation phase of treatment, usually in combination with 6-mercaptopurine. However, patients still relapse and develop drug resistance (i.e., are not as sensitive to the same drugs used previously), and as a consequence can only be salvaged in 40–50% of cases with high doses of drugs followed by allogenic or autologous or peripheral blood stem cell transplants.[2,3] In contrast, MTX is not usually employed in the treatment programs for acute myelocytic leukemia (AML), as response rates reported for this drug as a single agent in the treatment of this disease are 15% or less.[4] During the past decade, application of the advances in molecular biology have made it possible to study both intrinsic and acquired mechanisms of resistance to this drug. The study of ALL presents a unique opportunity to study acquired resistance to this drug, as relatively pure populations of blast cells can be obtained before treatment and at relapse, while the study of AML blasts offers an opportunity to study a disease in which intrinsic resistance is present.[5,6]

In experimental tumor systems the two common mechanisms of acquired resistance to MTX are decreased transport and amplification of the target gene, dihydrofolate reductase (DHFR).[5–7] We have shown that low level DHFR gene amplification is present in approximately 30% of patients with ALL who relapse after treatment with this drug.[8] In a previous study blasts from 2 of 4 patients with ALL believed to be clinically resistant to MTX had evidence of impaired transport, allowing the suggestion that MTX transport impairment may also be a mechanism of acquired resistance in this disease. To measure MTX transport in blasts, a competitive displacement flow cytometric assay was developed utilizing the fluorescent lysine analog of MTX, N^α-(4-amino-4-deoxy-N^{10}-methylpteroyl)-N^ϵ-(4'flouresceinthio-carbamyl)-L-lysine (PT430). This method is both sensitive and rapid, and is a useful method to detect MTX transport resistance.[9] This assay has also been used by other laboratories, to demonstrate decreased MTX transport may be a component of MTX resistance in childhood ALL.[10] The availability of a human cDNA for the reduced folate carrier (RFC) has also allowed us to measure RFC mRNA expression by Northern blot analysis and to develop a RT-PCR assay to quantitate RFC gene expression.[11–14] Our studies of MTX transport in the blasts of leukemia patients, will be described in this report.[15]

Correlating with the decreased MTX sensitivity, AML blasts accumulate less long chain MTX polyglutamates than pre-B ALL.[16] This polyglutamylation allows the MTX to be retained intracellularly in the absence of extracellular drug allowing prolonged inhibition of DHFR and the enzymes of purine biosynthesis.[17,18] The amount of long chain polyglutamates in cells is the result of the balance of the activity of two different enzymes, folylpolyglutamate synthetase (FPGS) which adds up to 4 glutamyl groups to MTX and gamma-glutamyl hydrolase (GGH), a lysosomal exopeptidase that hydrolyses MTX to the monoglutamate form.[19,20] We have investigated the possible causes for the reduced accumulation of MTX polyglutamates in AML blasts as compared to ALL.[20] Our studies investigating FPGS and GGH in the blasts of leukemia patients, will be described in this report.

3. MECHANISM OF MTX ACTION AND RESISTANCE IN EXPERIMENTAL TUMORS

Although for the most part MTX action is now understood we continue to learn more about this drug in relation to folate metabolism (Figure 1). MTX enters most cells through the RFC, which is a bi-directional anion exchanger.[21] Folate receptors which activate a endocytic process, as well as a low pH folate transport system may play a role in some systems.[21–23] Once inside the cell, MTX is polyglutamylated, i.e., additional glutamates (up to five) are added.[24] MTX and MTX polyglutamates bind tightly to dihydrofolate reductase (DHFR), thus inhibiting tetrahydrofolate formation, required for thymidylate biosynthesis. MTX polyglutamates as well as DHFR polyglutamates inhibit the enzymes of purine synthesis, including 5'-phosphoribosylglycinamide (GAR) and aminoimidazole carboxamide ribonucleotide (AICAR) transformylases. Polyglutamylation is also necessary for the intracellular retention of MTX.[17,18] Negatively charged polyglutamates enter lysosomes through a simple mobile carrier system with the property of exchange diffusion that appears to favor the transport of MTX polyglutamates with increasing gamma-glutamyl chain length.[25] In the lysosomes, GGH, an enzyme with exopeptidase activity (in humans) catalyzes the hydrolysis of intracellular polyglutamates of the folates as well as MTX.[19] Free MTX is effluxed through a separate energy dependent transport pathway.[21]

The knowledge of the mechanisms of MTX action also has allowed the elucidation of the various mechanisms by which cells are resistant to MTX. The four common mechanisms of MTX resistance in experimental systems are a decrease in transport, a decrease in retention due to defective polyglutamylation, an increase in DHFR enzyme activity, or a decrease in binding of MTX to DHFR.[5,6] The genetic basis for certain of these mechanisms in MTX-resistant cell lines has been recognized to be gene amplification and point mutations resulting in amino acid changes in DHFR.[7] The genetic basis for decreased transport or defective polyglutamylation (which could be synthesis or degradation) are only recently being elucidated. The recent cloning of the cDNA for human GGH, RFC and FPGS is allowing identification of the molecular basis for these resistant phenotypes in cell lines and patient samples.[11–14,26,27]

4. DECREASED TRANSPORT AS A MECHANISM OF ACQUIRED MTX RESISTANCE IN ALL

The PT430 competitive displacement assay was utilized to measure transport in 94 leukemic blast samples. Only 4 of 30 (13%) leukemic blast samples obtained from pa-

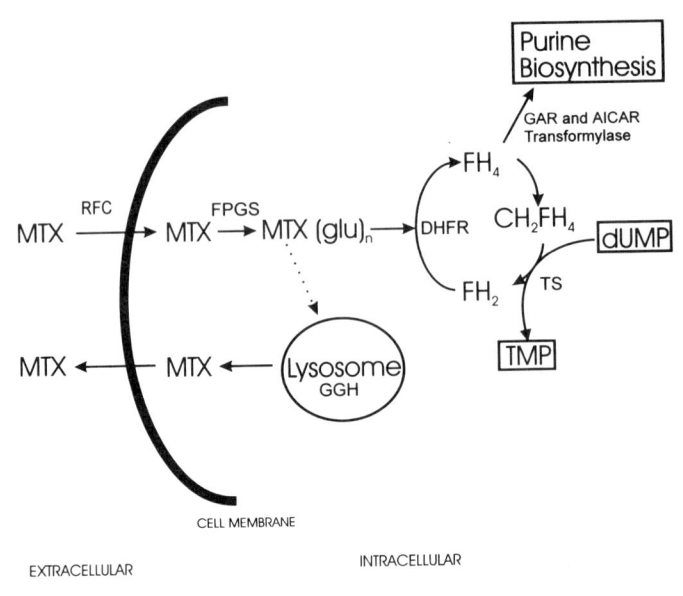

Figure 1. Methotrexate (MTX) metabolism and mechanism of action. MTX is taken up by mammalian cells predominantly by the reduced folate carrier (RFC). Once inside the cell MTX is polyglutamylated by the enzyme folylpolyglutamate synthetase (FPGS). Both MTX and MTX(glu)$_n$ act as potent inhibitors of dihydrofolate reductase (DHFR) and by depleting cells of tetrahydrofolate (FH$_4$) inhibits thymidylate synthesis. By inhibition of FH$_4$ formation as well as by direct inhibition of glycinamide ribonucleotide (GAR) and aminoimidazole carboxamide (AICAR) transformylase, MTX inhibits purine biosynthesis. MTX polyglutamates are transported into and hydrolyzed in the lysosome to monoglutamate forms by the enzyme GGH. Free MTX is rapidly effluxed through an energy dependent transporter.

tients with newly diagnosed ALL had less than 40% displacement of PT430 by MTX. In contrast, blasts from 25 of 35 patients (71%) with relapsed ALL had less than 40% displacement (p<0.0001). As expected, as trimetrexate (TMTX) does not utilize the RFC for uptake, only 10 of 35 (28%) patients with relapsed ALL had less than 40% displacement of PT430 by TMTX (compared to 2 of 27 untreated patients).[15] As TMTX has been reported to share in the multidrug resistance phenotype, it is possible that blasts from these patients were expressing p-glycoprotein, the product of the MDR-1 gene, as all had received therapy which could induce MDR expression.[28] In AML, 10 of 29 (34%) samples had less than 40% displacement of PT430 by MTX. Seven of the 20 (35%) patients with newly diagnosed AML and 3 of 9 (33%) with relapsed AML had less than 40% displacement. In AML failure to displace PT430 by TMTX (10 of 29, 34%) is more common than in ALL (2 of 27, 7%) (p=0.032).[15] In AML, previous studies have attributed intrinsic resistance to MTX to defects in polyglutamylation of this drug.[16] This provides evidence that defective MTX transport may also contribute to intrinsic resistance in AML, as impaired MTX transport was found in 35% of blasts from AML patients at the time of diagnosis. In addition, evidence of defective TMTX transport is also observed in 25% of AML patients at diagnosis. This also may be secondary to expression of p-glycoprotein as AML has been reported to have a high incidence of expression in untreated patients with this disease.[28,29]

In order to determine the basis for the impairment of MTX transport in blasts from ALL patients in relapse, considered to be clinically resistant to this drug, we measured expression of the RFC. There was only sufficient material available to perform Northern analysis and semiquantitative RT-PCR on RNA obtained from blasts of 9 patients with impaired transport as measured by PT430 displacement and in 15 patients not showing impaired transport of MTX. Of the nine transport defective samples 5 had decreased and one had no detectable RFC expression as compared to the RNA from the CCRF-CEM cell line. The remaining 3 transport defective samples tested had no decrease in RFC expression. Sequencing of the entire cDNA for the RFC in these 3 samples is currently in progress, to determine if there are mutations in the coding sequence that might explain the low level of MTX transport in these samples.[15] A mutation in the RFC of a murine L1210 leukemia cell line resulted in decreased MTX uptake and MTX resistance despite an approximately five fold increase in RFC message.[30] None of the 15 samples with normal MTX transport had decreased RFC mRNA expression. Defective MTX transport associated with decreased RFC expression is therefore common in relapsed ALL following treatment with MTX containing therapy.

5. ALTERATIONS IN FPGS AND GGH AS POTENTIAL BASES OF THE IMPAIRED MTX POLYGLUTAMYLATION OBSERVED IN AML

The cytotoxicity and polyglutamylation of MTX were measured in two lymphoid (CCRF-CEM, MOLT-3) and two myeloid (K562, HL60) cell lines.[31] The cytotoxicity correlated closely with the amount of long chain polyglutamates accumulated. To investigate the basis of the impaired polyglutamylation in the myeloid cell lines FPGS and GGH enzyme activity were measured. The observation that FPGS activity was not low and the GGH activity not high in the K562 cell line prompted an investigation of the enzyme kinetics of FPGS in the AML and ALL cell lines. FPGS in the two myeloid cell lines had a decreased affinity for MTX as a substrate (K_m was 92 and 89 µmol/L) as compared to the lymphoid cell lines (K_m was 44 and 23 µmol/L). This difference in K_m continued to be observed after FPGS was partially purified and after subcellular fractionation. To determine if this difference extended to leukemia patient samples, we compared the K_m of FPGS with MTX as a substrate in three AML samples to three ALL samples. As observed in the cell lines the AML samples (mean K_m = 86 ± 12 µmol/L) had a higher K_m than the ALL samples (mean K_m = 40 ± 12 µmol/L). This difference in K_m may partly explain the impaired MTX polyglutamylation observed in AML.[31] The difference in substrate affinity may be explained at the molecular level by studies performed by Chen, et al, in which alternative splice variants of FPGS were identified.[32] These additional splice variants may be responsible for the tissue-specific encoding of different isoforms of FPGS. This possibility is currently being investigated.

In order to determine the role of GGH in determining MTX polyglutamylation 15 blast samples from children with acute leukemias, eight with ALL and seven with AML, were studied.[20] The median accumulation of total MTX polyglutamates after 24h exposure to 10µM [^{3}H] MTX was 5 fold higher in ALL blasts (2276 pmol/10^7 cells) as compared to AML blasts (830 pmol/10^7 cells). The FPGS activity was 2.7 fold higher in ALL samples as compared to AML blasts; the AML blasts showed 1.8 fold higher GGH activity. A statistically significant correlation was observed in these 15 patient samples between the long chain polyglutamates/total polyglutamates ratio with the GGH/FPGS ratio (r = 0.81; p<0.001). We used the ratio of long chain polyglutamates/total polyglutamates to normalize for transport. This correlation was significant also in the subgroup of patients with ALL (r = 0.7, p < 0.05) but did not reach statistical significance in the subgroup of patients with AML ($r = 0.66$, $p = 0.1$). In the whole group of 15 patient samples FPGS activity alone did not show any significant correlation with long chain polyglutamates or total polyglutamates values or with their ratio. A slightly better correlation was present between GGH activity alone with the ratio long chain/total polyglutamates ($r = 0.63$; $p = 0.05$). Measurement of FPGS and GGH activities together was therefore better at predicting the accumulation of long chain MTX polyglutamates than measurement of either activity alone. These findings, together with previous studies showing that high levels of GGH may be associated with MTX resistance, emphasize the role of GGH as an important determinant of treatment outcome in acute leukemias.[20]

6. STRATEGIES TO OVERCOME MTX RESISTANCE

The finding that a decreased K_m of FPGS with MTX as a substrate, may partly explain the impaired polyglutamylation observed in AML, led to a laboratory investigation of Tomudex® in AML and ALL cell lines, as this compound is known to have a stronger binding affinity.[31] Tomudex® demonstrated near equivalent polyglutamylation and cytotoxicity in AML cell lines as ALL cell lines suggesting the efficacy in treating patients would be similar.[31,33] Based on this data a phase II trial of Tomudex® in the treatment of AML was initiated.

The finding that defective transport of MTX is a common resistance mechanism to MTX in relapsed ALL has led to an interest in drugs such as TMTX which do not utilize the reduced folate carrier for cell entry.[34] In addition, leukemic cells which are resistant to MTX on the basis of transport are collaterally sensitive to TMTX, possibly due to decreased uptake of folates.[35] The combination of TMTX and leucovorin (LV) is very active and non-toxic for the treatment of *pneumocystis carinii* infections in acquired immunodeficiency syndrome patients. The basis of this selectivity is that TMTX is transported by passive diffusion in this parasite, and LV can not rescue this organism because of lack of LV transport. With this combination, the side effects of TMTX on the host are eliminated as normal host cells are protected by LV.[36] We have applied this strategy to selectively target leukemia cells which developed resistance to MTX on the basis of transport. In vitro cytotoxicity studies showed that CCRF-CEM cells resistant to MTX because of defective transport are not protected from the cytotoxic effects of TMTX by LV. Severe combined immunodeficiency mice bearing MTX resistant transport defective CCRF-CEM ALL cells were then tested with the combination of TMTX and LV, and marked tumor regression occurred with limited toxicity.[37] These studies have prompted a study using TMTX with LV protection (not rescue) in relapsed ALL patients that demonstrate resistance to MTX associated with impaired uptake of this drug.

ACKNOWLEDGMENTS

Supported by American Cancer Society Grant No. BC-561C, the Charles A. Dana Foundation, and Grant No. CA09512 from the National Cancer Institute.

REFERENCES

1. Farber S, Diamond LK, Mercer RD, Sylvester RF Jr, Wolff JA. Temporary remissions in acute leukemia in children produced by folic acid antagonist, 4-aminopteroyl-glutamic acid (aminopterin). N Engl J Med 1948, 238, 787–793.
2. Pui CH. Childhood leukemias. N Engl J Med 1995, 332, 1618–1630.

3. Boulad F, Kernan NA. Treatment of childhood acute nonlymphoblastic leukemia: a review. Cancer Investigation 1993, 11, 534–553.
4. Bertino JR, Goker E. Drug resistance in acute leukemia. Leuk Lymph 1993, 11, 37–42.
5. Gorlick R, Goker E, Trippett T, Waltham M, Banerjee D, Bertino JR. Intrinsic and acquired resistance to methotrexate in acute leukemia. N Engl J Med 1996, 335, 1041–1048.
6. Bertino JR. Ode to methotrexate. J Clin Oncol 1993, 11, 5–14.
7. Schweitzer BI, Dicker AP, Bertino JR. Dihydrofolate reductase as a therapeutic target. FASEB J 1990, 4, 2441–2452.
8. Goker E, Waltham M, Kheradpour A, Trippett T, Mazumdar M, Elisseyeff, Y, Schnieders B, Steinherz P, Tan C, Berman E, Bertino JR. Amplification of the dihydrofolate reductase gene is a mechanism of acquired resistance to methotrexate in patients with acute lymphocytic leukemia and is correlated with p53 gene mutations. Blood 1995, 86, 677–684.
9. Trippett T, Schlemmer S, Elisseyeff Y, Goker E, Wachter M, Steinherz P, Tan C, Berman E, Wright JE, Rosowsky A, Schweitzer B, Bertino JR. Defective transport as a mechanism of acquired resistance to methotrexate in patients with acute lymphocytic leukemia. Blood 1992, 80,1158–1162.
10. Matherly LH, Taub JE, Ravindranath Y, Proefke SA, Wong SC, Gimotty P, Buck S, Wright JE, Rosowsky A. Elevated dihydrofolate reductase and impaired methotrexate transport as elements in methotrexate resistance in childhood acute lymphocytic leukemia. Blood 1995, 85, 500–509.
11. Williams FMR, Flintoff WF. Isolation of a human cDNA that complements a mutant hamster cell defective in methotrexate uptake. J Biol Chem 1995, 270, 2987–2992.
12. Moscow JA, Gong M, He R, Sgagias MK, Dixon KH, Anzick SL, Meltzer PS, Cowan KH. Isolation of a gene encoding a human reduced folate carrier (RFC1) and analysis of its expression in transport-deficient, methotrexate-resistant human breast cancer cells. Cancer Res 1995, 55, 3790–3795.
13. Wong SC, Proefke SA, Bhushan A, Matherly LH. Isolation of Human cDNAs that restore methotrexate sensitivity and reduced folate carrier activity in methotrexate transport-defective chinese hamster ovary cells. J Biol Chem 1995, 270, 17468–17475.
14. Prasad PD, Ramamoorthy S, Leibach FH, Ganapathy V. Molecular cloning of the human placental folate transporter. Biochem Biophys Res Comm 1995, 206, 681–687.
15. Gorlick R, Goker E, Trippett T, Steinherz P, Elisseyeff Y, Mazumdar M, Flintoff WF, Bertino JR. Defective transport is a common mechanism of acquired methotrexate resistance in acute lymphocytic leukemia and is associated with decreased reduced folate carrier expression. Blood 1997, 89, 1013–1018.
16. Lin JT, Tong WP, Trippett TM, Niedzwiecki D, Tao Y, Tan C, Steinherz P, Schweitzer BI, Bertino JR. Basis for natural resistance to methotrexate in human acute non-lymphocytic leukemia. Leukemia Res 1991, 15, 1191–1196.
17. Allegra CJ, Chabner BA, Drake JC, Lutz R, Rodbard D, Jolivet J. Enhanced inhibition of thymidylate synthase by methotrexate polyglutamates. J Biol Chem 1985, 260, 9720–9726.
18. Allegra CJ, Drake JC, Jolivet J, Chabner BA. Inhibition of phosphoribosylaminoimidazole carboxamide transformylase by methotrexate and dihydrofolic acid polyglutamates. Proc Natl Acad Sci USA 1985, 82, 4881–4885.
19. Galivan J, Johnson T, Rhee M, McGuire JJ, Priest D, Kesevan V. The role of folylpolyglutamate synthase and gamma-glutamyl hydrolase in altering cellular folyl- and antifolyl polyglutamates. Adv Enzyme Regul 1987, 26, 147–155.
20. Longo GSA, Gorlick R, Tong WP, Lin S, Steinherz P, Bertino JR. ((-Glutamyl hydrolase and folylpolyglutamate synthetase activities predict polyglutamylation of methotrexate in acute leukemias. Onc Res 1997, 9, 259–263.
21. Assaraf YG, Goldman ID. Loss of folic acid exporter function with markedly augmented folate accumulation in lipophilic antifolate-resistant mammalian cells. J Biol Chem 1997, 272, 17460–17466.
22. Antony AC. The biological chemistry of folate receptors. Blood 1992, 79, 2807–2820.
23. Anderson RG, Kamen BA, Rothberg KG, Lacey SW. Potocytosis: sequestration and transport of small molecules by caveolae. Science 1992, 255, 410–411.
24. Mcguire JJ, Hsieh P, Coward JK, Bertino JR. Enzymatic synthesis of folylpolyglutamates. Characterization of the reaction and its products. J Biol Chem 1980, 255, 5776–5788.
25. Barrueco JR, O'Leary D, Sirotnak FM. Metabolic turnover of methotrexate polyglutamates in lysosomes derived from S180 cells. J Biol Chem 1992, 267, 15356–15361.
26. Garrow TA, Admon A, Shane B. Expression cloning of a human cDNA encoding folylpoly ((-glutamate) synthetase and determination of its primary structure. Proc Natl Acad Sci USA 1992, 89, 9151–9155.
27. Yao R, Schneider E, Ryan TJ, Galivan J. Human gamma-glutamyl hydrolase: cloning and characterization of the enzyme expressed in vitro. Proc Acad Sci USA 1996, 93, 10134–10138.

28. Assaraf YG, Molina A, Schimke RT. Cross-resistance to the lipid-soluble antifolate trimetrexate in human carcinoma cells with the multidrug-resistant phenotype. J Natl Cancer Inst 1989, 81, 290–297.
29. Zochbauer S, Gaur A, Brunner R, Kyrle PA, Lechner K, Pirker R. P-glycoprotein expression as unfavorable prognostic factor in acute myeloid leukemia. Leukemia 1994, 8, 974–979.
30. Brigle KE, Spinella MJ, Sierra EE, Goldman ID. Characterization of a mutation in the reduced folate carrier in a transport defective L1210 murine leukemia cell line. J Biol Chem 1995, 270, 22974–22979.
31. Longo GSA, Gorlick R, Tong WP, Ercikan E, Bertino JR. Disparate affinities of antifolates for folylpolyglutamate synthetase from human leukemia cells. Blood 1997, 90, 1241–1245.
32. Chen L, Qi H, Korenberg J, Garrow TA, Choi YJ, Shane B. Purification and properties of human cytosolic folylpoly-(-glutamate synthetase and organization, localization, and differential splicing of its gene. J Biol Chem 1996, 271, 13077–13087.
33. Mauritz R, Bekkenk M, Pieters R, Veerman AJP, Peters GJ, Jansen G. Resistance to methotrexate and sensitivity for novel antifolates in different types of childhood leukemia. Blood 1994, 84, 45a.
34. Kamen BA, Eibl B, Cashmore A, Bertino JR. Uptake and efficacy of trimetrexate (TMQ, 2,2-diamino-5-methyl-6-[(3,4,5-trimethoxyanilino)methyl] quinazoline), a non-classical antifolate in methotrexate-resistant leukemia cells in vitro. Biochem Pharmacol 1984, 33, 1697–1699.
35. Jackson RC, Fry DW, Boritzki TJ, Besserer JA, Leopold WR, Sloan BJ, Elslager EF. Biochemical pharmacology of the lipophilic antifolate, trimetrexate. Adv Enz Reg 1984, 22, 187–206.
36. Allegra CJ, Chabner BA, Tuazon CU, Ogata-Arakaki D, Baird B, Drake JC, Simmons JT, Lack EE, Shelhamer JH, Balis F. Trimetrexate for the treatment of pneumocystis carinii pneumonia in patients with the acquired immunodeficiency syndrome. N Engl J Med 1987, 317, 978–985.
37. Lacerda JF, Goker E, Kheradpour A, Dennig D, Elisseyeff Y, Jagiello C, O'Reilly RJ, Bertino JR. Selective treatment of SCID mice bearing methotrexate-transport resistant human acute leukemia tumors with trimetrexate and leucovorin protection. Blood 1995, 85, 2675–2681.

60

LACK OF CROSS-RESISTANCE BETWEEN PREDNISOLONE AND METHOTREXATE IN CHILDHOOD ACUTE LYMPHOBLASTIC LEUKEMIA?

A Preliminary Analysis

I. R. H. J. Hegge,[1] G. J. L Kaspers,[1*] M. G. Rots,[1,2] G. Jansen,[2] R. Pieters,[1] and A. J. P. Veerman[1]

[1]Department of Pediatric Hematology/Oncology
[2]Medical Oncology
University Hospital Vrije Universiteit
De Boelelaan 11117, NL-1081 HV Amsterdam

Keywords: antifolates, glucocorticoids, leukemia, lymphoblastic, childhood, drug resistance.

1. ABSTRACT

We studied the cross-resistance between prednisolone (PRD) and methotrexate (MTX) in children with newly diagnosed acute lymphoblastic leukemia (ALL). This was done because of a previous observation that such patients could show a good clinical response to systemic PRD monotherapy plus intrathecal MTX, despite in vitro PRD resistant ALL cells (as determined with the MTT assay). This suggests an antileukemic effect of MTX, and thus the lack of cross-resistance between PRD and MTX. A systemic antileukemic effect of intrathecally administered MTX has been reported in the literature. Clinical good responders with PRD resistant ALL cells (n=15) did not show unfavorable MTX-polyglutamylation nor unfavorable low inhibition of thymidylate synthase by MTX,

---

* Correspondence to: G.J.L. Kaspers; Department of Pediatric Hematology/Oncology; University Hospital Vrije Universiteit; De Boelelaan 1117; NL-1081 HV Amsterdam; Phone: +31 - 20 444 2420; Fax: +31 - 20 444 2422; E-mail: gjl.kaspers@azvu.nl

as compared to a heterogenous group of newly diagnosed ALL children (n = 47). In addition, we did not find a significant correlation between these two parameters and in vitro PRD resistance within the clinical good responders with PRD resistant ALL cells. In conclusion, we did not find a significant cross-resistance between PRD and MTX in vitro. It therefore may be that the good clinical response to systemic PRD plus intrathecal MTX in patients with in vitro PRD resistant ALL cells was caused by a systemic antileukemic activity of the intrathecally administered MTX.

2. INTRODUCTION

We previously reported that clinically poor responders to an initial one week systemic monotherapy with predniso(lo)ne (PRD) had acute lymphoblastic leukemia (ALL) cells that are relatively resistant to PRD in vitro.[1] However, 26% of clinically good responders had ALL cells that were also in vitro PRD resistant. In this context, it is important that all patients received one intrathecal injection with methotrexate (MTX) at the start of treatment, in addition to the systemic PRD. It is well known that intrathecally administered MTX can have systemic antileukemic activity,[2,3] up to inducing a tumor-lysis syndrome.[4] Thyss et al. reported that the percentage of clinically good responders to PRD alone for 1 week was 70%, and increased to 90.4% if MTX had been delivered before day 2 of the therapeutic window.[5] Therefore, the good clinical response in our patients with in vitro PRD resistant ALL cells may be explained by an (at least additional) antileukemic effect of MTX. We therefore studied the sensitivity or resistance to MTX of in vitro PRD resistant ALL cells of clinically good responders to systemic PRD plus intrathecal MTX.

3. MATERIALS AND METHODS

3.1. Patients and Samples

A test group of 15 cryopreserved samples of clinically good responders with in vitro PRD resistant ALL cells (LC50>150 µg/ml, determined with the 4-days MTT assay) was compared with a reference group including all types of (up to 47) newly diagnosed ALL patients. All samples contained at least 80% leukemic cells, if necessary after removal of contaminating non-malignant cells by immunomagnetic beads.[6] It concerned children that had been treated according to Dutch Childhood Leukemia Study Group protocols ALL-7 or -8. The treatment included an initial 7 days systemic monotherapy with PRD (60 mg/m^2/day), with 1 intrathecal injection with MTX (dose age-dependent, maximum 12 mg) at day 1 of the so-called window. Patients were divided into good or poor clinical responders, based on their absolute PB blast count: <1000/µl PB and >=1000/µl PB respectively. The test group consisted of only clinically good responders that also should have had >1000 blasts per µl PB at the start of the window treatment. Immunophenotypic subgroups were defined as common or pre-B ALL (HLA-DR and CD19 positive, and CD10 and/or cytoplasmic µ positive), and T-cell lineage ALL (positive for terminal deoxynucleotidyl transferase, CD3 and CD7).

3.2. Methods

In vitro MTX resistance was studied by 1) polyglutamylation after 24 hrs in vitro exposure to 1 µM ^{3}H-MTX, expressed in pmol per 10^9 cells; 2) 50% inhibition by MTX of the thymidylate synthase-catalysed conversion of [5-^{3}H]-2'-deoxycytidine to dTMP and ^{3}H$_2$O (tritium release assay, IC50 values expressed in µM). In vitro PRD resistance was determined using the MTT assay, expressed as concentrations lethal to 50% of the cells (LC50 values) in µg/ml. The methods of these assays have been described previously.[7,8] We previously reported that resistance to MTX can not be tested in short-term total-cell kill assays such as the MTT assay.[9,10] Statistical analyses were done using the Mann-Whitney U test and the Spearman's rank correlation test.

4. RESULTS

The extent of long-chain nor total MTX-polyglutamates differed significantly between the two groups of patient samples (Figure 1). Similarly, the IC50 values obtained in the tritium release assay did not differ between the two patient groups. However, the ratio of IC50 values for MTX for short (3 hours, followed by 18 hours drug-free incubation) over continuous 21 hours exposure, reflecting intracellular MTX retention, was median 1.9-fold unfavorably higher in the reference group (Figure 2). As can be seen in Figure 2, samples of the test group did not show unfavorably high IC50 values at short exposure nor unfavorably high ratios of short over continuous exposure. These results were similar within the immunophenotypic subgroups.

Within the test group, we studied the extent of cross-resistance between in vitro PRD resistance (MTT assay, LC50 values) and in vitro MTX resistance (MTX long-chain and total polyglutamates in pmol/10^9, tritium release assay, IC50 values in µM). There was no significant cross-resistance between these two drugs in vitro (Table).

5. DISCUSSION

We previously reported that a subgroup of children with newly diagnosed ALL that responded good clinically to systemic PRD plus intrathecal MTX, had relatively resistant ALL cells in vitro.[1] One of the explanations of this phenomenon is that the good clinical response was due to a systemic antileukemic activity of the intrathecally administered

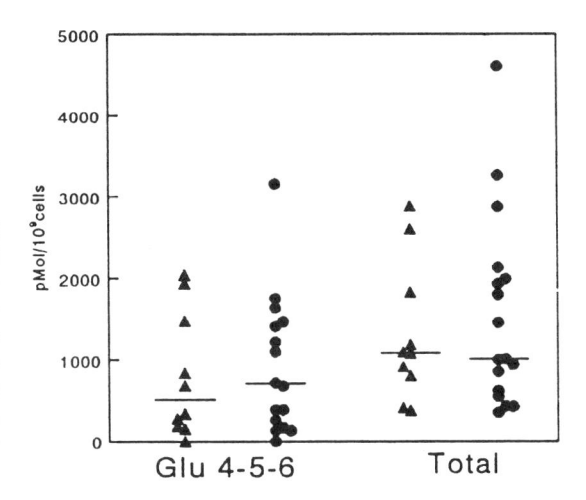

Figure 1. Comparison between clinically good responders to systemic PRD plus intrathecal MTX with in vitro PRD resistant ALL cells (triangles) and a reference group including a heterogenous group of untreated ALL patients (circles), with respect to the in situ MTX polyglutamylation: long-chain MTX-polyglutamates (Glu 4-5-6) and total MTX polyglutamylation. The lines indicate the group medians. Differences were not statistically significant.

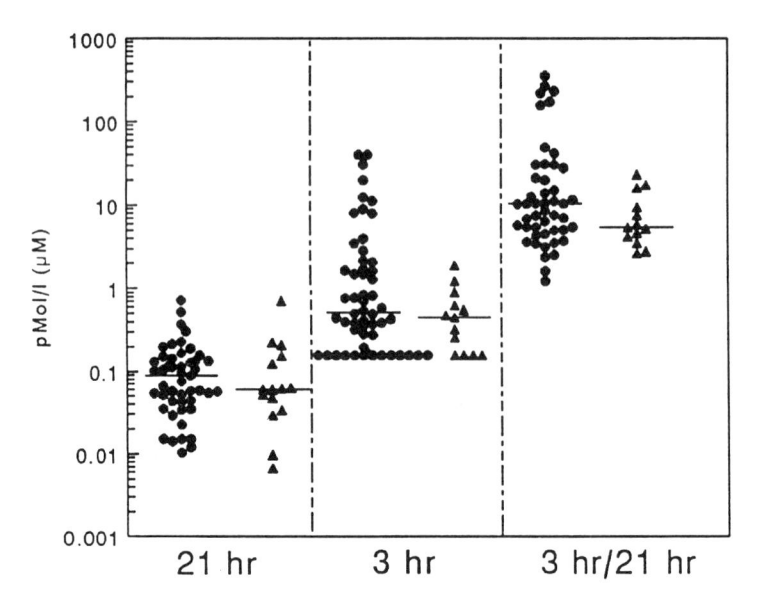

Figure 2. Comparison between clinically good responders to systemic PRD plus intrathecal MTX with in vitro PRD resistant ALL cells (triangles) and a reference group including a heterogenous group of untreated ALL patients (circles), with respect to the tritium release assay. The lines indicate group medians. Differences were not statistically significant.

MTX. Such an effect has been reported previously.[2-5] In that case, the ALL cells should be relatively sensitive to MTX. Ideally, we should have compared the extent of MTX sensitivity or resistance between clinically good and poor responders with in vitro PRD resistant ALL cells. However, the latter group comprises only 5-10% of cases, and we lacked material of these patients. Therefore, we compared the clinically good responders with in vitro PRD resistant ALL cells with a heterogenous group of newly diagnosed ALL patients. In this pilot study, we did not find a significant cross-resistance between PRD and MTX (MTX polyglutamylation and inhibition of thymidylate synthase in the tritium release assay) resistance within the clinically good responders with relatively PRD resistant ALL cells in vitro. This is in contrast to the general in vitro drug resistance that we reported previously in childhood ALL.[1] Moreover, we did not observe an increased MTX resistance in the clinically good responders with ALL cells resistant to PRD in vitro, as compared to the heterogenous group of newly diagnosed ALL patients. None of the pa-

Table 1. Lack of cross-resistance between in vitro PRD (MTT assay) and MTX (tritium release assay and MTX-polyglutamylation) resistance within children with newly diagnosed ALL that were clinically good responders to 1 week systemic PRD plus 1 injection with MTX, but with in vitro PRD resistant ALL cells

	Spearman's Rho	P-value	N
PRD LC50 vs IC50 3 hrs	0.21	0.49	13
PRD LC50 vs IC50 21 hrs	0.06	0.83	15
PRD LC50 vs MTX-Glu4-6	-0.52	0.12	10
PRD LC50 vs MTX-Glu(total)	-0.46	0.18	10

tients of the former group had unfavorably high IC50 values for MTX in the tritium release assays. Therefore, the good clinical response to systemic PRD plus intrathecal MTX in patients with in vitro PRD resistant ALL cells might indeed be explained by sensitivity to a systemic antileukemic effect of intrathecal MTX. This finding also suggests that the combination of PRD and MTX systematically is of clinical benefit to ALL patients, and lacks cross-resistance.

ACKNOWLEDGMENTS

This study was financially supported by the Dutch Cancer Society (VU 89-06 and 95-679).

REFERENCES

1. Kaspers GJL, Pieters R, Van Zantwijk CH, Van Wering ER, Van Der Does-Van Den Berg A, Veerman AJP. Prednisolone resistance in childhood acute lymphoblastic leukemia: vitro-vivo correlations and cross-resistance to other drugs. Blood 1998, 92: 259–266
2. Bleyer WA, Dedrick RL. Clinical pharmacology of intrathecal methotrexate: I. Pharmacokinetics in nontoxic patients after lumbar injection. Cancer Treatm Rep 1977, 61: 703–708
3. Jacobs SA, Bleyer WA, Chabner BA, Johns DG. Altered plasma pharmacokinetics of methotrexate administered intrathecally. Lancet 1975, 1: 465–466
4. Simmons ED, Somberg KA. Acute tumor lysis syndrome after intrathecal methotrexate administration. Cancer 1991, 67: 2062–2065
5. Thyss A, Suciu S, Bertrand Y, et al. Systemic effect of intrathecal methotrexate during the initial phase of treatment of childhood acute lymphoblastic leukemia. J Clin Oncol 1997, 15: 1824–1830
6. Kaspers GJL, Veerman AJP, Pieters R, Broekema GJ, Huismans DR, Kazemier KM, Loonen AH, Rottier MMA, Van Zantwijk CH, Hählen K, Van Wering ER. Mononuclear cells contaminating leukaemic samples tested for cellular drug resistance using the methyl-thiazol-tetrazolium assay. Br J Cancer 1994, 70: 1047–1052
7. Kaspers GJL, Veerman AJP, Pieters R, Van Zantwijk CH, Smets LA, Van Wering ER, Van Der Does-Van Den Berg A. In vitro cellular drug resistance and prognosis in childhood acute lymphoblastic leukemia. Blood 1997, 90: 2723–2729
8. Rots MG, Pieters R, Van Zantwijk CH, Veerman AJP, Noordhuis P, Peters GJ, Jansen G. Mechanisms of methotrexate resistance and its circumvention by novel antifolates in childhood leukemia. In: Chemistry and Biology of Pteridines and Folates. Pfleiderer W and Rokos H (editors). Blackwell Science, Berlin 1997: 175–180
9. Kaspers GJL, Pieters R, Van Zantwijk CH, De Laat PAJM, De Waal FC, Van Wering ER, Veerman AJP. In vitro drug sensitivity of normal peripheral blood lymphocytes and childhood leukaemic cells from bone marrow and peripheral blood. Br J Cancer 1991, 64: 469–474
10. Pieters R, Loonen AH, Huismans DR, Broekema GJ, Dirven MWJ, Heyenbrok MW, Hählen K, Veerman AJP. In vitro sensitivity of cells from children with leukemia using the MTT assay with improved culture conditions. Blood 1990, 76: 2327–2336

NEW DEVELOPMENTS IN THE TREATMENT OF ACUTE MYELOID LEUKEMIA

Mariëlle Smeets,* Theo de Witte, Netty van der Lely, Reinier Raymakers, and Petra Muus

University Hospital St. Radboud
Nijmegen, The Netherlands

Keywords: acute myeloid leukemia, anthracyclines, cytarabine, drug resistance, growth factors.

ABSTRACT

Remission induction therapy fails in 20–30% of the patients with acute myeloid leukemia (AML) despite dose intensification and the use of new and more effective drugs. Primary and acquired drug resistance, metabolic or kinetic are a fundamental problem. Expression of the P-glycoprotein in AML is correlated with therapeutic outcome. Randomized clinical studies with Pgp modulators are currently on-going. Ara-C and anthracyclines, are preferentially cytotoxic to proliferating cells. Proliferation induction of leukemia blasts with growth factors in vitro resulted in an increased toxicity of Ara-C and anthracyclines. Normal hematopoietic blast cells with a high Pgp expression are noncycling and less sensitive to anthracyclines, in contrast to the more proliferating cells with a low Pgp expression. Proliferation induction by growth factors results in a down regulation of Pgp expression. Priming of leukemic cells with growth factors in vivo might be promising and randomized clinical studies are warranted.

TREATMENT OF AML

Combination chemotherapy with standard dose anthracyclines and Cytarabine (Ara-C) given as remission induction therapy of de-novo untreated acute myeloid leukemia (AML) results in remission rates of 55% to 70% and possible cure rates of 25% to 30%.[1]

---

*Correspondence to: Mariëlle Smeets, Division of Hematology, University Hospital Nijmegen, PO Box 9101, 6500 HB Nijmegen, The Netherlands Telephone: 024-3614762; Fax: 024-3542080

Drug Resistance in Leukemia and Lymphoma III, edited by Kaspers *et al.*
Kluwer Academic / Plenum Publishers, New York, 1999.

Standard remission induction therapy resulted in a complete remission (CR) rate of 66% in the EORTC AML-8 trial. Twenty-five per cent of the patients showed a partial response, absolute resistance or leukemia regrowth after two courses of remission induction therapy.[2] The mechanisms which lead to treatment failure may be either selection or induction of leukemia clonogenic cells with metabolic drug resistance or escape of malignant stem cells from cytotoxic therapy due to their non-cycling status. Ara-C and anthracyclines are preferentially cytotoxic to proliferating cells.

CYTARABINE

Ara-C is a potent antileukemic drug. Its cytotoxic effect is mainly determined by the intracellular synthesis and retention of Ara-C triphosphate (Ara-CTP). In conventional dosage Ara-C acts primarily as an antimetabolite. When given in higher dosages, Ara-C may saturate the capacity of Ara-C inactivating enzymes, and prolong exposure of the leukemia cells to the active intracellular metabolite Ara-C-triphosphate. These effects may augment the inhibition of DNA synthesis further and overcome cellular resistance to standard dose Ara-C.[3] Uncontrolled studies of patients with previously untreated de-novo AML have reported CR rates of 50% to 81%.[4-5] A prospective randomized study of the Southwest Oncology Group compared high-dose Ara-C (HDAC) with daunorubicine (DNR) with standard-dose Ara-C (SDAC) with DNR for remission-induction of 723 previously untreated patients with AML.[6] The CR rate was slightly poorer with HDAC: 55% versus 58% with SDAC for patients aged less than 50, and 45% (HDAC) versus 53% (SDAC) for patients aged 50 to 64 years. Induction with HDAC was associated with a significantly increased risk of fatal (p = .003) and neurologic toxicity (p <.0001). A smaller randomized trial of 302 patients by the Australian Leukemia Study Group reported no change in remission rate, but an improved remission duration (36.9 versus 12.7 months).[7] Patients received either HDAC at $3g/m^2$ every 12 hours for eight doses, plus DNR at 50 mg/m^2 on days 1 to 3, and etoposide at 75 mg/m^2 on days 1 to 7 or a SDAC regimen of 100 mg/m^2/day for seven consecutive days with identical dosages of DNR and etoposide.

ANTHRACYCLINES

Since the introduction of anthracyclines in the treatment of AML the prognosis of patients with AML has improved markedly. Their cytotoxic effects have been attributed to the generation of reactive free radicals causing DNA strand scission, lipid peroxidation, and disruption of cell membrane functions and integrity. Intercalation of anthracyclines into DNA responsible for the inhibition of RNA and/or DNA synthesis is the most important mechanism. Additional interference and binding with topoisomerase II has also been proposed as a mechanism of cytotoxic action.[8]

Modification of the schedule and dose intensification improved the efficacy, but increased toxicity. Prolonged intravenous infusion of anthracyclines at adequate dose levels exposes leukemia cells longer to cytostatic drug, resulting in higher intracellular levels and avoiding excessive, potentially cardiotoxic, peak levels. The efficacy of continuous, longer interspaced administration of DNR in combination with standard dose Ara-C was established in 21 patients with relapsed primary AML or secondary AML. Twelve (57%) of the patients attained a complete or partial remission.[9] New drugs may offer additional improvement of treatment with respect to toxicity and/or efficacy of anthracyclines. The new anthracycline analogue 4-Demethoxydaunorubicin (Idarubicin: IDA) seems to be an especially interesting anthracycline, since the minor alteration at position 4 of the chromophore ring results in a prolonged half-life of the hydroxy derivative (idarubicinol), with more rapid cellular uptake, and more DNA single strand breaks in tumor cells. Idarubicinol has cytotoxic activity and thus both the parent drug and metabolite are active while daunorubicinol is an inactive compound. In view of the prolonged half-life of idarubicinol, the major metabolite if IDA, IDA may be administered on days 1, 3 and 5 instead of days 1–3. A randomized study performed by the Memorial Sloan Kettering Cancer Center in AML, comparing IDA to DNR in combination with standard dose Ara-C, has resulted in a significantly higher CR rate (80% vs 58%).[10] Two additional similar studies comparing IDA with DNR in standard dose remission-induction schedules of untreated patients with AML resulted in superior results for the IDA containing schedules.[11–12]

MULTI DRUG RESISTANCE

Drug resistance is related to overexpression of the MDR1-gene and production of a 170 Kd membrane-associated P-glycoprotein (P-gp).[13] P-gp expression in leukemic blasts of newly diagnosed and relapsed patients is closely related to clinical resistance.[14] Clinical importance of other resistance phenotypes such as the expression of the MRP and LRP proteins is currently investigated.

Pgp functions as an energy dependent efflux pump which transports many structurally unrelated compounds like vinca alkaloids, taxols, actinomycin D, epipodophyllotoxins, mitoxantrone and anthracyclines (Ling et al, 1992). Several agents, e.g. verapamil or ciclosporin A(CsA) are effective modulators of this efflux pump in vitro, probably by competitive binding to P-gp.[15–16] The cytotoxicity of Idarubicin appeared to be less dependent on P-glycoprotein expression.[17] Clinical pilot studies with CsA showed interesting results in poor-risk AML. Overall 69% of 42 patients with poor-risk AML achieved complete or partial remission after treatment with DNR and high dose Cytarabine in combination with CsA.[18] However, randomized studies are warranted.

Pgp is not only present on malignant cells, but also on peripheral blood cells (fractions of T and B cells) and on hematopoietic progenitor cells.[19–20] Several studies showed that the rhodamine efflux assay is also a sensitive method to study MDR-1 expression. Rhodamine retention has also been used to isolate pluripotent hematopoietic stem cells (HSC). Rhodamine uptake is minimal in HSC residing in the quiescent phases of the cell cycle (G0/G1). Chaudhary et al showed by double staining with rhodamine and MRK16, an inverse correlation between rhodamine retention and Pgp expression on normal human bone marrow cells. A low rhodamine retention corresponded also with a high CD34 expression and high clonogenic capacity of these cells.[21] The more rhodamine bright cells represent the more proliferating and more mature HSC. Rhodamine retention in HSC reflects Pgp expression rather than the mitochondrial content of the cells.

We have shown previously that within normal CD34+ a distinct subpopulation of 20–25% has a low rhodamine retention, which shows an increase in rhodamine retention in the presence of verapamil (Figure 1).[21] Sorting this rhodamine dull subfraction and the most rhodamine bright cells revealed that the rhodamine dull HSC were predominantly noncycling cells (S/G$_2$+M=4.5 ± 2.2%), whereas the rhodamine bright cells were more proliferating cells (S/G$_2$+M=21.5 ± 4.4%). In a clonogenic assay, these noncycling rhodamine dull cells were less sensitive to anthracycline toxicity compared to the rhodamine bright cells (Figure 2) In accordance with the high Pgp expression of the rhodamine dull

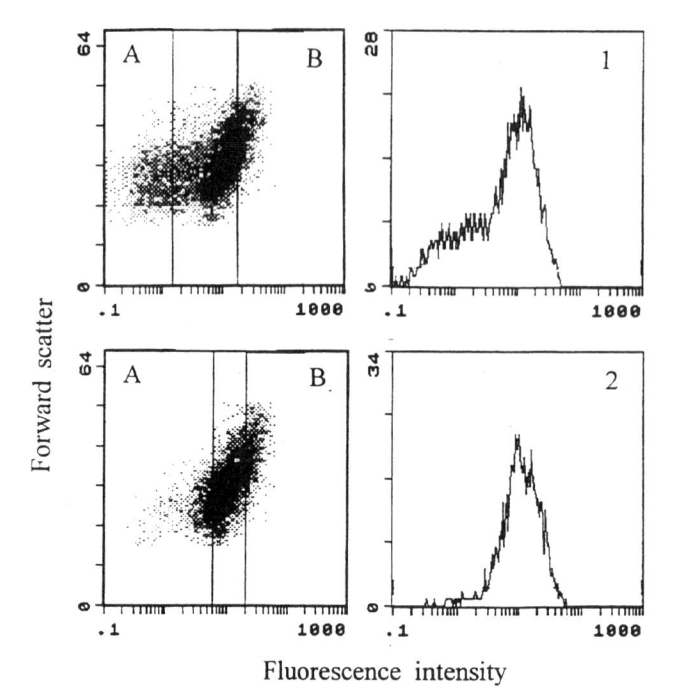

Figure 1. Rhodamine content of normal CD34+ cells after 2 hours efflux in dye free medium without (1) and with (2) verapamil. Sorting experiments were performed according to the gate setting A (25% of the most rhodamine dull cells) and B (25% of the most rhodamine bright cells).

cells, verapamil increased anthacycline toxicity only in the rhodamine dull HSC and not in the rhodamine bright cells (Figure 3).

HEMATOPOIETIC GROWTH FACTORS AND DRUG RESISTANCE

It is generally accepted that escape of quiescent malignant clonogenic cells from cytotoxic therapy might be an important mechanism for *in vivo* drug resistance. Hematopoietic growth factors (HGF) may induce proliferation of leukemia cells *in vitro* and presumably also *in vivo*. A higher proliferation may result in an increased sensitivity to cytostatic therapy. Prolongation of the Ara-C exposure time in vitro in the presence of a cocktail of HGF (GM-CSF, G-CSF and IL-3) from 5 to 10 days increased the cytotoxicity towards leukemia progenitor cells (CFU-L) (ID50: $0.8 \pm 0.6 \times 10^{-8}$M) but not towards normal CFU-GM (ID50: $5.7 \pm 2.8 \times 10^{-8}$M).[22] Significantly more CFU-L than normal CFU-GM were killed after 10 days of exposure to Ara-C in the presence of the cocktail of HGF (p = 0.04). These results indicated that leukemic clonogenic cells can be eradicated preferentially by prolonged exposure to low dosages of Ara-C in the presence of growth factors.[23]

A new in vitro iodeoxyuridine (IdUrd) labelling technique was developed to study whether HGF may influence the kinetics of CFU-L and their sensitivity to Ara-C. The median percentage of cycling CFU-L increased significantly (p = 0.009) from 8.5% without growth factors to 87.5% with growth factors. The relative percentage of IdUrd positive CFU-L (cycling CFU-L) decreased with increasing concentrations of Ara-C. Proliferation induction of leukemia blast resulted in a lower Ara-C ID50 (Table 1).[24]

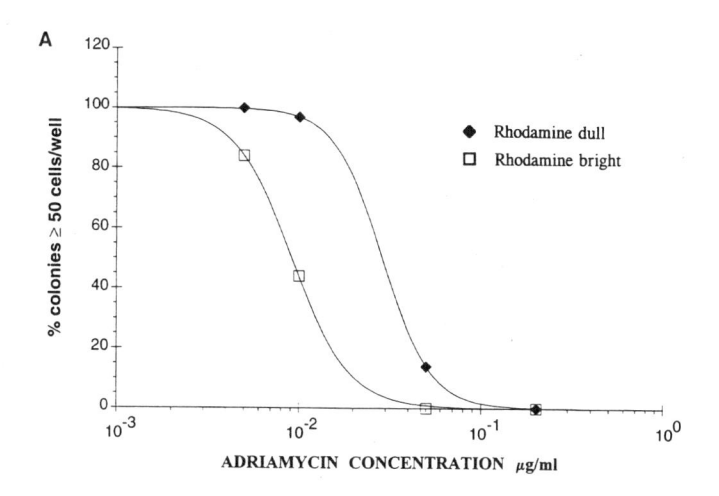

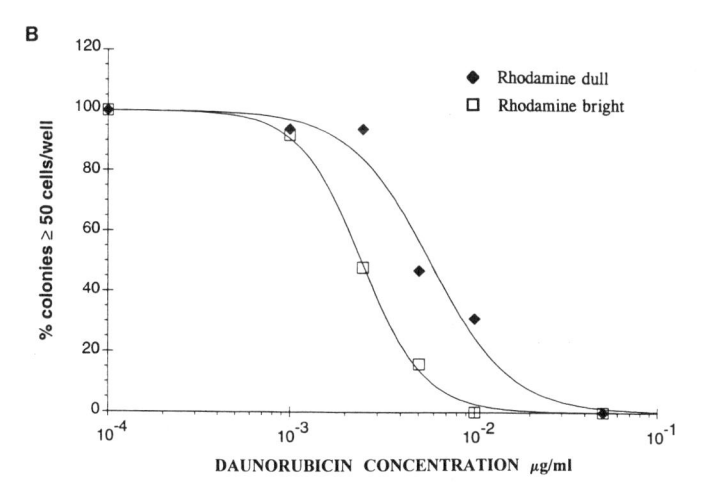

New Developments in the Treatment of Acute Myeloid Leukemia

Figure 2. Dose response curve of adriamycine (A) and daunorubicin (B), expressed as the % colonies (>50 cells/well) of the control. The ID50 values for rhodamine dull CD34+ cells is 0.03 µg/ml and for rhodamine bright cells 0.01 µg/ml. The ID50 values of daunorubicin are respectively 0.005 µg/ml and 0.0025 µg/ml.

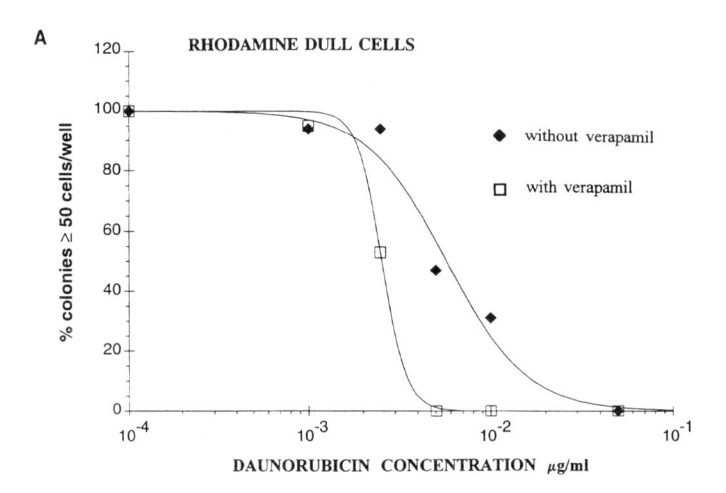

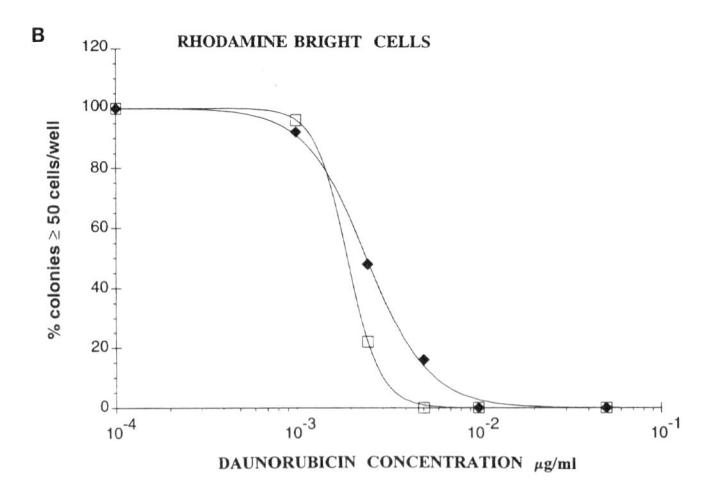

Figure 3. Dose response curve of daunorubicin for rhodamine dull (A) and bright (B) CD34+ cells without and with 10 μM verapamil (corrected for the mean intrinsic toxicity of verapamil <10%). A significant (p< 0.04) modulation of toxicity was measured only in the rhodamine dull cells.

Table 1. Ara-C sensitivity for IdUrd+ and IdUrd- clonogenic leukemic cells

Patient no.	Added factor[b]	Ara-C ID$_{50}$ × 10^{-8} M[a]		
		Overall	IdUrd	IdUrd⁻
1	GM-CSF	19.1	7.2	140
2	IL-3, GM-CSF+ G-CSF	4.6	3.5	>10
5	GM-CSF+ G-CSF	0.6	0.3	0.9
6	GM-CSF	0.6	0.4	>10

[a] Ara-C concentration that inhibited 50% of the CFU-L growth. The values were calculated from survival curves constructed after 3-days exposure to various concentrations of Ara-C.
[b] Growth factors added to liquid culture.

Preliminary results showed that induction of proliferation of AML blasts by granulocyte/macrophage colony-stimulating factor (GM-CSF) increased the cytotoxicity of DNR and adriamycin. cells. In contrast, idarubicin toxicity was not increased after incubation with GM-CSF.[25] Since noncycling rhodamine dull normal blasts are protected to anthracycline toxicity by a relatively high Pgp expression in contrast to the proliferating and more sensitive rhodamine bright blast, a down-regulation of MDR expression by triggering blast cells into cell cycle is suggested.

In most prospective randomized studies comparing G-CSF or GM-CSF with placebo the growth factor has been administered during and after chemotherapy or only after chemotherapy. This may obscure the positive contribution of the increased sensitivity of faster proliferating leukemic cells to cytostatic therapy, since HGF may stimulate leukemic growth and shorted the duration of neutropenia. Two studies described a higher CR rate which could be contributed to a lower leukemic resistance in one of these studies. The EORCT Leukemia Co-operative Group conducted a prospective, factorial 2 × 2 design, study comparing GM-CSF during and/or after chemotherapy with placebo in patients with untreated AML. The CR rate was significantly lower in patients who received GM-CSF after chemotherapy when compared to the control groups. The CR rate was not different whether or not the patients received GM-CSF during chemotherapy (Table 2).[26–31] The effects of growth factors on proliferation induction of leukemic blasts have not been reported in these studies. Moreover, sensitivity of leukemic blasts is different for G-CSF and GM-CSF. Randomized studies are necessary to analyze the effect of selective priming of leukemic blasts with growth factors on the outcome of remission induction regimen.

Table 2. G-CSF or GM-CSF during and/or after remission-induction of AML

	HGF	During/after	Number HGF/control	CR (%)
Ohno 1990	G-CSF	+/+	108	50/36
Stone 1995	GM-CSF	-/+	347	49/53
Dombret 1995	G-CSF	-/+	173	70/47*
Rowe 1995	GM-CSF	-/+	118	61/46
Zittoun 1996	GM-CSF	-/+	102	47/74
Zittoun 1996	GM-CSF	+/+	102	NS

*: $p < .05$

REFERENCES

1. Bennett, J.M., Andersen, J.W., Cassileth, P. (1991) Long term survival in acute myeloid leukemia: the Eastern Oncology group experience (ECOG). *Leukemia Research*, **15**, 223–7.
2. Zittoun, R.A., Mandelli ,F., Willemze, R., De Witte, T., Labar, B., Resegotti, L., Damasio, E,., Visani, G. Papa, G. (1995) The European Organisation for Research and Treatment of Cancer (EORTC) and the Gruppo Italiano Malattie Ematologiche Maligne dell'Adulto (GIMEMA) Leukemia Co-operative Groups. Autologous or allogeneic bone marrow transplantation compared with intensive chemotherapy in acute myelogenous leukemia. *New England Journal of Medicine*, **332**, 217–23.
3. Vogler, W.R., McCarley, D.I., Stagg, M., Bartolucci, A.A., Moore, J., Martelo, O., Omura, G.A. (1994) A phase III trial of high-dose cytosine arabinoside with or without etoposide in relapsed and refractory acute myelogenous leukemia. A Southeastern Cancer Study Group trial. *Leukemia*, **8**, 1847–53.
4. Phillips, G.L., Reece, D.E., Shepherd, J.D. (1991) High dose cytarabine and daunorubicin induction and postremission chemotherapy for the treatment of acute myelogenous leukemia in adults. *Blood*, **77**, 1429–35.
5. Harousseau, J.L., Milpied, N., Briere, J., Desablens, B., Leprise, P.Y., Ifrah, N., Gandhour, B., Casassus, P. (1991) Double intensive consolidation chemotherapy in adult acute myeloid leukemia. *Seminars of Hematology*, **28**, 80–3.
6. Weick, J.K., Kopecky, K.J., Appelbaum, F.R., Head, D.R., Kingsbury, L.L., Balcerzak, S.P., Bickers, J.N., Hynes, H.E., Welborn, J.L., Simon, S.R., Grever (1996) M. A randomized investigation of high-dose versus standard-dose cytosine arabinoside with daunorubicin in patients with previously untreated acute myeloid leukemia: a Southwest Oncology Group study. *Blood*, **88**, 2841–51.
7. Bishop, J.F., Young, G.A., Szer ,J., Matthew, J.P., Page, A. (1992) Randomized trial of high dose cytosine arabiniside (ARA-C) combination in induction of acute myeloid leukemia (AML). *Proceedings of the American Society of Clinical Oncology*, **11**, A849.
8. Sinha, B.K. and Politi, P.M. (1990) Anthracyclines. *Cancer Chemotherapy and Biological Response Modifiers*, **11**, 45–57.
9. Bär, B., De Witte, T., De Pauw, B.E., Haanen, C. (1990) Continuous intravenous administration of daunorubicin and Cytarabine for remission induction therapy of poor risk acute myelogenous leukemia and myelodysplastic syndromes. *Netherlands Journal of Medicine*, **36**, 19–24.
10. Berman, E., Heller, G., Santorsa, J.(1991) Results of a randomized trial comparing idarubicin and cytosine arabinoside with daunorubicin and cytosine arabinoside in adult patients with newly diagnosed acute myelogenous leukemia. *Blood*, **77**, 1666–74.
11. Vogler, W.R., Velez-Garcia, E., Weiner,R.S., Flaum, M.A., Bartolucci, A.A., Omura, G.A., Gerber, M.C., Banks, P.L. (1992) A phase III trial comparing idarubicin and daunorubicin in combination with Cytarabine in acute myelogenous leukemia: a Southeastern Cancer Study Group study. *Journal of Clinical Oncology*, **10**, 1103–11
12. Wiernik ,P.H., Banks, P.L.C., Case., D.C.,Jr., Arlin, Z.A., Periman, P.O., Toda, M.B., Ritch, P.S., Enk, R.E., Weitberg, A.B. (1992) Cytarabine plus idarubicin or daunorubicin as induction and consolidation therapy for previously untreated adult patients with acute myeloid leukemia. *Blood*, **79**, 313–9.
13. Ueda, K., Cornwell, M.M., Gottesman, M.M., Pastan, I. Roninson, I.B., Ling, V., Riordan, J.R. (1986) The mdr1 gene, responsible for multidrug-resistance, codes for P-glycoprotein. *Biochemical and Biophysical Research Communications*, **141**, 956–62.
14. Hunault, M., Zhou, D., Delmer, A., Ramond, S., Viguie, F., Cadiou, M., Perrot, J.Y., Levy, V., Rio, B., Cymbalista, F., Zittoun, R., and Marie, J.P. (1997) Multidrug resistance gene expression in acute myeloid leukemia: major prognosis significance for in vivo drug resistance to induction treatment. *Annals of Hematology.* **74**, 65–71.
15. List, A.F. (1996) Role of multidrug resistance and its pharmacological modulation in acute myeloid leukemia. *Leukemia*, **10**, 937–42.
16. Malayeri, R., Filipits, M., Suchomel, R.W., Zochbauer, S., Lechner, K., and Pirker, R. (1996) Multidrug resistance in leukemias and its reversal. *Leukemia and Lymphoma*, **23**, 451–458.
17. Berman, E. and McBride, M., (1992) Comparative cellular pharmacology of daunorubicin and idarubicin in human multidrug-resistant leukemia cells. *Blood*, **79**, 3267–73.
18. List, A.F., Spier, C., Green, J. (1992) Biochemical modulation of anthracycline resistance (MDR) in acute leukaemia with Cyclosporin A. *Proceedings American Soc Clin. Oncology.* **11**, 264a.
19. Chaudhary, P.M., Mechetner, E.B. and Roninson, I.B. (1992) Expression and activity of the multidrug resistance P-glycoprotein in human peripheral blood lymphocytes. *Blood*, **80**, 2735–9.

20. Chaudhary, P.M. and Roninson, I.B. (1991) expression and activity of P-glycoprotein, a multidrug efflux pump, in human hematopietic stem cells. *Cell*, **66**, 85–94.
21. Smeets, M., Raymakers, R., Vierwinden, G., Pennings, A., van de Locht, L., Wessels, H., Boezeman, J., and de Witte, T (1997) A low but functionally significant MDR1 expression protects primitive haemopoietic progenitor cells from anthracycline toxicity. *British Journal of Haematology*, **96**, 346–55.
22. Van Der Lely. N., De Witte, T., Muus, P., Raymakers, R., Preijers, P., Haanen, C. (1991) Prolonged exposure to cytosine arabinoside in the presence of hematopoietic growth factors preferentially kills leukemia versus normal clonogeneic cells. *Experimental Hematology*, **19**, 267–72.
23. Van Der Lely, N., Minderman, H., Wessels, J., Hillegers, M., Linssen, P., Pennings, A., Brons, P., Boezeman, J., De Witte, T. (1995) Detection of incorporated iodeoxyuridine in colonies by immunoperoxidase staining: a novel method to measure the proportion of cycling colony-forming cells. *Experimental Hematology*; **23**, 236–43.
24. Van Der Lely, N., Raymakers, R., Boezeman, J., De Witte, T. Hematopoietic growth factors increase the fraction of cycling leukemia clonogenic cells and reduce the kinetic resistance to cytosine arabinoside in vitro. (submitted)
25. Minderman, H., Linssen, P., Van der Lely, N., Wessels, J., Boezeman, J. de Witte, T. and Haanen, C. (1994) Toxicity of idarubicin and doxorubicin towards normal and leukemic human bone marrow progenitors in relation to their proliferative state. *Leukemia*, **8**, 382–7.
26. Ohno, R., Naoe, T., Kanamaru, A., Hiraoka, A., Kobayashi, T., Ueda, T., Minami, S., Morishima, Y., Saito, Y., Furusawa, S., Imai, K., Takemoto, Y., Miura, Y., Teshima, H., Hamajima, N., Kosheisho Leukemia Study group. (1994) A double-blind controlled study of granulocyte-colony stimulating factor started two before chemotherapy in refractory acute myeloid leukemia. *Blood*, **83**, 2086–92.
27. Rowe, J.M., Andersen, J.W., Mazza,J.J., Bennett, J.M., Pacetta, E., Hayes, F.A., Oette, D., Casseleth, P.A., Staatmaier, E.A., Wiernik, P.H. (1995) A randomized placebo-controlled phase III study of granulocyte-macrophage colony-stimulating factor in adult patients (>55 to 70 years of age) with acute myelogenous leukemia (AML). A study of the Eastern Cooperative Oncology Group (E1490). *Blood*, **86**, 457–62.
28. Stone, R.M,, Berg ,D.T, George, S.L., Dodge, R.K., Paciucci, P.A., Schulman, P., Lee, E.J., Moore, J.O., Powel, B.L., Schiffer, C.A. (1995) Granulocyte-macrophage colony-stimulating factor after initial chemotherapy for elderly patients with primary acute myelogenous leukemia. *New England Journal of Medicine*, **332**, 1671–7.
29. Dombret, H., Chastang, C., Fenaux, P., Reiffers, J., Bordessoule, D., Bouabdallah, R., Mandelli, F., Ferrant, A., Auzanneau, G., Tilly, H., Yver, A., Degosl, (1995). A controlled study of recombinant human granulocyte colony-stimulating factor in elderly patients after treatment for acute myelogenous leukemia. *New England Journal of Medicine*, **332**, 1678–83.
30. Löwenberg, B., Touw, I.T. (1993) Hematopoietic growth factors and their receptors in acute leukemia. *Blood*, **81**, 281–92.
31. Zittoun, R., Suciu ,S., Mandelli, F., de Witte, T., Thaler, J., Stryckmans, P., Hayat, M., Peetermans, M., Cadiou, M., Solbu, G., Pette, M.C., Willemze, R.(1996) Granulocyte-macrophage stimulating factor (molgramostim) associated to induction treatment of acute myelogenous leukemia. A randomized trial of the EORTC and GIMEMA Leukemia Cooperative Groups. *Journal of Clinical Oncology*, **7**, 2150–9.

62

APHIDICOLIN MARKEDLY INCREASES THE *IN VITRO* SENSITIVITY TO ARA-C OF BLAST CELLS FROM PATIENTS WITH AML

J.M. Sargent, A.W. Elgie, C.J. Williamson, and C.G. Taylor

Haematology Research
Pembury Hospital
Pembury, Kent, TN2 4QJ, United Kingdom

Keywords: ara-C, aphidicolin, AML, drug resistance, DNA repair.

1. ABSTRACT

Drug resistant cells often have an increased capacity to repair their DNA after damage by cytotoxic agents. Aphidicolin can inhibit this DNA repair. We describe a study of the effect of aphidicolin to modulate the sensitivity to cytotoxic drugs of blast cells from 13 patients with AML, 11 with *de novo* disease on presentation and 2 secondary to MDS. Three patients had relapsed following previous therapy and samples were received from 1 patient both on presentation and relapse. Blast cells were exposed to anthracyclines, antimetabolites or etoposide ± aphidicolin (15μM) for 48 hours. The MTT assay was used to measure cell survival and the LC_{50} (concentration of drug required for 50% cell kill) was calculated. Overall, there was a significant increase in sensitivity to ara-C on co-incubation with aphidicolin in 12/14 samples (p = 0.007). The median increase in sensitivity was 3.88-fold (range 1.26- to 80-fold). Interestingly, when patients were grouped according to *in vitro* sensitivity to ara-C, cells from resistant patients demonstrated the greatest increase in sensitivity (median 14-fold compared to 2-fold for the sensitive group, p = 0.02). Despite the documented evidence for altered DNA repair as a mechanism of resistance to the topoisomerase II inhibitors, we found no significant increase in sensitivity to daunorubicin, doxorubicin or etoposide on co-incubation with aphidicolin. Nevertheless, we believe the unparalleled modulation of ara-C warrants further investigation.

2. INTRODUCTION

Whilst prognosis has improved considerably in childhood ALL, this is not the case in adult AML and drug resistance remains a major reason for the failure of chemotherapy. Whilst initial remission induction rates are around 70–80%, most patients will relapse early and only <25% can expect to have a sustained long term survival.

These patients are usually treated with combination chemotherapy which almost invariably includes cytosine arabinoside (ara-C). Using chemosensitivity testing, we, and others, have shown that it is the *in vitro* sensitivity of the anthracycline in the combination that most often predicts response to treatment.[1] Initial resistance to ara-C, however, has been shown to correlate with early relapse in this disease.[2]

Resistance to ara-C can be conferred by many different mechanisms including alteration of DNA repair.[3 for review] Aphidicolin is an inhibitor of the DNA polymerases involved in this repair mechanism and the glycinate ester of aphidicolin has entered clinical trials where limited toxicity was seen.[4] However, the anti-tumour effect was minimal and combination studies with cisplatin were suggested. These clinical trials were never completed and therefore the true worth of this compound has never been established.

We have previously shown aphidicolin markedly increased the *in vitro* sensitivity of platinum drugs using cells from patients with ovarian cancer[5] and we have extended this study of inhibition of DNA repair to the blast cells from patients with AML.

3. MATERIALS AND METHODS

3.1. Patients

Fourteen samples, 7 bone marrows and 7 peripheral blood, were collected from 13 patients with AML. Eleven patients had *de novo* disease, 8 on first presentation and 3 on relapse following previous cytotoxic therapy. Two patients were secondary to MDS. Two samples were taken from one patient, on presentation and relapse.

3.2. Cell Preparation and Drug Exposure

Blast cells were separated using density gradient centrifugation and a cell suspension in RPMI 1640 plus 10% FCS and antibiotics was prepared. There were >80% blast cells in these final preparations as measured by May Grünwald Giemsa staining. Blast cells were exposed, in triplicate, in a microtitre plate to 4 concentrations of drugs ± aphidicolin at a fixed dose of 15µM for 48 hours at 37°C, 5% CO_2. Drugs included daunorubicin (DNR), doxorubicin (DOX), ara-C and etoposide. Experiments were controlled by cells incubated in medium ± aphidicolin.

3.3. MTT Assay

Drug exposure was followed by removal of the medium plus drug and a further 4 hour incubation in 2mg/ml MTT.[6] Acid/alcohol (0.04N HCl in isopropanol) was used to dissolve any formazan crystals and the plate was read at 570nm (reference 690nm). The LC_{50} (concentration required to kill 50% of the cells) was calculated for each experiment. The sensitivity ratio of the LC_{50} of drug over that for drug + aphidicolin gave a measure of any modulation effect.

3.4. Statistics

Non-parametric methods were employed. Wilcoxon signed rank test was used to compare paired data. Mann Whitney U test was used to compare groups of patients.

4. RESULTS

4.1. Chemosensitivity

When drugs were tested as single agents, there was a marked variation in their effect between patients. The LC_{50} values for ara-C ranged from 0.25–41µM, for DNR 0.09–3.9µM, for DOX 0.16–2.07µM and for etoposide 0.02–93µM. Using the criteria previously described,[6] 8 of the 14 samples tested were resistant to ara-C, 1 of 5 to DNR, 2 of 6 to DOX and 7 of 9 to etoposide.

4.2. Effect of Co-Incubation with Aphidicolin

Aphidicolin when tested alone was found to be non-cytotoxic up to 30µM. In combination with the cytotoxic drugs the greatest modulation effect was seen with ara-C (p = 0.007) with up to 80-fold increases in sensitivity and a median sensitivity ratio of 3.88 (Table 1). There was no significant increase overall in sensitivity to the topo II inhibitors on co-incubation with aphidicolin. When patients were grouped according to *in vitro* sensitivity to ara-C alone the greatest modulation effect was seen in the cells deemed resistant (median 14-fold increase in sensitivity compared to 2-fold for the sensitive group, p = 0.02).

5. DISCUSSION

We have previously demonstrated aphidicolin to be a potent inhibitor of DNA repair after cytotoxic attack in cells from patients with ovarian cancer.[5] This study confirms these results as aphidicolin showed a similar, marked, modulatory effect on *in vitro* sensitivity to ara-C. Up to 80-fold increases in sensitivity were seen. Furthermore, the greatest modulatory effects were seen in resistant cells agreeing with the theory that these cells often have an increased capacity to repair their damaged DNA.

As both aphidicolin and ara-C have been shown to inhibit DNA polymerases this questions the mode of action of this synergistic effect. Resistance to ara-C is normally attributed to alterations in the enzymes that influence the conversion of ara-C to ara-CTP. Our results suggest that either aphidicolin modulates the rate of intracellular accumulation

Table 1. Evidence for resistance modulation by aphidicolin

Drug	Number tested	Median LC_{50} µM	Median LC_{50} µM +aph	Increased cytotoxicity (n)	SR median	SR range
ara-C	14	5.02	0.92*	12	3.88	1.26-80
DOX	6	0.83	0.82	1	1.07	0.89-9.0
DNR	5	0.89	0.62	3	1.38	0.71-4.15
Etop	9	50.9	47.6	1	1.11	0.33-1.75

*p=0.007 SR: sensitivity ratio

of ara-CTP or, aphidicolin and ara-C inhibit DNA repair by different mechanisms. Mirzayans et al., using proliferating human fibroblasts, showed that the former did not appear to be the case [7]. Indeed, there is some evidence to suggest that ara-C may inhibit DNA polymerases indirectly by terminating DNA chain elongation and so preventing the addition of nucleotides whereas aphidicolin directly affects the enzymes themselves.[8]

We found limited modulation on combining aphidicolin with the the anthracyclines and this may be explained by the fact that very few samples from this group of patients were resistant *in vitro* to these drugs. Because increased capacity for modulation was found in cells resistant to ara-C, it may well be aphidicolin could show good effect in anthracycline resistant cells.

Aphidicolin did not increase the sensitivity to ara-C in every case. Indeed, 2 of the 14 samples tested had sensitivity ratios of around 1. This demonstrates the necessity to screen individual patients *in vitro* before attempting any drug resistance modulation regimens. It is possible that another mechanism of resistance to ara-C is evident in these patients.

These modulation results are the most encouraging we have ever seen after almost 10 years in the field and we believe they support the further development of this extremely interesting compound.

ACKNOWLEDGMENTS

This study was supported by the EB Hutchinson Trust and the Kent Leukaemia and Cancer Equipment Fund to whom we are extremely grateful.

REFERENCES

1. Sargent JM, Elgie AW, Taylor CG, Faulkner Pulsford J. Resistance patterns of anthracycline analogues in acute myeloid leukemia using the MTT assay. In: Kaspers G et al. (eds), Drug resistance in leukemia and lymphoma: the clinical value of laboratory studies, 1993, Harwood Academic, London, 285–291.
2. Klumper E, Ossenkoppele GJ, Pieters R, Huismans DR, Loonen AH, Rottier A, Westra G, Veerman AJP. *In vitro* resistance to cytosine arabinoside, not to daunorubicin, is associated with the risk of relapse in *de novo* acute myeloid leukaemia. Br J Haematol, 1996, 93, 903–910.
3. Peters GJ, Jansen G. Resistance to antimetabolites. In: Schilsky RL et al. (eds), Principles of antineoplastic drug development and pharmacology, 1996, Marcel Dekker Inc, New York, 543–585.
4. Sessa C, Zucchetti M, Davoli E, Califano R, Cavalli F, Fristaci S, Gumbrell L, Sulkes A, Winograd B, D'Incalci M. Phase I and clinical evaluation of aphidicolin glycinate. J Natl Cancer Inst, 1991, 83, 1160–1164.
5. Sargent JM, Elgie AW, Williamson CJ, Taylor CG. Aphidicolin markedly increases the platinum sensitivity of cells from primary ovarian tumours. Br J Cancer, 1996, 74, 1730–1733.
6. Sargent JM, Taylor CG. Appraisal of the MTT assay as a rapid test of chemosensitivity in acute myeloid leukaemia. Br J Cancer, 1989, 60, 206–210.
7. Mirzayans R, Enns L, Cubitt S, Karimian K, Radatus B, Paterson MC. Effect of DNA polymerase inhibitors on repair of γ ray-induced DNA damage in proliferating (intact versus permeable) human fibroblasts: evidence for differences in the modes of action of aphidicolin and 1-β-D-arabinofuranosylcytosine. 1994, Biochim Biophys Acta 1227, 92–100.
8. Plunkett W, Gandhi V. Cellular pharmacodynamics of anticancer drugs. 1993, Sem Oncol, 20, 50–63.

63

COMMON RESISTANCE MECHANISMS TO NUCLEOSIDE ANALOGUES IN VARIANTS OF THE HUMAN ERYTHROLEUKEMIC LINE K562

Charles Dumontet,[1*] Evelyne Callet Bauchu,[1] Krystyna Fabianowska,[2] Michel Lepoivre,[3] Dorota Wyczechowska,[2] Frédérique Bodin,[1] and Marie Odile Rolland[1]

[1]Laboratoire d'Immunochimie et Service d'Hématologie
Centre Hospitalier Lyon Sud
69495 Pierre Bénite Cedex, France
[2]Department of General Chemistry
Medical Institute of Lodz
Lindleya 6
90-131 Lodz, Poland
[3]ERS CNRS 571
Institut de Biochimie
Université de Paris Sud
91405 Orsay Cedex, France

ABSTRACT

Variants of the human K562 were developed against the nucleoside analogues cytosine arabinoside, 2 chlorodeoxyadenosine, fludarabine and gemcitabine. The resistant lines displayed a high degree of cross-resistance to all nucleoside analogues, with little or no cross resistance to other agents. There was a profound accumulation defect of the different nucleoside analogues in all of the variants. There was a strong overexpression of 5' nucleotidase, measured by rt-PCR and enzyme activity, in all resistant variants. There was a two fold increase of ribonucleotide reductase in the fludarabine resistant line and increased expression of purine nucleoside phosphorylase in the 2 chlorodeoxyadenosine se-

---

[*] Correspondence should be addressed to: Charles Dumontet, Service d'Hématologie, Centre Hospitalier Lyon Sud, 69495 Pierre Bénite Cedex, France. Tel 33 4 78 86 16 79, Fax 33 4 78 86 65 66, e-mail: cd@hematologie.univ-lyon1.fr

lected line. Karyotypic analysis revealed the loss of a 6(q16;q22) deletion present in the parental line in all of the resistant lines. This portion of chromosome 6 has been shown to contain the gene for 5'nucleotidase. Early events in the transport and metabolism appear to be involved in the resistance mechanisms to nucleoside analogues and are responsible for broad cross resistance to this family of compounds.

INTRODUCTION

Nucleoside analogues constitue an important class of antimitotic drugs in the treatment of hematological malignancies (1) This family includes the pyrimidine sugar modified analogue cytosine arabinoside, and the halogenated purines 2 chlorodeoxyadenosine (cladribine) and 2-fluoroadenine-β-D-arabinoside (fludarabine). Whereas aracytine has mostly been used in acute disorders (2), fludarabine and cladribine have mostly been indicated in low grade malignancies, with an antimitotic effect on nondividing cells (3, 4). Gemcitabine is a purine analogue which has been studied in solid tumors, with some promising preliminary results in Hodgkin's disease (5).

These therapeutic compounds essentially behave like the normal nucleoside compounds in terms of uptake and metabolism and are incorporated into nucleic acids. These analogues interfere with nucleic acid synthesis, both by inhibiting the synthesis of normal nucleotides by ribonucleotide reductase and by inhibiting nucleic acid polymerization, causing "chain termination". It has been shown that these compounds penetrate the cells thanks to nucleoside transporters which are normally expressed in the cell membrane and are activated by phosphorylation. Some of these compounds (fludarabine and cladribine) are resistant to degradation by adenosine deaminase.

A number of diverse resistance mechanisms to these agents have been described in cell lines, and in a few cases analyzed in clinical samples (6, 7). There are however relatively few data on the differences in resistance mechanisms to these difference agents in the same setting. We therefore sought to determine potential mechanisms of resistance to these compounds in variants of the human erythroleukemic cell line K562, exposed for prolonged periods of time to increasing exposures of aracytine, cladribine or fludarabine or gemcitabine. Our results suggest that early events in the metabolism of these drugs are involved in the development of drug resistance.

MATERIAL AND METHODS

Cell Lines and Development of Variants

The human erythroleukemic cell line K562 was purchased from the American Type Culture Collection. Resistant variants were developed using step wise increases of concentration of either cytosine arabinoside (K/araC), 2chlorodeoxyadenosine (K/2cdA), fludarabine (K/fluda) or gemcitabine (K/gem) over a 12-month period. The Pgp expressing variant of K562, K562/R7 was generously provided by B.I. Sikic (Stanford University, Palo Alto, CA) and used as an MDR-positive control.

Reagents

Drugs used for cell selection were clinical formulation for cytarabine (Aracytine, Upjohn, Paris), fludarabine (Fludara, Scherring), cladribine (Leustatine) and gemcitabine

(Gemzar, Lilly Laboratories). Compounds used for proliferation assays included bleomycin (Roger Bellon, Neuilly-sur-Seine), cis-platin (CISPLATYL, Roger Bellon), methotrexate (Roger Bellon), carmustine (BICNU, Bristol Myers Squibb, Paris), mafosfamide (Asta Laboratories), doxorubicin (Adriblastine, Pharmacia, St Quentin). Hydroxyurea, dipyridamole, nitrobenzylthioinosine (NBMPR) and fluoro adenine arabinoside were purchased from Sigma (Saint Quentin Fallavier, France). Labelled nucleoside analogues were purchased from Moravek Biochemicals (Brea, CA) except for tritiated gemcitabine which was generously provided by Lilly Laboratories. 2–^{3}H AMP was purchased from Amersham.

Drug Accumulation Assays

Cells grown free of drug for at least three passages were washed in serum-free media and incubated as 1×10^6 aliquots in a final volume of 1 ml, with 100,000 dpm of labeled compound. All incubation assays were performed for 1 hour at 37°C unless otherwise specified. Cells were then rapidly spun down at 10,000 g, washed thrice in ice-cold PBS, and lysed. The results were determined as the dpm/mg protein ratio.

Proliferation Assays

Drug resistance phenotype was measured by determination of the inhibitory concentration 50% (IC50) in a 72 hour MTT proliferation assay. Briefly, 10 000 cells, sampled from exponential cultures, were incubated with increasing concentrations of compounds in a 96-well plate. Semi-logarithmic cell growth curves were generated using an MTT colorimetric assay, after a 1 hour incubation in the presence of MTT.

Enzyme Assays

Assays for adenosine deaminase, 5'nucleotidase, purine phosphorylase and ribonucleotide reductase were performed on lysates of cells grown free of drug for at least three passages.

RESULTS

Resistance Phenotypes

Table 1 summarizes the resistance phenotype of the resistant variants K/araC, K/2cdA and K/fluda and K/gem. The results show high levels of cross-resistance to all nucleoside analogues tested. The ratios of the IC50 values of the resistant lines to the parental line were very high, in the order of 500 to 1000. Of note, the highest levels of resistance were not always observed with the selecting agent. Some degree of cross resistance to etoposide was observed in the K/araC line (10-fold) and in the K/2cdA (3-fold) line. No cross-resistance was observed against cis platin, bleomycin, 5 fluorouracil, methotexate, carmustine, paclitaxel, mafosfamide and hydroxyurea.

Drug Accumulation

Drug accumulation results are summarized in Figure 1. All of the resistant lines displayed accumulation defects for all of the analogues tested. The reduction in intracellular

Table 1. Sensitovity of K562 and resistant variant to various cytotoxic agents[a]

Drug	K562	K/araC	K/2cdA	K/flud	K/gem
AraC nM	15	1340	230	>10000	2500
2cdA nM	20	>100000	>100000	15000	8500
flud nM	600	20 000	15 000	2 000	7000
gem nM	1.5	45	13	>100	68
doxo nM	850	1300	1500	700	900
CDDP µg/ml	3	2.7	3.2	3.6	2.6
bleo µg/ml	250	320	280	230	260
taxol nM	100	85	120	118	105
BCNU ng/ml	550	1200	650	780	495
FU µg/ml	85	103	110	97	78
VP16 µg/ml	18	180	54	12	21
HU µg/ml	175	172	220	150	199

Doxo : doxorubicin ; CDDP : cisplatin ; bleo : bleomycin ; HU : hydroxyurea ; FU : 5 fluorouracil.
[a]Values shown are inhibitory concentrations 50% determined using a 72 hour MTT assay.

drug accumulation was in the order of 63–85% for cytarabine, 2cda and fludarabine and 35–52% for gemcitabine.

Enzyme Activities

The enzyme activities in the various cell lines are summarized in Table 2. The most remarkable alterations are the reduction of deoxycytidine kinase and the increase of 5' nucleotidase in the resistant lines. Purine nucleoside phosphorylase was increased in K/2cdA only and ribonucleotide reductase was increasedin K/fludarabine only.

Karyotypes, Chromosome Painting and FISH Results

As shown in Table 3, the parental cell line K562 contains a number of chromosomal abnormalities. Three of the resistant lines (K/araC, K/2cdA, K/fluda) shared some differ-

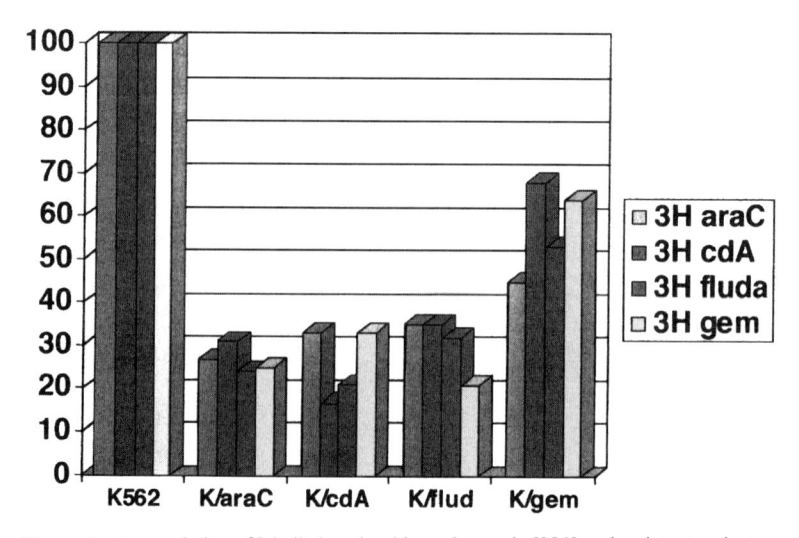

Figure 1. Accumulation of labelled nucleoside analogues in K562 and resistant variants.

Table 2. Enzymatic activities measured in K562 and variants resistant to nucleoside analogues

Activity	K562	K/AraC	K/2cdA	K/Fluda	K/Gem
5' Nucléotidase nmol/mg	38,8	145,5	405,8	180,9	556,2
Purine Phosphorylase ukat/kg	746	836	1434	859	725
Adénosine déaminase ukat/kg	166	159	111	136	193
Ribonucléotidyl réductase	11.5	8,05	10,9	20,7	n.d.

ences with the parental line, namely they did not have the deletion of 6q(q16q22), and had lost the second chromosome 20. Chromosome painting with a chromosome 6 probe confirmed the absence of the 6q deletion in these resistant lines (data not shown).

DISCUSSION

Nucleoside analogues have been an essential component in combination chemotherapy for patients with acute myelogenous leukemia and have been extensively used in patients with other hematologically malignancies. The sensitivity of hematopoietic cells is due among other factors to their requirement on exogenous nucleotides and hence the expression of membrane nucleoside receptors. The development of halogenated compounds which are resistant to early degradation by adenosine deaminase has enriched this class of compounds. The more recent analogue gemcitabine shows a broader spectrum of activity and is currently used in patients with solid tumors.

We have observed that all of the nucleosides tested selected variants with a marked decrease in intracellular drug accumulation. This decrease concerned all of the nucleoside analogues, although the accumulation defect was less pronounced in the case of gemcitabine. A number of nucleoside transporters, either sensitive or insensitive to NBMPR have described and cloned. The hENT1 pump, described by Griffiths et al. has been shown to transport therapeutic nucleoside compounds (8). Further analyses of the expression and function of the various nucleoside pumps in these cell lines are warranted.

Table 3. Karyotypic abnormalities in K562 and in variant lines resistant to nucleoside analogs

Karyotype of parental cell	X, -Xx2, t(1;18), -3, -4, dup(5)(q13q14), del6 (q16q22), add(6)(p21), add(7)(p22), -9, add(9)(p24), del(9)(p11), del(10)(p12), add(11)(p11), -13, add(13)(p11), -14, -15, -17, del(17)(p11), -261-63, 0, -21, dup(22)(q11q13), +mar
Differences common to K/araC, K/2cdA, K/fluda	Disappearance of del(6)(q16q22) -20 x 2
Differences specific to each variant	
K/araC	add(X)(p21), -X or -Y, -13 x 2, add(14)(p11)
K/2cdA	add(X)(p21), -X or -Y, del(17)(p11), +7, del(12)(q23), -21 x 2, add(11)(p15)
K/fluda	-12, -13 x 2
K/gem	-2, der(5)ins(5;?)(q23;?) HSR (5;?)(q23;?) del5 (q16,q22), add(7)(p13),-9, add9 (p24) del 9 (p11), -10, add(11)(p11), -12, dup (15)(q14,q21),-16, del(17)(p11) x 2, 21 x 2, add 21 (p11), -22, + 3-10 mar

araC : cytosine arabinoside; 2cdA: 2 chlorodeoxyadenosine; fluda: fludarabine; gem: gemcitabine

5' nucleotidase levels were found to be increased in all the resistant lines. These results suggests that the early step of phosphorylation, which is essential in drug activation, is crucial in developing cross resistance to this family of compounds. 5' nucleotidase may either be cytoplasmic or membrane bound, the latter form having been described as the cluster differentiation CD73 (9). Our assay analyzes total enzyme activity in cell extracts and it remains to be determined whether the increased activity is due to the cytoplasmic or the membrane bound enzyme, which is frequently expressed in acute leukemias. Remarkably the deletion of 6(q16;q22), which contains the gene for 5' nucleotidase, in the parental line is restaured in the resistant lines.

Some enzymatic abnormalities were observed specifically in one of the cell lines. The increase in purine nucleoside phosphorylase in the cladribine selected cell may result in the necessity for these cells to eliminate excess adenosine generated in the presence of cladribine. A two fold increase in ribonucleotide reductase was observed only in the fludarabine resistant line, although there was no significant cross resistance to hydroxyurea (10). Increased target content may thus also contribute to drug resistance in the case of fludarabine. Other enzymatic abnormalities involved in drug metabolism or drug-target interaction are also likely to be involved (11, 12).

The phenotype of the resistant lines demonstrate very high levels of cross resistance to other nucleoside analogues. There was no cross resistance to MDR related substrates, except for etoposide in the cytarabine and cladribine selected lines and the resistant cells did not express the *mdr1* gene (data not shown). The induction of cross resistance to nucleoside analogues may be important in the clinic, when considering the use of a nucleoside analogue for salvage therapy in patients having received prior treatment with this family of drugs. The low degree of cross resistance to etoposide may be due to alterations in DNA repair mechanisms.

Early events in cellular penetration and activation appear to play a critical role in resistance mechanisms to nucleoside analogues. Circumventing deficient intracellular drug delivery and inhibiting overexpressed enzymes involved in drug degradation, such as 5' nucleotidase, may constitute promising therapeutic options. Although downstream events involving drug target interactions and the signaling of apoptosis may be involved, achieving adequate intracellular concentrations of active triphosphorylated nucleoside compounds remains a prerequisite to cytotoxic activity.

REFERENCES

1. Cheson, B. D. New antimetabolites in the treatment of human malignancies, Semin Oncol. *19:* 695–706, 1992.
2. Ellison, R. R., Holland, J. F., and M., W. Arabinosyl cytosine: a useful agent in the treatment of acute leukemia in adults, Blood. *32:* 507–523, 1968.
3. Juliusson, G., Christiansen, I., Hansen, M. M., Johnson, S., Kimby, E., Elmhorn-Rosenborg, A., and Liliemark, J. Oral cladribine as primary therapy for patients with B-cell chronic lymphocytic leukemia, J Clin Oncol. *14:* 2160–2166, 1996.
4. Keating, M. J., O'Brien, S., Kantarjian, H., Plunkett, W., Estey, E., Koller, C., Beran, M., and Freireich, E. J. Long-term follow-up of patients with chronic lymphocytic leukemia treated with fludarabine as a single agent, Blood. *11:* 2878–2884, 1993.
5. Tesch, H., Santoro, A., Fiedler, F., Bonadonna, G., Bredenfeld, H., Oliva, C., Buksmaui, S., Sieber, M., and Diehl, V. Phase II study of gemcitabine in pretreated Hodgkin's disease results of a multicenter study. *In:* American Society of Hematology, San Diego, 1997.
6. Richel, D. J., Colly, L. P., Arkesteijn, G. J. A., Arentsen-Honders, M. W., Kerster, M. G. D., ter Riet, P. M., and Willemze, R. Substrate-specific deoxycytidine kinase deficiency in 1-b-D-arabinofuranosylcytosine-resistant leukemic cells, Cancer Res. *50:* 6515–6519, 1990.

7. Whelan, J., Smith, T., Phear, G., Rohatiner, A., Lister, A., and Meuth, M. Resistance to cytosine arabinoside in acute leukemia: the significance of mutations in CTP synthetase, Leukemia. *8:* 264–265, 1994.
8. Griffiths, M., Beaumont, N., Yao, S. Y. M., Sundaram, M., Boumah, C. E., Davies, A., Kwong, F. Y. P., Coe, I., Cass, C. E., Young, J. D., and Baldwin, S. A. Cloning of a human nucleoside transporter implicated in the cellular uptake of adenosine and chemotherapeutic drugs, Nature Med. *3:* 89–93, 1997.
9. Ujhazy, P., Berleth, E. S., Pietkiewicz, J. M., Kitano, H., Skaar, J. R., Ehrke, M. J., and Mihich, E. Evidence for the involvement of ecto-5'-nucleotidase (CD73) in drug resistance, Int J Cancer. *68:* 493–500, 1996.
10. Choy, B. K., Mc Clarty, G. A., Chan, A. K., Thelander, L., and Wright, J. A. Molecular mechanisms of drug resistance involving ribonucleotide reductase: hydroxyurea resistance in a series of clonally related mouse cell lines selected in the presence of increasing drug concentrations, Cancer Res. *48:* 2029–2035, 1988.
11. Warzocha, K., Fabianowska-Majewska, K., Blonski, J., Krykowski, E., and Robak, T. 2 chloro deoxyadenosine inhibits activity of adenosine deaminase and S-adenosylhomocysteine hydrolase in patients with chronic lymphocytic leukemia, Eur J Cancer. *33:* 170–173, 1996.
12. Gandhi, V., Huang, P., Chapman, A. J., Chen, F., and Plunkett, W. Incorporation of fludarabine and 1-β-D-arabinofuranosylcytosine 5'-triphosphates by DNA polymerase α: affinity, interaction and consequences, Clin Cancer Res. *3:* 1347–1355, 1997.

64

EXPRESSION OF DNA MISMATCH REPAIR PROTEINS IN ACUTE LYMPHOBLASTIC LEUKAEMIA AND NORMAL BONE MARROW

E. C. Matheson and A. G. Hall

LRF Molecular Pharmacology Group
CRU, Medical School
Newcastle-Upon-Tyne, NE2 4HH

Keywords: Mismatch repair, 6-thioguanine, drug, sensitivity.

1. ABSTRACT

Errors during normal DNA synthesis may produce mismatched base pairs. 6-Mercaptopurine (6MP), given during continuing therapy in acute lymphoblastic leukaemia (ALL), undergoes intracellular activation to give cytotoxic thioguanine nucleotides which are then incorporated into the DNA of dividing cells in place of guanine. Cell death is thought to result from futile attempts at mismatch repair. Previous work has shown that cell lines with a defect in this pathway develop tolerance to incorporated 6-thioguanine bases. In order to investigate the possible relevance of mismatch repair to the chemosensitivty of blasts to 6MP, relative to normal tissues, we have measured the expression of the mismatch repair proteins MLH1, MSH2, PMS2 and MSH6 in blasts from children and adults with ALL and in normal bone marrows, using western blotting. Fifty cases of childhood ALL, 22 cases of adult ALL and 7 normal marrows have been studied. Expression of MSH2, and of MLH1 in all but three cases, was detectable in all the blasts studied. Noticeably, expression of MLH1 was not detected in any of the normal marrow samples. MSH2 was detected in 4 of the normal marrows. Expression of PMS2 was not detected in 29 cases of ALL and, like MLH1, was absent from each of the normal marrow samples. In contrast, MSH6 was detected in all of the normal marrows and all but 16 of the cases of ALL. There was no difference in expression between adults and children. These results may help to explain the relative sensitivity of leukaemic blasts to thiopurines at presentation as compared to normal bone marrow.

Drug Resistance in Leukemia and Lymphoma III, edited by Kaspers *et al.*
Kluwer Academic / Plenum Publishers, New York, 1999.

2. INTRODUCTION

The chief mode of action of 6-MP and 6-TG is believed to be the fraudulent incorporation of thioguanine nucleotides into DNA, leading in turn to chromosome damage manifested by sister chromatid exchange. How this leads to cell death has only recently been determined. During replication 6-TG is incorporated in place of guanine but is unable to form stable thioguanine-cytosine base pairs. Mispairing with thymine occurs causing a base-pair mismatch (Figure 1).

Post-replicative mismatches are a common normal occurrence and cells have developed an efficient biochemical pathway for the recognition and correction of these defects. Studies were originally performed in *E.Coli* and yeast, although the details in eukaryotes are now beingdetermined.[1,2,3] In *E.Coli* mismatches are recognised by the MutS protein. This then binds to a second protein, MutL, and the complex binds to MutH which introduces a nick into the daughter DNA strand several bases away from the mismatch. A stretch of DNA is excised, including the mismatch and then resynthesised by DNA polymerase III. In *E.Coli* the daughter DNA strand is temporarily non-methylated allowing recognition by the post-replicative mismatch repair system of the correct strand. In humans it is not yet known how template and daughter strands are distinguished.

In humans the recognition of mismatched base pairs involves a dimer of MSH2 (human MutS homologue-2) and MSH6. Once bound to a mismatch a complex is formed with MLH1 (human MutL homologue-1) and PMS2 (Figure 2). Further details of the mismatch repair pathway in humans have yet to be determined.

The relevance of mismatch repair to carcinogenesis is demonstrated by the finding that MSH2 is mutated in many cases of hereditary non-polyposis coli (HNPPC). Most of the cases which do not have defects in MSH2 have mutations in MLH1. The relevance of mismatch repair to molecular pharmacology has been demonstrated by studies of DNA damage in cells treated with the agents N-methyl-N-nitrosourea (MNU) and N-methyl-N'-nitro-N-nitrosoguanidine (MNNG) which methylate guanine in the O^6 position. Cells resistant to these agents have been shown to display cross-resistance to 6-TG but not to other drugs.[4] Surprisingly, resistance in these cells is not associated with increased expression of O^6-methylguanine-DNA methyltransferase, a protein which removes methyl groups from methylated guanine, but appear instead to tolerate the presence of O^6-methyl or S^6-thioguanine/thymine mismatches. There is evidence that these cells have defects in the mismatch repair pathway as they also demonstrate microsatellite instability and in-

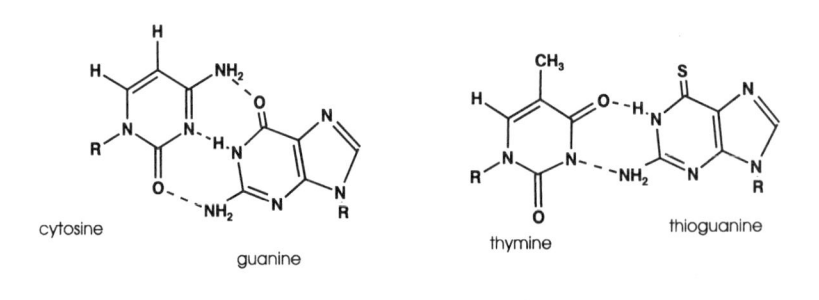

Figure 1. Thymine-thioguanine mismatches. The presence of a sulphur atom in place of oxygen in guanine disrupts the normal hydrogen bonding with cytosine and leads to mispairing with thymine.

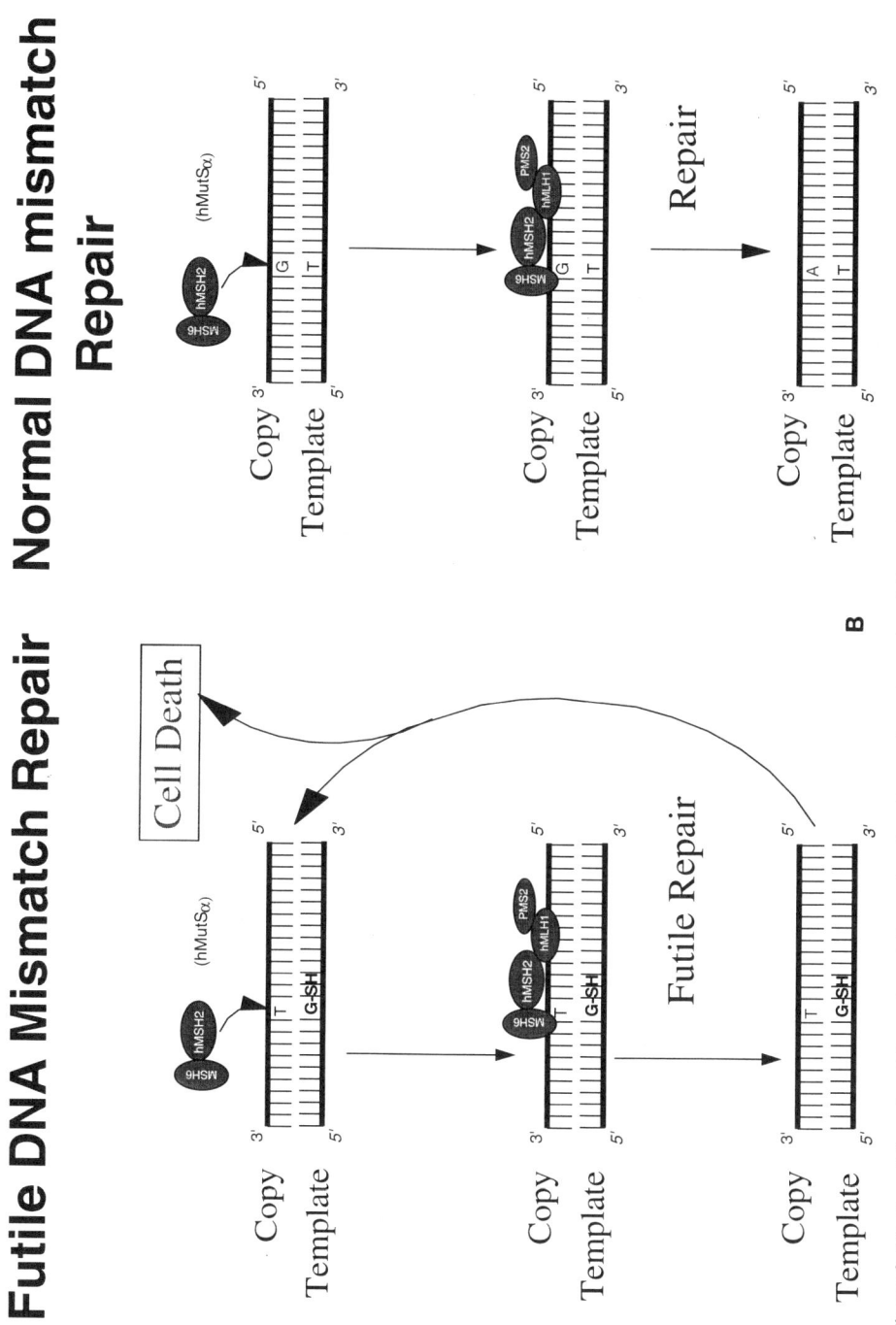

Figure 2. Binding of the mismatch repair proteins to thymine-thioguanine mismatches. Mismatches are recognised by a heterdimer formed by MSH2 and MSH6. A complex is subsequently formed with MLH1 and PMS2. In normal mismatches replacement of the mismatched base occurs (panel A). In cells with incorporated thioguanine in the template DNA futile repair cycles lead eventually to cell death as repair can only occur in the new DNA strand (panel B).

creased rates of mutation in selectable genes. The mutator phenotype and microsatellite instability are also features of tumour cells in patients with HNPPC.

The presence of O^6-methylguanine or S^6-thioguanine/thymine mismatches in DNA template strands is thought to trigger mismatch repair but this is unsuccessful due to the fact that repair can only take place in the daughter strand. Cell death ensues, possibly due to the introduction of double strand breaks or by stalling DNA replication. This model would fit with the delayed cytotoxicity characteristic of 6-thiopurines.

In this study we have documented the level of expression of the mismatch repair proteins in blasts obtained from children with ALL and marrow obtained from normal donors.

3. MATERIALS AND METHODS

Samples of bone marrow were obtained at presentation from 50 children and 20 adults with ALL and 7 normal bone marrow donors. Samples were collected according to local ethical guidelines. Mononuclear cells were separated by density gradient centrifugation using Lymphoprep. The level of expression of MLH1, MSH2, PMS2 and MSH6 was determined in cell lysates using western blotting with commercially available primary antibodies and enhanced chemoluminescence detection. Band intensity was determined by densitometry. Results were expressed relative to actin controls in order to eliminate variations due to loading artifacts.

4. RESULTS

Expression of MSH2, and of MLH1 in all but three cases, was detectable in all the blasts studied (Figure 3a and b) Noticeably, expression of MLH1 was not detected in any of the normal marrow samples. MSH2 was detected in 4 of the normal marrows, but only at a low level. The difference of expression of both MSH2 and MLH1 between ALL and normal marrow was highly statistically significant by the Mann-Whitney test ($p<0.0001$). Expression of PMS2 was not detected in 29 cases of ALL and, like MLH1, was absent from each of the normal marrow samples (Figure 3c). The diference in expression between blasts from children and normal marrow was not statistically significant, whereas the difference between blasts from adults and normal marrow did reach statistical significance ($p<0.001$). In contrast, MSH6 was detected in all of the normal marrows and all but 16 of the cases of ALL (Figure 3d). The difference in expression did not reach statistical significance. There was no difference in expression between adults and children for any of the 4 proteins studied.

5. DISCUSSION

The finding that the level of expression of mismatch repair proteins in normal bone marrow differs from that found in lymphoblasts suggests a possible explanation for the selectivity of thiopurine drugs used in the treatment of ALL. Cell line studies have demonstrated that cells with reduced expression of mismatch repair proteins have an increased tolerance to the incorporation of thiopurines into DNA. Conversely the high level of expression of these proteins, particularly MSH2 and MLH1, in leukaemic cells may be ex-

Expression of DNA Mismatch Repair Proteins

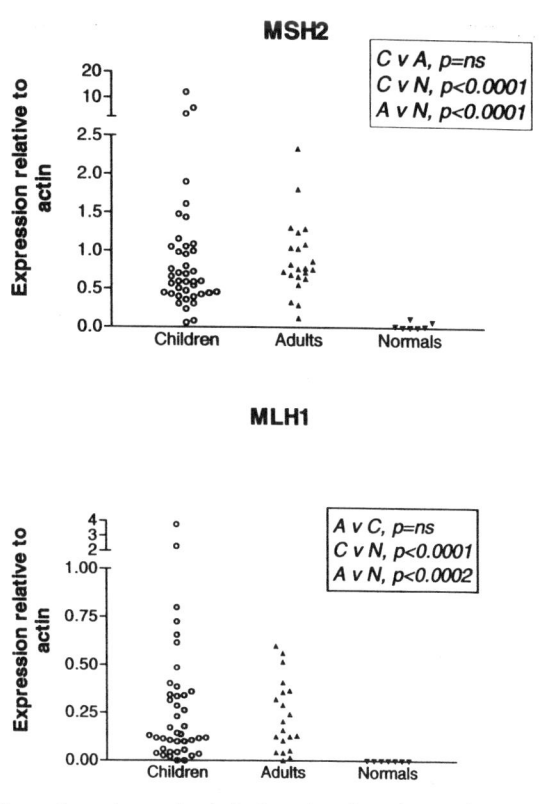

Figure 3. Expression of mismatch repair proteins in leukaemic cells and normal marrow. Scatter plots showing the expression of mismatch repair proteins relative to actin in normal marrow and blasts obtained from adults and children with ALL. Panel A: MSH2. Panel B: MLH1. Panel C: PMS2. Panel D: MSH6. Inset boxes indicate the results of the comparison of expression between the groups tested as analysed by the Mann-Whitney test. "A" = adults, "C" = children, "N" = normal bone marrow.

pected to render these cells particularly sensitive to drug incorporation. The cause of the difference in expression remains to be determined but may be due to hypomethylation in the cells which have undergone malignant transformation.

ACKNOWLEDGMENTS

The support of the Leukaemia Research Fund is gratefully acknowledged.

REFERENCES

1. Karran P and Bignami M: DNA damage tolerance, mismatch repair and genome instability. Bioessays. 1994, 16:833–839
2. Chung DC and Rustgi AK: DNA mismatch repair and cancer. Gastroenterology. 1995 109:1685–1699
3. Kolodner R: Biochemistry and genetics of eukaryotic mismatch repair. Genes Dev. 1996 10:1433–1442
4. Aquilina G, Giammarioli AM, Zijno A, Muccio AD, Dogliotti E, Bignami M: Tolerance to O^6-methylguanine and 6-thioguanine cytotoxic effects: a cross-resistant phenotype in N-methylnitrosourea-resistant Chinese hamster ovary cells. Cancer Res 1990, 50:4248–4253

65

EFFECTS OF CSFS AND THEIR COMBINATIONS WITH CHEMOTHERAPEUTIC AGENTS (CH) ON LEUKEMIC BLASTS (LB) IN CHILDREN (MTT-ASSAY)

E. Litvinova, K. Gurova, K. Chimishkian, and G. Mentkevich

Pediatric Oncology and Hematology Institute
Department of Bone Marrow Transplantation
Cancer Research Center
Kashirskoye sh. 24, Moscow, 115478 Russia

Keywords: Leukemia, growth factors, Ara-C, DOX, VP-16, MTT-assay.

1. ABSTRACT

Thirty five samples of bone marrow (BM) from 17 patients (pts) with ALL and 18 pts with AML (aged 9m-20yrs, median 7.7 yrs) were obtained. Using MTT-assay the sensitivity of LB to Ara-C, VP-16, DOX, G(GM)-CSF and their combinations was measured. LC50 was higher in pts with AML than with ALL: to Ara-C 1.94-fold ($p<0.05$), to VP-16 1.62-fold ($p=0.2$), to DOX 3.9-fold ($p<0.05$). Incubation with G-CSF increased the viability of ALL and AML LB—104.3% and 104.1% respectively (the viability of leukemic cells without CSF accepted as 100%). Incubation with GM-CSF decreased the viability of ALL LB (96.5%) and increased the viability of AML LB (139.1%) ($p = 0.08$). Combining Ara-C with G- or GM-CSF resulted in equal or increased LC50 (compared with LC50 of Ara-C alone) in 100% cases of AML. For ALL: LC50 of "Ara-C+G-CSF" was equal or increased in 63.6% cases; LC50 of "Ara-C+GM-CSF"- in 62.5%. For VP-16 and DOX all pts (ALL,AML) except two had equal or increased LC50 of "CH+CSF" (compared with LC50 of CH alone). These data show: 1) AML LB were less sensitive to the investigated CH than ALL LB. 2) The LC50 of "CH+CSF" was equal or increased compared to the LC50 of CH for the absolute majority of cases with VP-16 and DOX. The same results were obtained with AML and in about 60% cases of ALL. The effect of the increasing of cytototoxity of CH in presence of CSF probably exists mostly at higher concentrations of CH than those that can be achieved in clinical practice.

2. INTRODUCTION

Colony-stimulating factors (CSFs) are used in oncohematology to accelerate the hematopoietic recovery after chemotherapy and to enhance the cytotoxicity of CH. Increasing the proportion of leukemic cells in the S-phase of cell cycle enhances their vulnerability to phase-specific CH in vitro.[1,2] We tried to compare the sensitivity of lympho- and myeloblasts to CH, CSFs and their combinations and to determine the safety and effectiveness of combined application of CH and CSF in vitro on short-term culture of leukemic cells from children with ALL and AML.

3. MATERIALS AND METHODS

3.1. Patients

Leukemic cells from 35 patients (pts) were investigated. The age of pts was from 9 months to 20 years, median—7.7 years. Eighteen pts had AML (15 at initial diagnosis, 3 at first relapse) and seventeen pts had ALL (13 at initial diagnosis, 2 at first, 1 at second, 1 at third relapse). In all cases the percentage of blast cells in bone marrow was more than 60%.

3.2. Methods

Mononuclear cells were isolated by centrifugation in density gradient, washed twice and resuspended in RPMI 1640 with 15% FCS $2-3 \times 10^5$ cells per well in round bottom 96-well microculture plates. Cells were incubated without drugs (control), with growth factor alone (G-CSF (Neupogen®) or GM-CSF (Leukine®) in five duplicate concentrations, with CH alone in five (Ara-C, VP-16) or seven (DOX) duplicate concentrations or with combination "CSF+CH" in these cases G-CSF was used in concentration 30 ng/ml, GM-CSF—5 ng/ml. The investigated concentrations of drugs are shown in Table 1.

Plates were incubated for 72h in the humidified incubator at the 5% carbon dioxide at 37°C. Then 10 μl of MTT (3-[4,5-dimethyl thiazol]-2,5-diphenyl tetrazolium bromide) solution (5mg/ml PBS) was added and after shaking for 1 min the plates were incubated for 5h. Crystals of formazan were dissolved with 200 μl of DMSO. The optical density of the wells was measured with a multichannel microplate reader MR-5000 (Dynatech) at 550 nm. Leukemic cell survival (LCS) was calculated by the following equation: LCS = (OD treated well/mean OD control well) × 100%. The LC50 defined as the drug concen-

Table 1. The range of concentrations of the tested drugs

Drug	Range of the tested concentrations
Ara-C	0.02–200 μg/ml
DOX	0.00002–20 μg/ml
VP-16	0.02–200 μg/ml
GM-CSF	0.05–500 ng/ml
G-CSF	0.3–3000 ng/ml

tration that results in 50% LCS was derived by calculating the point where the dose response curve crosses the 50% LCS level.[3]

3.3. Statistics

Statistics was performed with Quattro.Pro and Easy Plot programs.

4. RESULTS

4.1. Comparison of the Sensitivity of ALL and AML Blasts to CH

Median LC50 of Ara-C for ALLs was 0.604 µg/ml, AMLs—1.174 µg/ml; median LC50 of VP-16 for ALLs—0.381 µg/ml, AMLs—0.616 µg/ml; median LC50 of DOX for ALLs—0.185 µg/ml, AMLs—0.716 µg/ml. Lymphoblasts were therefore more sensitive than myeloblasts: to Ara-C 1.94-fold (p<0.05); to VP-16 1.62-fold (p=0.2); to Dox 3.9-fold (p<0.05) (Figure 1).

4.2. Incubation of Leukemic Cells with Growth Factors Alone

If the viability of leukemic cells after three day incubation without CSF is accepted as 100% (control) then the viability of leukemic cells incubated during the same time with CSF was as follows: the viability of lymphoblasts incubated with G-CSF in concentration 30 ng/ml—104.3%; myeloblasts—104.1%; the viability of lymphoblasts incubated with GM-CSF in concentration 5 ng/ml—96.5%; myeloblasts with the same CSF—139.1% (p=0.08) (Figure 2). No dose-dependance was observed between the concentration of CSF and the viability of cells in all cases except in four cases (there were cases when AML cells were incubated with GM-CSF, one of these is shown on Figure 3).

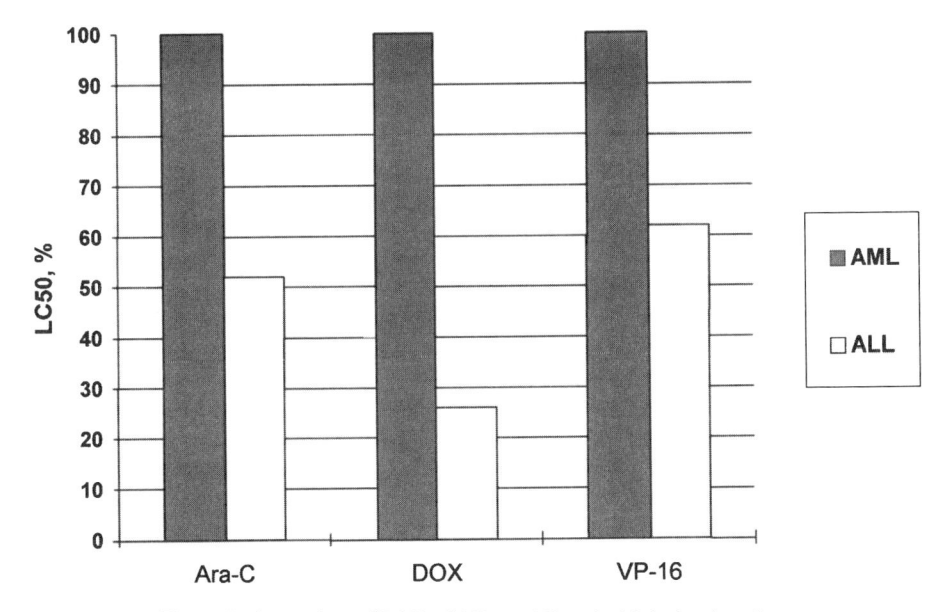

Figure 1. Comparison of LC50 of CH on AML and ALL leukemic cells.

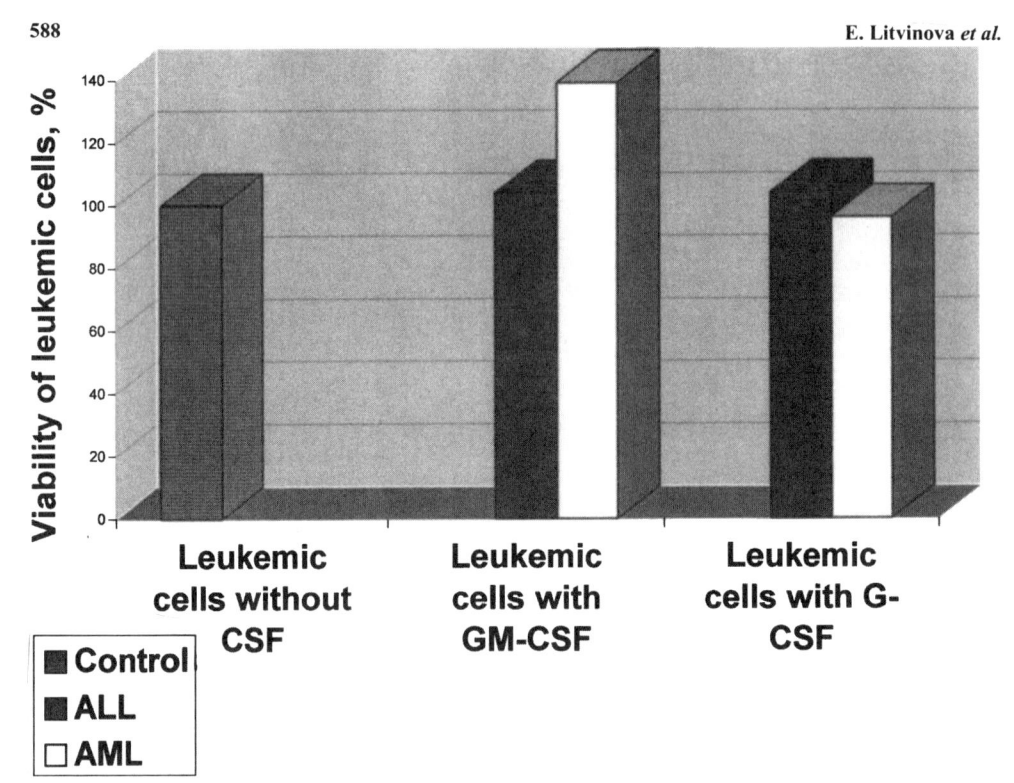

Figure 2. Effects of CSFs on AML and ALL leukemic cells.

4.3. Incubation of Leukemic Cells with CSF and CH

Ara-C with any CSF had equal or increased LC50 compared to Ara-C alone in 100% cases of AML. LC50 of combination "Ara-C+G-CSF" was lower than LC50 of Ara-C in 36.4% cases of ALL; LC50 of combination "Ara-C+GM-CSF" was lower than LC50 of Ara-C in 37.5% cases of ALL. LC50 was decreased in these cases an average of 37%.

VP-16 and DOX with CSFs had an increased or equal LC50 (compared with CH alone) in all cases of AML and ALL except two: these were patients with ALL. LB from the first patient had lower LC50 with "VP-16+G-CSF" and from the second patient—lower LC50 with "DOX+G-CSF" compared to CH alone (Figure 4).

The median values of increasing of LC50 "CH+CSF" compared with the LC50 of CH alone are in Table 2.

The viability of leukemic cells from the patient with AML related to Ara-C dose is shown on Figure 5. This is the same patient whose cells had a high proliferative response on GM-CSF with dose-dependant character that was shown on Figure 3.

5. DISCUSSION

As was already shown[4] fewer than half of AML leukemic blast cells are in S phase of cell cycle. Also it was found that patients with relapsed acute nonlymphocytic leukemia had longer duration of total cell cycle time than those at initial diagnosis. The subgroup of patients whose total cell cycle time was extremely long demonstrated clinically documented resistance in response to chemotherapy courses.[5]

Effects of CSFs and Their Combinations with Chemotherapeutic Agents

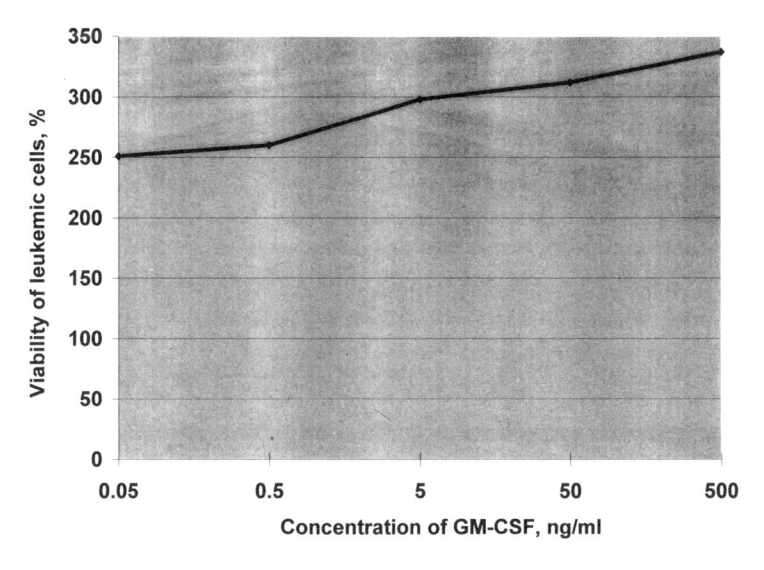

Figure 3. Effects of different doses of GM-CSF on leukemic cells from the patient with AML.

Though in ALL the growth fraction is more than 90% of cells the total cell cycle time is long too, probably due to a long G1-phase.[6] B-lineage and T-lineage ALL cells have a lower dividing capacity than their normal counterparts.[7]

It was shown in vitro that such cytokines as GM-CSF, G-CSF, Il-3 can recruit myeloblasts into the cell cycle and significantly increase their sensitivity to Ara-C, daunomycin,[8] mitoxantrone, VP-16.[9] This happens because more leukemic cells enter into S-phase of cell cycle and, therefore, overcome kinetic drug resistance.[10] Also, CSFs increase the phosphorylation of Ara-C to Ara-CTP[11] and potentiate Ara-C- induced programmed cell death in leukemic cells.[5] But some studies in vitro have shown increased Ara-C sensitivity in a presence of GM-CSF in only a minority patients.[12] It was also found that GM-CSF pro-

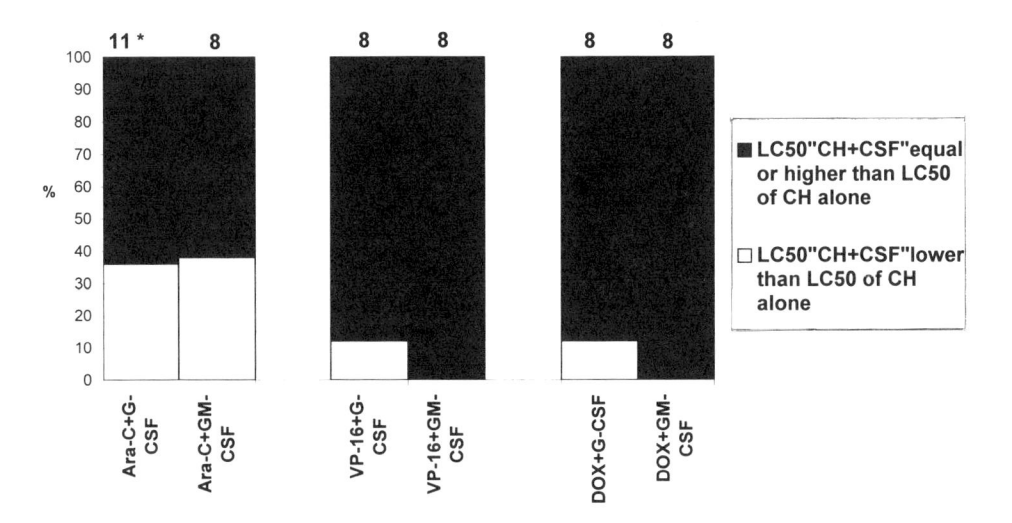

Figure 4. Effects of the combinations "CH+CSF" on ALL leukemic cells.

Table 2. Relative values of LC50 "CH+CSF" (in %) comparing with LC50 of CH alone accepted as 100% *

	LC of Ara-C with		LC of VP-16 with		LC of DOX with	
	G-CSF	GM-CSF	G-CSF	GM-CSF	G-CSF	GM-CSF
ALL	125.5%	168.5%	163.2%	123.5%	140.7%	127.4%
AML	277.2%	353.1%	940.2%	1209.1%	296.3%	445.1%

*In this table all cases were included for which LC50 "CH+CSF" was equal or increased than LC50 of CH alone.

tected blast cells from Ara-C toxicity[13] and GM-CSF and Il-3 protected leukemic cells against doxorubicin-induced apoptosis.[14] In vivo administration of GM-CSF, G-CSF in conjunction with chemotherapy in adults also had contradictory results.[15,16,17]

We studied the effects of CSFs applied together with chemotherapeutic agents in vitro on leukemic cells from chidren. According to our data CSFs did not influence significantly the viability of leukemic cells, except for the stimulatory effect of GM-CSF on myeloblasts. In the majority of cases CSFs increased the LC50 of chemotherapeutic agents—more significantly in AML than in ALL but it was observed in ALL too. The latter fact could be partly explained by the existance of restricted stem cells those were capable of differentiating into myeloid and B-lineage cells or myeloid and T-lineage cells.[18,19] Also it is known that some chromosomal abnormalities (such as 11q23, t(9;22)) are associated with bipotential lymphoid and myeloid differentiation capability.[20] Thus, lymphoid cells with "mixed" features may response to CSFs due to the presence of appropriate receptors on their surface. It was also found that primary adult T-cell leukemia cells can express G-CSF receptors and proliferate in vitro in response to G-CSF.[21]

We agree with Sundman-Engberg B. et al.,[9] that CSFs increase cytotoxicity of chemotherapy on leukemic cells but the stimulation of the remaining cells may offset the clinical benefit (so we can see the increasing of LC50 in majority of cases of our investigation).

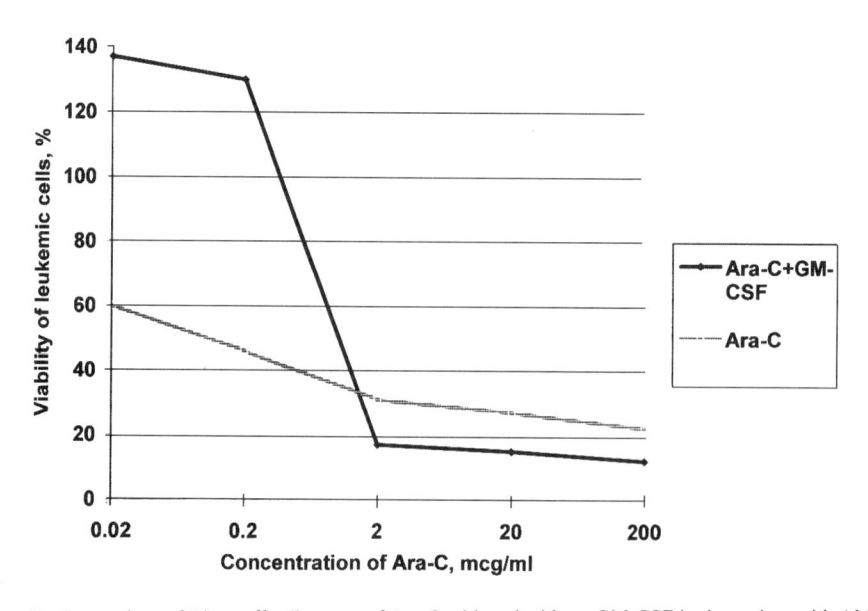

Figure 5. Comparison of "dose-effect" curves of Ara-C with and without GM-CSF in the patient with AML.

This phenomenon is the so called "regrowth resistance"—rapid regrowth of drug sensitive high proliferating cells which survive chemotherapy.[22] In one example of an AML patient with high proliferating response to GM-CSF (Figures. 3 and 5), we can see that at low concentrations of Ara-C the stimulating effect of GM-CSF on leukemic cells exceeded the cytotoxic effect of combination "Ara-C+GM-CSF" and "regrowth resistance" was observed, but at high concentrations of Ara-C the increasing of cytotoxic effect of Ara-C by GM-CSF was observed. However, these high concentrations of chemotherapeutic agents can be hardly achieved in clinical practice.

The decrease of the LC50 with the combination "CH+CSF" in some cases of ALL can be explained by the fact that lymphoblasts are more sensitive to the investigated chemotherapeutic agents than myeloblasts (as was shown above) and the effect of the enhancing cytotoxicity in presence of CSF can be achieved with lower doses of CH than in cases of AML. But we did not notice any dramatic decrease of LC50 CH in presence of CSF. Therefore, according to our preliminary data, we can conclude that simultaneous application of CSF and chemotherapeutic drugs with the purpose to enhancing the cytotoxicity of chemotherapy can be useful only in minority of cases in children with acute leukemia. These cases could be determined by in vitro methods.

REFERENCES

1. Koistinen P., Wang C., Yang GS, et al. OCI/AML-4 an acute myeloblastic leukemia cell line: Regulation and response to cytosine arabinoside. Leukemia 1991, 5, 704–711.
2. Tafuri A., Andreeff M. Kinetic rationale for cytokine-induced recruitment of myeloblastic leukemia followed by cycle-specific chemotherapy in vitro. Leukemia 1990, 4, 826–834.
3. Metelitsa L., Shmelev V., Shvedova E., Popov A., Mentkevich G. 25 Effects of cytokines and their combinations with Ara-C on short term culture of tumor cells from children with acute leukemia by the MTT-assay. In Pieters R., Kaspers G.J.L., Veerman A.J.P. (eds): "Drug resistance in Leukemia and Lymphoma II". Harwood academic publishers, 1997, 209–216.
4. Clarkson B., Strife A., Fried J., et al. Studies of cellular proliferation in human leukemia. IV. Behavior of leukemic cells in 3 adults with acute leukemia given continuous infusion of 3H-thymidine for 8 to 10 days. Cancer, 1970, 26, 1–19.
5. Raza A., Maheshwari Y., Preisler HD. Differences in cell cycle characteristics among patients with acute nonlymphocytic leukemia. Blood, 1987, 69(6), 1647–1653.
6. Hirt A., Antic V., Wang E., Luthy AR., Leibundgut R., et al. Acute lymphoblastic leukaemia in children: cell proliferation without rest. Br J Haematology 1997,96, 366–368.
7. Campana D., Janossy G.: Proliferatoin of normal and malignant human immature lymphoid cells. Blood, 1988, 71, 1201.
8. Cannistra SA, Groshek P., Griffin JD. Granulocyte-macrophage colony-stimulating factor enhances the cytotoxic effects of cytosine arabinoside in acute myeloblastic leukemia and on the myeloid blast crisis phase of chronic myelogenous leukemia. Leukemia, 1989, 3, 328–334.
9. Sundman- Engberg B., Tidelfelt U., Paul C. 24 In vitro studies of growth factors in combination with cytostatic drugs on human leukemia cells. In Pieters R., Kaspers G.J.L., Veerman A.J.P. (eds): "Drug resistance in Leukemia and Lymphoma II". Harwood academic publishers, 1997, 203–208.
10. Hederson E.S., Lister T.A., Greaves M.F. (eds): "Leukemia. Sixth edition",1996.
11. Bhalla K., Ibrado AM, Holladay C., Bullock G. Hemopoietic growth factors (HGFs) G-CSF and Il-3 improve the antileukemic selectivity of high-dose Ara-C (HIDAC). Blood 1991, 78 (Suppl 1), 425 (abstr).
12. Smith MA, Singer CRG, Pallister CJ, Smith JG. The effect of haemopoietic growth factors on the cell cycle of AML progenitors and their sensitivity to cytosine arabinoside in vitro. Br J Haematology, 1995, 90, 767–773.
13. Koistinen P., Wang C., Curtis JE, McCulloch EA. Granulocyte-macrophage colony-stimulating factor and interleukin-3 protect leukemia blast cells from Ara-C toxicity. Leukemia 1991, 5, 789–795.

14. Kaplinsky C., Lotem J., Sachs L. Protection of human myeloid leukemia cells against doxorubicin-induced apoptosis by granulocyte-macrophage colony-stimulating factor and interleukin-3. Leukemia, 1996, 10, 460–465.
15. Estey E., Thall PF, Kantarjian H., et al: Treatment of newly diagnosed acute myelogenous leukemia with granulocyte-macrophage colony-stimulating factor (GM-CSF) before and during continuous infusion high-dose Ara-C+daunorubicin: Comparison to patients treated without GM-CSF. Blood 1992, 79, 2246–2255.
16. Bettelheim P., Valent P., Andreeff M., Tafuri A., Haimi J., et al. Recombinant human granulocyte-macrophage colony-stimulating factor in combination with standard induction chemotherapy in de novo acute myeloid leukemia. Blood 1991, 77, 700–711.
17. Archimbaud E., Fenaux P., Reiffers J., Cordonnier C., Leblond V., Travade P., Troussard X., et al. Granulocyte-macrophage colony-stimulating factor in association to timed-sequential chemotherapy with mitoxantrone, etoposide and cytarabine for refractory acute myelogenous leukemia. Leukemia 1993, 7, 372–377.
18. DiGiusto D., Chen S., Combs J., et al. Human fetal bone marrow early progenitors for T, B, and myeloid cells are exclusively in the population expressing high levels of CD34. Blood 1994, 84, 421
19. Kurtzberg J., Waldmann TA, Davey MP, et al. CD7+, CD4-, CD8- acute leukemia: A syndrome of malignant pluripotent lymphohematopoietic cells. Blood 1989, 73, 381.
20. Serrano J., Roman J., Sanchez J., Torres A. Myeloperoxidase gene expression in acute lymphoblastic leukaemia. Br J Haematology 1997, 97, 841–843.
21. Matsushita K., Arama N., Ohtsubo H., Fujiwara H., et al. Granulocyte colony-stimulating factor-induced proliferation of primary adult T-cell leukemia cells. Br J Haematology 1996, 96, 715–723.
22. Preisler HD, Raza A., Larson R., Goldberg J., Tricot G., et al. Some reasons for the lack of progress in the treatment of acute myelogenous leukemia. Leuk Res 1991, 15(9), 773–780.

14. Kaplinsky C., Lotem J., Sachs L. Protection of human myeloid leukemia cells against doxorubicin-induced apoptosis by granulocyte-macrophage colony-stimulating factor and interleukin-3. Leukemia, 1996, 10, 460–465.
15. Estey E., Thall PF, Kantarjian H., et al: Treatment of newly diagnosed acute myelogenous leukemia with granulocyte-macrophage colony-stimulating factor (GM-CSF) before and during continuous infusion high-dose Ara-C+daunorubicin: Comparison to patients treated without GM-CSF. Blood 1992, 79, 2246–2255.
16. Bettelheim P., Valent P., Andreeff M., Tafuri A., Haimi J., et al. Recombinant human granulocyte-macrophage colony-stimulating factor in combination with standard induction chemotherapy in de novo acute myeloid leukemia. Blood 1991, 77, 700–711.
17. Archimbaud E., Fenaux P., Reiffers J., Cordonnier C., Leblond V., Travade P., Troussard X., et al. Granulocyte-macrophage colony-stimulating factor in association to timed-sequential chemotherapy with mitoxantrone, etoposide and cytarabine for refractory acute myelogenous leukemia. Leukemia 1993, 7, 372–377.
18. DiGiusto D., Chen S., Combs J., et al. Human fetal bone marrow early progenitors for T, B, and myeloid cells are exclusively in the population expressing high levels of CD34. Blood 1994, 84, 421
19. Kurtzberg J., Waldmann TA, Davey MP, et al. CD7+, CD4-, CD8- acute leukemia: A syndrome of malignant pluripotent lymphohematopoietic cells. Blood 1989, 73, 381.
20. Serrano J., Roman J., Sanchez J., Torres A. Myeloperoxidase gene expression in acute lymphoblastic leukaemia. Br J Haematology 1997, 97, 841–843.
21. Matsushita K., Arama N., Ohtsubo H., Fujiwara H., et al. Granulocyte colony-stimulating factor-induced proliferation of primary adult T-cell leukemia cells. Br J Haematology 1996, 96, 715–723.
22. Preisler HD, Raza A., Larson R., Goldberg J., Tricot G., et al. Some reasons for the lack of progress in the treatment of acute myelogenous leukemia. Leuk Res 1991, 15(9), 773–780.

This phenomenon is the so called "regrowth resistance"—rapid regrowth of drug sensitive high proliferating cells which survive chemotherapy.[22] In one example of an AML patient with high proliferating response to GM-CSF (Figures. 3 and 5), we can see that at low concentrations of Ara-C the stimulating effect of GM-CSF on leukemic cells exceeded the cytotoxic effect of combination "Ara-C+GM-CSF" and "regrowth resistance" was observed, but at high concentrations of Ara-C the increasing of cytotoxic effect of Ara-C by GM-CSF was observed. However, these high concentrations of chemotherapeutic agents can be hardly achieved in clinical practice.

The decrease of the LC50 with the combination "CH+CSF" in some cases of ALL can be explained by the fact that lymphoblasts are more sensitive to the investigated chemotherapeutic agents than myeloblasts (as was shown above) and the effect of the enhancing cytotoxicity in presence of CSF can be achieved with lower doses of CH than in cases of AML. But we did not notice any dramatic decrease of LC50 CH in presence of CSF. Therefore, according to our preliminary data, we can conclude that simultaneous application of CSF and chemotherapeutic drugs with the purpose to enhancing the cytotoxicity of chemotherapy can be useful only in minority of cases in children with acute leukemia. These cases could be determined by in vitro methods.

REFERENCES

1. Koistinen P., Wang C., Yang GS, et al. OCI/AML-4 an acute myeloblastic leukemia cell line: Regulation and response to cytosine arabinoside. Leukemia 1991, 5, 704–711.
2. Tafuri A., Andreeff M. Kinetic rationale for cytokine-induced recruitment of myeloblastic leukemia followed by cycle-specific chemotherapy in vitro. Leukemia 1990, 4, 826–834.
3. Metelitsa L., Shmelev V., Shvedova E., Popov A., Mentkevich G. 25 Effects of cytokines and their combinations with Ara-C on short term culture of tumor cells from children with acute leukemia by the MTT-assay. In Pieters R., Kaspers G.J.L., Veerman A.J.P. (eds): "Drug resistance in Leukemia and Lymphoma II". Harwood academic publishers, 1997, 209–216.
4. Clarkson B., Strife A., Fried J., et al. Studies of cellular proliferation in human leukemia. IV. Behavior of leukemic cells in 3 adults with acute leukemia given continuous infusion of 3H-thymidine for 8 to 10 days. Cancer, 1970, 26, 1–19.
5. Raza A., Maheshwari Y., Preisler HD. Differences in cell cycle characteristics among patients with acute nonlymphocytic leukemia. Blood, 1987, 69(6), 1647–1653.
6. Hirt A., Antic V., Wang E., Luthy AR., Leibundgut R., et al. Acute lymphoblastic leukaemia in children: cell proliferation without rest. Br J Haematology 1997,96, 366–368.
7. Campana D., Janossy G.: Proliferatoin of normal and malignant human immature lymphoid cells. Blood, 1988, 71, 1201.
8. Cannistra SA, Groshek P., Griffin JD. Granulocyte-macrophage colony-stimulating factor enhances the cytotoxic effects of cytosine arabinoside in acute myeloblastic leukemia and on the myeloid blast crisis phase of chronic myelogenous leukemia. Leukemia, 1989, 3, 328–334.
9. Sundman- Engberg B., Tidelfelt U., Paul C. 24 In vitro studies of growth factors in combination with cytostatic drugs on human leukemia cells. In Pieters R., Kaspers G.J.L., Veerman A.J.P. (eds): "Drug resistance in Leukemia and Lymphoma II". Harwood academic publishers, 1997, 203–208.
10. Hederson E.S., Lister T.A., Greaves M.F. (eds): "Leukemia. Sixth edition",1996.
11. Bhalla K., Ibrado AM, Holladay C., Bullock G. Hemopoietic growth factors (HGFs) G-CSF and Il-3 improve the antileukemic selectivity of high-dose Ara-C (HIDAC). Blood 1991, 78 (Suppl 1), 425 (abstr).
12. Smith MA, Singer CRG, Pallister CJ, Smith JG. The effect of haemopoietic growth factors on the cell cycle of AML progenitors and their sensitivity to cytosine arabinoside in vitro. Br J Haematology, 1995, 90, 767–773.
13. Koistinen P., Wang C., Curtis JE, McCulloch EA. Granulocyte-macrophage colony-stimulating factor and interleukin-3 protect leukemia blast cells from Ara-C toxicity. Leukemia 1991, 5, 789–795.

66

GLUCOCORTICOSTEROID THERAPY IN CHILDHOOD ACUTE LYMPHOBLASTIC LEUKEMIA

Paul S. Gaynon and Aaron L. Carrel

Division of Pediatric Hematology-Oncology
Division of Diabetes and Endocrinology
Department of Pediatrics
University of Wisconsin School of Medicine
Madison, Wisconsin 53792

Keywords: acute lymphoblastic leukemia; prednisone; dexamethasone; cortivazol; glucocorticosteroids.

1. ABSTRACT

Treatment of childhood acute lymphoblastic leukemia has included glucocorticosteroids for almost 50 years. Glucocorticoids are the subject of renewed interest. In one randomized trial, deferral of glucocorticosteroids from the initial month of induction therapy to the second month of therapy decreased event free survival despite preservation of remission induction rate. Dexamethasone in induction and maintenance provides a better event free survival than prednisone for standard risk patients in an isotoxic comparison even though all patients received dexamethasone in Delayed Intensification (protocol II). In a third report, patients with prior glucocorticosteroid therapy who achieved remission with subsequent multiagent therapy had a relapse rate similar to that of patients in second remission after failure of multiagent therapy. In vitro and in vivo response of leukemic cells to glucocorticosteroids is highly predictive of outcome. At relapse, loss of in vitro sensitivity to glucocorticosteroids is common and out of proportion to the loss of sensitivity to other agents. Glucocorticoid induced cell kill does not require p53 function. Investigation of leukemic cell lines finds that glucocorticosteroid resistance is most commonly linked to altered receptor number or function. Not all ligands are equivalent. Cortivazol, a pyrazolosteroid, may bind to altered receptor in some cases and induce apoptosis in dexamethasone resistant leukemic cells. Host response to exogenous glucocorticosteroid also

Drug Resistance in Leukemia and Lymphoma III, edited by Kaspers *et al.*
Kluwer Academic / Plenum Publishers, New York, 1999.

varies. Associations between host sensitivity, disease sensitivity, and glucocorticosteroid side effects like avascular necrosis of bone remain to be investigated.

2. INTRODUCTION

Acute lymphoblastic leukemia (ALL) is unique among hormone responsive neoplasms. Estrogens and androgens promote proliferation of breast cancer and prostate cancer, respectively and specific hormone withdrawal induces apoptosis (1). On the other hand, administration of glucocorticosteroids (GCS) induce apoptosis in ALL. As single agents, GCS induce remission in perhaps 60% of children with newly diagnosed ALL (2).

GCS seem unique among the various agents used in the therapy of ALL. A poor peripheral blood response after 7 days of GCS "monotherapy" [including prednisone and a single dose of intrathecal methotrexate] carries a strongly adverse prognostic significance despite subsequent administration of usually effective multiagent therapy (3–7). Comparison of a GCS-containing induction regimen, i.e., vincristine, prednisolone, and asparaginase with a GCS-free induction regimen, i.e., vincristine, cytosine arabinoside, cyclophosphamide, and asparaginase resulted in similar remission induction rates, namely, 91% and 94%. Patients who received no prednisolone during induction received a two week course of prednisolone during the following 'CNS prophylaxis' phase. However, they still had an inferior event free survival (EFS), namely, 52% vs 62% (8). Treatment of childhood ALL with multiagent therapy after prior treatment with single agent GCS for misdiagnosed arthritis or aplastic anemia resulted in a striking decrease in EFS similar to that found for patients in second remission after relapse despite multi-agent therapy but no decrease in the remission induction rate (9). In vitro GCS sensitivity is a consistent prognostic factor in the MTT assay (10–16).

The mechanisms of GCS resistance has been studied most commonly in multiply passaged, "professional" leukemic cell lines, such as CEM (17–26). Less work has been done with freshly obtained patient samples of leukemic blasts (27–31).

Host variability with regard to response to GCS therapy for autoimmune disease has been noted (33–36) while appreciation of population variability in host GCS-sensitivity and resistance is growing (33–40). Host variability with regard to response to GCS therapy for childhood ALL has not been examined to date. Possible associations between host and leukemic GCS-sensitivity and resistance and/or between host GCS-sensitivity and GCS related complications like avascular necrosis of bone (AVN) (41–43), a potentially devastating complication of GCS therapy in adolescents and adults, remain to be explored.

3. GLUCOCORTICOSTEROID RECEPTOR

Glucocorticoid function requires glucocorticoid receptor (GCS-R). The GCS-R gene is located at chromosome 5q31 (19). The gene is 10 exons, numbered 1–8 and 9a and 9b, which gives rise to mRNA of about 7 kb (18) and alternative splicing variants GCS-Rα and GCS-Rb. The GCS-Ra binds ligand and the GCS-Rß does not. The molecular weight is approximately 92 kda (18).

The GCS-R is 777 amino acids long. It has three domains, like other receptors in the steroid hormone receptor superfamily, namely, an N-terminal domain, a DNA-biding domain, and a C-terminal ligand binding domain. The three residues in closest proximity to bound ligand are 604 (methionine), 638 (cysteine), and 756 (cysteine) (35). Unliganded

GCS-R is present in the cytoplasm in noncovalent association with hsp 90, hsp 56 (immunophilin), often hsp 70, and other proteins (19, 26, 33,34).

Nazareth and coworkers found that leukemic cell death required an intact GSC-response element specific DNA binding domain. Deletion of the known transactivation, ligand binding, dimerazation, and/or nuclear translocation domains leaves a receptor fragment capable of inducing cell death (44).

4. GLUCOCORTICOSTEROID-INDUCED APOPTOSIS

GCS enter cells via passive diffusion and bind with the GCS-R causing a conformational change (19, 26, 33,34). Ligand binding is facilitated by receptor-associated heat shock protein 90 (hsp 90) (45) and receptor phosphorylation state (46,47). Binding is maximal in late G1 phase and S-phase with low basal receptor phosphorylation and high ligand induced phosphorylation. GCS sensitivity is reduced in G2 and M phase with high basal receptor phosphorylation and low ligand induced phosphorylation (47).

The receptor-ligand complex sheds chaperon proteins. such as hsp90, which unmasks domains responsible for nuclear translocation, dimerazation, DNA binding, and transactivation (19, 26, 33,34). Ligand bound monomers and dimers cross into the nucleus via recognition of their nuclear localization sequences by the proteins of the nuclear pore.

GCS-induced apoptosis requires interaction with specific DNA sequences, the GCS-response elements (GRE's), 15 base pair partial palindromes (TGTACAGGATGTTCT), and transactivation (19, 26, 33, 34). GCS-R dimers can promote transcription of GCS-responsive genes directly, can inhibit transcription of other genes by interaction with the response elements of other positive transcription factors, and can modulate expression of yet other genes by formation of intranuclear complexes with other transcription factors like c-jun and Rel A. Inhibitors of RNA and protein synthesis inhibit GCS-induced apoptosis. Ligand non-binding beta receptors may compete with ligand binding alpha receptors in the nucleus and explain differences in tissue sensitivity in part (26,34).

In vitro, GCS induced cell death requires continuous saturation of GCS-receptors for a substantial period of time, usually between 18 and 24 hours, but ranging up to 168 hours in some cell lines (17). In vivo, a divided dose daily schedule was more effective than the same total dose administered qod and q4d in support of the in vitro requirement for continuous saturation (2).

GCS-induced apoptosis requires down regulation of c-myc which is constituatively expressed in proliferating lymphoblasts (48,49). Introduction of c-myc driven by a non-GCS sensitive promoter provides protection from GCS induced cell killing (48). Suppression of c-myc mRNA by introduction of an antisense oligonucleotide induces cell kill in the absence of GCS (49). G1 arrest is closely linked to cell death. Induction of glutamine synthetase, a GCS induced enzyme, is not (22). Endonuclease activation and production of DNA oligomers of multiples of about 180 base pairs, i.e. DNA laddering, are typical, but not universal findings in GCS-induced apoptosis.

Smets contrasts glucocortoid induced apoptosis with apoptosis induced by DNA dmaaging agents (see Table 1). Although both share the final common step of DNA laddering, other differences are apparent (50). Glucocortoid induced apoptosis may be termed "premature senescence"—like apoptosis induced by withdrawl of tropic hormones or of growth factors. Apoptosis induced by DNA damaging agents is most apparent in cycling cells and has been termed "mitotic catastrophy." Apoptosis induced by DNA damaging agents is p53 dependent, unlike GCS induced apoptosis (51). High levels of BCL-2 pro-

Table 1. Glucocorticoid induced apoptosis vs apoptosis induced by DNA damaging drugs

	Glucocorticoid induced apoptosis	DNA damaging drug induced apoptosis
Process (50)	Premature senescence	Mitotic catastrophy
Target (50)	G_0-G_1 Growth inhibition	Cycling cells Irreversible G_2 arrest
p53 dependence (51)	No	Yes
New gene transcription (50)	Yes	No
RNA/protein synthesis (50)	Yes	No
Calcium fluxes (50)	Yes	no
Final common pathway	DNA laddering	DNA laddering

tect cells from GCS-induced cell death (52) and apoptosis induced by a variety of physical agents and anti-cancer drugs (53).

Calcium is a second messenger in glucocorticoid induced apoptosis. $P2X_1$ and IP_3R are induced in GCS-induced apoptosis. $P2X_1$, a purinergic receptor, functions as an ATP-gated calcium channel while IP_3R encodes an inositol 1,4,5-triphosphate receptor (IP_3R) that functions as an IP_3-gated calcium channel. $P2X_1$ receptors allow intracellular passage of extracellular calcium. Typically, IP_3 receptors span the endoplasmic reticulum(ER) and allow passage of calcium from the ER lumen into the cytoplasm. However in other experiments, high concentrations of calcium chelators or calmodulin inhibitors blocked GCS-induced endonuclease activation but did not prevent GCS-induced cell death (54).

Elevation of intracellular cyclic AMP or administration of meta-iodobenzyl guanidine enhances GCS effect (55, 56).

5. GLUCOCORTICOSTEROID RESISTANCE

5.1. Population Variability in GCS Sensitivity

Endogenous levels of plasma cortisol levels are regulated by negative feedback from the hypothalamo-pituitary-adrenal axis and vary widely in the population. A small number of number of kindreds with severe familial GCS-resistance have been studied (33–38). However, clinically inapparent abnormalities may be present with greater frequency. Lamberts and coworkers report that 6.6% of a normal population have increased sensitivity to GCS while 2.3% have relative resistance (33). Koper and coworkers found that 20/216 elderly non-hospitalized people had a reduced response to a 1 mg dexamethasone suppression test (9%). However, none had mutation of the GCS-R (39)

Familial GCS resistance is a rare condition in which abnormal receptor alters the feedback inhibition of the hypothalamo-pituitary-adrenal axis. Levels of ACTH and cortisol are increased without symptoms of Cushings disease because of GCS-resistance caused by decreased numbers or function of GCS-R. Symptomatology, if any, derives from overflow mineralocorticoid and androgen excess (33–35). Patients may be identified by a higher levels of plasma cortisol and inadequate cortisol suppression 12 hours after 1 mg of dexamethasone.

GCS-resistance has been linked to point mutations in the ligand binding domain at residues 641 (valine for aspartate) and 729 (isoleucine for valine) and to a 4 base pair deletion at the exon/intron boundary of intron 6. These abnormal receptors have 3–5 fold reduced affinity for dexamethasone (37,38).

Not all polymorphisms in the GCS-R are associated with GCS resistance (39). Two point mutations have been associated with GCS-hypersensitivity, namely residues 638 (glycine for cysteine) (35) and 363 (serine for asparagine) (40).

Huizenga and coworkers found that 13/216 non-hospitalized elderly people (6%) had the N36S polymorphism (serine for asparagine) and demonstrated an abnormal GCS-R hypersensitivity in terms of insulin response and decrease in plasma cortisol following dexamethasone administration. Elderly patients with the N363S polymorphism had increased body mass index, and decreased bone density (40).

5.2. In Vitro Glucocorticosteroid Resistance

Mechanisms of GCS-resistance have been examined in a number of GSC-resistant cell lines. In older studies, reversible H^3-dexamethasone binding assays were employed to assay receptor number and receptors with low affinity were not identified. More recent studies have assessed antibody recognized receptor or employed covalent dexamethasone binding. Some supposed differences in GCS-steroid receptors by DEAE cellulose chromatography and SDS-polyacrylamide electrophoreses arose from artifactual proteolysis (18).

Resistance to GCS may arise from a decreased number of apparently normal receptors, receptors with altered ligand binding, or receptors with decreased nuclear translocation. In addition, mdr-1 amplification can impede the intracellular accumulation of prednisolone and dexamethasone necessary for receptor saturation (21,57). In most systems studied, GCS-resistance is associated with a decreased number or altered function of the GCS-receptor (21, 24). The S49 murine cell line and the human CEM-C7 cell lines have one wild-type allele of the GSC-R and one mutant allele (21). GCS resistance emerges as a random event at a rate of 3.5 × 10^{-6}/cell/generation in the S49 cell line and 1 × 10^{-5}/cell/generation in the CEM cell line even in the absence of selective pressure. The WEHI-7 cell line has two wild type alleles and complete GCS-resistance is acquired in a two step process at a rate of 1 × 10^{-10}/cell/generation. Exposure to mutagenic agents may increase the frequency of GCS resistance 1000-fold in the WEHI7 cell line (18) and to a lesser extent in other systems (23).

5.2.1. Decreased Glucocorticosteroid-Receptor Number or Hormone Bindings. Eighty to ninety percent of GCS-resistant variants obtained from leukemia or lymphoma cell lines demonstrate negligible steroid binding because of decreased numbers of normal receptors or because relatively normal numbers of receptors with decreased steroid binding (21).

Almost all GCS-resistant S49 murine cells have been shown to have altered GCS-receptor with decreased GCS binding. Some GCS-resistant P1798 cells appear to have abnormal GCS-R with molecular weight 40 kd compared to 90 kd for GCS-sensitive P1798 cells (18).

CEM-1CR27 cell lines are derived from treatment of a GCS sensitive cell line with 1 μmolar dexamethasone. CEM-C1 cells have fewer than 10% of the GCS binding sites found in GCS sensitive CEM cell lines and were labelled receptor deficient. However, these cells express a steroid binding protein of the same molecular weight as wild type GCS-R, 92 kDa (24).

5.2.2. Altered Nuclear Translocation. Treatment of CEM-C7 cells with 1^{-10} μmolar dexamethasone gives rise to cells lines such as 3R7, 3R43, and 4R4, with decreased nuclear translocation, so called activation labile variants. Temperature unstable steroid-receptor complexes may or may not be stabilized by molybdate salts (22).

5.2.3. Altered DNA Binding or Transcriptional Activity. Variants of murine cell lines are recognized with steroid-receptor complexes with decreased DNA binding or with N-terminal truncated receptor lacking transactivational activity.

5.2.4. Other. The murine T-cell line SAK8 has functional GCS-receptor. Induction of resistance follows DNA methylation and restoration of sensitivity follows demethylation by 5-azacytidine. Hybrids of GSC-sensitive and resistant cells are GCS sensitive. Human CEM-C1 cell lines are GCS-resistant despite normal numbers of GCS-receptors and normal GCS binding. Glutamine synthetase is induced normally by GCS and the line is characterized as lysis defective. GCS sensitivity was restored with treatment with 5-azacytidine (18).

Kojika and coworkers examined 9 GCS-resistant cell lines with normal ligand binding. They found that 2 of these cell lines expressed normal GCS-receptor but aberrant hsp 90 and extremely low levels of hsp 70 (58).

Intracellular accumulation of dexamethasone and prednisolone is diminished by active extrusion by mdr1 (21, 57). S7CD-5 cells overexpressed the mdr1 gene relative to the parent MS23 cell line and exhibited verapamil reversible resistance to dexamethasone (57). Overexpression of p-glycoprotein conveyed resistance to some GCS and not others, e.g., triamcinolone and not triamcinolone acetonide.

5.3. In Vivo Glucocorticosteroid Resistance

5.3.1. In Vitro Sensitivity. In vitro sensitivity to GCS is a consistent adverse prognostic factor in childhood ALL (10–13). Similar significance is found only for daunorubicin and 6-thioguanine among a large panel of conventionally important agents tested by the MTT assay. In vitro sensitivity to prednisolone carries prognostic significance even among good responders to the Berlin Frankfurt Münster (BFM) *vorphase* (12). In vitro sensitivity to GCS distinguishes childhood and adult ALL (14), childhood and infant ALL (15), and newly diagnosed and relapsed ALL (16). In vitro comparisons of the LC_{50}'s for a variety of agents in newly diagnosed and relapsed ALL, show an increase of > 100-fold for prednisolone compared to < 3-fold for any other agent (12). This disproportionate loss of sensitivity suggests the existence and clinical importance of a specific mechanism of GCS resistance.

5.3.2. Glucocorticoid Receptors in Patient Specimens. A flurry of work in the mid 1980's sought to link the number of GCS receptors/cell and outcome in childhood ALL using tritiated dexamethasone assays. Such assays would not detect receptor that did not bind dexamethasone.

In one series of papers from St. Jude, receptor levels in patient specimens ranged from 2,248 to 79,664/cell (median 18,123/cell). T-cell patients and black patients had fewer receptors/cell (28). Lower receptor level was an adverse prognostic factor in univariate and multivariate analyses. Among 27 patients who received single agent GCS therapy in an upfront window, a high level of GCS receptors, > 10,000 receptors/cell was correlated with good response (29). Levels of GCS-receptor were lower in patients who relapsed while on therapy and those who failed re-induction (30).

In a study from the Pediatric Oncology Group, early pre-B patients had a median of 9,700 receptors/cell and pre-B patients had a median of 8,100 receptors/cell while T-lineage patients had a median of 4000 receptors./cell. Among early pre-B patients high receptor number was associated with successful remission induction (31). Follow-up showed a superior EFS for patients with more than 8,000 receptors/cell. This advantage was preserved in multivariate analyses after adjustment for clinical features, immunophenotype, and treatment. Assays were successful for about 60% of patients (32).

6. CLINICAL IMPLICATIONS

6.1. Dexamethasone and Prednisone

Dexamethasone may be more effective than the more commonly employed prednisone. Dexamethasone may have a longer duration of action than prednisone (2). Dexamethasone provides better CNS penetration than prednisone (59). In terms of GCS effect, dexamethasone 1 mg/m2 is said to be the equivalent of prednisone 6–7 mg/m^2 (13). However, dexamethasone was 26 times more potent in than prednisone in suppressing urinary 17-ketosteroids and 17 times more potent in suppressing endogenous cortisol at 8 hours after ingestion and 30 fold more potent at 14 hours (2). Kaspers and coworkers found that dexamethasone 16-fold more potent than prednisolone on the MTT assay (13). On the other hand, Ito and coworkers studied cells cultured on allogeneic bone marow-derived stomal cell layers and found dexamethasone only 5–6 fold more active than prednisolone, a ratio more in keeping with the conventional equa-efficacy ratio (60). Resistance to prednisolone and dexamethasone is generally shared (13).

Laboratory observations may have clinical consequences. Jones and coworkers found fewer CNS relapses with dexamethasone than with predisone although ultimate EFS was similar (61). Veerman and coworkers replaced prednisone with dexamethasone in the Dutch ALL Study VI and found benefit compared to historical controls from the Dutch ALL Study VI pilot (62).

Dexamethasone is a component of Protocol II as defined in the ALL-BFM '76 trial (63). Dexamethasone was retained in the Children's Cancer Group modification of this successful regimen (64). Protocol II or Delayed Intensification was shown to be the critical element in the CCG average risk trial, CCG-105 (65).

Bostrom and Children's Cancer Group coworkers randomly allocated 1060 children with ALL and Rome/NCI Standard risk patients (66,67) to receive prednisone 40 mg/m^2/day or dexamethasone 6 mg/m^2/day in induction, daily × 28 days + taper, and maintenance as 5 day pulses each 4 weeks. All patients received dexamethasone 10 mg/m2/day × 21 days + taper in Delayed Intensification (DI). Preliminary results show an advantage for dxm in terms of isolated CNS relapses, 15 vs 32 (3.1% vs 7.1%, p=0.009) and overall EFS, 91% vs 86% (3-year, p=0.014). Thus far 25 patients on dexamethasone and 34 patients on prednisone have suffered bone marrow relapse but further follow-up is needed as this standard risk population remains at risk for later relapses, especially late bone marrow relapses. Avascular necrosis of bone was not a problem in this younger population. Dexamethasone was responsible for transient steroid myopathy in induction in 2.3% of patients and more frequent hyperglycemia (68).

In 2000 in the next CCG trial, "standard risk" patients will receive dexamethasone in induction and maintenance, if differences persist as they have on the Dutch ALL Study VI (62). The situation for "higher risk" patients is more complex. Dexamethasone 6 mg/m^2/day was shown superior to prednisone 40 mg/m^2/day not 60 mg/m^2/day, the dose employed in regimens for Higher risk patients. For a subset of Standard risk patients, CCG-105 found no advantage for prednisone at 60 mg/m2 versus 40 mg/m2 among a number of other additions to induction and consolidation therapy (65). The Higher risk population includes older children, older than 10 years of age, who are at particular risk for AVN. The risk for AVN may be enhanced by dexamethasone. A randomized comparison of dexamethasone and prednisone has been proposed for the next CCG Higher risk trial in 2000.

6.2. Cortivazol

Loss of sensitivity to glucocorticoids is a hallmark of relapsed vs de novo ALL (16) and adult vs childhood ALL (14). In childhood ALL, the LC_{50} for prednisolone may increase by 2–3 $\log_{10}$ by the MTT assay while the LC_{50}'s of other agent changes by < 0.5 log10 (16). In clinical generalized inherited glucocorticoid resistance syndromes, the majority of mutations affect glucocorticoid binding (33,34).

Cortivazol (RU 3625) is a pyrazolosteroid that binds to glucocorticoid receptor with 2 site kinetics(69,70). It is 500–2000 times more potent than hydrocortisone in a granuloma assay and 20–50 times more potent than dexamethasone in inducing lysis of lymphoblasts (69–75). Cortivazol is more effective than dexamethasone in treating CNS leukemia in a SCID mouse model (72).

Cortivazol binds to altered receptor in several dexamethasone-resistant cell lines and kills several dexamethasone-resistant lymphoblastic leukemia cell lines, including, ICR27, C1, 4R4, and 3R43, (69, 73, 74). ICR27 has been classified as "receptor deficient" as determined by dexamethasone binding, but cortivazol identified functional glucocorticoid receptor (73). CEM C1 has been classified as "lysis defective" (69). 4R4 and 43R3 have been classified as activation labile (74). However, dexamethasone resistant cells require hiogher levels of cortivazol for lysis than dexamethasone sensitive cells for lysis (74).

Harmon and coworkers were unable to isolate stable deacylcortivazol-resistant mutants from dexamethasone sensitive C7 cells. However, stable deacylcortivazol-resistant mutants could be isolated from dexamethasone-resistant mutants with a frequency of $1-8 \times 10^{-4}$/cell/ generation similar to that of dexamethasone-resistance in dexamethasone-sensitive cell lines, i.e., $2-3 \times 10^{-5}$/cell/ generation (72).

Cortivazol and deacylcortivazol may be resistant to extrusion by mdr1 (76) and thus achieve adequate intracellular concentrations in the presence of over production of p-glycoprotein.

The question remains whether cortivazol and another ligand will provide clinical antileukemic activity for some proportion of patients with dexamethasone-resistant lymphoblasts. A clincal phase II trial may be of interest.

6.3. Host Glucocorticoid Resistance and Sensitivity

Host glucocorticoid sensitivity and resistance may affect disease outcome and GCS morbidities like avascular necrosis of bone. Host RBC acumulation of 6-thioguanine nucleotides has been shown predictive of outcome in childhood ALL(77, 78). Host formation of anti-asparaginase antibody is related to failure to respond to asparaginase containing therapy (79–81). Might variable host sensitivity or resistance to GCS be related the the GCS sensitivity or resistance of the leukemic clone or to the likelihood of steroid induced complications? Koper and coworkers found about 9% of people to exhibit relative resistance to exogenous GCS (39).

Among patients older than 10 years on CCG-1882, fully 15% had avascular necrosis of bone with prednisone in induction and maintenance and dexamethasone in Delayed Intensification. Unfortunately, with the addition of a second Delayed Intensification phase in the augmented regimen which included a second 21 day course of dexamethasone at 10 mg/m^2, the incidence of AVN increased to 23% among patients older than 10 years (82, 83).

Among older patients, AVN remains a major concern. The schedule of dexamethasone in current CCG trials has been changed from 10 mg/m^2/d × 21 plus taper to 10 mg/m2/d Days 0–6 and 14–20 with no taper for all patients who receive two Delayed Intensification phases (CCG-1952, and CCG-1961). An assessment of the efficacy of this modification is eagerly awaited but not yet available. Might patients who suffer AVN be among the 6% of people reported to have relatively increased sensitivity to GCS (33, 34)?

7. CONCLUSIONS

Despite their almost 50 year history in the treatment of childhood ALL, GCS may provide a new opportunities to improve the outcome of children with ALL. Dexamethasone may be more efective than prednisone. Simple substitution of dexamethasone for prednisone improved outcome in the Dutch Study VI (62). Simple substitution of dexamethasone for prednisone in induction and maintenance provided a therapeutic benefit for Standard risk patients on CCG-1922, even though all patients received dexamethasone in Delayed Intensification (68). The question remains open for Higher risk patients where prednisone is used at 60 mg/m^2 instead of 40 mg/m^2 in CCG trials and among older patients where AVN remains an issue.

GCS induced apoptosis is independent of p53 function (50, 51). Although abnormalities of p53 function are rare at diagnosis in childhood ALL (84, 85), abnormalities of p53 (/mdm-2) function may be more common among patients with induction failure (86) and at relapse (87, 88). Alternative ligands like cortivazol or deacylcortivazol may circumvent multidrug resistance mediated by mdr1 (76). GCS may induce apoptosis in p53 deficient cells (51) and prevent the emergence of a multidrug resistant population.

GCS resistance may be marked at relapse (16). Known mutations most frequently affect the GCS receptor and affect ligand binding (21–24). Novel ligands like cortivazol may bind to altered receptor and induce apoptosis, although at higher concnetrations than in sensitive cells (69–76). Demethylation may restore GCS sensitivity in some instances of GCS resistance (18).

Host variability in GCS -sensitivity is substantial may be related to the sensitivity of the leukemic cell populationand the propensity for GCS complications like AVN. As much as 9% of the normal population may have relative GCS resistance (38) while 6% is hypersentive (39). Future data may warrant dose individualization.

ACKNOWLEDGMENTS

Grant support through the Children's Cancer Group from the Division of Cancer Treatment, National Cancer Institute of Health, Department of Health and Human Services, United States of America

REFERENCES

1. Thompson Brad E: Apoptosis and steroid hormones. Mol Endocrinol; 1994; 8: 665–673.
2. Gaynon PS and Lustig RH: The use of glucocorticoids in acute lymphoblastic leukemia of childhood. J Pediatr Hematol Oncol 1995; 7:1–12, 1995.

3. Riehm H, Reiter A, Schrappe M, Berthold F, Dopfer R, Gerein V, Ludwig R, Ritter J, Stollmann B, and Henze G: Die corticosteroid-abhängige Dezimierung der Leukämiezellzahl im Blut als Prognosefaktor bei der akuten lymphoblastischen Leukämie im Kindesalter (Therapiestudie ALL-BFM 83). Klin Pädiatr 1986; 199:151–60.
4. Riehm H, Feickert H-J, Schrappe M, Henze G, Schellong G. Therapy results in five ALL-BFM studies since 1970: Implications of risk factors for prognosis. Hamatol Bluttransfus 1987; 30:139–46.
5. Riehm H, Gadner H, Henze G, Kornhuber B, Lampert F, Niethammer D, Reiter A, Schellong G: Results and significance of six randomized trials in four consecutive ALL-BFM studies. Haematol Blood Transfus 1990; 33: 439–450.
6. Schrappe M, Reiter A, Sauter S, Ludwig WD, Wörmann B, Harbott J, Bender-Götze C, Dörffel W, Dopfer R, Frey E, Havers W, Henze G, Kühl J, richter R, Ritter J, Treuner J, Zintl F, Odenwald E, Welte K, and Riehm J: Konzeption und Zwischenergebnis der Therapiestudie ALL-BFM 90 zur Behandlung der akuten lymphoblastischen Leukämie bei Kindern und Jugendlichen: die Bedeutung des initialen Therapieansprechens in Blut und Knochenmark. Klin Pädiatr 1994; 206: 208–21.
7. Aricò M, Basso G, Mandelli F, Rizzari C, Colella R, Barisone E, Zanesco L, Rondelli R, Pession A, Masera G: Good steroid response in vivo predicts a favorable outcome in children with T-cell acute lymphoblastic leukemia. Cancer 1995; 75: 1995, 1684–93.
8. Ekert H, Waters KD, Matthews RN, Smith PJ, O'Regan P, Rice M, Toogood I, Mauger D, and Tauro G: A randomized trial of corticosteroid and non-corticosteroid containing regimens in induction therapy of childhood ALL. Cancer Ther Control 1990; 1:87–95.
9. Revesz T, Kardos G, Kajtar P, Schuler D: The adverse effect of prolonged prednisolone pretreatment in children with acute lymphoblastic leukemia. Cancer 1985; 55:1637–1640.
10. Pieters R, Kaspers GJL, Klumper E, and Veerman AJP: Clinical relevance of in vitro drug resistance testing in childhood acute lymphoblastic leukemia: the state of the art. Med Pediatr Oncol 22:299–308, 1994.
11. Hongo T, Yajima S, Sakurai M, Horikoshi Y, and Hanada R: In vitro drug sensitivity testing can predict induction failure and early relapse of childhood acute lymphoblastic leukemia. Blood 1997; 89:2959–2965.
12. Pieters R, Kaspers GJL, van Wering ER, van der Does-van den Berg A, Veerman AJP: Prospective study of the in vitro prednisolone resistance in childhood acute lymphoblastic leukemia: A new risk factor in BFM-oriented treatment. Blood 1993; 82:194a (abstract #762).
13. Kaspers GJL, Veerman AJP, Popp-Snijders C, Lomecky M, Van Zantwijk CH, Swinkels LMJW, van wering ER, Pieters R:. Comparison of the antileukemic activity in vitro of dexamethasone and prednisolone in childhood acute lymphoblastic leukemia. Med Pediatr Oncol 27:114–121, 1996.
14. Maung ZT, Reid MM, Matheson E, Taylor PRA, Proctor SJ, and Hall AG: Corticosteroid resistance is increased in lymphoblasts from adults compared with children: preliminary results of the in vitro drug sensitivity study in adults with acute lymphoblastic leukemia. Br J Haematol 1995; 91:93–100.
15. Pieters R, den Boer ML, Durian M, Janka G, Schmiegelow K, Kaspers GJL, van Wering ER, Veerman AJP: Infants acute lymphoblastic leukemia cells are highly resistant to prednisolone and asparaginase in vitro but highly sensitive to cytosine arabinoside (AraC). Med Pediatr Oncol 1997; 29:335 (abstract #O70).
16. Klumper E, Pieters R, Veerman AJP, Huismans DR, Loonen AH, Hählen K, Kaspers GJL, van Wering ER, Hartmann R, and Henze G: In vitro cellular drug resistance in children with relapsed/refractory acute lymphoblastic leukemia. Blood 86:3861–3868, 1995.
17. Thompson EB and Harmon JM: Glucocorticoid receptors and glucocorticoid resistance in human leukemia in vivo and in vitro. In Chrousos GP, Loriaux DL, Lipsett MB, eds. Steroid Hormone Resistance, Newe York: Plenum Publishing, 1986:111–127.
18. Harmon JM and Thompson EB: Glucocorticoid resistance in leukemic cells. In Kessel D, ed. Boca Raton: CRC Press, Inc, 1988:385–402.
19. Norgaard P and Skovgaard Poulsen H: Glucocorticoid receptors in human malignancies. Ann Oncol 1991; 2:541–557.
20. Kaspers GJL, Pieters R, Klumper E, de Waal FC, Veerman AJP: Glucocorticoid resistance in childhood leukemia. Leukemia Lymph 1994; 13:187–201.
21. Moalli PA and Rosen ST: Glucocorticoid receptors and resistance to glucocorticoids in hematologic malignancies. Leukemia Lymph 1994; 15:363–374.
22. Schmidt TJ: Analyses of glucocorticoid receptor structure and function using the human CEM acute lymphoblastic leukemia T-cell line. In Gametchu B(ed): Glucocorticoid Receptor Structure and Leukemic Cell Responses, R.G. Landes Co., 1995: 125–154.
23. Palmer LA, Hukku B, Harmon JM: Human glucocorticoid receptor gene following exposure to cancer chemotherapeutic drugs and chemical mutagens. Cancer Res 1992; 52: 6612–6618.

24. Powers JH, Hillmann AG, Tang DC, and Harmon JM: Cloning and expression of mutant glucocortioid receptors from glucocorticoid-sensitive and resistant human leukemic cells. Cancer Res 1993; 53: 4059–4065.
25. Strasser-Wozak EMC, Hattmannstorfer R, Hala M, Hartmann BL, Fiegel M, Geley S, Kofler R: Splice site mutation in the glucocorticoid receptor gene causes resistance to glucocorticoid-induced apoptosis in a human acute leukemic cell line. Cancer Res 1995; 55: 348–353.
26. Ray DW: Molecular mechanisms of glucocorticoid resistance. 1996; 149:1–5.
27. Distelhorst CW, Benutto BM, Grffith RC: A single common electrophoretic abnormality of glucocortioid receptors in human leukemia cells. Blood 1985; 66: 679–685.
28. Costlow ME and Pui CH: Glucocorticoid receptors in childhood acute lymphocytic leukemia. Cancer Res 1982; 42:4801–4806.
29. Pui CH, Dahl GV, Rivera G, Murphy SB, and Costlow ME: The relationship of blast cell glucocorticoid receptor levels to response to single agent steroid trial and remission response in children with acute lymphoblastic leukemia. Leukemia Res 1984; 8:579–585.
30. Pui CH and Costlow ME: Sequential studies of lymphoblast glucocorticoid receptor levels at diagnosis and relapse in childhood leukemia: an update. Leukemia Res 1986; 10:227–229.
31. Quddus FF, Leventhal BG, Boyett JM, Pullen DJ, Crist WM, and Borowitz MJ: Glucocorticoid receptors in immunological subtypes of childhood acute lymphoblastic leukemia cells: a Pediatric Oncology Group study. Cancer Res 1985; 45:6482–6486.
32. Kato GJ, Quddus FF, Shuster JJ, Boyett J, Pullen JD, Borowitz MJ, Whitehead VM, Crist WM, Leventhal BG: High glucocorticoid receptor content of leukemic blasts is a favorable prognostic factor in childhood acute lymphoblastic leukemia. Blood 1993; 82:2304–2309.
33. Lamberts SWJ, Huizenga ATM, de Lange P, de Jong FH, and Koper JW: Clinical aspects of glucocorticoid sensitivity. Steroids 1996; 61:157–160.
34. Chrousos GP, Castro M, Leung DYM, Webster E, Kino T, Bamberger C, Elliot S, Stratakis C, and Karl M: Molecular mechanisms of glucocorticoid resistance/ hypersensitivity. Am J Resp Crit Care Med 1996; 154; s39-s44.
35. Bronnegard M, and Carlstedt-Duke J: The genetic basis of glucocorticoid resistance. Trends Endocrinol Metab 1995; 6:160–164.
36. Werner S and Brönnegård M: Molecular basis of glucocorticoid resistance syndromes. Steroids 1996; 61:216–221.
37. Hurley DM, Accili D, Stratakis CA, Karl M, Vamvakopoulos N, Rorer E, Constantine K, Taylor SI, and Chrousos GP: Point mutation causing a single amino acid substitution in the hormone binding domain of the glucocorticoid receptor in familial glucocorticoid resistance. J Clin Invest 1991; 87: 680–687.
38. Karl M, Lamberts SWJ, Detera-Wadleigh SD, Encio IJ, Statakis CA, Hurley DM, Accili D, and Chrousos GP: Familial glucocortioid resistance caused by a splice site deletion in the human glucocortioid receptor gene. J Clin Endocrinol Metab 1993; 76: 683–689.
39. Koper JW, Stolk RP, de Lange P, Huizenga NATM, Molijn GJ, Pols HAP, Grobbee DE, Karl M, de Jong FH, Brinkmann AO, Lamberts SWJ: Lack of association between five polymorphisms in the human glucocorticoid receptor gene and glucocorticoid resistance. Hum Genet 1997; 99:663–668.
40. Huizenga NATM, Koper JW, de Lange P, Pols HAP, Stolk RP, Burger H, Grobbee DE, Brinkmann AO, de Jong FH, and Lamberts SWJ: A polymorphism in the glucocortoid receptor gene may be associated with an increased sensitivity to glucocorticoids in vivo. J Clin Endocrinol Metab 1998; 83:144–151.
41. Murphy RG and Greenberg ML. Osteonecrosis in pediatric patients with acute lymphoblastic leukemia. Cancer 1990; 65:1717–1721.
42. Hanif I, Mahmoud H, and Pui C-H. Avascular femoral head necrosis in pediatric cancer patients. Med Pediatr Oncol1993; 21:655–660.
43. Chan-Lam D, Prentice AG, Copplestone JA, Weston M, Williams M, and Hutton CW. Avascular necrosis of bone following intensified steroid therapy for acute lymphoblastic leukaemia and high-grade malignant lymphoma. Br J Haematol 1994; 86:227–230.
44. Nazareth LV, Harbour DV, and Thompson EB: Mapping the human glucocorticoid receptor for leukemic cell death. J Biol Chem 1991; 266: 12976–12980.
45. Baulieu EE; The connection between steroid receptors and stress proteins (hsp 90). In Jasmin G, Proschek L (eds): Stress Revisited 2. Systemic Effects of Stress. Methods Achieve Exp Pathol. Basel Karger 1991, vol 15, pp104–125.
46. Distelhorst CW, Benutto BM, and Bergamini RA: Effect of cell cycle position on dexamethasone binding by mouse and human lymphoid cell lines: correlation between an increase in dexamethasone binding during S phase and dexamethasone sensitivity. Blood 1984; 63:105–113.

47. Bodwell JE, Hu JM, Hu LM, Munck A: Glucocorticoid receptors: ATP and cell cycle dependence, phosphorylation, and hormone resistance. Am J Resp Crit Care Med 1996; 154:52–56.
48. Thompson EB, Nazareth LV, Thulasi R, Ashraf J, Harbour D, and Johnson BH: Glucocorticoids in malignant lymphoid cells: gene regulation and the minimum receptor fragment for lysis. J Steroid Biochem Molec Biol 1992; 41:273–282.
49. Thulasi R, Harbour DV, and Thompson EB: Suppression of c-myc is a critical step in glucocorticoid-induced human leukemic cell lysis. J Biol Chem 1993; 268: 18306–18312.
50. Smets L: Programmed cell death (apoptosis) and response to anticancer drugs. Anti-Cancer Drugs 1994;5:3–9
51. Annun YA: Apoptosis and the dilemma of cancer chemotherapy. Blood 1997; 89:1845–1853.
52. Alnemri ES, Fernandes TF, Haldar S, Croce CM, Litwack G: Involvement of BCL-2 in glucocorticoid-induced apoptosis of human pre-B-leukemias. Cancer Res 1992; 52:491–495, 1992.
53. Lotem J, Sachs L: Regulation by bcl-2, c-myc, and p53 of suseptibility to induction of apoptosis by heat shock and cancer chemotherapy compounds in differentiation-competent and -defective myeloid leukemic cells. Cell Growth & Differentiation 1993;4:41–47.
54. Distelhorst CW and Dubyak G: Role of calcium in glucocorticosteroid-induced apoptosis of thymocytes and lymphoma cells: resurrection of old theories by new findings. Blood 1998, 91;731–734.
55. McConkey DJ, Orrenius S, Okret S, Jondal M: Cyclic AMP potentiates glucocorticoid-induced endogenous endonulease activation in thymocytes. FASEB J 1993; 7: 580–585.
56. Pieters R, Klumper E, Veerman AJP: Can nonradioactive meta-iodobenzylguanidine (MIBG) restore resistance to glucocorticoids in lymphoblastic leukemia? Med Pediatr Oncol 1996; 27:229 (abstract #O72).
57. Gruol DJ and Bourgeois S: Expression of the mdr1 p-glycoprotein gene: a mechanism of escape from glucocorticod-induced apoptosis. Biochem Cell Biol 1994; 72: 561–571.
58. Kojika S, Sugita K, Inukai T,Saito M, Iijima K, Tezuka T, Goi K, Shirashi K, Mori T, Okazaki T, Kagami K, Ohyama K, and Nakazawa S: Mechanisms of glucocorticoid resistance in human leukemic cells: implications of abnormal 90 and 70 kDa heat shock proteins. Leukemia 1996; 10:994–999.
59. Balis FM, and Poplack DG. Central nervous system pharmacology of antileukemic drugs. Am J Pediatr Hematol/Oncol 1989; 11:74–86.
60. Ito C, Evans WE, McNinch L, Coustan-Smith E, Mahmoud H, Pui CH, and Compana D: Comparative cytotoxicity of dexamethasone and prednisolone in childhood acute lymphoblastic leukemia. J Clin Oncol 1996; 14:2370–2376.
61. Jones B, Freeman AI, Shuster JJ, Jacquillat C, Weil M, Pochedly C, Sinks L, Chevalier L, Maurer HM, Koch K, Falkson G, Patterson R, Seligman B, Sartorius J, Kung F, Haurani F, Stuart M, Burgert EO, Ruymann F, Sawitsky A, Forman E, Pluess H, Truman J, Hakami N, Glidewell O, Glicksman AS, and Holland JF: Lower incidence of meningeal leukemia when prednisone is replaced by dexamethasone in the treatment of acute lymphocytic leukemia. Med Pediatr Oncol 1991; 19:269–275.
62. Veerman AJP, Hählen K, Kamps WA, Van Leeuwen EF, de Vaan GAM, Van Wering ER, Vasnderdoes-Vanderberg A, Solbu G, and Suciu S:. Dutch Childhood Leukemia Study Group: Early results of Study ALL VI (1984–1988) Haematol Blood Transfus 1990; 33:473–477.
63. Henze G, Langermann H-J, Brämswig J, Breu H, Gadner H, Schellong G, Welte K, and Riehm H. Ergebnisse der Studie BFM 76/79 zur Behandlung der akuten lymphoblastischen Leukämie bei Kindern und Jugendlichen. Klin Pädiat 1981; 193:145–154.
64. Gaynon PS, Bleyer WA, Steinherz PG,Finklestein JZ, Littman PS, Miller DR, Reaman GH, Sather HN, and Hammond GD: Modified BFM therapy for children with previously untreated acute lymphjoblastic leukemia and unfavorable presenting features: report fo the Children's Cancer Study Group Study CCG-193P. Am J Pediatr Hematol Oncol 1988; 10:42–50.
65. Tubergen DG, Gilchrist GS, O'Brien RT, Coccia PF, Sather HN, Waskerwitz MJ, and Hammond GD. Improved outcome with delayed intensification for children with acute lymphoblastic leukemia and intermediate presenting features: A Childrens Cancer Group Phase III trial. J Clin Oncol 1993; 11:527–537.
66. Mastrangelo R, Poplack D, Bleyer A, Riccardi R, Sather H, and D'Angio G. Report and recommendations of the Rome Workshop concerning poor-prognosis acute lymphoblastic leukemia in children: Biologic bases for staging, stratification, and treatment. Med Pediatr Oncol 1986; 14:191–194.
67. Smith M, Arthur D. Camitta B, Carroll W, Crist W, Gaynon P, Hgelber R, Heerema N, Korn EL, Link M,Murphy S, Pui CH, Pullen J, Reaman G, Sallan SE, Sather H, Shuster J, Simon R, Trigg M, Tubergen D, Uckun F, and Ungeleider R: Uniform approach for risk classification and treatment assignment for children with acute lymphoblastic leukemia. J Clin Oncol 1996;14:14–18.
68. Bostrom B, Gaynon PS, Sather H, Gold S, Hutchinson RJ, Provisor A, and Trigg M: Dexamethasone (DEX) decreases central nervous system (CNS) relapse in lower risk acute lymphoblastic leukemia (ALL). Proc Am Soc Clin 1998; 17:5270 (abstract #2024).

69. Thompson EB, Srivastava D, and Johnson BH: Interactions of the phenylpyrazolo-steroid cortivazol with glucocorticoid receptors in steroid-sensitive and -resistant human leukemic cells. Cancer Res 1989; 49 (suppl): 2253s-2258s.
70. Srivastava D and Thompson EB: Two glucocorticoid binding sites on the human glucocortoicoid receptor. Endocrinol 1990; 127: 1770–1778.
71. Harmon JM, Schmidt TJ, and Thompson EB: Deacylcortivazol acts through glucocorticoid receptors. J Steroid Biochem 1981; 14:273–279.
72. Harmon JM, Schmidt TJ, and Thompson EB: Non-glucocorticoid receptor-mediated effects of the potent glucocorticoid deacylcortivazol. Cancer Res 1982; 42:2110–2114.
73. Schlechte JA and Schmidt TJ: Use of [3H]cortivazol to characterize glucoorticoid receptors in a dexamethasone-resistant human leukemic cell line. J Clin Endocrinol Metab 64:441–446, 1987.
74. Ashraf J, Kunapuli S, Chilton D, and Thompson EB: Cortivazol mediated induction of glucocorticoid messenger ribonucleic acid in wild-type and dexamethasone-resistant human leukemic (CEM) cell lines. J Steroid Biochem Molec Biol 38:561- 568, 1991.
75. Juneja HS, Harvey WH, Brasher WK, and Thompson EB: Successful in vitro purging of leukemia blasts from marrow by cortivazol, a pyrazolosteroid: a preclinical study for autologous transplantation in acute lymphoblastic leukemia and non-Hodgkin's lymphoma. Leukemia 9:1771–1778, 1995.
76. Kralli A, Bohen SP, Yamamoto KR: LEM1, and ATP-binding-cassette transporter, selectively modulates the biological potency of steroid hormones. Proc Natl Acad Sci (USA) 1995; 92: 4701–4705.
77. Lilleyman JS and Lennard L. Mercaptopurine metabolism and risk of relapse in childhood lymphoblastic leukaemia. Lancet 343:1188–1190, 1994.
78. Bostrom B and Erdmann GR. Association of relapse with mercaptopurine (6MP) cellular pharmacokinetics (CPK) in children with acute lymphoblastic leukemia (ALL). Proc Am Soc Clin Oncol 1992; 11:278.
79. Cheung N-KV, Chau IY, and Coccia PF. Antibody response to Escherichia coli L-asparaginase. Am J Pediatr Hematol Oncol 1986; 8:99–104.
80. Kurtzberg J, Asselin B, Pollack B, Bernstein M, Buchanan G, and the Pediatric Oncology Group. Peg-L-asparaginase (PEGasp) vs Native E coli asparaginase (asp) for reinduction of relapsed acute lymphoblastic (ALL): POG #8866 Phase II trial. ASCO Proc 1993; 12:325.
81. Abshire T, Pollock B, Billett A, Bradley P, and Buchanan G. Weekly polyethylene glycol conjugated (PEG) L-asparaginase (ASP) produces superior induction remission rates in childhood relapsed acute lymphoblastic leukemia (rALL): A Pediatric Oncology Group (POG) study 9310. ASCO Proc 1995; 14:344.
82. Nachman J, Sather HN, Gaynon PS, Lukens JN, Wolff L, and Trigg ME: Augmented Berlin-Frankfurt-Münster therapy abrogates the adverse prognostic significance of slow early response to induction chemotherapy for children and adolescents with acute lymphoblastic leukemia and unfavorable presenting features: a report from the Children's Cancer Group. J Clin Oncol 1997; 15:2222–2230, 1997.
83. Nachman J, Sather H, Lukens J, Gaynon P, Wolff L, Cherlow J, and Trigg M: Augmented Berlin-Frankfurt-Münster (a-BFM) chemotherapy improves event free survival (EFS) for children with acute lymphoblastic leukemia and unfavorable presenting features who show a slow early response (ser) to induction therapy. Blood 1997; 90:558a, 1997.
84. Imamura J, Miyoshi I, and Koeffler HP: p53 in hematologic malignancies. Blood 1994; 84:2412–2421.
85. Harris CC: Structure and function of the p53 tumor suppressor gene: clues for rationale cancer therapeutic strategies. J Natl Cancer Inst 1996; 88:1422–1455.
86. Marks DI, Kurz BW, Link MP, Ng E, Shuster JJ, Lauer SJ, Brodsky I, and Haines DS: High incidence of potential p53 inactivation in poor outcome childhood acute lymphoblastic leukemia at diagnosis. Blood 1996; 87:1155–1161.
87. Diccianni MB, Yu J, Hsiao M, Mukherjee S, Shao L-E, Yu AL. Clinical significance of p53 mutations in relapsed T-cell acute lymphoblastic leukemia. Blood 1994; 84:3105–3112.
88. Kawamura M, Kikuchi A, Kobayashi S, Hanada R, Yamamoto K, Horibe K, Shikano T, Ueda K, Hayashi K, Sekiya T, and Hayashi Y: Mutations of the p53 and ras genes in childhood t(1;19)-acute lymphoblastic leukemia. Blood 1995; 85:2546–2552.

GLUCOCORTICOID INDUCED APOPTOSIS IN LEUKEMIA

Lou A. Smets, Gajja Salomons, and Joop van den Berg

Department of Experimental Therapy
The Netherlands Cancer Institute/Antoni van Leeuwenhoek Huis
121 Plesmanlaan, NL-1066 CX, Amsterdam

Keywords: Apoptosis, Leukemia, Resistance, Bcl-2, Mitochondria, Glucocorticoids.

1. ABSTRACT

Lymphoid and leukemic cells are uniquely sensitive to the lytic actions of glucocorticoid hormones which activate a programmed cell death in these cells. The response to glucocorticoids is sensitive to modulations at each step of hormone action: cellular uptake, binding and activation of cytosolic receptors, nuclear translocation and transcriptional activity of the activated receptor and the expression levels of pro- and anti-apoptotic genes. This review, based mainly on our studies with leukemic cells in tissue culture and on clinical observations in childhood acute lymphoblastic leukemia, summarizes the potential impact of these checkpoints in the treatment of this disease. In addition, we will discuss interventions that may reverse resistance or promote sensitivity to apoptosis of leukemic cells by glucocorticoid hormones.

2. INTRODUCTION

Apoptosis or programmed cell death is a special form of cellular demise for the removal of unwanted or redundant cells. In lymphoid tissues apoptosis controls the elimination of unstimulated or selfreactive thymocytes and the downregulation of immune responses. It has been postulated that for these functions lymphoid cells are primed by a default apoptotic mechanism.[1] This propensity may be also responsible for the marked chemosensitivity of their malignant counterparts leukemia and lymphoma. Cytostatic treatment frequently induces apoptotic cell death which is delayed or blocked by manipulation of apoptosis-regulating genes. The expression levels and mutational status of pro-

and anti-apoptotic genes are therefore considered by many as a major determinant of the intrinsic sensitivity of malignant disease to cytostatic treatment.

Lymphoid and leukemic cells are not only generally prone to apoptosis but also uniquely sensitive to the lytic action of glucocorticoid hormones (GC). Binding of GCs activates cytosolic receptors, a process involving dissociation of two heat-shock proteins from the large, heteromeric GC receptor complex which results in the exposure of nuclear localization and DNA binding motifs on the monomeric, 96 kDa receptor. The activated GC receptor translocates to the nucleus and interacts with GC-responsive elements. How the transcriptionally active receptor initiates apoptosis is largely unknown but would seem to involve both transcriptional activation and repression. GC-signaling to apoptosis is essentially different from that by cytostatic drugs or ionizing radiation. GCs can kill their sensitive target cells only by inducing a programmed cell death whereas the contribution of apoptosis to the total level of cell kill by cytostatic drugs and radiation is a matter of debate.[2] Consequently, each step in the initiation and execution of the death program is a potential checkpoint in the sensitivity of leukemic cells to glucocorticoid treatment.

3. FACTORS AFFECTING APOPTOSIS BY GLUCOCORTICOIDS

3.1. Glucocorticoid Uptake and Binding

It is generally accepted that lipophilic glucocorticosteroids enter the cells by passive diffusion through the plasma membrane to bind their cognate, cytosolic receptors. There is increasing evidence that several corticosteroids can be substrates for MDR-mediated export.[3] So far, there is little evidence for an important role of active export as a cause of GC resistance, however. This may relate to the dose-effect relationship in GC action, which is essentially different from that of most other cytostatic drugs. Whereas GCs only have to bind their receptors in a saturating concentration of about 10^{-7}M, other drugs usually display a linear relationship between intracellular concentration and cytotoxic potential. Likewise, this non-linear relationship may be responsible for the limited importance of the number of functional receptors in the response to GC. Induction of apoptosis in responsive cells requires only binding of a critical minimum of about 5,000 receptors out of a total of 20,000 to 40,000 per cell.

Gross alterations in the number of GC receptors are an infrequent cause of intrinsic or acquired GC resistance in acute leukemia.[4] Differences observed in receptor density of leukemic blasts are often due to variations in sample quality, notably in metabolic condition and cell cycle distribution. In addition, routine laboratory assays performed on cell lysates at ambient temperature, may not accurately reflect receptor properties in intact cells, as will be discussed in the next paragraph.

3.2. Receptor Activation

Activation of GC receptors in cytosolic preparations, conveniently determined as the acquisition of DNA-binding capacity, is rapid, quantitative and irreversible. By contrast, receptor activation in intact cells at physiological temperature is a highly dynamic and reversible process. Even in very sensitive cells only a subset of all receptors is translocated to the nucleus during drug exposure and these rapidly reassume their native configuration and cytoplasmic localization after removal of the steroid[5]. The most important cause of this discrepancy between *in vitro* and *in situ* observations is the temperature sensitivity of the interaction between GC and receptor. At 28 °C or lower this interaction appears to be much more stable and activation-effective than at physiological temperature.[6] Other *in vitro* artefacts, that include low ATP content and dilution of activation-inhibiting cytosolic factors, may be involved as well. The repercussion of this could be that some potential types of clinical resistance escape detection in assays that probe GC binding or receptor activation under these conditions.

Model studies suggest that GC resistance can indeed be a consequence of impaired or insufficient receptor activation. Selection of cells resistant to dexamethasone (DEX) frequently results in so-called "deathless phenotypes", *i.e.*, cells that display normal hormone binding and sometimes even DEX-mediated growth inhibition but that fail to enter apoptosis subsequently.[7,8] Deathless phenotypes have unchanged sensitivity to apoptosis by cell penetrating ceramide analogues or Ca^{++}-mobilizing agents, indicating that their apoptotic machinery is basically intact. By contrast, they are cross-resistant to physiological inducers such as cAMP analogues or growth factor deprivation. The observations in deathless cells have been interpreted by us[8] to reflect an increased threshold for receptor activation, not only by DEX but also by physiological stress. These findings attribute a novel function to the GC receptor in the regulation of lymphoid and leukemic cell numbers. The deathless phenotype also offers a possible model of high-risk ALL, presenting with very high blast counts. Impaired receptor activation would not only account for a poor response to GC therapy but also for an increased survival capacity of the leukemic blasts in the face of unfavorable physiological conditions such as a poor supply of oxygen, nutrients and growth factors.

In deathless variants, resistance to DEX can be abrogated by using more potent GC agonist, *e.g.* cortivasol. Mono-ADP-ribosylation is a posttranslational modification of heat-shock proteins which release ADP-ribose moieties in response to stress conditions. Because inhibitors of mono-ADP-ribosylation can sensitize deathless cells to DEX and physiological stress,[6,8] we have speculated that increased ADP-ribosylation of GC receptor-associated heat-shock proteins may be involved in resistance to hormone-dependent and -independent receptor activations.

3.3. Cell Proliferation

Non-proliferating lymphoid cells such as prothymocytes are rapidly committed to apoptosis by a brief exposure to GCs. Conversely, GC-mediated lysis of proliferating cells is preceded by an induction phase of several hours during which GC action is reversible.[9,10] The duration of the induction phase is grossly proportional to cell cycle time and functions to arrest the cells in G_1/G_0, a necessary but not a sufficient condition for apoptosis. The notion that active cell proliferation and GC-action are mutually antagonistic is strongly supported by the frequently observed phenomenon of "mitogenic rescue" from GC action by serum, exogenous growth factors or immune stimulations[11] and by GC-induced repression of the IL-6 gene in multiple myeloma cell lines.[12] We therefore suggest (Figure 1) that GCs synchronize proliferating cells in G_1/G_0 by repressing autocrine growth factor production whereas the activation of killer genes is restricted to cell-cycle arrested cells.

The *in vitro* established requirement for leukemic cell synchronization prior to lysis is in agreement with the strategy in many current ALL protocols of frequent administration of glucocorticoids. Moreover, the favorable prognosis associated in earlier ALL studies with a low %S-phase index and with hyperdiploidy, a condition associated with a tendency for cell cycle exit, are both consistent with a preferential sensitivity of non-cycling leukemic cells to GCs.[14]

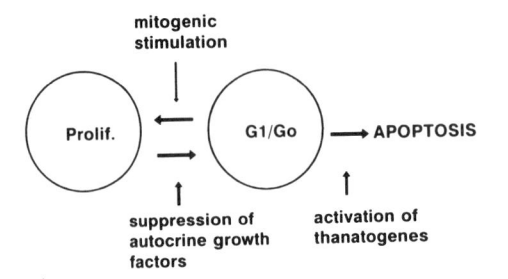

Figure 1. Proposed role of cell proliferation in the induction of apoptosis by glucocorticoid hormones. During a reversible induction phase, proliferating leukemic blasts are synchronized by the transcriptionally active GC receptor into G_1/G_0 phase, which is the effector phase of GC-mediated apoptosis. These cells can be rescued from GC action by mitogenic stimulations.

Protection by growth/survival factors has been reported also for several non-hormonal apoptotic triggers,[13] indicating that other mechanisms can be also involved in mitogenic rescue, for instance the upregulation of apoptosis-inhibiting proteins or protection against non-hormonal GC receptor activation.

3.4. Survival Controlling Proteins

Apoptosis is under control of several promoting and inhibiting genes that are often deregulated in cancer cells. Of these, p53 is of paramount importance in the induction of apoptosis by DNA damaging agents but not so in case of GC-mediated cell death.[15] By contrast, the protective role of anti-apoptotic Bcl-2 against GC-mediated apoptosis has been amply demonstrated in several cell systems, mostly by transfection of the *bcl-2* gene. Also in non-manipulated leukemic cell lines there is a inverse relationship between Bcl-2 protein content and GC sensitivity.[16] Although the precise site of Bcl-2 action is a matter of intense research, it is clear that the protein acts on distal steps of the apoptotic cascade and confers therefore resistance to a wide array of triggers. However, from a therapeutic point of view blocked apoptosis by elevated Bcl-2 would seem much more problematic in case of glucocorticoids than with cytostatic, mostly DNA-damaging, drugs. Cells whose apoptosis is blocked after GC treatment are true survivors whereas blocked apoptosis from many cytostatic drugs yields "undeath" cells which eventually die by other mechanisms, *e.g.* mitotic failure.

4. BCL-2 AND BAX IN ACUTE LYMPHOBLASTIC LEUKEMIA

4.1. Variable Expressions

Bcl-2 belongs to a large and expanding family of related pro- and anti-apoptotic proteins that can form homo- and heterodimers. Bcl-2 typically dimerizes with pro-apoptotic Bax and the Bcl-2:Bax ratio is therefore considered to act as a pre-set rheostat whose setting determines survival or death after cytotoxic insult.[17] Because in model studies the relevant genes are either completely knocked out or highly overexpressed by gene transfer techniques, we have addressed two trivial but relevant questions with regard to the role of Bcl-2:Bax in childhood ALL. First, we investigated the interpatient variation of Bcl-2:Bax by quantitative western blotting. The results[18] revealed large, up to 25-fold differences in the level of either Bcl-2 or Bax protein, ranging from very low values as observed in normal lymphocytes to very high levels, exceeding those in t(14;18)-positive lymphoma cells. This large variation, which may be similar in AML, differs from that in B-CLL or lymphoma in which Bcl-2 is usually overexpressed. In case of ALL variation in protein levels could not be attributed to mutations in the coding regions of the *bcl-2* or *bax* gene.[19] The next question was if the variations in Bcl-2:Bax in blasts from ALL patients affected the sensitivity to the synthetic glucocorticoid dexamethasone. Transfection of *bax* into leukemic cells and analysis of thymocytes from *bcl-2* and *bax* transgenic mice both confirmed that a moderate increase in Bax protein significantly stimulated GC-mediated apoptosis.[20] Moreover, the variations in Bcl-2:Bax in ALL blasts spanned the full range of protein levels relevant for DEX response in the experimental models.[18]

4.2. Prognostic Value of Bcl-2:Bax in Acute Leukemia

Because an elevated setting of Bcl-2:Bax blocks GC action and confers, according to some authors, a special form of multidrug resistance, one would expect it to correlate with (poor) outcome of treatment. This prediction has not been consistently confirmed in clinical studies of leukemia and solid tumors. In fact, in ALL the levels of Bcl-2 bear either no obvious relationship with treatment outcome or are associated with a favorable prognosis.[18,21,22] Moreover, the high Bcl-2 levels in follicular lymphoma, in which t(14;18) deregulates the *bcl-2* gene, do not prevent the response to standard therapy which includes GCs.

Similar discrepancies between predictions from *in vitro* studies and clinical observations have been encountered in studies involving p53 status or cytological markers of apoptosis in solid tumors. Collectively, these observations indicate that the prognostic impact of apoptosis-regulating genes is context dependent. In case of Bcl-2, this context is obviously defined by the relative levels of counteracting Bax, but a role for other members of the Bcl-2 family should be considered as well. In cell lines Bcl-2 has anti-proliferative potential[16,23] and studies with thymocytes from transgenic mice have confirmed that Bcl-2 inhibits G_0 to G_1 transition which is stimulated by an excess of Bax.[24] The proliferation-suppressing function of Bcl-2 may reside in a domain different from that encoding the anti-apoptosis capacity.[25] Despite overall large variation in Bcl-2 protein levels in pediatric ALL, there is an obvious clustering of high levels in B-lineage ALL with low blasts counts on the one hand and of low Bcl-2 in high-risk patients with elevated WBC values on the other[18]. The anti-proliferative function of Bcl-2, by mitigating blast cell production and stimulating GC-sensitivity (cf 3.3), may account for the paradoxical association of high Bcl-2 levels with a favorable prognosis in some studies. Conversely, in high-risk ALL mitogenic rescue from low Bcl-2:Bax could decrease the sensitivity to GC, thereby outweighing its pro-apoptotic effect. While admittedly speculative, the concept of balanced and context-dependent Bcl-2/Bax actions (Figure 2), being dependent on relative protein content, tissue type and cytostatic agents, may be pertinent to the conflicting or unexpected clinical observations regarding the prognostic impact of these apoptosis-regulating genes.

5. MODULATION OF SENSITIVITY TO GLUCOCORTICOIDS

Enhanced export, a frequent cause of multidrug resistance to amphipatic compounds, may include glucocorticoids as well. If confirmed, the use of suitable MDR reversal agents could be considered. Defects in GC receptor activation, either by inappropriate hormone binding or by an increased threshold of receptor activation in deathless phenotypes is frequently encountered in model studies. So far, the inadequacy of most laboratory assays in revealing subtle difference in GC-receptor activation *in vitro* has prevented realistic estimates of the frequency of deathless mutations in acute leukemia. More potent GC agonists and pharmacological sensitization of GC receptor activation with inhibitors

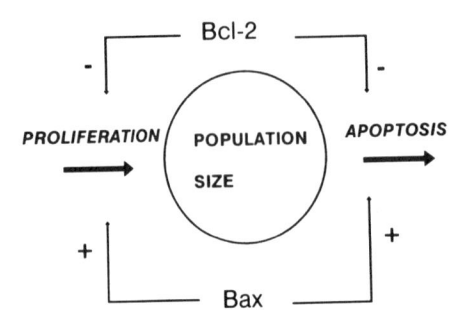

Figure 2. Opposing actions of Bcl-2 and Bax on cell proliferation and apoptosis. Bcl-2 inhibits both cell proliferation and apoptosis and is antagonized by Bax. The sensitivity to GC-mediated apoptosis is the balance of Bcl-2:Bax action on cell cycle exit, which increases GC sensitivity, and its protective effect by inhibition of apoptosis.

of mono-ADP-ribosylation, can possibly revert this type of GC resistance. Cell kinetic resistance, defined as the insensitivity of proliferating and mitogenically stimulated cells to the acute induction of apoptosis by GCs, has been amply demonstrated in model studies. Treatment schedules of ALL that involve frequent administration of GC are most probably adequate in circumventing proliferation-associated insensitivity. Enforcing the synchronizing activity of GCs (Figure 1) by promoting cell cycle exit with negatively acting recombinant growth factors and cytokines, should be considered for patients who still fail on such schedules.

Pro-apoptotic strategies, especially those interfering with Bcl-2 and Bax functions, could conceivably promote the effectiveness of GC-based therapies. However, because of the conflicting results of clinical studies, it is obvious that we need much more knowledge of the precise role of a given setting of the Bcl-2: Bax ratio in acute leukemia, notably ALL. Ongoing studies, in which the expression levels of several members of the Bcl-2 family are being compared with drug sensitivity in MTT assays and follow-up data, may provide interesting clues. Antisense strategies to repress apoptosis-inhibiting genes and oligonucleotides that interfere with homo-and hetero-dimerizations are currently being explored for clinical applications. Finally, the role of mitochondria is a recurrent theme in apoptosis research. It is becoming increasingly clear that this organelle is the bottleneck in apoptosis signaling or the execution of the death program and the playground of Bcl-2 and Bax. Accordingly, mitochondrial inhibition could interfere with various functions attributed to Bcl-2, *e.g.* by preventing Bcl-2 protection of mitochondrial dysfunction[26] or by decreasing ATP levels required for Bcl-2's alledged functions in Ca^{++} homeostasis and anti-oxidant activities.[16] Potentiation of GC action by mitochondrial inhibitors has been demonstrated in a Bcl-2 overexpressing lymphoma cell line with functional, translocation-competent GC receptors[27] and in GC-resistant, relapsed ALL in MTT assays.[28]

6. CONCLUDING REMARKS

Resistance to glucocorticoids in childhood ALL, detected either by appropriate *ex vivo* assays[29] or inferred from a poor response to GC monotherapy, is an important cause of treatment failure. Model studies with leukemic cells in tissue culture have hinted at several mechanisms of GC resistance and also at interventions that may reverse it. Unfortunately, the clinical relevance of these observations remains to be established and as yet, not a single case of clinical resistance has been unambiguously attributed to any of them. Studies that address this question, combined with the rapidly expanding knowledge and analytical possibilities in apoptosis research, are likely to produce meaningful answers soon.

ACKNOWLEDGMENTS

Part of the studies described in this review was funded by a grant NKI 94–808 of the Dutch Cancer Foundation. The authors gratefully acknowledge the collaborations with the Dutch Childhood Leukemia Study Group, The Hague (head: Dr. A. van der Does - van den Berg) and with the departments of pediatric oncology of the Emma Children Hospital/Amsterdam Medical Center (head: Prof. P. Voûte) and of the Academic Hospital, Free University, Amsterdam (head: Prof. A. Veerman) in the course of these investigations.

REFERENCES

1. Gregory, C., and Milner, A. Regulation of cell survival in Burkitt lymphoma: implications from studies of apoptosis following cold-shock treatment. Int. J. Cancer 1994, **57**, 419–426.
2. Smets, L. Programmed cell death (apoptosis) and response to anti-cancer drugs. Anti-Cancer Drugs 1994, **5**, 3–9.
3. Schinkel, A. The physiological function of drug-transporting P-glycoproteins. Seminars in Cancer Biology 1997, **8**, 161–170.
4. Kaspers, G., Pieters, R., Klumper, E., De Waal, F., and Veerman, A. Glucocorticoid resistance in childhood leukemia. Leukemia and Lymphoma 1994, **13**, 187–201.
5. Van den Berg, J., Smets, L., Hutchinson, K., Van Rooij, H., and Van den Elshout, M. High levels of non-activated receptors in glucocorticoid-sensitive S49^{wt} mouse lymphoma cells incubated with dexamethasone. J. Steroid Biochem. Molec. Biol. 1994, **51**, 33–40.
6. Van den Berg, J., Smets, L., Van den Elshout, M, Van Geel, I., and Janssen, M. Temperature dependence of glucocorticoid binding in sensitive and refractory murine leukaemia cells. Leuk. Res. 1993, **17**, 263–269.
7. Dowd, D. and Miesfeld, R. Evidence that glucocorticoid- and cyclic AMP-induced apoptotic pathways share distal events. Mol. Cell Biol. 1992, **12**, 3600–3608.
8. Smets, L., Salomons, G., Van Rooij, H., and Van den Berg, J. Involvement of the glucocorticoid receptor in stress-induced apoptosis of leukemic cells. Leukemia 1998, **12**, 406–413.
9. Harmon, J., Norman, M., Fowlkes, B., and Thompson, E. Dexamethasone induces irreversible G_1 arrest and death of a human lymphoid cell line. J. Cell. Physiol. 1979, **98**, 267–278.
10. Smets, L., Bout, B., Brouwer, M., and Tulp, A. Cytotoxic effects of dexamethasone restricted to non-cycling, early G1-phase cells of L1210 leukemia. J. Cell Physiol. 1983, **116**, 397–403.
11. Smets, L. and Van den Berg, J. Bcl-2 expression and glucocorticoid-induced apoptosis of leukemic and lymphoma cells. Leukemia and Lymphoma 1996, **20**, 199–205.
12. Hardin, J. McLeod, S., Grigoriva, A., Chang, R., Barlogie, B., Xiao, H. and Epstein, J. Interleukin-6 prevents dexamethasone-induced myeloma cell death. Blood 1994, **84**, 3063–3070.
13. Sachs, L., and Lotem, J. Control of programmed cell death in normal and leukemic cells: new implications for therapy. Blood 1993, **82**, 15–21.
14. Smets, L., Slater, R., Van Wering, E., Van der Does- van den Berg, A., Hart, A., Veerman, A., and Kamps, W. DNA index and %S-phase cells determined in acute lymphoblastic leukemia of children: a report from studies ALL V, ALL VI and ALL VIII (1979–1991) of the Dutch Childhood Leukemia Study Group and The Netherlands Workgroup on Cancer Genetics and Cytogenetics. Med. Pediatr. Oncol. 1995, **25**. 437–444.
15. Clarke, A., Purdie, C., Harrison, D., Morris, R., Bird, C., Hooper, M., and Wyllie, A. Thymocyte apoptosis induced by p53-dependent and independent pathways. Nature 1993, **362**, 894 852.
16. Smets, L., van den Berg, J., Acton, D., Top, B., Van Rooij, H., and Verwijs-Janssen, M. BCL-2 expression and mitochondrial activity in leukemic cells with different sensitivity to glucocorticoid-induced apoptosis. Blood 1994, **84**,1613–1619.
17. Reed, J. Bcl-2 and the regulation of programmed cell death. J. Cell Biol. 1994, **124**, 1–6.
18. Salomons, G., Brady, H., Verwijs-Janssen, M, Van den Berg, J., Hart, A., Van den Berg, H., Behrendt, H., Hählen, K., and Smets, L. The Baxα:Bcl-2 ratio modulates the response to dexamethasone in leukemic cells and is highly variable in childhood acute leukemia. Int. J. Cancer 1997, **71**, 959–965.
19. Salomons, G., Buitenhuis, C., Martinez Muñoz,C., Verwijs-Janssen, M., Behrendt, H., Zsiros, J., and Smets, L. Mutational analysis of bax and bcl-2 in childhood acute lymphoblastic leukemia. Int. J. Cancer 1998 **179**, 273–277.

20. Brady, H., Salomons, G., Bobeldijk, R. and Berns, A. T cells from baxα transgenic mice show accelerated apoptosis in response to stimuli but do not show restored DNA-damage-induced cell death in the absence of p53. EMBO J. 1996, **15**, 1221–1230.
21. Uckun, F., Yang, Z., Sather, H., Steinherz, P., Nachman, J., Bostrom, B., Crotty, L., Sarquis, M., Ek, O., Zeren, T., Tubergen, D., Reaman, G., and Gaynon, P. Cellular expression of antiapoptotic Bcl-2 oncoprotein in newly diagnosed childhood acute lymphoblastic leukemia: a children's cancer group study. Blood 1997, **89**, 2506–2509.
22. Coustan-Smith, E., Kitanaka, A, Pui, C., McNinch, L., Evans, W., Raimondi, S., Behm, F., Arico, M., and Campana, D. Clinical relevance of Bcl-2 over-expression in childhood acute lymphoblastic leukemia. Blood 1996, **87**, 1140–1146.
23. Pietenpol, J., Papadopoulos, N, Markowitz, S., Willson, J., Kinzler, K., and Vogelstein, B. Paradoxical inhibition of solid-tumor cell growth by bcl2. Cancer Res. 1994, **54**, 3714–3717.
24. Brady, H., Gil-Gomez, G., Kirberg, J., and Berns, A. Baxα perturbs T cell development and affects cell cycle entry of T cells. EMBO J. 1996, **15**, 6991–7001.
25. Huang, D., O'Reilly, A., Strasser, A., and Cory, S. The anti-apoptosis function of Bcl-2 can be genetically separated from its inhibitory effect on cell cycle entry. EMBO J. 1997, **16**, 4628–4638.
26. Decaudin, D., Geley, S., Hirsch, T., Castedo, M., Marchetti, P., Macho, A., Kofler, R., and Kroemer, G. Bcl-2 and Bcl-XL antagonize the mitochondrial dysfunction preceding nuclear apoptosis induced by chemotherapeutic agents. Cancer Res. 1997, **57**, 62–67.
27. Van den Berg, J., Smets, L., and Van Rooij, H. Agonist-free transformation of the glucocorticoid receptor in human B-lymphoma cells. J. Steroid Biochem. Mol. Biol. 1996, **57**, 239–249.
28. Klumper, E. Thesis 1995, Free University, Amsterdam.
29. Kaspers, G., Veerman, A., Pieters, R., Van Zantwijk, C. Smets, L., Van Wering, E., and Van der Does-Van den Berg, A. In vitro cellular drug resistance and prognosis in newly diagnosed childhood acute lymphoblastic leukemia. Blood 1997, **90**, 2723–2729.

GLUCOCORTICOID RESISTANCE AND THE AP-1 TRANSCRIPTION FACTOR IN LEUKAEMIA

S. Bailey,[1] A.G. Hall,[1] A. D. J. P. Pearson,[1] M. M. Reid,[2] and C. P. F. Redfern[3]

[1]Department of Child Health
[2]Department of Medicine
[3]Department of Haematology
University of Newcastle upon Tyne, England

1. ABSTRACT

Glucocorticoids have been used in the treatment of acute lymphoblastic leukaemia (ALL) for many years, initially as the only agent and then as part of multiagent chemotherapy. In ALL 20% of patients are resistant to glucocorticoids at presentation but this rises to greater than 70% on relapse. It has recently been reported that the glucocorticoid receptor inhibits activity of the AP-1 transcription factor by the ligand-dependant binding of glucocorticoid receptor (GR) to the fos and jun components of AP-1. Since AP-1 is necessary for cell proliferation, the upregulation or over-expression of AP-1 may be a mechanism of resistance to glucocorticoids. The aim of the study was to investigate whether AP-1 levels correlate with *in vitro* glucocorticoid resistance. *In vitro* sensitivity to glucocorticoids was measured using the MTT assay. AP-1 levels were quantified using gel shift analysis: a consensus sequence for the AP-1 binding site was synthesised, labelled with ^{32}P and incubated with nuclear extracts of leukaemic blasts from 14 ALL and 26 CLL patients. Leukaemic blasts were treated with prednisolone or with vehicle alone before preparation of nuclear extracts. The gels were dried and bands quantified using a phosphorimager, using an appropriate internal standard and correcting for protein loading and cytoplasmic contamination of nuclear extracts. The patient samples fell into two distinct groups with respect to their sensitivity to glucocorticoids: AP-1 levels were significantly higher ($p<0.02$) in sensitive blasts than resistant ones. There was no significant change in AP-1 levels after treating blasts for 4 hours with 0.2 mM prednisolone. No change was seen in CLL samples. These data show that glucocorticoid resistance is not associated with increased AP-1. Conversely, glucocorticoid resistance in these samples was apparently associated with decreased AP-1 levels in ALL samples. Whether this has any causal relationship to glucocorticoid resistance is unknown. Clearly, further studies on the role of

AP-1 and related transcription factors is essential for understanding the control of proliferation and apoptosis in ALL.

2. INTRODUCTION

Glucocorticoids are used extensively in the management of haematological malignancies, especially in acute lymphoblastic leukaemia (ALL) and chronic lymphocytic leukaemia (CLL). In ALL glucocorticoids are used both at the initiation of treatment as well as in the intensification and maintenance phases of treatment. Glucocorticoids are able to induce a short lived remission when used as monotherapy.[1] In CLL prednisolone is used in short bursts usually in conjunction with the alkylating agent chlorambucil to bring the disease under control.

The majority of patients with childhood ALL are initially sensitive to glucocorticoids (80%) but at relapse the majority are resistant (65%).[2] The development of resistance has important implications for the treatment of these patients but the aetiology is unknown.

Glucocorticoids exert their action via a 97 kD receptor which is present in the cytosol in an unliganded form associated with a number of chaperone proteins including heat shock proteins (reviwed by Ashraf and Thompson[3]). After binding of ligand the complex dissociates and the glucocorticoid receptor (GR) is translocated as a dimer into the cell nucleus. The GR dimer binds to specific DNA binding sites (glucocorticoid response element or GRE) where it either positively or negatively regulates gene transcription ultimately leading to apoptosis in sensitive lymphoblasts. It has recently been reported that the GR inhibits the activity of the AP-1 transcription factor.[4,5] AP-1 is a dimer of fos and jun proteins and is an important regulator of cell proliferation.[6] Glucocorticoid inhibition of AP-1 activity is thought to be mediated by the ligand-dependant interaction between the fos and jun components of AP-1. Apoptosis in response to glucocorticoids may thus result from an inhibition of AP-1 activity and the upregulation or over-expression of AP-1 could be a mechanism of steroid resistance.

3. MATERIALS AND METHODS

Fourteen patients with ALL were studied (adults and children) and 26 patients with CLL. The spectrum covered patients both resistant and sensitive to *in vitro* glucocorticoids. *In vitro* sensitivity to glucocorticoids was tested by the MTT test as well as scoring apoptosis in response to glucocorticoids. Receptor number was determined by ligand binding assay and AP-1 activity was determined by gel shift analysis.

For the MTT assay blasts were incubated with increasing concentrations of glucocorticoid in a 96 well plate for 4 days. MTT (Sigma) was then added and the optical density measured at 492 nm. LC 50 values were calculated from dose response curves.

To measure the extent of apoptosis scoring cells were stained with Hoescht 33258 to identify apoptotic cells. LC50 values were calculated from a dose response curve for the percentage of apoptotic cells.

Free GR receptor concentrations were measured in whole cell extracts from 1×10^8 cells using ^{3}H dexamethasone (Amersham) with and without an excess of unlabelled dexamethasone. The number of binding sites per milligram of protein and affinity for glucocorticoid receptor (Kd) was estimated by non-linear curve fitting to the binding data.

Nuclear protein extracts were made from blasts with or without treatment with glucocorticoids *in vitro*. Synthetic oligonucleotides corresponding to the AP-1 consensus sequence[7] were end-labelled with γ^{32} P dATP (Amersham) and incubated with nuclear protein extracts. The samples were run on a 5% non denaturing polyacrylamide gel which were then dried and exposed to a phosphorimager to identify and quantify shifted bands. To compare AP-1 activity in samples from separate patients, the phosphorimager data were corrected for protein loading, for inter-gel variability by internal standards (CCRF-CEM) and for cytoplasmic contamination by measurement of the lactate dehydrogenase (LDH) levels.

4. RESULTS

The patients were divide into 2 distinct groups with regard to *in vitro* sensitivity to glucocorticoids (Figure 1) using the MTT test. The number of binding sites per milligram of protein showed less spread and were within previously reported limits [8,9] (ALL median = 7.4×10^{10} binding sites/mg of protein range, range $1.8 \times 10^{10} - 7.1 \times 10^{11}$ and CLL median = 1.7×10^{11}, range $8.7 \times 10^{9} - 1.4 \times 10^{12}$). There was no correlation between the number of receptor sites (or Kd) and *in vitro* sensitivity using the MTT test for ALL (p=0.65) or CLL (p=0.24).

AP-1 bands identified on gel shift analysis were excessed out with an 500 fold excess of cold unlabelled AP-1 oliginucleotide but not by the unrelated oligonucleotide Retinoic Acid A Receptor (RAR). This band was also supershifted with AP-1 antibody (Santa Cruz) and was induced in NIH 3T3 cells by phorbol ester.[6]

There was no correlation between the change in AP-1 activity in response *in vitro* glucocorticoids and glucocorticoid sensitivity (MTT) in both ALL (p = 0.9) and CLL (p = 0.54) or apoptosis scoring (ALL, p = 0.25, CLL p = 0.9). No correlation was found between receptor number and AP-1 activity in ALL (p = 0.24) or CLL (p = 0.8). There was also no correlation between AP-1 activity in those blasts treated with glucocorticoid and steroid sensitivity (MTT) for ALL (p = 0.394) or CLL (p = 0.221). In ALL blasts not treated with prednisolone AP-1 levels were higher in patient samples sensitive to *in vitro* glucocorticoids (p=0.02) (Figure 2) but this was not the case in CLL blasts (p=0.662) (Figure 3).

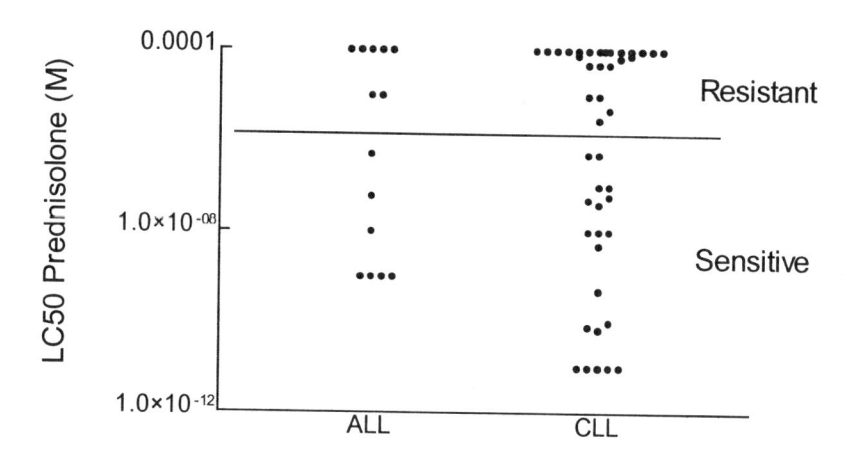

Figure 1. MTT LC50 values (M) for prednisolone in ALL and CLL patient blasts.

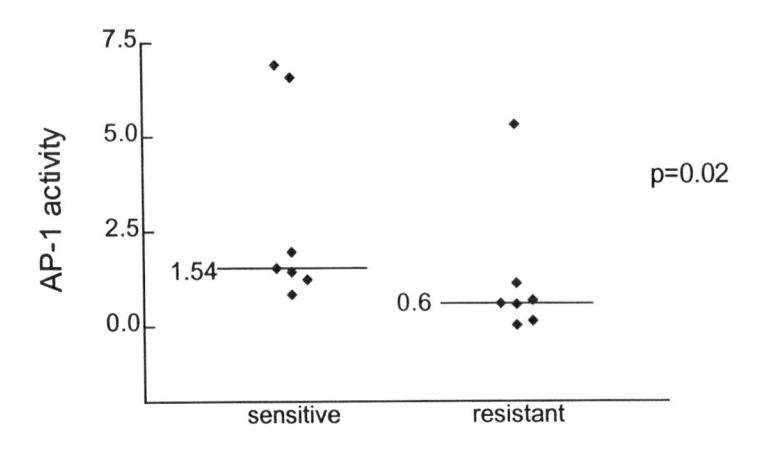

Figure 2. AP-1 activity in ALL blasts sensitive and resistant to *in vitro* prednisolone using the MTT test. Median values are shown.

5. DISCUSSION

The specific band on the gel shift was shown to be AP-1 by a number of methods as described above. The change in AP-1 activity induced by *in vitro* glucocorticoid treatment was not related to measures of glucocorticoid sensitivity or to receptor number. In the basal state AP-1 activity in ALL was inversely related to glucocorticoid resistance as measured by the MTT test, this was in contrast to the hypothesis we had formulated based on suggestions that GR interfered with AP-1 activity.[5,10] It may be that in lymphoblasts AP-1 activity is not related to *in vitro* sensitivity and that our result was due to either small numbers involved or a doubtful biological significance of the difference in AP-1 levels. It is

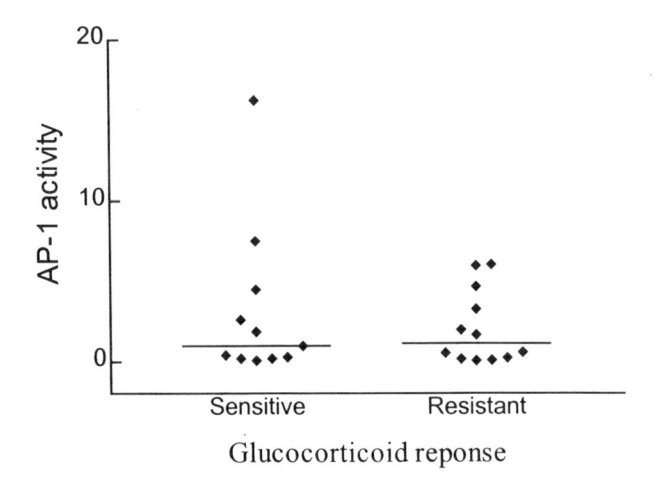

Figure 3. AP-1 activity in CLL blasts sensitive and resisitant to *in vitro* glucocorticoid treatment (MTT). Median values are shown.

also possible that AP-1 is still able to bind to its DNA binding sites (TRE) but not enhance transcription whilst interacting with GR, the gel shift assay would be unable to detect this. It is therefore unlikely that the development of resistance to glucocorticoids is due to AP-1 induction. Alternatively in ALL cells AP-1 activity may be necessary for the induction of apoptosis as suggested by some groups.[11,12] Further work is needed in this field to determine the mechanism of resistance in glucocorticoid induced apoptosis in leukaemia in order to address this clinically important question.

ACKNOWLEDGMENTS

We would like to thank Dr J. Wallis and Dr P. Saunders for providing the patient material and Dr A.W. Skillen for helping with the LDH analysis and The Tyneside Leukaemia Research Fund for funding this research.

REFERENCES

1. Wolff JA, Brubaker CA, Murphy ML, Pierce MI, Severo N. Prednisone therapy of acute childhood leukemia: Prognosis and duration of response in 330 treated patients. *Journal of Pediatrics* 1967; 70:627–631.
2. Kaspers GJL, Pieters R, Klumper E, De Waal FC, Veerman AJP. Glucocorticoid resistance in childhood leukaemia. *Leukemia and Lymphoma* 1994; 13:187–201.
3. Ashraf J, Thompson EB. Glucocorticoid receptors in leukaemias, lymphomas and myelomas of the young and old. In: Yang S S, Warner H R, eds. *The underlaying molecular, cellular, and immunological factors in cancer and aging*. New York: Plenum Press, 1993; 241–269.
4. Helmberg A, Auphan N, Caelles C, Karin M. Glucocorticoid-induced apoptosis of human leukemic cells is caused by the repressive function of the glucocorticoid receptor. *EMBO J* 1995; 14:452–460.
5. Yang-Yen HF, Chambard J, Sun Y, et al. Transcriptional Interference between c-Jun and the Glucocorticoid Receptor: Mutual Inhibition of DNA Binding Due to Direct Protein-Protein Interaction. *Cell* 1990; 2:1205–1215.
6. Angel P, Karin M. The role of Jun, Fos and the AP-1 complex in cell-proliferation and transformation. *Biochemica et Biophysica Acta* 1991; 1072:129–157.
7. Beato M. Gene regulation by steroid hormones. *Cell* 1989; 56:335–344.
8. Costlow ME, Pui C, Dahl GV. Glucocorticoid receptors in childhood acute lymphocytic leukemia. *Cancer Research* 1982; 42:4801–4806.
9. Pui C, Ochs J, Kalwinsky DK, Costlow ME. Impact of treatment efficacy on the prognostic value of glucocorticoid receptor levels in childhood acute lymphoblastic leukemia. *Leukemia Research* 1984; 8:345–350.
10. Helmberg A, Auphan N, Caelles C, Karin M. Glucocorticoid-induced apoptosis of human leukaemic cells is caused by the repressive function of the glucorticoid receptor. *EMBO J* 1995; 14:453–460.
11. Zhou F, Thompson EB. Role of c-jun Induction in the Gluccorticoid -Evoked Apoptotic Pathway in Human Leukemic Lymphoblasts. *Molecular Endocrinology* 1996; 10:306–316.
12. Bossy-Wetzel E, Bakiri L, Yaniv M. Induction of apoptosis by the transcription factor c-Jun. *EMBO J* 1997; 16:1695–1709.

69

THE THREE ASPARAGINASES

Comparative Pharmacology and Optimal Use in Childhood Leukemia

Barbara L. Asselin[*]

Associate Professor of Pediatrics and Oncology
The Children's Hospital at Strong and the Cancer Center at the University of
  Rochester Medical Center
Rochester, New York

Keywords: asparaginase, acute lymphoblastic leukemia, childhood leukemia, pharmacology, hypersensitivity, and drug resistance.

1. ABSTRACT

Asparaginase (ASP) is a standard component of the antileukemia armamentarium. There are currently 3 preparations of asparaginase available: (1) *E. coli* (ASP, Elspar™); (2) the enzyme derived from *Erwinia chrysanthemi* (ERW, Erwinase™); (3) pegaspargase (PEG, Oncaspar™), the *E. coli* enzyme modified by covalent attachment of polyethylene glycol. This report describes the findings of 3 pharmacologic end points: ASP enzyme activity in patients' sera, depletion of asparagine and the development of anti-ASP antibodies. Pharmacokinetics and pharmacodynamic studies in a group of naive children with newly diagnosed ALL demonstrate a significant difference in apparent half-life (1.24 days *E. coli* vs. 0.65 ERW vs. 5.73 PEG; $p < 0.001$) and days of asparagine depletion (14–23 E. coli vs. 7–15 ERW vs. 26–34 PEG; $p < 0.01$) for the 3 different preparations. Data from Pediatric Oncology Group (POG) Protocol #8866 show that high antibody levels correlated with rapid ASP clearance and a significantly lower response rate (NR = 26% vs. CR + PR+64%). The pharmacologic characteristics of ASP in terms of clearance of enzyme

---

[*] Children's Hospital at Strong, University of Rochester School of Medicine & Dentistry, 601 Elmwood Avenue, Box 777, Rochester, NY 14642, Tel: (716) 275-2981, Fax: (716) 273-1039, Email: basselin@mail.urmc.rochester.edu

activity and ability to deplete serum asparagine was dependent upon the nature of the enzyme and are significantly altered in patients who develop anti-ASP antibodies regardless of their clinical status. In addition, these data demonstrate that ASP pharmacokinetics are directly related to its anti-leukemic effect. In order to maximize the therapeutic benefits of ASP, the optimal dose and schedule of treatment should be determined based on pharmacologic testing rather than by clinical criteria alone. Future studies will focus on the role of "silent hypersensitivity" as a mechanism of resistance to ASP and strategies to maximize the therapeutic efficacy of ASP as part of ALL therapy.

2. INTRODUCTION

Thirty-five years ago, J.D. Broome discovered that the L-asparaginase of guinea pig serum is responsible for its antilymphoma effects.[1] In 1998, asparaginase is a standard component of the antileukemia armamentarium for childhood acute lymphoblastic leukemia (ALL), which effects 2,000 new children annually, and is gaining acceptance as part of ALL therapy in 1,500 adults diagnosed each year within the United States. There are currently 3 preparations of ASP available: (1) *E. coli* (ASP) Elspar™), (2) the enzyme derived from *Erwinia chrysanthemi* (ERW, Erwinase™); (3) pegaspargase (PEG, Oncaspar™), the *E. coli* enzyme modified by covalent attachment of polyethylene glycol.

As an enzyme, asparaginase hydrolyzes the nonessential amino acid, asparagine, into aspartic acid and ammonia, thus depleting the circulating pool of serum asparagine. As a chemotherapy, asparaginase has a unique mechanism of action as it selectively starves the leukemia cells which are unable to synthesize adequate amounts of asparagine and normally rely on serum asparagine as their source for protein synthesis. The most common dose-limiting toxicity of asparaginase is clinical hypersensitivity reactions which are reported in up to two-thirds of patients receiving intensive schedules of the native forms of the enzyme.[2-5] Additional patients develop anti-asparaginase antibodies without clinical evidence of hypersensitivity reactions, i.e., silent hypersensitivity.[2, 6-8] These antibodies may diminish asparaginase efficacy by neutralizing asparaginase activity and/or increasing the rate of clearance. Thus, silent hypersensitivity may be an important yet previously unrecognized mechanism of drug resistance among patients receiving L-asparaginase therapy.

This report describes the findings of 3 pharmacologic end points: ASP enzyme activity in patient serum, depletion of asparagine and the development of anti-ASP antibodies. The discussion specifically focuses on the effect of the nature of the enzyme, the effect of hypersensitivity reactions, the phenomenon of silent hypersensitivity, and the relationship between these measurable end points and disease control. The improved understanding of mechanisms of asparaginase sensitivity and resistance that results from these studies is vital to maximize the therapeutic efficacy of ASP and improve patient outcomes in treatment of ALL.

3. MATERIALS AND METHODS

3.1. Patient Populations

We studied patients with childhood ALL on protocols that included intramuscular (IM) asparaginase during remission induction and/or for at least 20 weeks after achieving remission. After obtaining informed consent, children with newly diagnosed or relapsed ALL were treated according to one of a series of treatment protocols between 1987 and 1995, sponsored by the Dana-Farber Cancer Institute Leukemia Consortium or the Pediatric Oncology Group. As part of pharmacologic studies of ASP, we measured ASP enzyme activity, asparagine levels and anti-ASP antibody titers in serum samples obtained from these patients at various time intervals during their therapy with ASP.

3.2. Materials

All 3 ASP preparations were pharmaceutical grade. The *E. coli* enzyme (Elspar™) was obtained from Merck, Sharp and Dohme, Inc., West Point, PA. The Erwinia-derived ASP is manufactured by the Center for Applied Microbiology and Research, Salisbury, England, and supplied through the National Cancer Institute (National Service Center #106977) for investigational use or provided by Speywood Pharmaceuticals, Ltd., Berkshire, England. Enzon, Inc. (Piscataway, NJ) provided the Enzon EKA-kit and the PEG product (Oncaspar), which is the Elspar™ *E. coli* enzyme modified by covalent attachment of PEG.

3.3. Specific Assay Methods

ASP activity in patient serum is measured by a kinetic spectrophotometric assay[9] and these data are used to calculate rate of enzyme clearance (apparent half-life), area under the curve (AUC), and peak concentrations (C max). Asparagine concentration following treatment with asparaginase is measured in patients' deproteinized sera using a high performance liquid chromatography method[10] with a limit of detection of 1 μM. Anti-ASP antibodies (IgG type) are detected using a semiquantitative ELISA method with horseradish peroxidase conjugated anti-human immunoglobulin.[5] Interested readers are referred to the cited references for detailed descriptions of sample collection and assay methods.[5,9,10]

4. RESULTS

4.1. Effect of Asparaginase Preparation and Repeated Doses on Serum Asparaginase Activity

Between 1987 and 1991, patients treated according to Dana-Farber Cancer Institute protocol 87–001 were randomized to receive 1 of the 3 preparations of asparaginase as a single IM injection on the first day of therapy as part of a 5 day investigative window. The dose was administered as follows: *E. coli* 25,000 IU/m^2, Erwinia 25,000 IU/m^2, or PEG-asparaginase 2,500 IU/m^2. Serial serum samples were drawn throughout the 26 day induction period and analyzed for ASP enzyme activity and asparagine. These pharmacokinetic and pharmcodynamic properties of the 3 different preparations are shown in Table 1 as apparent half-life and days of asparagine depletion.[9] Statistical analysis using student t-test showed the half-life of Erwinia to be significantly shorter than the half-life for *E. coli* ASP ($p < 0.001$). The half-life for PEG ASP was significantly greater than the half-life of native *E. coli* ASP ($p < 0.0001$). The 3 preparations were also significantly different when analyzed by student t-test for the duration of asparagine depletion ($p < 0.01$). Of note, asparaginase activity was measurable (> 0.01 IU/ml) in the sera of patients receiving PEG ASP for the entire 26 day observation period whereas the enzyme activity had disappeared by days 8 and 13 for Erwinia and *E. coli* ASP, respectively.

Table 1. Pharmacologic properties of different asparaginase preparations in naïve patients

Asparaginase type	Erwinia (n = 10)	E. coli (n = 17)	PEG (n = 10)
T ½ (days ± SD)	0.65[a] (± 0.13)	1.28 (± 0.35)	5.73[b] (± 3.24)
Asparagine Depletion (days)	7–15	14–23	26–34

[a] half-life significantly shorter than E. coli (p < 0.001).
[b] half-life significantly greater than E. coli (p < 0.0001) Asselin et al. J Clin Oncol, 1993.

Induction therapy was followed by multiple drug intensification therapy, featuring administration of intensive E. coli ASP 25,000 IU/m² IM weekly for at least 20 weeks. For middle and last-dose studies, blood was obtained on each of 4 or 5 days in the one week interval following one of the doses of asparaginase (middle dose was defined as between the 3rd and 15th dose) and in the same manner following the last dose of asparaginase (usually the 20th to 30th dose of weekly asparaginase). Figure 1 shows the apparent serum half-life of E. coli ASP as a function of repeated doses.[9] We studied 9 patients following one of their intensification doses and the last dose of intensification asparaginase. Comparison of t-1/2 showed no difference between half-lives after the first dose, middle dose or the last dose (1.28 days vs.1.21 vs.1.14, p > 0.3, respectively).

4.2. ASP Activity following Hypersensitivity Reaction

Table 2 describes the results of 10 patients studied following hypersensitivity reaction to E. coli ASP.[9] Five patients were evaluated with 1 or more ASP levels obtained in the week following an apparent hypersensitivity reaction varying in severity from minor redness, swelling and pain at the injection site to disseminated urticaria. In this group of 5 patients, asparaginase activity was markedly decreased when compared with predicted values making it impossible to calculate an apparent half-life. Five patients with a history of hypersensitivity reaction to the E. coli preparation were studied following a dose of PEG ASP. As shown in Table 2, enzyme activity decreased with an apparent t-1/2 of 1.82 days. This rate of clearance is significantly faster than that observed in patients treated with PEG who had not previously received any form of asparaginase (p < 0.01).

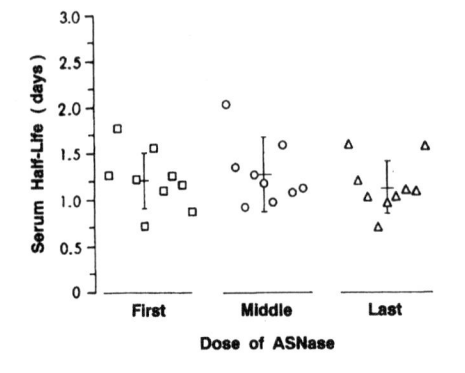

Figure 1. Serum half-life as a function of repeated doses. Dose intervals indicated as First (□, dose administered on day 0 of therapy); Middle (O, studies performed at approximately third to fifteenth dose); and Last (∇, studies performed at twentieth to thirtieth dose). The mean serum half-life ± SD is indicated for each group.

Table 2. Half-lives of asparaginase in patients with a previous hypersensitivity reaction to *E. coli*

Asparaginase type	Dose (IU/m^2)	Half-life (days)
E. coli (n = 5 patients)	25,000	Undetectable
PEG (n = 5 patients)	2,500	1.82 ± 0.3

p value < 0.01 compared to patients with no history of hypersensitivity.
Asselin et al. *J Clin Oncol*, 1993.

4.3. Effect of the Presence of Antibody on Pharmacology

The pharmacokinetics of PEG ASP were evaluated in 51 patients, previously treated with native *E. coli* ASP, some of whom had previous hypersensitivity (HS) reactions. PEG ASP was administered intramuscularly at 2,500 IU/m^2 to patients previously hypersensitive to native ASP on an every 7 day or every 14 day schedule, nonhypersensitive patients previously exposed to ASP and ASP naive patients on an every 14 day schedule. In patients with low antibody titers, the mean t-1/2 of PEG was 7.05 days compared to 2.59 days in high titer patients (p=0.0003).[7] The number of days that ASP was detectable in the serum was analyzed by anti-ASP antibody levels as shown in Table 3.[8] High antibody levels correlated with reduced days of ASP in the serum and with a lower number of days of asparagine depletion. High antibody levels were measured in 5 out of 6 patients without continuous asparagine depletion. These altered pharmacokinetics with high antibody levels were observed in both clinically hypersensitive and nonhypersensitive patients.

4.4. Effect of Altered Pharmacokinetics on Clinical Outcome

In Protocol #8866, the Pediatric Oncology Group evaluated the efficacy and toxicity of PEG ASP as compared to native *E. coli* ASP, combined with a standard 4 week vincristine plus prednisone induction, in children with ALL in second bone marrow relapse.[6] Of the 74 fully evaluable patients, 35 patients without prior hypersensitivity were randomized to treatment with either PEG ASP 2,500 IU/m^2 every 2 weeks or native *E. coli* ASP (Elspar™) 10,000 IU/m^2 three times per week. Thirty-nine patients with a history of hypersensitivity to native ASP were directly assigned to treatment with PEG ASP. Response rates were not significantly different between the 3 treatment groups with overall response rates (CR+PR) of 55–61%. Subsets of patients with high IgG antibody titers to ASP (n=23) cleared asparaginase more rapidly and had a response rate of 26% (see Figure 2). Those with low titers (n=14) cleared ASP slowly and had a significantly higher response rate, 64% (p=0.02). The absence of prior clinical hypersensitivity did not necessarily correlate with

Table 3. Duration of PEG asparaginase enzyme activity in patients previously treated with the *E. coli* and/or erwinia preparation

Patient group	Days ASP measurable low antibody (mean + SD)	Days ASP measurable high antibody (mean + SD)
Hypersensitive	13.3 + 0.6	4.0 + 1.4
Non-hypersensitive	12.2 + 1.4	6.0 + 0.0
ASP naïve	13.8 + 1.5	Not Applicable

Kurtzberg et al. *Proc Am Soc Clin Oncol*, 370A, 1994.
The dosing schedule for all patients was PEG ASP 2,500 IU/m^2 given every 14 days.

[Bar chart showing Anti-ASP Antibodies: Low titer group - 64% (clear bar, no response) and 26% (hatched bar, responding); High titer group - 36% (clear bar) and 74% (hatched bar).]

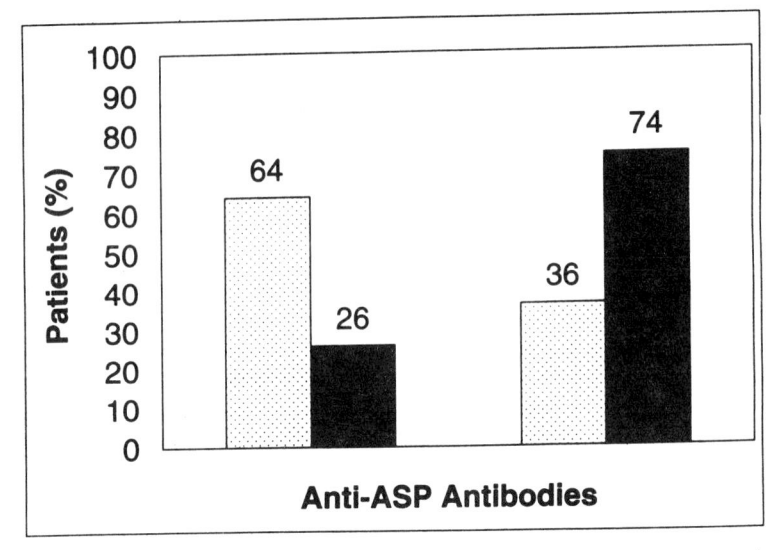

Figure 2. Response rates as a function of anti-ASP antibody titers – Low vs. High. The % patients with no response are shown in clear bar and % patients responding (complete and partial remissions) are shown by the hatched bar.

low antibody titers. Sixty-three percent of patients without a history of clinical hypersensitivity to *E. coli* ASP had high titers at study entry. There was one severe grade III allergic reaction to ASP, but none to PEG ASP. The conclusions from this clinical experience were that PEG ASP is safe and effective in relapsed patients regardless of prior hypersensitivity status, however, development of an antibody response to ASP, which is not necessarily predictable by the patients' past clinical history, is associated with decreased efficacy.

The next study of the Pediatric Oncology Group #9310 compared weekly versus every other week PEG ASP in combination with prednisone, vincristine, doxorubicin and triple intrathecal therapy for reinduction in patients with ALL in first bone marrow or extramedullary relapse. Remission induction rates are given in Table 4 based on mean ASP levels and dosing schedule.[11] Low ASP levels significantly correlated with high titers of ASP antibody. Response significantly correlated with mean ASP levels. These data again suggest that ASP pharmacokinetics and the presence of antibody are directly related to its anti-leukemic effect.

Table 4. Remission rates in relapsed childhood ALL

PEG asparaginase dose	Remission rate
Weekly	97%
Every other week	82%
All (n = 128)	87%

p value = 0.02 Abshire et al. Proc Am Soc Clin Oncol, 1038A, 1995
Following reinduction with combination chemotherapy including PEG ASP. All patients received vincristine, prednisone, and doxorubicin. PEG 2,500 IU/m^2 was given every week or every other week based on randomization

5. DISCUSSION

Multiple clinical trials have demonstrated the importance of ASP therapy as part of combination chemotherapy for ALL.[12-15] Early experience at the Dana-Farber Cancer Institute showed that patients receiving intensive weekly ASP as part of intensification treatment for newly diagnosed ALL had significantly better event-free survival compared to those treated without ASP (63% vs. 44%; p < 0.05). As part of ongoing investigations of the biology of ASP, by the Dana-Farber Cancer Institute Leukemia Consortium, we examined the pharmacokinetic and pharmacodynamic properties of the 3 ASP preparations available in the United States. The mean t-1/2 in the PEG treated group was three to five times greater than the t-1/2 for native *E. coli* which was two times greater than the t-1/2 for ERW treated group. Not surprisingly, these differences in half-lives were reflected in significant differences in the duration of serum asparagine depletion. European investigators have also reported significant differences in ASP activity and asparagine depletion following treatment with two different *E. coli* preparations (Asparaginase medac™ and Crasnitin™) and Erwinia preparations.[16,17] These observations of significantly different pharmacologic profiles have important clinical implications with regard to appropriate dose and schedule when alternate preparations are being used. These data suggest that the clinical practice of substitution of different asparaginases according to the same dose and schedule for the *E. coli* enzyme Elspar is not reasonable or effective.

Other investigators have reported that patients with symptoms of hypersensitivity to ASP had markedly shortened half-lives following and sometimes before the overt allergic reaction.[2,4,18,19] Our results demonstrate a similar phenomenon in the five patients who had a hypersensitivity reaction, even a minor localized one, the serum enzyme activity was significantly decreased or undetectable. Therefore even though ASP treatment might be safely continued the antileukemia effect would likely be diminished. These findings suggest that the clinical practice of premedication with antihistamines prior to an ASP dose in order to prevent overt symptoms of allergy is not appropriate since the risk: benefit ratio is so high. These patients are being exposed to the risk of adverse effects without benefit of the desired biologic effect.

The Dana-Farber Cancer Institute studies demonstrated that the t-1/2 of *E. coli* ASP in 9 children was not affected by repeated doses.[9] Boos et al report that three of five children had inadequate asparagine depletion after repeated exposure to ERW.[20] Interpretation of these results is limited due to the small numbers of patients. We hypothesize that if a large enough group of patients was followed longitudinally that a cohort of patients would demonstrate decreased enzyme activity with repeated doses related to the appearance of anti-ASP antibodies without clinical signs of allergy. It is not possible from the available data to estimate the incidence of such alterations in pharmacokinetics among patients on front-line studies.

Previous studies from the POG have shown that up to 73% of patients exposed to ASP during induction and consolidation developed hypersensitivity reactions to *E. coli* ASP and approximately 24% of these patients also became HS to ERW preventing further ASP therapy.[3] The results of POG #8866 and #9310 showed that PEG ASP could be safely given to a majority of patients with a history of prior hypersensitivity to either *E. coli* and/or Erwinia ASP, allowing continuation of ASP as part of effective combination chemotherapy. In these and other studies[2,4,5,18,19] the association between HS reactions, anti-ASP antibodies and altered pharmacokinetics is clear. Of particular clinical significance in the #8866 study was the observation that 63% of patients without a history of clinical hypersensitivity to ASP had high antibody titers at study entry. High antibody levels in this study were associated with decreased serum enzyme activity and decreased efficacy. The presence or development of antibodies is not necessarily predictable by the patients' past clinical history, a phenomenon termed as "silent hypersensitivity". Like HS reactions which are associated with rapid enzyme clearance, and suboptimal asparagine depletion, "silent hypersensitivity" is also associated with rapid enzyme clearance, and suboptimal asparagine depletion and thus diminished antileukemic efficacy.

The results of these two POG protocols also demonstrate the negative impact of altered pharmacokinetics on clinical outcomes. Development of anti-ASP antibodies which diminish ASP efficacy by causing immune clearance of the enzyme therefore is a mechanism *of resistance to ASP therapy*. In #9310 the weekly schedule of PEG administration appeared to circumvent the potential impact of decreased ASP levels on ASP response with significantly better remission rates compared to the every other week schedule. The frequency of this "silent hypersensitivity" as a mechanism of resistance remains to be explored. Further characterization of this phenomenon should lead to the development of improved schedules of ASP delivery based on pharmacologic endpoints. Another strategy for overcoming this type of immune-mediated drug resistance is use of PEG and Erwinia ASP as part of front-line chemotherapy in patients with newly diagnosed ALL. Studies are currently underway to examine the relative efficacy and toxicity, especially hypersensitivity in these naïve patients. Future studies will test whether targeting of pharmacologic endpoints will positively influence disease outcome.

REFERENCES

1. Broome JD. "Evidence that the L-asparaginase of guinea pig serum is responsible for its antilymphoma effects" Nature 1961, 191:1144–1115.
2. Killander D, Dohlwitz A, Engstedt L, Franzen S, Gahrton G, Gullbring B, Holm G, Holmgren A, Hoglund S, Killander A, Lockner D, Mellstedt H, Moe PJ, Palmblad J, Reizenstein P, Skarberg KD, Swedberg B, Uden AM, Wadman B, Wide L, Ahstrom L. Hypersensitivity reactions and antibody formation during L-asparaginase treatment of children and adults with acute leukemia. Cancer 1976, 37:220–228.
3. Land VJ, Shuster JJ, Pullen J, Harris M, Krance RA, Castleberry R, Akabutu J, Barbosa JL and Rosen D. Unexpectedly high incidence of allergic reactions with high dose weekly asparaginase consolidation therapy in children with newly diagnosed non-T, non-B acute lymphoblastic leukemia: A Pediatric Oncology Group Study. Proc Am Soc Clin Oncol 1989, 8:215,A834.
4. Cheung NKV, Chau IY, Coccia PF. Antibody response to *Escherichia coli* L-asparaginase. Am J Pediatr Hematol/Oncol 1986, 8(2):99–104.
5. Fabry U, Korholz D, Jurgens H, Gobel U, and Wahn V. Anaphylaxis to L-asparaginase during treatment for acute lymphoblastic leukemia in children - evidence of a complement-mediated mechanism. Pediatr Res 1985, 19:400–408.
6. Kurtzberg J, Asselin B, Pollack B, Bernstein M, Buchanan G, and the Pediatric Oncology Group. PEG L-asparaginase vs native E. coli asparaginase for reinduction of relapsed acute lymphoblastic leukemia: POG #8866 phase II trial. Proc ASOC 1993, 12:p325, 1079A.
7. Kurtzberg J, Asselin B, Poplack D, Grebanier A, Chen R, Franklin A, Scudiery D and Fisherman J. Antibodies to asparaginase alter pharmacokinetics and decrease enzyme activity in patients on asparaginase therapy. Proc AACR 1993, 34:p304, 1807A.
8. Kurtzberg J, Asselin B, Pollack B, Ettinger L, Ravindranath Y, Faucey J and Fisherman J. PEG-L-asparaginase pharmacology in pediatric patients with acute lymphoblastic leukemia. Proc ASCO 1994, 13:p144, 370A.
9. Asselin BL, Whitin JC, Coppola DJ, Rupp IP, Sallan SE and Cohen HJ. Comparative pharmacokinetic studies of three asparaginase preparations. J Clin Oncol 1993, 11(9):1780–1786.
10. Asselin BL, Lorenson My, Whitin JC, Coppola DJ, Kende AS, Blakley RL and Cohen HJ. Measurement of serum L-asparagine in the presence of L-asparaginase requires the presence of an L-asparaginase inhibitor. Cancer Res 1991, 51:6568–6573.

11. Abshire T, Pollock B, Billett A, Bradley P, and Buchanan G. Weekly polyethylene glycol conjugated L-asparaginase produces superior induction remission rates in childhood relapsed acute lymphoblastic leukemia: A Pediatric Oncology Group Study 9310. Proc ASCO 1995, 14:p344, 1038A.
12. Jones B, Holland JF, Glidewell O, Jacquillat C, Weil M, Pochedly C, Sinks L, Chevalier L, Maurer HM, Koch Kjell, Falkson G, Patterson R, Seligman B, Sartorious J, Kung F, Haurani F, Stuart M, Burgert EO, Ruymann F, Sawitsky A, Forman E, Pluess H, Truman J, Hakami N. Optimal use of L-asparaginase (NSC - 109229) in acute lymphocytic leukemia. Med Pediatr Oncol 1977,3:387–400.
13. Ertel IJ, Nesbit ME, Hammond D, Weiner J, and Sather H. Effective dose of L-asparaginase for inductio of remission in previously treated children with acute lymphoblastic leukemia: A report for the Children's Cancer Study Group. Cancer Res 1979, 39:3893–3896.
14. Sallan SE, Hitchcok-Bryan S, Gelber R, Cassady JR, Frei III E, and Nathan DG. Influence of intensive asparaginase in the treatment of childhood non-T-cell acute lymphoblastic leukemia. Cancer Res 1983, 43:5601–5607.
15. Clavell LA, Gelber RD, Cohen HJ, Hitchcock-Bryan S, Cassady JR, Tarbell NJ, Blattner SR, Tantravahi R, Leavitt P, and Sallan SE. Four-agent induction and intensive asparaginase therapy for treatment of childhood acute lymphoblastic leukemia. N Engl J Med 1986, 315:657–663.
16. Boos J, Werber G, Verspolh E, Nowak-Goth U, Jurgens H. Asparagine levels in children on *E. coli* and *Erwinia* - asparaginase therapy. Haematol Blood Transfusion 37: *Acute Leukemias V* - Hiddemann et al (eds) Springer-Verlag Berlin Heidelberg, 1996, p67–69.
17. DiBenedetto SP, DiCataldo A, Ragusa R, Meli C and Lo Nigrio L. Levels of L-asparagine in CSF after intramuscular administration of asparaginase from *Erwinia* in children with acute lymphoblastic leukemia. J Clin Oncol 1995, 13:339–344.
18. Ohnuma T, Holland JF, Freeman et al. Biochemical and pharmacological studies with asparaginase in man. Cancer Res 1970, 30:2297–2305.
19. Capizzi RL, Bertino JR, Skeel RT, et al. Clinical, biochemical, pharmacological and immunological studies. Ann Intern Med 1971, 74:893–901.
20. Boos J, Nowak-Gottl U, Jurgens H, Fleischhack G, Bode U. Loss of activity of *Erwinia* asparaginase on repeat applications (Letter). J Clin Oncol 1995, 13:2474–2475.

INDEX

Page numbers followed by '*t*' refer to tables; page numbers in *italics* refer to figures

Acute lymphoblastic leukemia (ALL), drug resistance, 391–394, 423–428; *see also* Leukemia
  adult
    MDR1 expression in, 7, 8*t*
    Ph/BCR+ phenotype in, 489–497
  AP-1 transcription factor in, 615–619
  apoptotic fraction in
    DNA *in situ* labeling of, 281–287
    white cell count and, 305–312
  asparaginase treatment in, 621–628
  BCL-2 expression in, 325–332, 386
    glucocorticoid-induced apoptosis and, 610–613
    remission and, 177–184
  CD95 antigen as prognostic marker in, 251–258
  cell surface reactivity in, 15–17
  cross-resistance of drugs in, 551–555
  cyclosporin modulation of, 453–459
  dexamethasone treatment in, 461–470
  DNA excision repair activity in: *see* DNA excision repair activity
  DNA ploidy in, 297–303, 383–384
  E2A-PBX1 fusion in, 385–386
  ETV6-CBFA2 fusion in, 384–385
  glucocorticoid treatment in, 593–601
    AP-1 transcription factor in, 615–619
    BCL-2 modulation of, 610–613
  glutathione activity in, 211–215
  growth factor modulation of, 585–591
  hyperdiploidy in, 297–303, 383–384
  in vitro drug effects and, 423–428; *see also* In vitro drug sensitivity
  interferon modulation of, 453–459
  MDR1 expression in, 5–18, 6*t*, 71–75
    remission and, 177–184
  mechanisms of, 543–548
  methotrexate treatment in: *see* Methotrexate
  MLL rearrangement in, 385
  mRNA gene expression and remission in, 177–184
  MRP gene expression and remission in, 177–184

Acute lymphoblastic leukemia (ALL) (*cont.*)
  PCNA, Ki-67 and Frag-EL in, 289–295
  P-glycoprotein expression and function in, 11–18, 112–117
  Ph/BCR+ phenotype in, 489–497
  prednisolone treatment in, 461–470
  proliferative fraction in, 289–312
  tumor suppressor genes in, 386
  white cell count and proliferative fraction in, 305–312
Acute myeloid leukemia (AML), drug resistance, 557–563; *see also* Leukemia
  adult
    in vitro drug sensitivity in, 437–443, 445–451
    MDR1 gene expression in, 2–4
    other protein expression in, 4–5
  anthracycline treatment in, 558–559
  aphidicolin modulation of, 567–570
  BCL-2 expression in
    in vitro sensitivity to Ara-C and 6TG and, 335–339
    remission and, 177–184
  childhood
    growth factor modulation of, 585–591
    in vitro drug sensitivity in, 327–443, 415–420, 429–434
    in vivo pharmacokinetics in, 429–434
    MDR1 expression in, 5–7, 6*t*
  cross-resistance to nucleoside analogs in, 571–576
  cytarabine treatment in, 558
  developments in research in, 557–563
  Down syndrome and cytarabine sensitivity in, 409–414
  flow cytometric assays of: *see* Flow cytometric assay(s)
  genes involved in, 2*t*, 78
  glutathione activity in, 205–208, 211–215
    MRP1 gene expression and, 187–194
  growth factors modulation of, 560–563, 585–591

631

Acute myeloid leukemia (AML) (cont.)
  immunocytochemical assay(s) of, 57–62; see also Immunocytochemical assay(s)
  LRP expression in, 133–138
  MDR1 expression in, 2–7, 71–75, 559–560
    remission and, 177–184
  methotrexate treatment in, 543–548
  mRNA gene expression and remission in, 177–184
  MRP/MRP1 gene expression in, 134, 141–148, 161–174
    GSH activity and, 187–194
    remission and, 177–184
  nucleoside analog treatment in, 571–576
  P-glycoprotein expression and function in, 29–33, 112–117, 161–174, 559–560
  prognostic role in
    LRP gene expression in, 133–141
    MDR1 and MPR1 expression in, 168–172
    MDR1 expression in, 3–4, 3t
  PSC833 in clinical trials in, 47–53
  remission and mRNA activity in, 177–184
Anthracycline(s)
  apoptosis by, in MDR1+phenotype, 313–323
  cytofluorometric assay of, 313–323
  HHT alkaloid as, 157–158
  sensitivity to, 29–33
    adult Ph/BCR+phenotype in ALL and, 489–497
    childhood AML and, 415–420
    natural fluorescence imaging detection of, 89–94
  in treatment of AML, 558–559
Anticancer drugs; see also Anthracycline(s); Glucocorticoids
  induction of CD95 expression by, 237–248, 256–258
  inhibition of fas/fas-ligand and apoptosis by, 259–265
  PARP inhibitors and apoptosis by, 267–276
  topoisomerase I inhibitors and, 355–362, 445–451
Antifolates, 543–548, 551–555
AP-1 transcription factor, 615–619
Apafs (Apoptosis activating factors), 227–228
Aphidicolin, and Ara-C activity in AML, 567–570
Apoptin®, induction of apoptosis by, 245–248
Apoptosis, drug-induced, 217–229, 246
  anthracyclines in, 313–323
  anticancer drugs in, 237–241
  Apoptin® in, 245–248
  BCL-2 regulation of, 221–229, 325–332, 335–339, 610–613
  BCR-ABL fusion protein effect on, 477–487
  biochemical pathway of, 219–221
  CD95 system and induction of, 219–221, 251–258
    inhibition of, 259–265
  in childhood ALL: see ALL; Apoptotic fraction
  cytofluorometric assay of, in MDR1+ phenotype, 313–323
  DNA ploidy and, 281–285, 297–303
  fas/fas-ligand inhibition of, 259–265
  glucocorticoids induction of, 595–596, 607–613
  glutathione activity in, 199–203

Apoptosis (cont.)
  mitochondrial changes in, 226–227
  modulation of, 228–229; see also Resistance modulating agent(s)
  oncogene expression in, 365–379
  PARP inhibition of, 267–276
  PCNA expression in, 289–295
  vs. proliferation in cell cycle, 289–295
  regulators of, 221–229
  TNF/receptor family molecules in, 219–221; see also CD95 expression
  topoisomerase I inhibitors in, 355–362
  triggers of, 219
Apoptosis activating factors (Apafs), 227–228
Apoptotic fraction, in childhood ALL
  DNA in situ labeling of, 281–287
  PCNA expression in, 289–295
  white cell count and, 305–312
Ara-C (arabinosylcytosine)
  Down syndrome response to, in AML, 409–414
  sensitivity to
    BCL-2 expression and, 335–339
    growth factor modulation of, 585–591
    in vitro, 399, 400–401, 402–406
      childhood AML and, 415–420, 585–591
      childhood leukemia and, 325–332, 335–339, 585–591
    PSC833 treatment in AML and, 47–53
  in treatment of AML, 557–563
Artificial neural networks (ANN), resistance modulating agents and, 95–105
Asparaginase(s), 621–628
  development of treatment with, 622
  in vitro sensitivity to, 399, 401, 402–406
  pharmacokinetics of, 623–627
  preparations of, 621, 623
Assay(s), 78–79; see also In vitro drug sensitivity
  agarose gel electrophoresis of DNA fragments, 369–370
  of asparaginase activity, 623
  cytofluorometric, of DNA, 254
  DISC-, 439
  of DNA repair activity, 501–505, 505–509
  flow cytometric: see Flow cytometric assay
  fluorescence imaging, natural: see Fluorescence imaging
  fluorometric microculture cytotoxicity assay, 154, 430–431
  functional: see Calcein-AM; Rhodamine-123
  gel electrophoretic: see Single cell gel electrophoresis
  of glutathione S-transferase expression, 206–207
  immunocytochemical: see Immunocytochemical assay(s)
  immunofluorescent, for antigen expression, 253
  in situ labeling of DNA in apoptotic cells, 281–285
  laser scanning microscopic: see Confocal laser scanning microscopy
  of microsatellite instability, 517–525

Index

Assay(s) (cont.)
  microspectrofluorometric, 154, 430–431; see also Confocal laser scanning microscopy
  MTT: see In vitro drug sensitivity; MTT assay
  of retention of anthracyclines: see Rhodamine-123
  Reverse transcriptase-PCR analysis: see Reverse transcriptase-PCR analysis
  Western blot, 370
Autocrine suicide, of T cells, 239

BAX expression
  and glucocorticoid-mediated apoptosis, 610–613
  and in vitro sensitivity to anthracyclines, 335–339
B-cell lymphoma: see Cutaneous lymphoma
BCL-2 expression
  Apoptin®-induced apoptosis and, 245–248
  in transformed cells, 247
  and changes in mitochondria, 226–227
  in childhood ALL, 177–184, 325–332, 386
  and glucocorticoid-mediated apoptosis, 610–613
  immunoblot assay of, 358
  and in vitro drug resistance, 325–332, 335–339
  post transcriptional modification of, 225–226
  and regulation of apoptosis, 221–229, 238
  in remission of leukemia, 177–184
  vs. spontaneous apoptosis, 325–332
  topoisomerase I inhibitors and, 355–362
BCL-2 proteins, structure and function of, 222–225
B-CLL: see Chronic lymphocytic leukemia
BCR-ABL expression, 377–378
  Apoptin® and, 245–248
  in chronic myeloid leukemia, 477–487
Burkitt lymphoma, microsatellite instability in, 517–525
Butyrolactone I, 346–347

Calcein-AM assay, 162
  for MPR1 and MDR1 expression, 164–167, 192–193
Camptothecin (CPT), 355–362
CD4/CD8 phenotype, as prognostic indicator, 119–131
CD27 ligand, 219–221
CD30 ligand, 219–221
CD30 phenotype, as prognostic indicator, 121
CD34 phenotype, as prognostic indicator, in AML, 168–174, 557–563
CD40 ligand, 219–221
CD95 expression, 219–221
  in chronic myeloid leukemia, 477–487
  in drug-induced apoptosis, 259–265
  induction of apoptosis by, 219–221, 238–241, 372
    PARP inhibition of, 267–276
  as prognostic marker in ALL, 251–258
CdA, fas/fas-ligand inhibition and apoptosis by, 259–265
CDK inhibitors: see Cyclin dependent kinase inhibitors
Cell culture: see In vitro drug sensitivity
Cell cycle; see also Apoptotic fraction; Growth factors; Proliferative fraction
  in multidrug resistant CD34 phenotype, 559–563
  progression of, effect of PARP on, 267–276
  S-phase link between proliferation and drug agent, 289–295

Cell death: see Apoptosis
Cell proliferation, and glucocorticoids, 609–610
CH11, 260
Chemosensitivity Index Ci, 439
Chemotherapeutic agents: see Anticancer drugs
Childhood leukemia: see ALL; AML
2-Chlorodeoxyadenosine, and mechanisms of cross resistance, 571–576
Chronic lymphocytic leukemia (CLL); see also Leukemia
  AP-1 transcription factor in, 615–619
  B-cell
    CD95 phenotype and drug-resistance in, 238–241, 256–258
    in vitro sensitivity to vinorelbine in, 473–475
    MDR1 and MDR3 expression in, 65–69; see also Leukemia
  glucocorticoids in, sensitivity to, 615–619
  MDR1 expression in, 65–69, 71–75
Chronic myeloid leukemia (CML), drug resistance, 477–487
CLL: see Chronic lymphocytic leukemia
CLSM: see Confocal laser scanning microscopy
CML: see Chronic myeloid leukemia
Colony stimulating factors (CSFs): see Growth factors
Comet tail analysis, 527–535
Confocal laser scanning microscopy, 368–369
  marrow sample analysis by, 501–505, 509–515
  optimization of, 527–535
Cortivazol treatment, in childhood ALL, 600–601
CPT (camptothecin), 355–362
Cross-resistance
  common mechanisms of, in K562 variants, 571–576
  between prednisolone and methotrexate, 551–555
Cutaneous lymphoma, drug resistance, 119–131
Cyclin dependent kinase inhibitors
  cytokine-derived, 347–350
  synthetic, 341–350
Cyclosporin modulation
  MTT assay of, 453–459
  of P-glycoprotein expression, 29–33, 320–323
Cystathionine B-synthase activity, in Down syndrome and AML, 410–414
Cytarabine: see Ara-C
Cytofluorometric assay
  of apoptosis, 313–323
  of DNA, 254
  two-color, 480
Cytosine arabinoside, in cross resistance, 571–576; see also Ara-C
Cytosolic pH
  daunorubicin treatment effect on, 375
  essential, for cell death, 378

Daunorubicin, sensitivity to; see also Anthracycline(s)
  apoptosis and, 377
    MDR1+ phenotype and, 313–323
  DNA fragmentation and, 372
  genes linked to, 411–413

Daunorubicin (*cont.*)
  liposomes and, 509–515
  MDR1 and MPR1 expression and, 164–167
  MDR1 expression and
    flow cytometry assay of, 79–87
    in K-H30 and K-H300 cells, 154–159
    Rhodamine-123 efflux assay of, 60–62, 73–74, 109–110
  oncogene expression and, 365–379
Dexamethasone, sensitivity to
  in childhood ALL, 599–601
  differential kinetics of, 461–470
  in vitro, 325–332, 461–470; *see also* Glucocorticoids
Differential kinetics, of drug resistance
  dexamethasone and, 461–470
  prednisolone and, 461–470
  SCGE/CLSM analysis of, 501–505
DISC assay, 439
DNA excision repair activity, 289–295
  in acute lymphoblastic leukemia, 579–583
  aphidicolin inhibition of, 567–570
  direct assessment of, 501–505, 527–535
    in Burkitt lymphoma, 517–525
    in childhood leukemia, 509–515
    in non Hodgkin lymphoma, 517–525
DNA *in situ* labeling, of ALL apoptotic fraction, 281–287
DNA ploidy, in childhood ALL, 383–384
  apoptosis-corrected proliferative fraction and, 297–303
  apoptosis-related, 281–287
  drug resistance and, 383–384
  methotrexate intracellular disposition and, 540–541
Down syndrome, and AML, 409–414
Doxorubicin, sensitivity to; *see also* Anthracycline(s)
  CD95 expression and, 239–240
  growth factor modulation of, 585–591
  induction of CD95 expression and, 257
  natural fluorescence imaging and, 89–94
  PARP inhibitors and, 267–276
Drug sensitivity assay: *see In vitro* drug sensitivity

E2A-PBX1 fusion, in childhood ALL, 385–386
Etoposide, sensitivity to
  fas/fas-ligand inhibition and, 259–265
  in vitro, 400, 401–406
  PARP inhibitors and, 267–276
  PSC833 treatment of AML and, 47–53
ETV6-CBFA2 fusion, in childhood ALL, 384–385

F-ara-A, PARP inhibitors and apoptosis by, 267–276
FAS/APO-1 antigen: *see* CD95 expression
Fas/fas-ligand, inhibition of, 259–265
Flavopiridol, 344–346
Flow cytometric assay
  of BCL-2 expression, 327, 337
  in cell cycle analysis, 269, 357
  of Fas expression, 367–377
  of MDR1 and MPR1 expression, 164–167
  of MDR1 expression, 59–62, 77–87, 108–109, 357, 367–377

Fludarabine, fas/fas-ligand inhibition by, 259–265; *see also* Nucleoside analogs
Fluorescence imaging, natural, for anthracyclines, 89–94
FMCA (fluorometric microculture cytotoxicity assay), 430–431
Folylpolyglutamate synthetase, and sensitivity to methotrexate, 543–548
Frag-EL expression, in proliferative phase, 289–295
Free-Wilson analysis
  combined Hansch and, 102–104
  data matrix and chemistry of, 96
  nonlinear, 101–102

Gamma-glutamyl hydrolase, 543–548
Gel electrophoresis: *see* Single cell gel electrophoresis
Gemcitabine, and mechanisms of cross resistance, 571–576
GF120918, modulation of P-gp expression by, 29–33
Gld (generalized lymphoproliferative disease), 220, 239
Glucocorticoids, sensitivity to, 596–599
  AP-1 transcription factor and, 615–619
  apoptosis and, 595–596, 607–613
  factors affecting, 608–610
  cell proliferation and, 609–610
  in childhood ALL, 593–601
  in vitro cellular, 393–394, 461–470; *see also* Prednisolone
  modulation of, 611–613
  receptors and, 594–595, 608–609
Glutathione (GSH) activity, 191–192
  in acute myeloid leukemia, 205–208
  apoptosis by, regulation of, 199–203
  detoxification of electrophilic drugs by, 199–201
  induction of, 192
  MRP expression and, 151–159
    MRP1 homologue in, 187–194
  and related enzymes, 191
Glutathione S-transferases (GSTs)
  in acute myeloid leukemia, 205–208
  as binding proteins, 199–201
GM-CSF (Granulocyte/macrophage colony stimulating factor): *see* Growth factors
Growth factors, as resistance modulators; *see also* Cell cycle
  in AML, 560–563
  in leukemic blasts, 585–591
GSH: *see* Glutathione (GSH) activity
GSTs: *see* Glutathione S-transferases

Hansch/Free-Wilson analysis, of resistance modulating agents, 102–105
H+ATPase pump, vacuolar, 151–159
HHT alkaloid, 157–158
Hyperdiploidy, and drug resistance, 383–384; *see also* DNA ploidy
Hypersensitivity, in asparaginase treatment of ALL, 621–628

Index

IAPs (Apoptosis inhibitory proteins), 228
Idarubicin, apoptosis by
  fas/fas-ligand inhibition and, 259–265
  in MDR1+ leukemic cells, 313–323
  PARP inhibitors and, 267–276
Immune-mediated drug resistance, 621–628
Immunocytochemical assay(s)
  of MRP, 125, 357; *see also* MRP/MRP1 gene expression
  of MRP, LRP and P-gp, 125; *see also* LRP gene expression; MRP/MRP1 gene expression; P-glycoprotein
  of P-glycoprotein, 14–15, 57–62, 65–69; *see also* P-glycoprotein
Immunofluorescence assay, of antigen expression, 253, 479
In situ labeling, of apoptotic fraction in ALL, 281–287
In vitro drug sensitivity
  in ALL, 325–332, 391–394, 423–428, 461–470
    cyclosporin modulation of, 453–459
    interferon modulation of, 453–459
  in AML, 335–339
    aphidicolin modulation of, 567–570
    cyclosporin modulation of, 453–459
    in adults, 437–443, 445–451
    in children, 415–420, 429–434
    interferon modulation of, 453–459
  aphidicolin modulation of, 567–570
  BAX protein synthesis and, 335–339
  in B-cell chronic lymphocytic leukemia, 473–475
  BCL-2 expression in, 325–332, 335–339
  cyclosporin modulation of, 453–459
  to dexamethasone, 461–470
  to glucocorticoids, 597–598
  growth factor modulation of, 585–591
  interferon modulation of, 453–459
  MTT assay for: *see* MTT assay
  pharmacokinetics of, 397–406
  to prednisolone, 461–470
  prognostic value of, 391–392
In vivo pharmacokinetics, in childhood ALL, 429–434, 598–599
Interferon modulation, MTT assay of, 453–459
Iodeoxyuridine (IdUrd) labeling, 560–563

K562 cell line, nucleoside analog cross resistance in, 571–576
Karyotype abnormality: *see* DNA ploidy
Ki-67 expression, in proliferative phase, 289–295
Kinetic spectrophotometric assay, 623

Large cell lymphoma: *see* Cutaneous lymphoma; Non Hodgkin lymphoma, malignant
Laser scanning microscopy: *see* Confocal laser scanning microscopy
Leukemia, acute, drug resistance; *see also* ALL; AML; Lymphoma
  apoptosis in, regulation of, 228–229, 237–241
    fas/fas-ligand inhibition and, 259–265

Leukemia (*cont.*)
  C95 antigen as prognostic marker in, 251–257
  CD95 expression in, 238–241
  cytofluorometric assay of apoptosis in, 313–323
  flow cytometric assay of, 77–87
  glucocorticoid-induced apoptosis in, 607–613
  glutathione activity in, 211–215
  growth factor modulation of, 585–591
  in vitro drug sensitivity in, 423–428, 453–459; *see also In vitro* drug sensitivity
  and intracellular methotrexate disposition, 540–541
  MDR1 expression in, 1–7, 66–67, 71–75; *see also* MDR1 expression
  MDR3 expression in, 66–67
  mRNA gene expression and remission in, 177–184
  MRP and MDR phenotypes in, 151–159
  natural fluorescence imaging in, 89–94
  PARP inhibition and apoptosis in, 267–276
  P-glycoprotein in; *see also* MDR1 expression; P-glycoprotein
    function of, 107–117
    prognosis by, 1–7, 21–27
Lpr (lymphoproliferation), 220, 239; *see also* Proliferative fraction
LRP gene expression
  flow cytometric assay of, 82–87
  in acute myeloid leukemia, 133–138
    adult, 4–5
    prognostic role of, 133–141
  in cutaneous lymphoma, 119–131
Lung resistance protein: *see* LRP gene expression
Lymphoma, drug resistance
  B-cell: *see* Cutaneous; Non Hodgkin
  Burkitt, microsatellite instability in, 517–525
  cutaneous, 119–131
  large cell: *see* Cutaneous
  malignant non Hodgkin, 517–525
  MDR1 expression in, 71–75
  MRP/MRP1 gene expression in, 119–131
  non Hodgkin
    B-cell, MDR1 and MDR 3 expression in, 68, 69
    malignant, microsatellite instability in, 517–525
    MDR1 expression in, 71–75
Lymphotoxin, 219–221

Malignant non Hodgkin lymphoma (MNHL), 517–525
MDR1 expression; *see also* MDR3 expression
  in acquired drug resistance, 24–25, 370–371
  in acute leukemia, 107–117
    anthracycline-induced apoptosis and, 313–323
    tumor remission and, 177–184
  in ALL, 5–18, 11–18, 71–75, 393–394
    prognostic value of, 17–18
  in AML, 29–33, 559–560
    Calcein-AM assay for MPR1 expression and, 161–174
  in B-cell leukemia, 65–69
  in chronic myeloid leukemia, 477–487
  in cutaneous lymphoma, 119–130

MDR1 expression (cont.)
  modulation of: see Resistance modulating agent(s)
  in myelodysplastic syndrome, 35–44
  in primary drug resistance, 24–25
  as prognostic factor, 25
    in acute leukemia, 1–7
    in childhood leukemia, 17–18, 21–27
  promoter gene mutation and, 71–75
  and regulation of drug resistance, 26–27
  and remission in acute leukemia, 177–184
  topoisomerase I inhibitors and, 355–362
  in vincristine resistant cells, 355–362
MDR3 expression, in B-cell leukemia, 65–69
MDS: see Myelodysplastic syndrome
Membrane transport proteins, function of, 26
Methotrexate (MTX)
  cross-resistance between prednisolone and, 551–555
  disposition of, in leukemic cells, 539–540
  induction of CD95 expression by, 257
  optimal dosage of, in childhood ALL, 537–541
  resistance to, in ALL, 393–394
    mechanisms of, 543–548
Microsatellite instability, 517–525; see also DNA excision repair activity
Microspectrofluorometry, 154; see also Confocal laser scanning microscopy
Mismatch repair, in ALL, 579–583
Mitochondrial membrane, in apoptosis, 375–377, 378
Mitoxantrone, and PSC833 treatment of refractory AML, 47–53
MLH1/MLH2 expression, in ALL, 579–583
MLL rearrangement, in childhood ALL, 385
MNHL (Malignant non Hodgkin lymphoma), 517–525
Modulation, of drug resistance; see also specific genes, e.g. BCL-2; MDR1
  agents used for: see Resistance modulating agent(s)
  Apoptin® in, 245–248
  CD95 expression and, 237–241
  by regulation of apoptosis, 228–229
MRP/MRP1 gene expression
  in AML, 141–148, 161–174, 187–194
  in cutaneous lymphoma, 119–131
  flow cytometric measurement of, 82–87
  functional activity of, 26
    MDR phenotype and, 151–159
  functional analysis of, 192–193
  glutathione activity and, 151–159, 201
  MRP1 homologue in, 187–194
  homologues of MRP in, 187–194
  phenotype of, 190
    vs. P-glycoprotein function, 161–174
  promoter gene mutation and, 71–75
  regulation of, 190–191
  remission in acute leukemia and, 177–184
  topoisomerase I inhibitors and, 355–362
  in vincristine resistant cells, 355–362
MSH6 expression, in ALL, 579–583

MTT (Methyl-thiazol-tetrazolium salt) assay, 30–31, 153, 327–328, 336, 464; see also In vitro drug sensitivity
  in adult AML, 445–451
  cyclosporin and interferon modulation of, 453–459
  of resistance modulation by growth factors, 585–591
Multidrug resistance protein (MRP): see MRP/MRP1 gene expression
Mycosis fungoides: see Cutaneous lymphoma
Myelodysplastic syndrome (MDS), drug resistance
  P-glycoprotein in, 35–44
  quinine modulation of, 35–44
    patient response to, 38, 40, 41, 42
    toxicity of, 40, 42, 43t

Natural fluorescence imaging, for anthracyclines, 89–94
NOK1, 260
Non Hodgkin lymphoma (NHL); see also Leukemia
  B-cell, MDR1 and MDR 3 expression in, 68, 69
  malignant, microsatellite instability in, 517–525
  MDR1 expression in, 71–75
Nucleoside analogs, and cross-resistance in K562 variants, 571–576

Oncogene expression, in drug resistant cells, 365–379
Oxazaphosphorines, in vitro cellular sensitivity to, 398–399, 400, 402–406
Oxygen radical generation, in Down syndrome and AML, 409–414

P53 tumor suppressor expression
  apoptosis independent of, 245–248
  in childhood ALL, 386
  mutation of, and resistance to drugs, 237–238
Paracrine death, of T cells, 239
PARP (Poly(ADP-ribose) polymerase), inhibitors of, in drug-induced apoptosis, 267–276
PCNA expression, in apoptotic phase, 289–295
P-glycoprotein (P-gp)
  expression of: see MDR1 expression; MDR3 expression
  flow cytometric assay of, 59–62, 77–87
  fluorescence imaging detection of, 89–94
  functional activity of, 25–26, 26t, 32–33
    in AML and ALL, 112–117
  expression of and, 107–117
  MRP phenotype and, 151–159
  MRP1 phenotype and, 161–174
  rhodamine-123 efflux detection of, 60–62, 559–560
  immunocytochemical assays of, 57–62
Pharmacokinetics
  of in vitro drug sensitivity, 397–406
  in vivo, in childhood AML, 429–434
PMS2 expression, in ALL, 579–583
Polyglutamylation, and sensitivity to methotrexate, 543–548, 551–555
Poly(ADP-ribose) polymerase: see PARP

Index

Prednisolone
  cross-resistance between methotrexate and, 551–555
  in vitro sensitivity to, 325–332, 461–470; *see also* Glucocorticoids
  sensitivity to, in childhood ALL, 599–601
Prognostic factor(s)
  BCL-2 expression as, in childhood ALL, 326–332, 611
  CD4/CD8 phenotype as, 119–131
  CD30 phenotype as, 121
  CD34 phenotype as, in AML, 168–172, 557–563
  CD95 phenotype as, 251–258, 259–265, 267–276
  cell cycle fraction as: *see* Apoptotic fraction; Proliferative fraction
  cytofluorometric assay of apoptosis as, 313–323
  DNA ploidy as, in childhood ALL, 540–541
  DNA repair activity as, 501–505, 527–535
    in Burkitt lymphoma, 517–525
    in childhood leukemia, 509–515
    in non Hodgkin lymphoma, 517–525
  glutathione activity as
    in acute leukemia, 211–215
  in vitro drug sensitivity as
    in adult AML, 437–443, 445–451
    in B-cell CLL, 473–475
    in childhood ALL, 391–394, 423–428, 453–459, 461–470
    in childhood AML, 415–420, 429–434, 453–459
  LRP gene expression as, in AML, 133–141
  lymphoblast lineage as, in childhood ALL, 540–541
  microsatellite instability as
    in Burkitt lymphoma, 517–525
    in malignant non Hodgkin lymphoma, 517–525
  MRP1 expression as
    in acute leukemia, 1–7
    in AML, 3–4, 3*t*
    in CML, 477–487
    MPR1 expression and, 168–172
  P-glycoprotein as, 25
    in childhood leukemia, 17–18, 21–27
    in CML, 477–487
    in leukemia, 1–7, 21–27
  Ph/BCR+phenotype as, in adult ALL, 489–497
  white cell count as, 305–312
Programmed cell death (PCD): *see* Apoptosis
Proliferative fraction, in childhood ALL
  apoptotic fraction vs., 289–295
  karyotype and apoptosis-corrected, 297–303
  white cell count and, 305–312
Promoter gene mutation, and MDR1 expression, 71–75
Propafenone, as resistance modulating agent, 95–105
PSC833 (Valspodar)
  P-glycoprotein expression modulated by, 29–33, 48–53
  in treatment of refractory AML, 47–53

Quinine, P-glycoprotein expression modulated by, 35–44

Reduced folate carriers, 543–548
Resistance modulating agent(s), 48–49
  in AML, 559–563
  cyclosporin as, 29–33, 320–323, 453–459
  GF120918 as, 29–33
  growth factors as, 585–591
  interferon as, 453–459
  predicting activity of, 95–105; *see also* Prognostic factor(s)
  propafenone as, 95–105
  PSC833 (Valspodar) as, 29–33, 49–53
  quinine as, 35–44
Resistance testing: *see* DNA excision repair activity; *In vitro* drug sensitivity
Reverse transcriptase-PCR analysis, 153, 154
  of BCL-2 expression, 179–180
  of BCR-ABL hybrid gene, 479
  of cellular RNA, 357
  of MDR1 expression, 164–167, 179–180
  of MRP expression, 179–180
  of MRP1 expression, 164–167
Rhodamine-123 efflux, for detection of
  MDR1 and MRP1 expression, 164–167
  MDR1 expression, 192–193, 480–481
  P-glycoprotein function, 60–62, 73–74, 109–110, 559–560
RT-PCR: *see* Reverse transcriptase-PCR analysis

Single cell gel electrophoresis (SCGE), of marrow sample, 501–505, 509–515
  optimization of, 527–535
6TG, sensitivity to, BCL-2 expression and, 335–339
SN-38, 355–362
Structure-activity relationship, in drug resistance, 95–105

T-cell leukemia, CD95 phenotype in, 238–241
Thiopurines, sensitivity to, in childhood ALL, 393–394
TNF (Tumor necrosis factor), 219–221, 238; *see also* CD95 expression
Tomudex®, in treatment of ALL and AML, 548
Topoisomerase I, immunoblot assay of, 358
Topoisomerase I inhibitors
  in vincristine-resistant cells, 355–362
  and *in vitro* drug sensitivity assays in adult AML, 445–451
TRAIL (TNF-related apoptosis-inducing ligand), 219–221
TRAJAN software, 99–100
Translocation variants, BCR-ABL, 477–487, 489–497
Transport, decreased, in resistance to methotrexate, 543–548
Trimetrexate, in treatment of ALL and AML, 548
Tumor suppressor gene(s), expression in childhood ALL, 386; *see also* 2-chlorodeoxyadenosine, and mechanisms of cross resistance; P53 tumor suppressor expression

Vault proteins: *see* LRP gene expression
Vinblastine, apoptosis by
  fas/fas-ligand inhibition and, 259–265
  PARP inhibitors and, 267–276

Vincristine-resistant cells
　oncogene expression in, 365–379
　topoisomerase I inhibitors and apoptosis in, 355–362
Vinorelbine, *in vitro* activity of, in B-cell CLL, 473–475

VP-16, growth factor modulation of resistance to, 585–591

White cell count, related to proliferative/apoptotic fraction, 305–312